Textbook of Type 2 Diabetes

To C. Ronald Kahn, an extraordinary mentor, who fostered our career interests in the molecular pathogenesis of diabetes and its complications

To our families for their love and support

To our patients, who suffer with the restrictions imposed by diabetes on their daily lives, with hope that this book will help alleviate their burden

Textbook of Type 2 Diabetes

Edited by

Barry J Goldstein MD PhD
*Professor of Medicine, Biochemistry and Molecular Pharmacology and Director
Division of Endocrinology, Diabetes and Metabolic Diseases
Department of Medicine
Jefferson Medical College of Thomas Jefferson University
Philadelphia, USA*

Dirk Müller-Wieland MD
*Professor of Clinical Biochemistry and Director
Department of Clinical Biochemistry and Pathobiochemistry
German Diabetes Center
Leibniz Institute at the Heinrich-Heine University Düsseldorf
Düsseldorf, Germany*

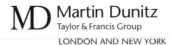
Martin Dunitz
Taylor & Francis Group
LONDON AND NEW YORK

© 2003 Martin Dunitz Ltd, a member of the Taylor & Francis Group

First published in the United Kingdom in 2003
by Martin Dunitz, a member of the Taylor & Francis Group,
11 New Fetter Lane, London EC4P 4EE

Tel.: +44 (0) 20 7583 9855
Fax.: +44 (0) 20 7842 2298
E-mail: info@dunitz.co.uk
Website: http://www.dunitz.co.uk

Although every effort has been made to ensure that drug doses and other
information are presented accurately in this publication, the ultimate responsibility
rests with the prescribing physician. Neither the publishers nor the authors can be
held responsible for errors or for any consequences arising from the use of
information contained herein. For detailed prescribing information or instructions
on the use of any product or procedure discussed herein, please consult the
prescribing information or instructional material issued by the manufacturer.

Although every effort has been made to ensure that all owners of copyright material
have been acknowledged in this publication, we would be glad to acknowledge in
subsequent reprints or editions any omissions brought to our attention.

A CIP record for this book is available from the British Library.

ISBN 1 84184 109 9

Distributed in the USA by
Fulfilment Center
Taylor & Francis
10650 Tobben Drive
Independence, KY 41051, USA
Toll Free Tel.: +1 800 634 7064
E-mail: taylorandfrancis@thomsonlearning.com

Distributed in Canada by
Taylor & Francis
74 Rolark Drive
Scarborough, Ontario M1R 4G2, Canada
Toll Free Tel.: +1 877 226 2237
E-mail: al_fran@istar.ca

Distributed in the rest of the world by
Thomson Publishing Services
Cheriton House
North Way
Andover, Hampshire SP10 5BE, UK
Tel.: +44 (0)1264 332424
E-mail: salesorder.tandf@thomsonpublishingservices.co.uk

Composition by Scribe, Gillingham, Kent, UK
Printed and bound in Spain by Grafos SA.

Contents

Contributors

William E Benson, MD
Retina Service
Wills Eye Hospital
840 Walnut Street
Philadelphia, PA 19107, USA

D John Betteridge BSc, PhD, MD, FRCP
Department of Medicine
Sir Jules Thorn Institute
The Middlesex Hospital
Mortimer Street
London WIN 8 AA, UK

Michael Camilleri, MD
Consultant Physician
Division of Gastroenterology and Hepatology
Mayo Clinic Rochester
200 First Street S.W.
Rochester, MN 55901, USA

Ramachandiran Cooppan, MBChB, FRCPC, FACE
Joslin Diabetes Center
One Joslin Place
Boston, MA 02215, USA

Philip E Cryer, MD
Irene E. and Michael M. Karl Professor of
Endocrinology and Metabolism
Washington University School of Medicine
Chief of Endocrinology, Diabetes and
Metabolism
Barnes-Jewish Hospital
Campus Box 8127
660 South Euclid Avenue
St. Louis, MO 63110, USA

Jaime A Davidson, MD, FACP, FACE
Endocrinologist in Private Practice at Medical
City Dallas Hospital
Clinical Associate Professor of Internal
Medicine
University of Texas Southwestern Medical
School, Dallas, Texas
Endocrine & Diabetes Associates of Texas
7777 Forest Lane, Suite C-204
Dallas, Texas 75230, USA

Cyrus Desouza MD
Fellow in Endocrinology, Diabetes and
Metabolism
Department of Medicine, SL-53
Section of Endocrinology, Diabetes and
Metabolism
Tulane University Health Sciences Center
1430 Tulane Avenue
New Orleans, LA 70123, USA

Vivian A Fonseca, MD
Professor of Medicine
Director, Diabetes Program
Department of Medicine, SL-53
Section of Endocrinology, Diabetes and
Metabolism
Tulane University Health Sciences Center
1430 Tulane Avenue
New Orleans, LA 70123, USA

Ruchira Glaser MD
Department of Medicine
Hospital of the University of Pennsylvania
9015 E. Gates Building
3400 Spruce Street
Philadelphia, PA 19104, USA

Barry J Goldstein, MD, PhD
Professor of Medicine, Biochemistry and
Molecular Pharmacology and Director
Division of Endocrinology, Diabetes and
Metabolic Diseases
Department of Medicine
Jefferson Medical College of Thomas Jefferson
University
1020 Locust Street, Suite 349
Philadelphia, PA 19107, USA

Markolf Hanefeld MD PhD
Centre for Clinical Studies - Metabolism and
Endocrinology
Technical University Dresden, Germany
Fiedlerstrasse 34
01307 Dresden, Germany

Elise Hardy MD
Fellow
Division of Endocrinology, Diabetes &
Metabolic Diseases
Thomas Jefferson University
211 South 9th Street, Suite 600
Philadelphia, PA 19107, USA

Hans-Ulrich Häring MD
Department of Medicine
Division of Endocrinology, Metabolic and
Vascular Medicine
University of Tübingen
Ottfried-Müller-Strasse 10
72076 Tübingen, Germany

Hans Hauner, MD
German Diabetes Research Institute
Heinrich-Heine Universität
Auf'm Hennekamp 65
40225 Düsseldorf, Germany

Arthur E Helfand, DPM
Professor Emeritus
Temple University School of Podiatric Medicine
Institute of Aging and Center for Public Health
9 Hansen Court
Narberth, PA 19072, USA

Helen B Holt BM MRCP(UK)
Research Registrar
Southampton University Hospitals NHS Trust
Southampton General Hospital
Tremona Road
Southampton SO16 6YD, UK

Serge A Jabbour, MD
Assistant Professor of Medicine
Division of Endocrinology, Diabetes &
Metabolic Diseases
Thomas Jefferson University
211 South 9th Street, Suite 600
Philadelphia, PA 19107, USA

Alan M Jacobson, MD
Behavioral and Mental Health Research
Joslin Diabetes Center
One Joslin Place
Boston, MA 02215, USA

Jeffrey I Joseph, DO
Director
The Artificial Pancreas Center
Department of Anesthesiology
Jefferson Medical College
Thomas Jefferson University
111 South 11th Street
Philadelphia, PA 19107, USA

Jörg Kotzka
Department of Clinical Biochemistry and
Pathobiochemistry
German Diabetes Center
Leibniz Institute at the Heinrich-Heine
University Düsseldorf
Auf'm Hennekamp 65
40225 Düsseldorf , Germany

Andrew J Krentz, MD, FRCP
Lead Consultant in Diabetes & Endocrinology
Honorary Senior Lecturer in Medicine
Southampton University Hospitals NHS Trust
Southampton General Hospital
Tremona Road
Southampton SO16 6YD, UK

Wilhem Krone, MD
Klinik II und Poliklinik für Innere Medizin
University of Cologne
Kerpener Strasse 62
50924 Cologne, Germany

Markku Laakso, MD
Professor and Chair
Department of Medicine
University of Kuopio
Kuopio University Hospital
70210 Kuopio, Finland

M James Lenhard, MD
Clinical Director
Diabetes and Metabolic Diseases Center
Christiana Care
Christiana Hospital
PO Box 6001
Newark, DE 19718, USA

Anthony L McCall, MD, PhD
James M Moss Professor in Diabetes in Internal
Medicine
Department of Internal Medicine
Division of Endocrinology & Metabolism
UVa Health System
PO Box 800770
Charlottesville VA 22908
USA

Jim I Mann
Department of Human Nutrition
University of Otago
PO Box 56
Dunedin, New Zealand

Stephan Matthaei, MD
Department of Medicine
Division of Endocrinology, Metabolic and
Vascular Medicine
University of Tübingen
Ottfried-Müller-Strasse 10
72076 Tübingen, Germany

Carolé Mensing, RN, MA, CDE
Coordinator
Diabetes Education Program
University of Connecticut Health Center
263 Farmington Avenue - Dowling South
Farmington, CT 06030, USA

Carl Erik Mogensen
Professor of Medicine
Department M - Diabetes & Endocrinology
Aarhus Kommunehospital
DK-8000 Aarhus C, Denmark

Kathryn Mulcahy, RN MSN CDE
3973 Acorn Ridge Court
Fairfax, VA 22033, USA

Dirk Müller-Wieland, MD
Professor of Clinical Biochemistry and Director
Department of Clinical Biochemistry and
Pathobiochemistry
German Diabetes Center
Leibniz Institute at the Heinrich-Heine
University Düsseldorf
Auf'm Hennekamp 65
40225 Düsseldorf , Germany

Maureen D Passaro, MD
Director
MedStar Clinical Research Center
650 Pennsylvania Avenue, Suite 50
Washington, DC 20003, USA

Merri Pendergrass MD PhD
Associate Professor of Medicine
Department of Medicine, SL-53
Section of Endocrinology, Diabetes and
Metabolism
Tulane University Health Sciences Center
1430 Tulane Avenue
New Orleans, LA 70123, USA

Andreas FH Pfeiffer
Medical Center Benjamin Franklin at the Free
University of Berlin
Department of Endocrinology, Diabetes and
Nutrition
Hindenburgdamm 30
D-12200 Berlin
Germany

Robert E Ratner, MD
Vice President of Scientific Affairs
MedStar Research Institute
650 Pennsylvania Avenue, Suite 50
Washington, DC 20003, USA

Carl D Regillo, MD FACS
Associate Professor of Ophthalmology
Thomas Jefferson University
Director, Clinical Retina Research and
Fellowship Training
Wills Eye Hospital
840 Walnut Street
Philadelphia, PA, 19107 USA

Matthew C Riddle, MD
Head, Section of Diabetes
Oregon Health Sciences University
3181 SW Sam Jackson Park Rd
Portland, OR 97201, USA

Brett Rosenblatt, MD
Vitreoretinal Fellow,
Barnes Retina Institute
Washington University
St Louis, MO 63110, USA

Arlan L Rosenbloom, MD
Distinguished Professor Emeritus of Pediatrics
Children's Medical Services Center
1701 SW 16th Avenue, Building B
Gainesville, FL 32608-1153, USA

Julio Rosenstock, MD
Clinical Professor of Medicine
University of Texas Southwestern Medical
Center at Dallas, and
Dallas Diabetes and Endocrine Center
7777 Forest Lane, C-618
Dallas, TX 75230, USA

Guntram Schernthaner
Head of the Department of Medicine I
Rudolfstiftung Hospital-Vienna
Juchgasse 25
A-1030 Vienna, Austria

Michael Stumvoll MD
Department of Medicine
Division of Endocrinology, Metabolic and
Vascular Medicine
University of Tübingen
Ottfried-Müller-Strasse 10
72076 Tübingen, Germany

Monika Toeller, MD
German Diabetes Research Institute
Heinrich-Heine Universität
Auf'm Hennekamp 65
40225 Düsseldorf, Germany

Adrian Vella, MD MRCP
Senior Associate Consultant
Division of Endocrinology
Mayo Clinic Rochester
200 First Street SW
Rochester, MN 55905, USA

Garry Welch, PhD
Behavioral and Mental Health Research
Joslin Diabetes Center
One Joslin Place
Boston, MA 02215, USA

Katie Weinger PhD
Behavioral and Mental Health Research
Joslin Diabetes Center
One Joslin Place
Boston, MA 02215, USA

Susan E Wiegers, MD FACC
Associate Professor of Medicine
Director of Clinical Echocardiography
Hospital of the University of Pennsylvania
9015 E. Gates Building
3400 Spruce Street
Philadelphia, PA 19104, USA

Kathleen Wyne, MD, PhD
Assistant Professor
Division of Endocrinology and Metabolism
Department of Internal Medicine
University of Texas Southwestern Medical
School
5323 Harry Hines Blvd
Dallas, Texas 75390, USA

Dan Ziegler
German Diabetes Research Institute
Heinrich-Heine Universität
Auf'm Hennekamp 65
40225 Düsseldorf, Germany

Foreword

Although diabetes mellitus was first described over 4000 years ago, the need for increasing our understanding of this disease has never been greater. There is a virtual epidemic of type 2 diabetes sweeping the world, coupled to an equally worrisome epidemic of obesity. Indeed, these medical problems are not only increasing dramatically in incidence, but also moving into younger and younger age groups. In many large cities in the USA, for example, up to one-third of the new cases of diabetes seen at children's hospitals and clinics are cases of type 2 diabetes. Since the major health risks of diabetes relate to the long-term complications which usually do not appear until after 10 or 20 years of disease, the increasing prevalence of the disease and shift to younger populations, predict a second epidemic of diabetes complications in the next two decades. At the same time, major clinical trials in the USA, Canada, Europe and Asia have demonstrated the importance of tight blood glucose control in reducing the risk of long-term complications. Thus, the need for early diagnosis, improved metabolic control, and long-term management present a challenge to the entire medical community.

In *Textbook of Type 2 Diabetes*, Drs Goldstein and Müller-Wieland and their international team of distinguished contributors consider all aspects of this disease. They examine the epidemiology of the dramatic increase in diabetes worldwide and how this relates to the pathogenesis and prevention of the disease. In the second section, there are five important chapters on the non-pharmacological management of the disease. Although this is among the oldest approaches to type 2 diabetes, recent research, including the US Diabetes Prevention Program, has re-inforced just how important these approaches can be. Indeed, it has been estimated that 50-80% of obese type 2 diabetic patients could be managed without pharmacological intervention, if effective diet and exercise regimens could be employed. Perhaps more importantly, when these lifestyle interventions are appropriately employed in individuals who are at high risk for this disease (pre-type 2 diabetes), the disease risk rate can be reduced by 58%.

The other major change over the past decade has been both the definitive demonstration that good glucose control reduces risk of complications in type 2 diabetes and the introduction of new pharmacological agents that can help achieve this goal. In addition, there is increased recognition of the need to use multiple drugs in many patients to achieve this goal. This use of polypharmacy in the treatment of type 2 diabetes has increased the challenge to the general practitioner and internist who now need to be aware of the different mechanisms of action of the various pharmacological agents and how they can be used singly or in combination to achieve the best possible glucose control. Chapters 8 through 13 explore the old and new insulin secretagogues, insulin sensitizers, alpha-glucosidase inhibitors and the use of insulin in type 2 diabetes.

When it comes to perception of diabetes, the general public is usually most sympathetic to the picture of the child with type 1 diabetes injecting herself with insulin. Physicians and public health officials know, however, that the major burden of disease and the greatest cost to society are in fact due to the long-term complications of the disease, especially in the very large population of people with type 2 diabetes. Type 2 diabetes is the major cause of end-stage renal failure requiring dialysis or transplantation, the major cause of non-traumatic amputation, and one of the major causes of blindness and peripheral neuropathies in adults. In Section IV, the authors deal with each of these issues in a scholarly and useful way, discussing the pathogenesis, clinical features and medical approach to these problems.

The final sections of this volume deal with a number of special situations, such as gestational diabetes and type 2 diabetes in children and adolescents. In addition, it examines the link between type 2 diabetes, insulin resistance and a number of other common metabolic problems, such as obesity, hyperlipidemia, hypertension, and accelerated atherosclerosis for a metabolic syndrome, sometimes referred to as Syndrome X. This link is not only important to recognize from a diagnostic perspective: it is now clear that management of patients is most effective when all of these problems are addressed. Indeed, reducing blood pressure in patients with type 2 diabetes can have as much or more effect on reducing the risk of long-term complications as reducing blood glucose. Overt and silent cardiovascular disease remains the major cause of death in people with type 2 diabetes, and must be addressed if one is to increase the quantity and quality of life of patients with this disease.

There are other special considerations which are needed when dealing with type 2 diabetes in adolescents and children and in geriatric populations. Hispanic, Asian, Indian and Black populations also present unique challenges, since they have a higher prevalence of type 2 diabetes and are at increased risk of complications, even given the same level of glucose control. Furthermore, since management of type 2 diabetes involves many lifestyle adjustments, it is critical to approach these in a manner that is most suitable for each ethnic group. Finally, one must also be aware of how to manage diabetic patients during surgery and anesthesia; how type 2 diabetes mellitus can occur secondary to drugs, hormones and other endocrinopathies; and what new devices and drugs are on the horizon.

Textbook of Type 2 Diabetes provides a rich picture of the multidimensional nature of type 2 diabetes with a strong emphasis on the practical issues regarding management of the disease. With the high and rising prevalence of this disease in the population, this is important information for every practitioner of medicine.

C. Ronald Kahn
Joslin Diabetes Center
Harvard University Medical School,
Boston, MA, USA

Preface

The incidence and prevalence of type 2 diabetes mellitus have increased dramatically in modernized and developing nations over the past few decades, and this 'epidemic' shows no signs of abating. Physicians and other healthcare professionals worldwide are well aware of this growing burden. The pathogenesis and the management of the hyperglycemia of diabetes and its associated risk factors and morbidities, especially involving cardiovascular complications, must be fully understood by all of the many providers that care for patients with diabetes.

Patients are always asking, 'Isn't there anything new to help manage my diabetes, doctor?', reflecting the relative inadequacies of many of our attempts at lifestyle change, as well as some of the shortcomings of currently available medications for the long-term management of this disorder. Certainly, changes in lifestyle are highly effective, but extremely difficult to implement over a long time period. Diabetes patient management is often implemented later in the course of the disease, since the disease can be asymptomatic and go unrecognized for many years. Recent studies have shown clearly that the onset of diabetes can be prevented or delayed, and more aggressive, earlier treatment may also help to alter its course and, possibly, also its chronic complications. Large clinical trials will help to answer these questions in the future.

In this volume, we have provided a current review of type 2 diabetes from an international perspective in a manner directed at primary care physicians: those that see the majority of patients with this and related disorders. The entire clinical field is covered in succinct chapters written by recognized experts, from a current perspective on diabetes demographics and epidemiology, pathophysiology, disease monitoring, approaches to glucose control, monitoring and management of micro- and macrovascular complications of diabetes, and ending with a look at new drugs and devices on the future horizon.

We hope this book will be used frequently and successfully in the management of this complex but widely prevalent disorder.

Barry J Goldstein
Dirk Müller-Wieland

1

Epidemiology and diagnosis of type 2 diabetes

Markku Laakso

INTRODUCTION

Diabetes mellitus refers to a number of disorders that share the common feature of elevated blood glucose levels. It affects about 3–5% of western populations and its prevalence is rapidly increasing, particularly among the elderly. There is a marked variation in the prevalence of diabetes among many national and ethnic populations. The spectrum ranges from a very low prevalence, of about 1%, in tribes in Papua New Guinea, Eskimos, or Chinese living in mainland China, to extremely high rates, of 20–45% among Australian aborigines, the Nauruans of Micronesia, and Pima Indians of Arizona[1]. The variation in prevalence is even marked within nations. For example, in the USA, African–Americans have a two-fold, Mexican–Americans 2.5-fold and Native Americans a five-fold increase in risk of development of type 2 diabetes over Caucasians[2]. The large variation in prevalence of type 2 diabetes in different populations probably results from environmental, as well as genetic determinants.

Although diabetes has been recognized for centuries, our understanding of the etiology and pathogenesis of the disease is still incomplete. This is particularly true for type 2 diabetes, a subtype of diabetes that comprises about 80–90% of all cases. Type 2 is a heterogenous, polygenic disorder; the genes responsible have been identified in only selected subtypes of the disease.

Type 2 diabetes is preceded by a long period of asymptomatic hyperglycemia, which may last for years. In this prediabetic state, postprandial or postglucose levels are mildly elevated, whereas fasting blood glucose can usually be maintained within the near-normal range. The elevation of postglucose levels is used to define impaired glucose tolerance (IGT), a non-specific reversible stage. About 30% of subjects with IGT progress to overt diabetes within 10 years[3]. Beta-cells compensate for insulin resistance in some individuals by increasing insulin secretion, and in these cases type 2 diabetes does not develop. However, in a large number of prediabetic individuals, multiple defects in insulin action and/or insulin secretion gradually lead to sustained hyperglycemia. As a consequence of insulin resistance, the beta-cells produce increased amounts of insulin, and compensatory hyperinsulinemia maintains normoglycemia. When beta-cell compensation to insulin resistance fails, decompensated hyperglycemic state develops. Thus, type 2 diabetic subjects have relative (rather than absolute) insulin deficiency. Usually, these individuals do not need insulin treatment to survive.

The chronic hyperglycemia of diabetes is associated with long-term complications, especially in the eyes, kidneys, nerves, heart, and blood vessels. Individuals with undiagnosed type 2 diabetes are at high risk of coronary heart disease, stroke and peripheral vascular disease.

More than half of type 2 diabetic patients die of cardiovascular causes.

DIAGNOSIS AND CLASSIFICATION OF DIABETES

Criteria for diagnosis of type 2 diabetes have changed considerably over the last 20 years. In 1979 the National Diabetes Data Group[4] and in 1980 the World Health Organization (WHO)[5] aimed to standardize the classification and criteria for diabetes. A new subtype, IGT, was created. This described subjects whose fasting glucose levels were normal, but whose 2 h post-glucose challenge levels were elevated, although not diabetic. The cut-off point between IGT and diabetes was based on an increased risk of developing diabetic complications, primarily retinopathy, for subjects with diabetes. In 1985, a WHO Study Group proposed a revised classification, which was adopted internationally[6]. Classification and diagnosis of diabetes have been debated for 20 years, and current recommendations by the American Diabetes Association (ADA) and WHO still differ.

The 1985 WHO Study Group proposal was a compromise between clinical and etiological classifications[6]. The glucose criteria for the diagnosis of diabetes was still based on microvascular complications known to be associated with hyperglycemia. The 2 h 75 g oral-glucose tolerance test was recommended as the international standard for diabetes diagnosis. IGT was defined as fasting glucose < 7.8 mmol L^{-1} and 2 h plasma glucose 7.8–10.9 mmol L^{-1}. Diabetes was defined as fasting plasma glucose ≥ 7.8 mmol L^{-1} or 2 h plasma glucose ≥ 11.0 mmol L^{-1}. The problem with this classification was that fasting plasma glucose was too high in comparison with the 2 h value.

At about the same time, the Whitehall study showed an increased risk of cardiovascular disease when the 2 h level exceeded 5.5 mmol L^{-1}, albeit after a 50 g glucose load[7]. This study, together with several other population-based studies indicated that the risk for macrovascular complications started at considerably lower levels of glycemia than was included in the definition of diabetes.

The diagnostic criteria for diabetes mellitus and glucose intolerance have recently been modified by the ADA[8] and WHO[9]. The main difference between these new criteria is that the ADA does not recommend the use of an oral glucose-tolerance test. The fasting glucose criteria for diagnosis were considered by the ADA to have good reproducibility, small variability, and easy application in clinical practice. Both the ADA and WHO recommend a fasting plasma glucose concentration of 7.0 mmol L^{-1} for the diagnosis of diabetes but, according to the WHO criteria, diabetes can also be diagnosed if the 2 h glucose concentration is at least 11.1 mmol L^{-1}. For the asymptomatic person, at least one additional glucose test result with a value in the diabetic range is essential, from a random (casual) sample, or from the oral glucose tolerance test. The ADA (but not the WHO) recommended that, in epidemiological studies, estimates of diabetes prevalence and incidence should be based only on fasting glucose criteria.

IGT is defined by WHO as a 2 h plasma glucose concentration of 7.8–11.0 mmol L^{-1}. The ADA also introduced a category of impaired fasting glucose (IFG), defined as a fasting plasma glucose level of 6.1–6.9 mmol L^{-1}, to replace IGT. IFG and IGT were considered to be metabolic stages intermediate between normal glucose homeostasis and diabetes. However, it is possible that IFG differs from IGT with respect to the relative contribution of insulin secretory defect, and hepatic and peripheral insulin resistance. Normoglycemia is defined as plasma fasting glucose < 6.1 mmol L^{-1} and 2 h glucose < 7.8 mmol L^{-1} in an oral glucose-tolerance test. The changes in diagnostic criteria for diabetes[10] recognized results from epidemiological studies that indicated that the risks of both retinopathy and cardiovascular disease start to increase at fasting plasma glucose values of about 6.0 mmol L^{-1}.

The new classification accepted by the ADA and WHO combines both the clinical stages of hyperglycemia and the etiological types. Two main subtypes of diabetes are type 1, either autoimmune or idiopathic, and type 2, caused by insulin resistance, insulin secretory defects,

Table 1.1 Etiologic classification of diabetes mellitus

Type 1 diabetes
Beta-cell destruction, usually leading to absolute insulin deficiency
Immune mediated
Idiopathic

Type 2 diabetes
May range from predominantly insulin resistance with relative insulin deficiency to a predominantly secretory defect with insulin resistance

Other specific types
Genetic defects in beta-cell function
Genetic defects in insulin action
Diseases of the endocrine pancreas
Endocrinopathies
Drug- and chemical-induced
Infections
Uncommon forms of immune-mediated diabetes
Other genetic syndromes sometimes associated with diabetes
Gestational diabetes

or both (Table 1.1). The terms 'insulin-dependent diabetes mellitus' and 'non-insulin-dependent diabetes mellitus' and their acronyms 'IDDM' and 'NIDDM' were eliminated. Both these diabetes types include clinical stages ranging from normal glucose tolerance to diabetes. The same disease process can cause IFG and/or IGT, without fulfilling the criteria for the diagnosis of diabetes. IFG and IGT are not clinical entities, but rather risk categories for future diabetes and/or cardiovascular disease. Hyperglycemia in diabetes is subcategorized as being not insulin requiring, insulin requiring for control, and insulin requiring for survival (type 1 diabetes). Patients with maturity-onset diabetes in the young (MODY), now appear under 'other specific types', and are not

categorized as having type 2 diabetes. Similarly, latent autoimmune diabetes in adults (LADA) falls within type 1 autoimmune diabetes, instead of being classified as type 2 diabetes.

The WHO[9] also suggested a working definition for the metabolic syndrome (Syndrome X, the insulin resistance syndrome) because people with hypertension, central obesity and dyslipidemia, with or without hyperglycemia, are at increased risk of macrovascular disease:

- IFG, IGT or diabetes
- Insulin resistance (under hyperinsulinemic euglycemic conditions, glucose uptake lies below the lowest quartile for the background population under investigation)
- Raised arterial pressure $\geq 160/90$ mmHg
- Raised plasma triglycerides (≥ 1.7 mmol L^{-1}) and/or low HDL cholesterol (< 0.9 mmol L^{-1} for men; 1.0 mmol L^{-1} for women)
- Central obesity (waist to hip ratio > 0.90 for men; waist to hip ratio > 0.85 for women) and/or body mass index (BMI) > 30 kg m^{-2}
- Microalbuminuria (urinary albumin excretion rate ≥ 20 µg min^{-1} or albumin/creatinine ratio ≥ 20 mg g^{-1})

A person has the metabolic syndrome if he/she has abnormal glucose tolerance and insulin resistance and two or more of the other components listed above.

A number of studies summarized by Shawn et al.[11] have compared the new fasting criteria and 2 h criteria. These studies demonstrate both an increase and a decrease in people with nearly diagnosed diabetes, depending on the population studied. A recent study has shown that, compared with the WHO criteria, fasting glucose-based ADA criteria under-estimate glucose abnormalities more in older than in younger people[12]. The Cardiovascular Health Study has also demonstrated a 50% under-estimation of diabetes prevalence in older adults (> 65 years) when comparing the ADA criteria with the WHO criteria[13]. Furthermore, recent studies have shown the higher sensitivity of IGT over IFG for predicting progression to type 2 diabetes[14].

In general, the fasting criterion identifies different people as being diabetic compared with those identified by the 2 h criterion[15]. In subjects without previously diagnosed diabetes, the DECODE study group of 16 different European populations[16] found that of all subjects diagnosed by either the fasting or 2 h criteria, only 29% qualified as diabetic according to both criteria. This result was confirmed in the DECODA study group[17], which included existing epidemiological data from 11 population-based studies collected from Asian people ($n = 17\,666$) between 30 and 89 years of age. The authors concluded that it would be inappropriate to use the ADA criteria alone for screening diabetes in Asian populations.

CRITERIA FOR TYPE 2 DIABETES AND LONG-TERM COMPLICATIONS

Early diagnosis of diabetes aims to prevent long-term complications. Cardiovascular disease is the main complication of type 2 diabetes, recent studies have therefore investigated the capability of new criteria to predict these complications.

The association of hyperglycemia and cardiovascular disease is a crucial one with which to test the validity of new criteria. The DECODE study[18] showed that the 2 h criteria was better at identifying people who are at increased risk of total and cardiovascular mortality than the ADA fasting criteria.

The DECODE study[18] analyzed 10 prospective European cohort studies, including 15 388 men and 7126 women, aged 30–89 years, who all had undergone a 2 h oral-glucose tolerance test. The median follow-up was 8.8 years, and hazard ratios for deaths from all causes, cardiovascular disease, coronary heart disease, and stroke were estimated. Multivariate Cox regression analyses showed that the inclusion of fasting glucose did not add significant information to the prediction value of the 2 h glucose alone, whereas the addition of a 2 h glucose test to fasting glucose criteria significantly improved the prediction. Table 1.2 reports adjusted hazard ratios for deaths from cardiovascular disease, coronary heart disease, stroke, and all causes with fasting and 2 h categories. IFG did not predict mortality. Diabetes based on fasting criteria predicted total mortal-

---

Table 1.2 Adjusted hazard ratios from cardiovascular disease (CVD), coronary heart disease (CHD), stroke, and all causes with fasting and 2 h glucose categories in the same model: the DECODE Study[a]

	CVD	CHD	Stroke	All causes
Fasting glucose criteria[b]				
IFG	1.01 (0.84–1.22)	1.01 (0.77–1.31)	1.00 (0.66–1.59)	1.03 (0.93–1.14)
Diabetes	1.20 (0.88–1.64)	1.09 (0.71–1.67)	1.64 (0.88–3.07)	1.21 (1.01–1.44)
2 h glucose criteria[c]				
IGT	1.32 (1.12–1.56)	1.27 (1.01–1.58)	1.21 (0.84–1.74)	1.37 (1.25–1.51)
Diabetes	1.40 (1.02–1.92)	1.56 (1.03–2.36)	1.29 (0.66–2.54)	1.73 (1.45–2.06)
Known diabetes[b]	1.96 (1.62–2.37)	1.94 (1.51–2.50)	1.73 (1.12–2.68)	1.82 (1.60–2.06)

[a]Adjusted for age, sex, center, total cholesterol, BMI, systolic blood pressure, and smoking.
[b]Using fasting plasma glucose < 6.1 mmol L^{-1} as reference group.
[c]Using 2 h plasma glucose < 7.8 mmol L^{-1} as reference group.

ity, but 2 h glucose criteria predicted mortality much better than fasting glucose criteria. IGT and diabetes predicted cardiovascular and coronary heart disease mortality, as well as coronary heart disease mortality and total mortality. The highest hazard ratios for all categories of death were observed in known diabetic patients. The largest number of excess cardiovascular deaths was found in subjects with IGT who had a normal fasting glucose level, supporting the notion that IGT has prognostic importance.

The Funaka Diabetes Study in Japan demonstrated that subjects with IGT had higher cardiovascular disease mortality than subjects with IFG[19]. In contrast to these findings, the Hoorn Study recently reported no clear differences in mortality risks for subjects classified as IGT, IFG, or newly diagnosed diabetes according to either set of criteria[20].

EPIDEMIC OF TYPE 2 DIABETES

Epidemiological studies have been crucial in the identification of the 'diabetes epidemic' already noticed in the 1970s. The extraordinarily high prevalence of type 2 diabetes was reported among Pima Indians[21] and in the Micronesian Nauruans in the Pacific[22], and subsequently in other Pacific and Asian island populations[23]. These studies showed that transition from a traditional lifestyle to the Western way of life resulted in obesity, lack of exercise, profound changes in the diet and, finally, to type 2 diabetes. The potential for a future global epidemic of diabetes was highlighted. Since the 1970s several other studies have shown that type 2 diabetes has reached epidemic proportions in several developing countries, e.g. among Australian aboriginals[24], African–Americans and Mexican–Americans[25].

Table 1.3 shows the trends in the number of diabetic patients worldwide[26]. A significant increase in the number of type 1 diabetic patients was expected, but the doubling in the number of diabetic patients in the following 10 years was due to a huge increase in the number of type 2 diabetic patients. Diabetes-related complications are therefore expected to emerge as a major health problem worldwide. Diabetes

Table 1.3 Estimates of the number of type 1 and type 2 diabetic patients (millions) worldwide for the years 1997–2010 (adapted from Reference 11)

Type of diabetes	1997	2000	2010
Type 1	3.5	4.3	5.3
Type 2	119.2	147.2	212.9
Type 1 + Type 2	122.8	151.2	218.3

is already among the five leading causes of death in most countries.

The prevalence of type 2 diabetes has also considerably increased in Western countries. The National Health and Nutrition Surveys (NHANES) have shown a substantial increase in the prevalence of diabetes in the USA. In the NHANES II (1976–80) the prevalence of diagnosed plus undiagnosed diabetes was 8.9%, but in the NHANES III (1988–94) it was 12.3% among the population 40–74 years of age[27]. The prevalence of IFG increased from 6.5% to 9.7%. Figure 1.1 demonstrates a large difference in diabetes prevalence between ethnic groups in the US population ≥ 20 years of age. The prevalence of diabetes (known plus undiagnosed) was particularly high in Mexican–American men (13.1%) and women (14.5%). IFG or diabetes was present in about 20% of Mexican–Americans. Diabetes has become one of the most common chronic diseases in the USA. In subjects ≥ 60 years of age the prevalence is already 18.8%.

The epidemic of type 2 diabetes is determined not only by an increase in the incidence, but also by mortality rates. Although cardiovascular complications in nondiabetic subjects have significantly reduced in the USA during the last decade, this is not the case in diabetic patients, particularly women, as shown recently by Gu et al.[28]. No reliable data on mortality rates are available from populations living in developing countries.

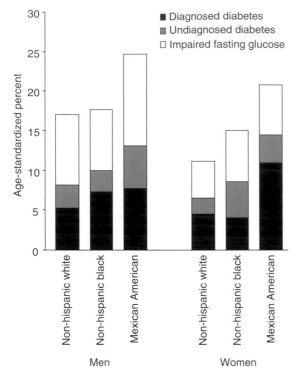

Figure 1.1 Age-standardized prevalence of diagnosed and undiagnosed diabetes and impaired fasting glucose in the US population > 20 years of age, presented according to sex and racial or ethnic group, based on NHANES III. Adapted from Harris et al.[27]; © 1998 American Diabetes Association. Reprinted with permission.

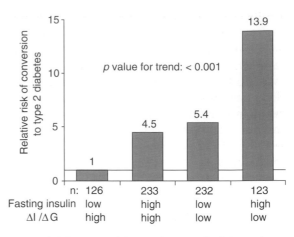

Figure 1.2 The risk of developing type 2 diabetes by fasting insulin concentration and insulin secretion (change in insulin divided by change in glucose concentrations over the first 30 min of an oral glucose tolerance test [$\Delta I_{30}/\Delta G_{30}$]). Adapted from Haffner et al.[30]; © 1996 American Diabetes Association. Reprinted with permission.

INSULIN RESISTANCE AND IMPAIRED INSULIN SECRETION AS PREDICTORS OF TYPE 2 DIABETES

Type 2 diabetes is caused by impaired insulin action (insulin resistance) and/or impaired insulin secretion. Insulin resistance is a characteristic metabolic defect in the great majority of patients, and it precedes the development of frank hyperglycemia. Impaired insulin action is observed in several tissues, e.g. skeletal muscle, adipose tissue and the liver. It leads to increased insulin secretion from the pancreas to overcome the impaired action. Compensatory hyperinsulinemia maintains glucose levels within the normal range but, in individuals destined to develop diabetes, beta-cell function eventually declines, leading to a hyperglycemic diabetic state. In a minority of subjects, diabetes develops

as a consequence of a primary defect in insulin secretion. Between 2 and 14% (on average about 5%) of people with IGT progress to type 2 diabetes each year[29]. Age, ethnicity and the degree of glucose intolerance influence the progression rate.

The degree of insulin resistance varies between different ethnic groups. For example, in the Insulin Resistance Atherosclerosis Study[30], which included 1100 healthy subjects, African–Americans and Mexican–Americans had a lower insulin sensitivity than non-Hispanic Caucasians. The first study to demonstrate that a combination of insulin resistance and impaired insulin secretion predicts type 2 diabetes studied Pima Indians. Lillioja et al.[31] showed that low insulin secretory response and increased insulin resistance were both predictors of type 2 diabetes. Furthermore, both impaired insulin secretion and insulin resistance acted as an independent risk factor. Similar results were published on Mexican–Americans. Baseline high fasting insulin level (indicator of insulin resistance) predicted the conversion to diabetes during the 7-year follow-up[32]. Furthermore, low insulin secretion, assessed by insulin response (30 min insulin minus fasting insulin divided by 30 min glucose minus fasting glucose) also predicted the development of diabetes. When these two parameters were combined, they had an additive effect on the risk of developing diabetes. High degree of insulin resistance and normal insulin secretion increased the risk by 4.5-fold, and high insulin sensitivity but low insulin secretion increased the risk by 5.4-fold; the combination of these two increased the risk by 13.9-fold (Figure 1.2).

RISK FACTORS FOR TYPE 2 DIABETES

The identification of risk factors is essential for the successful implementation of primary prevention programs. Risk factors for type 2 diabetes can be classified as modifiable and non-modifiable (Table 1.4). Subjects who subsequently develop diabetes have multiple adverse changes in risk-factor levels. A good example is our study of 892 elderly Finnish subjects followed for 3.5 years[33]. As shown in Figure 1.3, the highest risk of developing diabetes was associated with IGT and hyperinsulinemia.

Table 1.4 Risk factors for Type 2 diabetes	
Modifiable	**Nonmodifiable**
Obesity	Ethnicity
Central obesity	Age
Lack of physical activity	Sex
Smoking	Genetic factors
Alcohol abstinence	Family history of Type 2 diabetes
Low fiber in the diet	Prior gestational diabetes
High saturated fat in the diet	Previous glucose intolerance
	History of hypertension
	History of dyslipidemia
	Low birth weight

Furthermore, hypertriglyceridemia, central obesity, low HDL cholesterol, high BMI, hypertension, and a family history of diabetes were risk factors for diabetes.

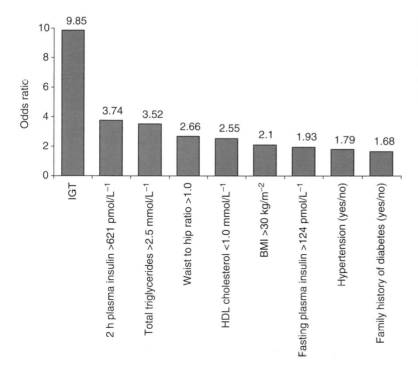

Figure 1.3 Odds ratio of developing type 2 diabetes in elderly Finnish subjects. Adapted from Mykkänen et al.[33]; © 1990 American Diabetes Association. Reprinted with permission.

Modifiable risk factors

Recently, Hu et al.[34] published results from the Nurses' Heath Study, which included 84 941 female nurses followed from 1980 to 1996. These women were free of diagnosed cardiovascular disease and diabetes at baseline. During the 16 years follow-up 3300 new cases of type 2 diabetes were diagnosed. As shown in Figure 1.4, obesity was the single most important predictor of diabetes. Women whose BMI was at least 35.0 kg m⁻² had almost 40-fold risk of becoming diabetic compared with women whose BMI was < 23.0 kg m⁻². Weekly exercise for at least 7 h per week reduced the risk of type 2 diabetes by 39% compared with women who exercised < 0.5 h per week. Smoking > 14 cigarettes per day increased diabetes risk by 39%, but alcohol intake > 10 g per day reduced the risk by 41%. The study also indicated that a diet high in cereal fiber and polysaturated fat, and low in saturated and trans fats and glycemic load, reduced the risk of developing diabetes. A combination of several lifestyle factors, including low BMI (< 25 kg m⁻²), a diet high in cereal fiber and polysaturated fat, and low in saturated fat and trans fats and glycemic load, regular exercise, abstinence from smoking and moderate alcohol intake, was associated with a reduction of type 2 diabetes incidence by 90% compared with women without these factors.

Recent studies have demonstrated that greater visceral adiposity precedes the development of type 2 diabetes. Boyko et al.[35] showed in their study of Japanese–Americans that CT-measured intra-abdominal fat area remained a significant predictor of diabetes incidence, even after adjust-

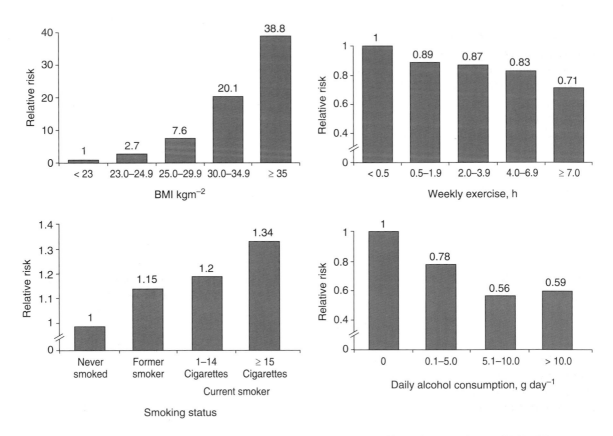

Figure 1.4 Relative risk of type 2 diabetes among 84 941 women in the Nurses' Health Study, 1980–96. Adapted with permission from Hu et al.[34] © 2001 Massachusetts Medical Society. All rights reserved.

ment for BMI, total body fat area, subcutaneous fat area and other risk factors for diabetes. Interestingly, high insulin resistance and low insulin secretion predicted diabetes independently of directly measured visceral adiposity, suggesting that visceral adiposity could contribute to the development of diabetes through actions independent of its effect on insulin sensitivity. Van Dam et al.[36] showed that in Dutch subjects the association between abdominal obesity (waist circumference) and hyperglycemia was stronger in the presence of a parental history of diabetes.

Physical inactivity is a major risk factor for the development of type 2 diabetes. Physical activity reduces insulin resistance, and total and visceral fat mass[37]. In contrast, the association of total dietary fat with type 2 diabetes or insulin sensitivity is less consistent. Meyer et al.[38] studied the relation between dietary fatty acids and diabetes in a prospective cohort study of 35 988 older women who initially did not have diabetes. Altogether, 1890 new cases of diabetes occurred during 11 years of follow-up. Diabetes risk was negatively associated with dietary polysaturated fatty acids, vegetable fat, and trans fatty acids. Even after adjustment for confounding factors, dietary vegetable fat remained a significant predictor for new diabetes.

Non-modifiable risk factors

The prevalence and incidence of type 2 diabetes are strongly related to age. In fact, about 50% of all type 2 diabetic patients are over 60 years old. Ethnicity is a strong determinant of diabetes occurrence. Among the Chinese the prevalence of type 2 diabetes is 1%, whereas among Pima Indians it affects > 50% of the adult population, probably as a result of a genetic influence, or due to interaction between genes and environment. No systematic effect of gender on the prevalence and incidence of type 2 diabetes has been observed, but in some ethnic groups the occurrence of diabetes might depend on gender. Previous abnormality of glucose tolerance, a history of gestational diabetes, and a family history of type 2 diabetes are all strong predictors of type 2 diabetes. Interestingly, the presence of other disease states or conditions, for example hypertension and dyslipidemia, also increase the risk of type 2 diabetes. In recent years interest has also focused on low birth-weight as a risk factor for type 2 diabetes.

Associations between low birth-weight and increased risk of type 2 diabetes in adult life have been reported in various populations[39,40]. Several explanations for this relationship have been presented. Long-term effects of nutritional deprivation in utero could affect fetal growth and the development of the endocrine pancreas. Genetic factors could cause both low birth-weight and later abnormalities of insulin secretion or insulin sensitivity. Whether the relationship between diabetes and low birth-weight is mediated through impaired insulin sensitivity or secretion still remains to be determined[39]. Recent analysis of five studies regarding birth-weight and the incidence of diabetes in adult subjects concluded that impaired fetal growth accounts for a minority of type 2 diabetes cases[41].

PREVENTION OF TYPE 2 DIABETES: IMPLICATIONS FOR SCREENING

Screening for diabetes may be appropriate under certain circumstances because early detection and prompt treatment may reduce the burden of type 2 diabetes and its complications. However, widespread screening of asymptomatic individuals for type 2 diabetes can not be recommended. Screening may be appropriate if the subjects have one or more of the risk factors listed in Table 1.4. But the rationale for screening for type 2 diabetes must be based on the presence of factors that have a significant effect on the risk of developing diabetes. Screening for diabetes is warranted only if diabetes can be prevented by normalizing modifiable risk factors. Recent clinical trials have demonstrated the efficacy of lifestyle-intervention programs in the prevention of type 2 diabetes. Da Qing's study from China[42] showed that exercise and diet resulted in a decrease of 42–46% in the incidence of type 2 diabetes among 577 subjects with IGT. The Finnish Diabetes Prevention Program demonstrated that weight loss and regular exercise reduced the incidence of type 2 diabetes by 58%[43]. Similarly, the preliminary results from the Diabetes Prevention Study in the USA showed that diet and regular exercise reduced the incidence of type 2 diabetes by 58% among 3234 subjects with IGT[44]. Lifestyle intervention works equally well in men and women, and in all ethnic groups. The present state of knowledge therefore suggests that lifestyle intervention is highly successful, and screening should be targeted at subjects with a high risk of developing diabetes.

The ADA has recommended the plasma fasting glucose measurements as a screening test because it is easier and faster to perform, more convenient and acceptable to patients, and less expensive[45]. In contrast, the WHO criteria for diabetes still includes a 2 h oral-glucose tolerance test, which might be used in the screening of high-risk individuals. Recent studies indicating that 2 h glucose is better than fasting glucose values in identifying individuals at high risk of cardiovascular disease favors the use of the 2 h oral-glucose tolerance test. However, this test has a high within-test variability, of up to 25%. According to different studies when subjects were retested after an interval of up to 3 months, 35–75% of the subjects who were IGT at the first test had reverted to normal when retested.[46]

CONCLUDING REMARKS

In the next 20 years we will face a global epidemic of type 2 diabetes. Although the numbers of new cases may depend somewhat on the glucose criteria used to define diabetes, there has already been a true increase in the incidence and prevalence of type 2 diabetes. The epidemic has emerged as a result of an increasing prevalence of obesity worldwide and the incidence of diabetes in a population is closely linked to the average weight of that population. Type 2 diabetes does not only cause micro- and macro-vascular complications, excess mortality and morbidity, but it is also an expensive health problem. Socio-economic, behavioral, nutritional and public-health issues relating to the epidemic of obesity and type 2 diabetes should therefore be addressed.

More funds are needed for continuing research aimed at solving issues of pathophysiology and genetics of type 2 diabetes. Extremely important areas of research will be the identification of the genes responsible for the predisposition to type 2 diabetes, and the identification of environmental factors which bring out this predisposition. Once these issues have been solved we will better understand the 'epidemic' of type 2 diabetes, and be able to target our non-pharmacological and pharmacological treatment modalities more effectively, to prevent this continuously growing health problem and its devastating complications.

REFERENCES

1 King H, Rewers M. WHO *Ad Hoc* Diabetes Reporting Group: global estimates for prevalence of diabetes mellitus and impaired glucose tolerance. *Diabetes Care* 1993;16:157–77.

2 Haffner SM. Epidemiology of type 2 diabetes: risk factors. *Diabetes Care* 1998;21 (Suppl. 3):C3–C6.

3 Valsania P, Micossi P. Genetic epidemiology of non-insulin-dependent diabetes. *Diabetes Metab Rev* 1994;10:385–405.

4 National Diabetes Data Group. Classification and diagnosis of diabetes mellitus and other cat-

egories of glucose intolerance. *Diabetes* 1979;28:1039–57.

5 World Health Organization Expert Committee on Diabetes Mellitus. *Second Report. Technical Report Series 646*. Geneva: WHO, 1980.

6 World Health Organization Study Group on Diabetes Mellitus. *Technical Report Series 727*. Geneva: WHO, 1985.

7 Fuller J, Shipley MJ, Rose G *et al*. Mortality from coronary heart disease and stroke in relation to degree of glycaemia: the Whitehall Study. *Br Med J* 1983;287:867–70.

8 The Expert Committee on the Diagnosis and Classification of Diabetes Mellitus. Report of the Expert Committee on the Diagnosis and Classification of Diabetes Mellitus. *Diabetes Care* 1997;20:1183–97.

9 Alberti KGMM, Zimmet PZ, for the WHO Consultation. Definition, diagnosis and classification of diabetes mellitus and its complications. Part 1: diagnosis and classification of diabetes mellitus. Provisional report of a WHO Consultation. *Diabetic Med* 1998;15:539–53.

10 Balkau B, Eschwege E, Tichet J, Marre M. Proposed criteria for the diagnosis of diabetes: evidence from a French epidemiological study. *Diabetes Metab* 1997;23:428–34.

11 Shaw JE, Zimmet PZ, McCarthy D, de Couten M. Type 2 diabetes worldwide according to the new classification and criteria. *Diabetes Care* 2000;23 (Suppl. 2):B5–B10.

12 Resnick HE, Harris MI, Brock DB, Harris TB. American Diabetes Association diabetes diagnostic criteria, advancing age, and cardiovascular disease risk profiles. Results from the Third Health and Nutrition Examination Survey. *Diabetes Care* 2000;23:176–80.

13 Wahl PW, Savage PJ, Psaty BM *et al.* Diabetes in older adults: comparison of 1997 American Diabetes Association classification of diabetes mellitus with 1985 WHO classification. *Lancet* 1998;352:1012–15.

14 Shaw JE, Zimmet PZ, de Courten M *et al.* Impaired fasting glucose or impaired glucose tolerance. What best predicts future diabetes in Mauritius? *Diabetes Care* 1999;22:399–402.

15 Shaw JE, de Courten M, Boyko E, Zimmet PZ. Impact of new diagnostic criteria for diabetes on different populations. *Diabetes Care* 1999;22:762–6.

16 DECODE Study Group. Is fasting glucose sufficient to define diabetes? Epidemiological data from 20 European studies. *Diabetologia* 1999;42:647–54.

17 Qiao Q, Nakagami T, Tuomilehto J *et al.* Comparison of the fasting and the 2-h glucose criteria for diabetes in different Asian cohorts. *Diabetologia* 2000;43:1470–5.

18 The DECODE Study Group, on behalf of the European Diabetes Epidemiology Group. Glucose tolerance and cardiovascular mortality. Comparison of fasting and 2-hour glucose criteria. *Arch Intern Med* 2001;161:397–404.

19 Tominaga M, Eguchi H, Manaka H *et al.* Impaired glucose tolerance is a risk factor for cardiovascular disease, but not impaired fasting glucose: the Funagata Diabetes Study. *Diabetes Care* 1999;22:920–4.

20 De Vegt F, Dekker JM, Stehouwer CDA *et al.* Similar 9-year mortality risks and reproducibility for the World Health Organization and American Diabetes Association glucose tolerance categories. *Diabetes Care* 2000;23:40–44.

21 Bennett PH, Burch TA, Miller M. Diabetes mellitus in American (Pima) Indians. *Lancet* 1971;ii:125–8.

22 Zimmet PZ, Taft P, Guinea A *et al.* The high prevalence of diabetes mellitus on a Central Pacific island. *Diabetologia* 1977;13:111–15.

23 Zimmet PZ. Kelly West Lecture. Challenges in diabetes epidemiology: from West to the rest. *Diabetes Care* 1992;15:232–52.

24 O'Dea K. Westernisation, insulin resistance and diabetes in Australian Aborigines. *Med J Aust* 1991;155:258–64.

25 Burke JP, Williams K, Haffner SM *et al.* Elevated incidence of Type 2 diabetes in San Antonio, Texas, compared with that of Mexico City, Mexico. *Diabetes Care* 2001;24:1573–8.

26 De Courten M, Bennett PH, Tuomilehto J, Zimmet P. Epidemiology of NIDDM in non-europids. In: Alberti KGMM, Zimmet P, DeFronzo RA, editors. *International textbook of diabetes mellitus*. 2nd edn. Chichester; Wiley, 1997: 143–70.

27 Harris MI, Flegal KM, Cowie CC *et al.* Prevalence of diabetes, impaired fasting glucose, and impaired glucose tolerance in U.S. adults. *Diabetes Care* 1998;21:518–24.

28 Gu K, Cowie CC, Harris MI. Diabetes and decline in heart disease mortality in US adults. *J Am Med Assoc* 1999;281:1291–7.

29 Yudkin JS, Alberti KGMM, McLarty DS, Swai H. Impaired glucose tolerance. Is it a risk factor for diabetes or a diagnostic ragbag? *Br Med J* 1990;301:397–401.

30 Haffner SM, D'Agostino R, Saad MF *et al.* Increased insulin resistance and insulin secretion in nondiabetic African–Americans and Hispanics compared with non-Hispanic whites: the Insulin Resistance Atherosclerosis Study. *Diabetes* 1996;45:742–8.

31 Lillioja S, Mott DM, Spraul M *et al.* Insulin resistance and insulin secretory dysfunction as precursors of non-insulin-dependent diabetes mellitus: prospective studies of Pima Indians. *N Engl J Med* 1993;329:1988–92.

32 Haffner SM, Miettinen H, Gaskill SP, Stern MP. Decreased insulin secretion and increased insulin

resistance are independently related to the 7-year risk of NIDDM in Mexican–Americans. *Diabetes* 1995;44:1386–91.

33 Mykkänen L, Laakso M, Uusitupa M, Pyörälä K. Prevalence of diabetes and impaired glucose tolerance in elderly subjects and their association with obesity and family history of diabetes. *Diabetes Care* 1990;13:1099–105.

34 Hu FB, Manson JE, Stampfer MJ. Diet, lifestyle, and the risk of type 2 diabetes mellitus in women. *N Engl J Med* 2001;345:790–7.

35 Boyko EJ, Fujimoto WY, Leonetti DL, Newell-Morris L. Visceral adiposity and risk of type 2 diabetes. A prospective study among Japanese Americans. *Diabetes Care* 2000;23:465–71.

36 Van Dam RM, Boer JMA, Feskens EJM, Seidell JC. Parental history of diabetes modifies the association between abdominal adiposity and hyperglycemia. *Diabetes Care* 2001;24:1454–9.

37 Kriska AM, Pereira MA, Hanson RL *et al.* Association of physical activity and serum insulin concentrations in two populations at high risk for type 2 diabetes but differing by BMI. *Diabetes Care* 2001;24:1175–80.

38 Meyer K, Kushi LH, Jacobs DR, Folsom AR. Dietary fat and incidence of type 2 diabetes in older Iowa women. *Diabetes Care* 2001;24:1528–35.

39 Hales CN, Barker DJP. Type 2 (non-insulin-dependent) diabetes mellitus: the thrifty phenotype hypothesis. *Diabetologia* 1992;35:595–601.

40 McCance DR, Pettitt DJ, Hanson RL *et al.* Birth weight and non-insulin-dependent diabetes: thrifty genotype, thrifty phenotype, or surviving small baby genotype? *Br Med J* 1994;308:942–5.

41 Boyko EJ. Proportion of type 2 diabetes cases resulting from impaired fetal growth. *Diabetes Care* 2000;23:1260–4.

42 Pan X-R, Li G-W, Wang J-X *et al.* Effects of diet and exercise in preventing NIDDM in people with impaired glucose tolerance: the Da Qing IGT and Diabetes Study. *Diabetes Care* 1997;20:537–44.

43 Tuomilehto J, Lindström J, Eriksson JG *et al.* Prevention of type 2 diabetes mellitus by changes in lifestyle among subjects with impaired glucose tolerance. *N Engl J Med* 2001;344:1343–50.

44 Diet and exercise dramatically delay type 2 diabetes. [Press release of the National Institute of Diabetes and Digestive and Kidney Diseases.] August 8, 2001. http://www.niddk.nih.gov/welcome/releases/8_8_01.htm) Accessed August 22, 2001.

45 American Diabetes Association. Screening for type 2 diabetes. *Diabetes Care* 1998;21 (Suppl 1):S20–S22.

46 Alberti KGMM. Impaired glucose tolerance—fact or fiction. *Diabet Med* 1996;13:S6–S8.

2

Pathogenesis of type 2 diabetes

Dirk Müller-Wieland, Jörg Kotzka and Barry J. Goldstein

INTRODUCTION

Diabetes mellitus type 2 is one of the most frequently encountered endocrine metabolic disorders and affects about 5–10% of most populations in the developed world[1]. Late complications as a result of micro- and macro-angiopathy are an enormous health economic burden. Accordingly, diabetes is one of the major causes of blindness, renal insufficiency and amputation of the lower extremities. Furthermore, patients with type 2 diabetes have a 3–5-fold increased cardiovascular risk.

From the pathogenic point of view, type 2 diabetes is a heterogeneous group of disorders, which are diagnosed by an established level of blood glucose elevation. This hyperglycemia is due to a decreased action or secretion of insulin. This chapter focuses on some molecular mechanisms involved in the pathogenesis of insulin resistance and type 2 diabetes, which have been recognized to be of clinical significance for the diagnosis of type 2 diabetes and influence strategies for therapeutic interventions.

PATHOPHYSIOLOGY

Although clinical manifestations of type 2 diabetes occur most frequently at an age > 40 years and are associated with increased body weight, genetic factors appear to play a predominant role in the pathophysiology. It has been shown that there is a very high concordance rate in twins, meaning that if one of a pair of twins has type 2 diabetes, in spite of growing up in socially different environments, the second twin has a high probability of developing clinically overt type 2 diabetes in later years[2]. Genetic disposition is therefore a major pathogenic determinant and environmental factors may only have a modulatory role in determining the diabetic phenotype. However, lifestyle and other social factors have great clinical importance; they have been shown to sharply affect the onset of disease and offer the possibility of preventive strategies.

With regard to glucose homeostasis, clinically overt type 2 diabetes is characterized by three pathophysiological phenomena that typically develop in the following sequence and might represent different phases of the disease process:

- Reduced insulin sensitivity or insulin resistance
- Dysfunction of pancreatic beta-cells with relative insulin deficiency
- Increased hepatic glucose production.

Several epidemiological studies in different populations have shown that increased hepatic glucose production with elevated fasting blood sugar levels is a relatively late phenomenon of type 2 diabetes. This increased hepatic glucose production is most likely caused by an altered ratio of hepatic insulin to glucagon action, regulating liver metabolism and leading to an increased rate of hepatic gluconeogenesis.

Insulin secretion by pancreatic beta-cells stimulated by glucose is characterized by two phases, one rapid and the other a slow continuous insulin release. Insulin is released in a pulsatile fashion. Absence of the first phase of insulin secretion and an alteration in the pulsatility of insulin secretion are early signs of beta-cell dysfunction in the development of type 2 diabetes and can often be detected before clinical manifestations of the disease.

Reduced insulin-stimulated glucose uptake or insulin resistance is the earliest detectable dysfunction in the development of type 2 diabetes. For example, in a prospective study Martin et al.[3] investigated the pattern of insulin secretion as well as insulin sensitivity in children of families in which both parents were afflicted with type 2 diabetes. The children were examined every 5 years and the investigators showed that reduced insulin sensitivity was already detectable 20 years before their type 2 diabetes was clinically manifest. However, alterations in insulin secretion were detectable only 3–5 years prior to the onset of overt hyperglycemia. Both abnormalities, reduced insulin action as well as defects in insulin secretion, must be present before type 2 diabetes can be diagnosed. This is important because patients with even severe levels of insulin resistance can maintain glucose levels within the normal range, if they are able to mount a sufficiently elevated level of insulin secretion.

Insulin resistance is a key phenomenon not only in the development of glucose intolerance and type 2 diabetes – which depends on the pancreatic insulin response – but also in the development of the constellation of cardiovascular risk factors, including abdominal (visceral) obesity, lipid disorders and essential hypertension that comprise insulin resistance or the 'metabolic' syndrome. This is discussed in more detail in Chapter 22.

Decreased insulin sensitivity is detected clinically as a reduced insulin-stimulated glucose uptake. However, at the cellular level, insulin resistance is defined as reduced insulin action, which can affect not only glucose uptake, but also other cellular responses to insulin action. Different defects and disorders in various signaling pathways, multiple cells and tissues can develop in diverse combinations over time, contributing to the heterogeneous clinical phenotype of these patients[4,5]. The characterization of these different disorders of insulin action at the genetic, cellular and clinical level may lead to new subclassifications, and diagnostic and therapeutic approaches in the management of type 2 diabetes in the future.

MOLECULAR MECHANISMS OF INSULIN ACTION

One approach towards the understanding of the relation between insulin resistance and type 2 diabetes is the elucidation of complex cellular signaling networks mediating not only insulin-stimulated glucose uptake but also many other cellular effects, including gene regulatory networks affecting cell growth and differentiation.

The principal mechanisms of signal transduction by insulin are similar to other members of the growth factor family, all of which appear to stimulate receptors at the cell surface[6–8]. Activation of these receptors by hormone binding leads to autophosphorylation at tyrosine residues on the receptor protein, which activates the intrinsic kinase activity of the receptor. The activated receptor kinase phosphorylates substrates within the cell at tyrosine residues. The tyrosine phosphorylated substrates act as 'docking' or 'adapter' proteins, since they in turn bind other molecules and generate physical complexes of signaling proteins. These signaling complexes regulate the activity of different signaling cascades in diverse areas of cellular function, including glucose uptake and gene regulation. Thus, signaling networks (Figure 2.1) are generated by protein–protein interactions, which are regulated by phosphorylation, subcellular localization, and the abundance or availability of each signaling molecule. Each signaling step or component protein appears to be a potential candidate for genetic as well as regulatory defects of insulin action, which might

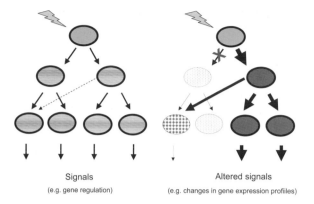

Signals
(e.g. gene regulation)

Altered signals
(e.g. changes in gene expression profiiles)

Figure 2.1 The activated receptor kinase phosphorylates substrates within the cell at tyrosine residues. The tyrosine phosphorylated substrates act as 'docking' or adapter proteins by binding other signaling molecules, thereby generating signaling complexes. These complexes regulate activity of different signaling cascades in diverse cellular functions, including glucose uptake and gene regulation. Signaling networks are therefore generated by protein-protein interactions, which are regulated by phosphorylation, subcellular localization, and abundance of each signaling molecule. Each signaling step or protein appears to be a potential candidate for genetic, as well as regulatory defects of insulin action, which might play a role in various forms of insulin resistance.

play a role in various forms of insulin resistance. This chapter therefore focuses on some of the principal mechanisms of insulin signaling, glucose uptake, and gene regulation.

Signal transduction pathways of insulin

The insulin receptor consists usually of two extracellular alpha-subunits and two transmembrane beta-subunits, which are processed from a single precursor protein. Two different insulin receptor isotypes can be generated by alternative splicing of the receptor mRNA, which generates isoforms that differ in the existence or absence of 12 amino acids close to the C-terminal region of the receptor alpha-subunit. The two alpha-subunits generate the extracellular binding region of the receptor, whereas the intracellular domain of the beta-subunit contains the

enzymatic tyrosine kinase domain. Binding of insulin leads to an alteration in the conformation of the receptor protein and the process of trans-autophosphorylation of several tyrosine residues in the cytoplasmic region of the beta-subunit. Tyrosine 960 in the juxtamembrane region plays a pivotal role in signal transduction, facilitating the interaction with postreceptor signaling molecules, such as the insulin receptor substrates. Tyrosine phosphorylation of insulin receptor substrates leads to binding and activation of downstream signaling elements: for example, the binding and activation of different phospatidylinositol (PI) 3-kinases or signaling proteins regulating mitogen-activated protein (MAP) kinases that play a role in glucose uptake and gene regulation, respectively.

Insulin-stimulated glucose uptake

A disease-defining phenomenon of type 2 diabetes is impaired insulin-stimulated glucose uptake and consumption in muscle and fat tissue. Insulin-dependent glucose transport is mediated by glucose transport proteins[9,10]. The family of glucose transporters consists of 11 different proteins and facilitates the transport of the D-glucose energy independent of the concentration gradient into the cell.

Insulin-dependent glucose transport is mediated mainly by the isoform GLUT4, which is the predominant glucose transporter in fat tissue and skeletal muscle. Transporter activity is regulated by reversible distribution of glucose transporters from inside the cell to the plasma membrane, by regulated vesicle transport. Most of the GLUT4 glucose transporters in unstimulated adipocytes are found within an intracellular reservoir, which appears to be associated with the *trans*-Golgi network. Insulin stimulation leads to an increase in the exocytosis rate of GLUT4 vesicles. There is thus an insulin-mediated translocation of GLUT4 to the plasma membrane. GLUT4 transporters at the plasma membrane are internalized continuously and hormone-independently into an endosomal sorting compartment[11]. The precise mechanisms of insulin-mediated sorting and translocation of GLUT4-containing vesicles to the plasma membrane are still unclear. However, identification of regulatory proteins involved in the process, and characterization of the respective pathways will reveal novel potential targets for the understanding of drug therapy and insulin resistance.

Insulin-related gene regulation

Insulin action is not only related to the uptake of glucose, but also to the regulation of many different genes, inducing alterations in gene regulatory networks affecting cell growth, differentiation of adipocytes, composition of metabolic active and inactive muscle fibers, mitochondrial respiration rate or energy expenditure, insulin secretion and insulin sensitivity. Alterations in gene expression might therefore play a role not only in cellular insulin resistance, but also in molecular changes related to the development of other clinical features associated with insulin resistance, such as obesity, lipid disorders, hypertension, and increased cardiovascular risk. It is therefore very likely that proteins involved in gene regulatory pathways, such as transcription factors, might be a gene regulatory link between insulin sensitivity, obesity and other cardiovascular risk factors.

Transcription factors could be altered in their abundance and activity primarily or secondary as a consequence of altered insulin action and/or other metabolic features. One of the best examples of transcription factors integrating cellular information induced by nutrients, metabolites, hormones, growth factors, inflammatory signals and drugs on insulin sensitivity as well as on intracellular lipid metabolism are peroxisomal proliferator activator receptors (PPARs) and sterol-regulatory element binding proteins (SREBPs)[12].

PPARs have different isoforms, such as PPARalpha, PPAR beta/delta, and PPARgamma[13]. PPARalpha is mainly expressed by the liver, plays a central role in fatty acid metabolism and is a target for the fibrate drugs. PPAR beta/delta is expressed in many different tissues and appears to be regulated by some fatty acids. PPARgamma is a key player in the control of adipogenesis and insulin sensitivity[14–16].

PPARgamma is also a target for the class of insulin sensitizers called glitazones (thiazolidinediones). The precise mechanisms by which glitazones or PPARgamma-activity affect insulin sensitivity are still not entirely clear, but appear to involve several potential alterations, including redistribution of visceral fat to subcutaneous fat, increasing lipid catabolism and reducing lipotoxicity, and affecting fat-cell size, as well as via the secretion of various adipokines[17,18].

PPARgamma is controlled by coactivators, of which the PPARgamma coactivator-1 (PGC-1) has become of increasing interest. Spiegelman's group showed that PGC-1alpha plays a central role in controlling PPARgamma activity and thereby adipogenesis, but can also interact with other transcription factors controlling muscle differentiation and hepatic gluconeogenesis. PGC-1alpha is therefore an example of how a single signaling step controlling gene expression and cellular differentiation networks affects diverse cells and biological phenomena, e.g. fat-cell differentiation, muscle cell differentiation, hepatic gluconeogenesis and energy expenditure[19–24]. Clearly, alterations in any of these several functions can have an impact on glucose metabolism and type 2 diabetes.

Another upstream regulator of the gene regulatory network controlled by PPARgamma is the sterol regulatory element-binding protein (SREBP)-1c, which has been shown to also promote adipocyte differentiation. Interestingly, over-expression of the nuclear form of SREBP-1c in adipose tissue of transgenic mice under the control of the adipocyte-specific aP2 enhancer causes a syndrome with lipoatrophy, marked insulin resistance, and overt diabetes mellitus[25]. SREBP-isoforms, SREBP-1a and SREBP-1c, as well as SREBP-2, belong to the family of bHLH proteins and their intranuclear abundance is controlled by intracellular sterol levels[26–28]. It has been shown that SREBP-2 is one of the main regulators of cholesterol synthesis, whereas SREBP-1c affects predominantly synthesis of fatty acids, and SREBP-1a affects both pathways. In addition, many other genes appear to be targets of SREBPs. We have shown recently that transactivity of SREBPs can be controlled by insulin, growth factors and cytokines, thereby providing a gene regulatory link for metabolites, hormones and inflammatory signals[29–31].

MOLECULAR MECHANISMS OF INSULIN RESISTANCE

Information flux at the cellular level via different signaling pathways and networks depends on many factors underlying complex regulation. Regulatory mechanisms can affect abundance and thereby stoichiometry of interacting signaling proteins, specificity and time course of tyrosine phosphorylation events, subcellular localization and trafficking of signal mediators, etc. Furthermore, activity and function of signaling proteins involved in insulin action can be influenced by interaction with inhibitory proteins, serine phosphorylation and tyrosine phosphatases.

Regulatory mechanisms reducing insulin sensitivity

Cell and animal studies have shown, for example, that the insulin signal can be inhibited at the receptor level by specific tyrosine phosphatases. Protein tyrosine phosphatases (PTPases) that function as negative regulators of the insulin signaling cascade have been identified as novel targets for the therapeutic enhancement of insulin action in insulin-resistant disease states[32,33]. Recent studies have provided compelling evidence that one of the main functions of the intracellular enzyme PTPase 1B (PTP1B), and perhaps to a lesser extent the transmembrane PTPase leukocyte antigen-related (LAR), is to suppress insulin action[34]. Reducing PTP1B abundance not only enhances insulin sensitivity and improves glucose metabolism, but has also been shown to effectively protect against obesity induced by high-fat feeding in rodent models.

Increased phosphorylation at serine residues of the insulin receptor or insulin receptor substrates has been shown to be another type of modification associated with decreased insulin signaling[35]. The detailed mechanisms are still unclear, but serine phosphorylation might

impair transferase activity of protein tyrosine kinases, phospho-tyrosine-dependent protein–protein interactions, or accelerate the dissociation of signaling complexes. Insulin-resistant states induced by inflammatory signals, hyperglycemia, free fatty acids, catecholamines and cytokines, including tumor necrosis factor alpha (TNFalpha), have been related to molecular mechanisms associated with increased serine phosphorylation of signaling proteins involved in insulin action, such as the insulin receptor or insulin receptor substrates[36–40].

Another secondary mechanism might be the role of regulatory proteins, such as the recently identified Grb7 family and PC-1. PC-1 is a large membrane glycoprotein whose function is unknown, but which can act as an inhibitor of insulin receptor tyrosine kinase activity[41,42]. PC-1 is over-expressed in cells from insulin-resistant subjects, including patients with type 2 diabetes. Searching for new proteins able to bind to the intracellular domain of the insulin receptor led to the identification of a new protein family, the Grb7 family of molecular adapters[43,44]. These proteins (Grb7, Grb10, Grb14) possess a C-terminal domain that can interact with different signaling proteins, and a family-specific domain for interaction with the insulin receptor. For example, recently it has been shown that Grb14 is a direct inhibitor of the catalytic activity of the insulin receptor and can be considered to be a modulator of insulin signaling. The detailed function of these proteins in modulating the insulin receptor in different tissues of patients with type 2 diabetes is still unclear. However, alterations in regulatory proteins might play a key role in the development of insulin resistance and type 2 diabetes, and regulatory proteins are therefore potential new therapeutic targets for anti-diabetic therapy.

Transgenic mouse models of insulin signaling pathways

The potential clinical relevance and role of cellular signaling proteins in the pathophysiology of insulin resistance and type 2 diabetes can be best tested in transgenic mice models[45–47]. Although it is still unclear whether the physiology of mice

Table 2.1 Transgenic mice models of insulin receptor (IR) and insulin receptor substrates (IRS): monogenic and tissue selective knockout (KO) animals are shown

Monogenic knockout mice	Phenotype
IR$^{-/-}$	Early post-natal death by ketoacidosis
IR$^{+/-}$	Diabetes in 10% of adults
IRS-1$^{-/-}$	Growth retardation
	Insulin resistance, normoglycemia
	Beta-cells hyperplasia, altered insulin secretion
IRS-2$^{-/-}$	Severe insulin resistance
	Beta-cells hypoplasia, decreased insulin secretion
	Diabetes in early life

Tissue-specific knockout mice	Phenotype
MIRKO (skeletal muscle)	Normal glucose and insulin levels
	Dyslipidemia and increased adiposity
LIRKO (liver)	Severe insulin resistance
	Fasting hyperglycemia
	Hyperplastic islets
BIRKO (beta-cell)	Loss of glucose-induced first-phase insulin release
	Age-dependent glucose intolerance
	Decreased islet size and pancreas insulin content
	Diabetes in obese mice
FIRKO (adipose tissue)	Protection against obesity and
	obesity-related glucose intolerance
NIRKO (neuronal)	Diet-induced obesity, insulin resistance, dyslipidemia
	Dysregulation of LH secretion, impaired spermatogenesis
	Impaired ovarian follicule maturation

and the alterations induced by transgenic technology are comparable with human diabetes, this model can help with the generating and testing of clinical hypotheses and with delineating different components in complex systems (see Table 2.1).

The pivotal role of insulin, as well as the fact that absolute insulin deficiency leads to the development of ketoacidosis, was proven in transgenic mice lacking the insulin receptor[48,49]. These mice died shortly after birth as a result of severe ketoacidosis. However, most of the heterozygous animals were clinically normal.

This corresponds with the clinical observation of patients with genetic syndromes of severe insulin resistance. These patients, in whom two defective alleles of the insulin receptor can be identified, died soon after birth. The parents, however, who apparently have heterozygous alterations of the insulin receptor gene, are clinically silent, or show only a mild glucose intolerance. Adding a defective allele of the insulin receptor substrate-1 to these heterozygous insulin-receptor knockout mice increased insulin resistance, by adding a post-receptor defect, and resulted in the clinical manifestation of diabetes. This is an example of a transgenic polygenic disease model[50].

The clinical observation that skeletal muscle is responsible for most postprandial insulin-stimulated glucose uptake has always affected the current hypothesis that insulin resistance in skeletal muscle plays an essential role in the development of clinically overt type 2 diabetes. It was surprising, therefore, that transgenic mice, in which the insulin receptor was deleted specifically in skeletal muscle, did not have clinically overt hyperglycemia, growth alteration or even glucose intolerance, but only mild insulin resistance with slightly elevated levels of insulin and plasma triglycerides[51]. Further studies showed that glucose was redistributed to adipose tissue[52]. Mice deficient in the liver insulin receptor develop overt diabetes due to increased hepatic gluconeogenesis[53]. Insulin receptor knockout mice exhibit defects in insulin secretion from the beta-cells of the pancreas similar to those occurring in early stages of type 2 diabetes[54,55]. These data provided evidence for the first time that the insulin resistance of beta-cells can be associated with reduced glucose-stimulated insulin secretion. Insulin resistance can lead, therefore, not only to reduced insulin-stimulated uptake of glucose and increased glucose production, but also to impaired insulin secretion, i.e. all biochemical features of type 2 diabetes.

Mice with fat-specific disruption of the insulin receptor gene are protected against age-related and hypothalamic lesion-induced obesity, and obesity-related glucose intolerance[56]. In this context it is also interesting to note that insulin receptor deficiency in the central nervous system leads to hyperphagia, with obesity, insulin resistance and elevated triglyceride levels[57].

Mice deficient in the insulin receptor substrate protein IRS-1 exhibit insulin resistance with glucose intolerance, hypertriglyceridemia and low HDL-cholesterol levels, as well as an elevated blood pressure, which is reminiscent of the metabolic syndrome in human subjects[58-62]. Furthermore, these animals show a reduced embryonal and postnatal growth rate, and a body weight reduced by 40–50%. The insulin resistance is compensated for by an increased insulin production of the beta-cells. IRS-2-deficient mice have severe insulin resistance in liver and muscle[63,64]. However, in these animals insulin resistance cannot be compensated for by increased insulin production, since insulin secretion by the beta-cells is decreased, associated with reduced neogenesis of beta-cells.

These types of transgenic mouse studies have provided insights relevant to type 2 diabetes in human subjects, demonstrating multiple lines of communication in the metabolic relationship between various tissues involved in glucose and lipid homeostasis. Decreased insulin action in one tissue can induce profound alterations and insulin resistance in others, revealing multiple sites of potential intervention in ameliorating the insulin resistance of diabetes and its consequences.

IDENTIFICATION OF TYPE 2 DIABETES GENES

Type 2 diabetes is not only clinically but also genetically a heterogeneous and multifactorial disease. Accordingly, clinical manifestation of type 2 diabetes is the result of not only genes that appear to be altered primarily, but also of genes whose expression rate is altered secondary to initial pathophysiologically relevant mechanisms.

Interestingly, it has been observed that low birth-weight appears to be associated with an increased risk of developing insulin resistance and its clinical consequences, such as type 2 diabetes or syndrome X in later life. This points to the possibility that intrauterine nutritive components can alter the underlying genetic programming (e. g. imprinting)[65].

When blood glucose levels increase above certain diagnostic criteria, type 2 diabetes can be diagnosed. However, since blood glucose levels are a physiological parameter, it is likely that different genetic alterations or events combine in their contribution to the overall level of blood glucose, which is a continuum. This makes genetic characterization difficult, since the phenotype of type 2 diabetes is not a simple pathophysiological state or a clinical homogeneous entity. This heterogeneous clinical phenotype makes it quite difficult to identify major genes in genetic associations or linkage studies. Most genetic studies of the common 'garden' variety of type 2 diabetes have shown that it is not due to a single major gene alteration, but is the result of changes at many gene loci, i.e. a polygenic disorder[66–68].

SYNDROMES RELATED TO INSULIN RESISTANCE AND TYPE 2 DIABETES

Syndromes related to insulin resistance or diabetes, for example polycystic ovarian (PCO) syndrome, rare genetic syndromes of severe insulin resistance, and genetic defects affecting the regulation of insulin secretion – termed maturity-onset diabetes of the young (MODY) – may be relevant to the identification of novel candidate genes and pathogenic mechanisms.

Insulin resistance and PCO

Stein and Leventhal initially reported the major characteristics of PCO in 1935. The essential characteristics of PCO are unaltered LH-/FSH-relation, elevated androgen plasma levels, chronic anovulation associated with insulin resistance and hyperinsulinemia[69–72]. The major clinical signs are amenorrhea, hirsutism and obesity. Morphological features are a thickened tunica albuginea, a hyperplasia of theca interna, a thick corticostroma and multiple follicles of different developmental stages. The syndrome appears to be a heterogeneous disorder and is very frequently the cause of unovulatory infertility. The cardinal clinical features are often manifested during puberty or adolescence, and have been attributed to an elevated synthesis and secretion of androgens by the ovaries and adrenals. The elevated androgen production may also be caused or enhanced by insulin resistance, and result, at least in part, from the effect of high circulating insulin levels, which can stimulate androgen production by activating the receptor for insulin-like growth factor (IGF)-1 in ovary and adrenal cells.

Hyperandrogenism and acanthosis nigricans are also cardinal features of patients with rare inherited syndromes of severe insulin resistance (see below). Insulin resistance-related androgen production, as well as estrogen generation, can be aggravated by overweight. Several studies have shown an amelioration of all the essential clinical, endocrine and biochemical features of PCO by weight reduction, as well as by the use of drugs that increase insulin sensitivity, such as metformin and thiazolidinediones[73–75].

Rare syndromes of severe insulin resistance

As described above, genetic defects can appear in each step of the insulin signaling cascade. Syndromes of severe insulin resistance, which are caused by alterations of the insulin receptor gene, can therefore be differentiated from syndromes associated with 'postreceptor' defects, the molecular etiology of which remains unknown[76]. Combinations of both might also play a role in the development of the presenting clinical findings, which are mainly determined by the extent or degree of disturbance in different insulin signaling pathways. Other cellular biological alterations, beside the insulin action pathway, may play a role in the clinical appearance, for example in the case of sisters with the same genetic mutation in the insulin receptor gene who have been shown to have different clinical phenotypes[76].

Patients with the 'type A' syndrome of insulin resistance have a heterozygous mutation in the kinase domain of the insulin receptor and associated severe hyperinsulinemia and hyperglycemia. Most of these patients have an acanthosis nigricans, which is a velvety thickening and darkening of skin typically in the axilla and the back of the neck. Acanthosis nigricans appears to correlate with the degree of insulin resistance. Female patients with type A syndrome are often virilized, and have cystic ovaries because of a hyperandrogenemia that appears to be the result of stimulated androgen production of the ovaries. In the ovaries, androgen production is controlled by the IGF-1-receptor, which might be activated in the state of high insulin levels. Patients with a leprechaunism or Rabson–Mendenhall syndrome are very rare and are diagnosed as young children. These patients suffer frequently from a homozygous or compound heterozygous mutation of the insulin receptor gene, associated with severe cellular and clinical insulin resistance. These patients also have reduced subcutaneous fat and often a hepatomegaly. In addition, patients with Rabson–Mendenhall syndrome have specific features, including multiple rows of teeth and alterations in the nails.

Patients with congenital lipoatrophy have no genetic defect in the insulin receptor gene, but apparently have postreceptor defects affecting gene regulatory pathways. It is interesting to note that the complete lack of white adipose tissue is associated with insulin resistance, comparable to patients with obesity[77]. One linking pathophysiological feature appears to be lipotoxicity (see below). This lipotoxicity might also play a role in the recently more frequently observed lipodystrophy associated with the use of protease inhibitors in HIV-positive patients. This lipodystrophy is characterized by a loss of subcutaneous adipose tissue from the extremities and face, combined with increased fat accumulation in the neck and trunk. This clinical feature is associated with insulin resistance, elevated blood glucose levels and dyslipidemia. There is a reduced adipocyte differentiation rate and HIV-protease inhibitors also affect the cleavage of sterol regulatory element-binding proteins, such as SREBP-1c. SREBP-1c plays a role in the rate of adipocyte differentiation and can enhance the effects of PPARgamma, most likely by inducing endogenous ligands.

A family of patients with lipoatrophy has been described; they show different features of the insulin resistance syndrome, such as dyslipidemia, hyperglycemia and hypertension, and have a homozygous mutation in the nuclear receptor PPARgamma-2. PPARgamma-2 is a major regulator of adipocytes and the target of the glitazone class of insulin-sensitizing drugs. Treatment of lipodystrophic patients with leptin can also improve insulin sensitivity[78]. Leptin not only regulates food intake at the level of the hypothalamus, but also has significant peripheral effects and can stimulate lipid oxidation in non-adipose tissue. Reduction of lipid accumulation

within skeletal muscle cells and liver might therefore explain the improvement in insulin sensitivity (lipotoxicity; see below) by leptin treatment in patients with congenital lipoatrophy[78].

Clinical features and genetic defects in patients with MODY

MODY represents a group of clinically and genetically heterogenous familial disorders resembling early-onset type 2 diabetes (Table 2.2)[79,80]. The main clinical features are nonketotic diabetes mellitus with an onset before age of 25 years, autosomal dominant inheritance with a family history of diabetes in several generations, absence of obesity, and a lack of autoimmune phenomena. A primary defect in pancreatic beta-cell function is present and usually causes mild hyperglycemia due to moderately reduced insulin secretion. In most cases, mutations in six different genes have been identified and related to six distinct clinical phenotypes (Table 2.2). One of the genes codes for glucokinase, a glucose sensor for the beta-cells (MODY2), while the other genes code for transcription factors that play key roles in the development and function of beta-cells and pancreatic islets. MODY2 and MODY3 are the most frequently found mutations, while MODY1 and MODY4–6 are rare.

More than 130 mutations have been found in the glucokinase gene in MODY2. These genetic defects impair the glucose-sensing function of this enzyme in the beta-cell, causing an upward shift in the plasma glucose threshold for stimulation of insulin secretion. Fasting and postprandial hyperglycemia is therefore mild in most cases, with satisfactory control of blood sugar levels by diet alone. These patients need to control their body weight and perform regular physical activity, to maintain peripheral insulin sensitivity and not stress the limited insulin secretion available from the pancreas. About half of the female carriers of MODY2 may present with gestational diabetes during pregnancy.

MODY3 is also frequent, representing up to two-thirds of MODY patients. MODY3 is caused by mutations in the transcription factor hepatocyte nuclear factor (HNF)-1alpha. More than 120 mutations have been already found in this gene.

Table 2.2 MODY-related genes and associated clinical phenotypes

MODY type	Gene	Clinical features of heterozygous state	Most common treatment	Distribution (% of MODY families)	Age at diagnosis
MODY 1	HNF-4α	Diabetes, microvascular complications (in many cases); reductions in serum concentration of triglycerides, apolipoproteins AII and CIII, and Lp(a) lipoprotein	Oral hypoglycemic agent, insulin	Rare	Postpubertal
MODY 2	Glucokinase	Impaired fasting glucose tolerance, diabetes, normal proinulin-to-insulin ratio in serum	Diet and exercise	8–63	Childhood
MODY 3	HNF-1α	Diabetes, microvascular complications (in many cases); renal glycosuria, increased sensitivity to sulfonylurea drugs, increased proinsulin-to-insulin ratio in serum	Oral hypoglycemic agent, insulin	21–64	Postpubertal
MODY 4	IGP-1	Diabetes	Oral hypoglycemic agent	Rare	Early adulthood
MODY 5	HNF-1β	Diabetes, renal cysts and other abnormalities of renal development; progressive nondiabetic renal dysfunction, leading to chronic renal insufficiency and failure; internal genital abnormalities (in female carriers)	Insulin	Unknown	Postpubertal
MODY 6	NeuroD1 or BETA2	Diabetes	Insulin	Rare	Early adulthood
MODY X	Unknown	Unknown/heterogeneous?	–	10–20% in Europe	Heterogeneous

Despite mild elevations in fasting plasma glucose concentrations to a similar degree as in patients with MODY2, 2-h post-challenge glucose levels are higher. Since HNF-4alpha regulates the expression of HNF-1alpha, the clinical phenotype of the rare MODY1 subtype, which is caused by mutations in the HNF-4alpha gene, is similar to MODY3. In contrast to MODY2, the development of diabetes with hyperglycemia in MODY3 is more rapid or aggressive over time, therefore tighter control of these individuals is warranted. Furthermore, patients with MODY3 have reduced tubular reabsorption of glucose and a decreased glucose threshold for glycosuria.

MODY4–6 are rare syndromes. About one-fifth of European individuals presenting with typical clinical features of MODY do not have mutations in any of the identified six MODY genes, indicating that there may still be several additional genes and pathways waiting to be discovered in MODY families.

MODY: a history of bench-to-bedside genetics

The history of MODY is a paradigm example of bench-to-bedside genetics in the elucidation of complex polygenic multifactorial disorders, like type 2 diabetes. The distinct clinical phenotype of MODY as a familial early-onset type of non-insulin-dependent diabetes mellitus was known for many years. Careful clinical characterization led to the discovery of glucokinase mutations in some families. Searches for additional defects in glucokinase in many other MODY families later proved negative. Increased interest in beta-cell biology revealed novel candidates and mutations were identified in different transcription factors. Careful observation of the clinical features in MODY individuals has also revealed clinically different MODY subtypes, and this may lead to improved individual care of patients with these syndromes. Similarly, it is likely that patients with type 2 diabetes could also be classified into many subtypes, each presenting with distinct clinical manifestations and different courses of disease natural history, and requiring individualized treatment strategies. Genetic approaches may enable these determinations to be made.

LIPOTOXICITY: A NOVEL LINK BETWEEN INSULIN RESISTANCE AND FAT

Several studies regarding the role of adipose tissue in insulin-resistant states have altered our understanding of the role of this tissue in the pathogenesis of abnormal glucose metabolism. Perhaps the most surprising finding is that adipose tissue is not only a simple reservoir for energy stored as triglycerides, but also a very active endocrine organ, which secretes several peptides and cytokines (TNFalpha, leptin, adiponectin, resistin, etc.). These peptides and cytokines regulate energy metabolism in liver and muscle, as well as energy intake and insulin sensitivity[81,82]. Furthermore, fat tissue is also a source of inflammatory molecules, like interleukin 6 and TNFalpha, and can release mediators affecting blood pressure level and coagulation. One area of active research involves determining how the endocrine activity of fat tissue is altered in different localities, e.g. subcutaneous versus visceral fat and invasive fat cells within different organs.

The hypotheses of 'lipotoxicity' or excess lipid 'supply', generated by the groups of McGarry and Unger[83,84] and Kraegen and colleagues[85], postulate that increased intracellular lipid accumulation impairs certain cellular signaling pathways and functions, and can contribute markedly to insulin resistance. Tissue lipid accumulation in liver and skeletal muscle cells, as well as the pancreatic islets, has been identified in mouse models that lack white adipose tissue. This intracellular accumulation of lipids is associated with reduced insulin sensitivity. For example, Kim et al.[86] showed in transgenic lipo-atrophic mice that insulin-stimulated PI3 kinase activation was greatly reduced in liver, as well as in skeletal muscle. Interestingly, the cellular insulin resistance was restored to a large extent by transplantation of small amounts of adipose tissue, which caused a redistribution of lipid stores, with a reduction in the lipid content in liver and skeletal muscle. These findings and other studies have provided evidence that white adipose tissue is not just a passive reservoir for lipids, but also a very active endocrine organ, with a strong influence on insulin action and glucose metabolism in other tissues[87].

A very active area of current research is to determine whether the effect of white adipose tissue on lipid accumulation and insulin action is more closely related to the secretion of adipokines (leptin, TNFalpha, adiponectin) by white fat cells, or the distribution of tissue triglyceride stores in the body. Most likely a combination of these effects accounts for the important influence of obesity on insulin action, and glucose and lipid metabolism in the body.

Insulin sensitivity and lipid metabolism have been shown to be improved by leptin treatment in patients with lipodystrophy. Patients with congenital lipodystrophy and insulin resistance have greatly increased levels of lipids within skeletal muscle cells[88]. This is in accordance with the hypothesis that insulin-stimulated glucose uptake, or insulin sensitivity, correlates much stronger with intramural cellular lipid content than with body-mass-index (BMI). Lipotoxicity might therefore be a mechanism that can shed light onto the intricate relationship between body weight and insulin sensitivity[89,90]. Many basic and important clinical questions could be answered. Why does insulin sensitivity not correlate with the amount of subcutaneous fat? Why is insulin sensitivity greatly increased by a body weight reduction of only 5–10%? Why are not all obese individuals insulin-resistant, and why is it that patients lacking white adipose tissue are not insulin-sensitive? Several animal and human studies have suggested that intramyocellular lipid accumulation correlates best with a degree of insulin-stimulated glucose uptake of the body. Mobilization or decrease of intramyocellular lipid appears to be more sensitive to weight reduction than fat of subcutaneous tissue. Similar observations have been made regarding the amount of visceral fat. The amount of visceral fat might then be an indicator or marker of the amount of lipid accumulation outside of white subcutaneous tissue.

Clinical studies have recently shown that the intracellular lipid content of liver may also be a feature of the metabolic syndrome, i.e. be associated with insulin resistance[91,92]. Data from several types of experimental studies have also provided evidence that intracellular lipid metabolism of pancreatic beta cells might also play a role in the regulation of insulin secretion[93]. Primary or secondary alterations of intracellular lipid homeostasis therefore can be a cause of insulin resistance and its associated features, such as type 2 diabetes.

PREVENTION OF TYPE 2 DIABETES

One major aim of trying to prevent the development of clinical overt type 2 diabetes is not only to reduce the incidence of this metabolic disease, but also to reduce associated micro- and macrovascular complications[94]. Undoubtedly, different kinds of lifestyle intervention can reduce or delay the development of type 2 diabetes (see Chapter 1).

Since lifestyle alterations are difficult to sustain, there is a growing worldwide interest in the prevention of type 2 diabetes by pharmacological intervention. This interest is based on the intention to reduce the incidence of this disease, as well as to reduce early microvascular complications. Between 20 and 30% of individuals already suffer from retinopathy, nephropathy, or neuropathy at the time of diagnosis. In order to improve these dismal statistics, there needs to be a shortening of the time to diagnosis, or initiation of rigorous treatment of glucose intolerance much earlier than at the onset of the clinical criteria we currently use for type 2 diabetes. Even today, it is still unclear what the relation is between blood glucose levels, reduced insulin sensitivity and the development of atherosclerotic plaques and their acute complications, including myocardial infarction (MI), stroke, unstable angina and sudden death. It is therefore of great interest to determine whether pharmacological prevention trials reduce not only type 2 diabetes, but also other features of the metabolic syndrome, including hypertension and cardiovascular complications. The Diabetes Prevention Program research group[95] showed a significant reduction in the incidence of type 2 diabetes in a large group of patients with impaired glucose tolerance (IGT) with lifestyle intervention (58%), and with metformin therapy (31%). In the study to prevent non-insulin dependent diabetes mellitus (STOP-NIDDM) trial[96], acarbose was also shown to be effective in reducing the risk of the incidence of type 2 diabetes by 25%. Some of the initial data regarding the incidence of cardiovascular complications were recently presented for the STOP-NIDDM trial, and revealed that the treated group had a significant reduction in the incidence of hypertension, as well as a significant reduction in cardiovascular events. These interesting preliminary findings suggest that preventing diabetes and improving some of the parameters of the metabolic syndrome could reduce the cardiovascular risk that is so prevalent in this syndrome.

CONCLUSIONS AND PERSPECTIVES

The testing of different hypotheses and candidate pathways in transgenic mice has identified complex communication pathways between different tissues controlling insulin sensitivity, and interrelationships between glucose and lipid homeostasis. Elucidation of novel signaling networks within the cell, mediating and affecting insulin action, will reveal many novel genes and drug targets that might be of clinical relevance in the future[97]. We anticipate that the future of diabetes care will involve the elucidation of many different molecular subtypes of type 2 diabetes, enabling us to identify individuals at risk, perform effective prevention, and also treat and care for patients as specifically as possible, by targeting the abnormalities that constitute the underlying pathogenesis of their particular form of diabetes.

REFERENCES

1 Zimmet P, Alberti KGMM, Shaw J. Global and societal implications of the diabetes epidemic. *Nature* 2001;414:782–91.

2 Medici F, Hawa M, Ianari A, Leslie REG. Concordance rate for type 2 diabetes mellitus in monozygotic twins: actuarial analysis. *Diabetologia* 1999;42:145–50.

3 Martin BC, Warram JH, Krolewski AS et al. Role of glucose and insulin resistance in development of type 2 diabetes mellitus: results of a 25-year follow-up study. *Lancet* 1992;340:925–9.

4 Saltiel AR. New perspectives into the molecular pathogenesis and treatment of type 2 diabetes. *Cell* 2001;104:517–29.

5 De Fronzo RA. Pathogenesis of type 2 diabetes: metabolic and molecular implications for identifying diabetes genes. *Diabetes Rev* 1997;5:177–269.

6 Saltiel AR, Kahn CR. Insulin signaling and the regulation of glucose and lipid metabolism. *Nature* 2001;414:799–806.

7 Avruch J. Insulin signal transduction through protein kinase cascades. *Mol Cell Biochem* 1998;182:31–48.

8 Ullrich A, Schlessinger J. Signal transduction by receptors with tyrosine kinase activity. *Cell* 1990;20:203–12.

9 Kahn BB. Lilly lecture 1995. Glucose transport: pivotal step in insulin action. *Diabetes* 1995;45:1644–54.

10 Joost HG, Thorens B. The extended GLUT-family of sugar/polyol transport facilitators: nomenclature, sequence characteristics, and potential func-

tion of its novel members. *Mol Membr Biol* 2002;18.247–56.

11 Ploug T, van Deurs B, Ai H et al. Analysis of GLUT4 distribution in whole skeletal muscle fibers: identification of distinct storage compartments that are recruited by insulin and muscle contractions. *J Cell Biol* 1998;142:1428–46.

12 Auwerx J, Mangelsdorf D. X-ceptors, nuclear receptors for metabolism. In: Stemme S, Olsson AG, editors. *Atherosclerosis XII.* Amsterdam: Elsevier Science B.V. 2000; 21–39.

13 Ziouzenkova O, Perrey S, Marx N et al. Peroxisome proliferator-activated receptors. *Curr Atheroscler Rep* 2002;4:59–64.

14 Muller E, Drori S, Aiyer A et al. Genetic analysis of adipogenesis through peroxisome proliferator-activated receptor gamma isoforms. *J Biol Chem* 2002;277:41925–30.

15 Rosen ED, Walkey CJ, Puigserver P, Spiegelman BM. Transcriptional regulation of adipogenesis. *Genes Dev* 2000;14:1293–307.

16 Yamauchi T, Oike K, Kamon J et al. Increased insulin sensitivity despite lipodystrophy in *Crebbp* heterozygous mice. *Nat Gen* 2002;30:221–6.

17 Goldstein BJ. Possible vascular-protective effects of antidiabetic agents such as the thiazolidinediones (TZDs). *Clin Ther* 2002;24:1358–60.

18 Goldstein BJ. Insulin resistance as the core defect in type 2 diabetes mellitus. *Am J Cardiol* 2002;90 (5A):3G-10G.

19 Yoon JC, Puigserver P, Chen G et al. Control of

hepatic gluconeogenesis through the transcriptional coactivator PGC-1. *Nature* 2001;413:131–8.

20 Michael LF, Wu Z, Cheatham RB *et al.* Restoration of insulin-sensitive glucose transporter (GLUT4) gene expression in muscle cells by the transcriptional coactivator PGC-1. *Proc Natl Acad Sci USA* 2001;98:3820–5.

21 Herzig S, Long F, Jhala US *et al.* CREB regulates hepatic gluconeogenesis through the coactivator PGC-1. *Nature* 2001;413:179–83.

22 Puigserver P, Rhee J, Lin J *et al.* Cytokine stimulation of energy expenditure through p38 MAP Ki activation of PPARγ coactivator-1. *Mol Cell* 2001; 8:971–82.

23 Rosen ED, Hsu CH, Wang X *et al.* C/EBPa induces adipogenesis through PPARγ: a unified pathway. *Genes Dev* 2002;16:22–6.

24 Lin J, Wu H, Tarr PT *et al.* Transcriptional co-activator PGC-1alpha drives the formation of slow-twitch muscle fibres. *Nature* 2002;418:797–801.

25 Shimomura I, Hammer RE, Richardson JA *et al.* Insulin resistance and diabetes mellitus in transgenic mice expressing nuclear SREBP-1c in adipose tissue: model for congenital generalized lipodystrophy. *Genes Dev* 1998;12:2182–3194.

26 Horton JD, Goldstein JL, Brown MS. SREBPs: activators of the complete program of cholesterol and fatty acid synthesis in the liver. *J Clin Invest* 2002;109:1125–31.

27 Brown MS, Goldstein JL. The SREBP pathway: regulation of cholesterol metabolism by proteolysis of a membrane-bound transcription factor. *Cell* 1997;89:331–20.

28 Brown MS, Goldstein JL. A proteolytic pathway that controls the cholesterol content of membranes, cells, and blood. *Proc Natl Acad Sci USA* 1999;96:11041–8.

29 Müller-Wieland D, Kotzka J. SREBP-1: Gene regulatory key to syndrome X? *Ann NY Acad Sci* 2002;967:19–27.

30 Kotzka J, Müller-Wieland D, Roth G *et al.* Sterol regulatory element binding proteins (SREBP)-1 and SREBP-2 are linked to the MAP-kinase cascade. *J Lipid Res* 2000;41:99–108.

31 Roth G, Kotzka J, Kremer L *et al.* MAP kinases Erk1/2 phosphorylate sterol regulatory element-binding protein (SREBP)-1a at serine 117 *in vitro*. *J Biol Chem* 2000;275:33302–7.

32 Goldstein BJ. Protein-tyrosine phosphatases: emerging targets for therapeutic intervention in type 2 diabetes and related states of insulin resistance. *J Clin Endocrinol Metab* 2002;87:2472–80.

33 Wu X, Hoffstedt J, Deeb W *et al.* Depot-specific variation in protein–tyrosine phosphatase activities in human omental and subcutaneous adipose tissue: a potential contribution to differential insulin sensitivity. *J Clin Endocrinol Metab* 2001;86:5973–80.

34 Goldstein BJ, Bittier-Kowalczyk A, White MF, Harbeck M. Tyrosine dephosphorylation and deactivation of insulin receptor substrate-1B. Possible facilitation by the formation of a ternary complex with the Grb2 adaptor protein. *J Biol Chem* 2000;275:4283–9.

35 Al-Hasani H, Eisermann B, Tennagels N *et al.* Identification of Ser-1275 and Ser-1309 as autophosphorylation sites of the insulin receptor. *FEBS Lett* 1997;400:65–70.

36 Yu C, Chen Y, Cline GW *et al.* Mechanism by which fatty acids inhibit insulin activation of IRS-1 associated phosphatidylinositol 3-kinase activity in muscle. *J Biol Chem* 2002;Nov 14.

37 Kim YB, Shulman GI, Kahn BB. Fatty acid infusion selectively impairs insulin action on Akt1 and protein kinase C lambda/zeta but not on glycogen synthase kinase-3. *J Biol Chem* 2002;277:32915–22.

38 Aguirre V, Werner ED, Giraud J *et al.* Phosphorylation of Ser307 in insulin receptor substrate-1 blocks interactions with the insulin receptor and inhibits insulin action. *J Biol Chem* 2002;277:1531–7.

39 Yuan M, Konstantopoulos N, Lee J *et al.* Reversal of obesity- and diet-induced insulin resistance with salicylates or targeted disruption of Ikkbeta. *Science* 2001;293:1673–7.

40 Evans JL, Goldfine ID, Maddux BA, Grodsky GM. Oxidative stress and stress-activated signaling pathways: a unifying hypothesis of type 2 diabetes. *Endocrinol Rev* 2002;23:599–622.

41 Li M, Youngren JF, Dunaif A *et al.* Decreased insulin receptor (IR) autophosphorylation in fibroblasts from patients with PCOS: effects of serine kinase inhibitors and IR activators. *J Clin Endocrinol Metab* 2002;87:4088–93.

42 Goldfine ID, Maddux BA, Youngren JF *et al.* Role of PC-1 in the etiology of insulin resistance. *Ann NY Acad Sci* 1999;892:204–22.

43 Jahn T, Seipel P, Urschel S, Peschel C, Duyster J. Role for the adaptor protein Grb10 in the activation of Akt. *Mol Cell Biol* 2002;22:979–91.

44 Bereziat V, Kasus-Jacobi A, Perdereau D *et al.* Inhibition of insulin receptor catalytic activity by the molecular adapter Grb14. *J Biol Chem* 2002;277:4845–52.

45 Mauvais-Jarvis F, Kulkarni RN, Kahn CR.

Knockout models are useful tools to dissect the pathophysiology and genetics of insulin resistance. *Clin Endocrinol* 2002;57:1–7.

46 Terauchi Y, Kadowaki T. Insights into molecular pathogenesis of type 2 diabetes from knockout mouse models. *Endocr J* 2002;49:247–63.

47 Kadowaki T. Insights into insulin resistance and type 2 diabetes from knockout mouse models. *J Clin Invest* 2000;106:459–65.

48 Accili D, Drago J, Lee EJ et al. Early neonatal death in mice homozygous for a null allele of the insulin receptor gene. *Nat Gen* 1996;12:106–9.

49 Joshi RL, Lamothe B, Cordonnier N et al. Targeted disruption of the insulin receptor gene in the mouse results in neonatal lethality. *EMBO J* 1996;15:1542–7.

50 Bruning JC, Winnay J, Bonner-Weir S et al. Development of a novel polygenic model of NIDDM in mice heterozygous for IR and IRS-1 null alleles. *Cell* 1997;88:561–72.

51 Bruning JC, Michael MD, Winnay JN et al. A muscle-specific insulin receptor knockout exhibits features of the metabolic syndrome of NIDDM without altering glucose tolerance. *Mol Cell* 1998;2:559–69.

52 Kim JK, Michael MD, Previs SF et al. Redistribution of substrates to adipose tissue promotes obesity in mice with selective insulin resistance in muscle. *J Clin Invest* 2000;105:1791–7.

53 Michael MD, Kulkarni RN, Postic C et al. Loss of insulin signaling in hepatocytes leads to severe insulin resistance and progressive hepatic dysfunction. *Mol Cell* 2000;6:87–97.

54 Kulkarni RN, Bruning JC, Winnay JN et al. Tissue-specific knockout of the insulin receptor in pancreatic beta cells creates an insulin secretory defect similar to that in type 2 diabetes. *Cell* 1999;96:329–39.

55 Mauvais-Jarvis F, Virkamaki A, Michael MD et al. A model to explore the interaction between muscle insulin resistance and beta-cell dysfunction in the development of type 2 diabetes. *Diabetes* 2000;49:2126–34.

56 Bluher M, Michael MD, Perone OD et al. Adipose tissue selective insulin receptor knockout protects against obesity and obesity-related glucose intolerance. *Dev Cell* 2002;3:25–38.

57 Bruning JC, Gautam D, Burks DJ et al. Role of the brain insulin receptor in control of body weight and reproduction. *Science* 1998;299:2122–5.

58 Abe H, Yamada N, Kamata K et al. Hypertension, hypertriglyceridemia and impaired endothelium-dependent vascular relaxation in mice lacking insulin receptor substrate-1. *J Clin Invest* 1998;101:1784–8.

59 Shirakami A, Toyonaga T, Tsuruoe K et al. Heterozygous knockout of the IRS-1 gene in mice enhances obesity-linked insulin resistance: a possible model for the development of type 2 diabetes. *J Endocrinol* 2002;174:309–19.

60 Araki E, Lipes MA, Patti ME et al. Alternative pathway of insulin signaling in mice with targeted disruption of the IRS-1 gene. *Nature* 1994;372:186–90.

61 Kulkarni RN, Winnay JN, Daniels M et al. Altered function of insulin receptor substrate 1–deficient mouse islets and cultured beta-cell lines. *J Clin Invest* 1999;104:R67–R75.

62 Tamemoto H, Kadowaki T, Tobe K et al. Insulin resistance and growth retardation in mice lacking insulin receptor substrate-1. *Nature* 1994;372:182–6.

63 Kubota N, Tobe K, Terauchi Y et al. Disruption of insulin receptor substrate 2 causes type 2 diabetes because of liver insulin resistance and lack of compensatory ß-cell hyperplasia. *Diabetes* 2000;49:1880–9.

64 Withers DJ, Gutierrez JS, Towery H et al. Disruption of IRS-2 causes type 2 diabetes in mice. *Nature* 1998;391:900–4.

65 Lindsay RS, Dabelea D, Rournan J et al. Type 2 diabetes and low birth weight. The role of paternal inheritance in the association of low birth weight and diabetes. *Diabetes* 2000;49:445–9.

66 Stern MP. The search for type 2 diabetes susceptibility genes using whole-genome scans: an epidemiologist's perspective. *Diabetes Metab Res Rev* 2002;18:106–13.

67 Kahn CR. Insulin action, diabetogenes and the cause of type 2 diabetes. *Diabetes* 1994;43:1066–84.

68 Kalm CR, Vicent D, Doria A. Genetics of non-insulin-dependent (type 2) diabetes mellitus. *Annu Rev Med* 1996;47:509–31.

69 Silfen ME, Shackleton CH, Manibo AM et al. 5 alpha-reductase and 11 beta-hydroxysteroid dehydrogenase activity in prepubertal Hispanic girls with premature adrenarche. *J Clin Endocrinol Metab* 2002;87:4647–51.

70 Schofl C, Horn R, Schill T et al. Circulating ghrelin levels in patients with polycystic ovary syndrome. *J Clin Endocrinol Metab* 2002;87:4607–10.

71 Homburg R. What is polycystic ovarian syndrome? A proposal for a consensus on the definition and diagnosis of polycystic ovarian syndrome. *Hum Reprod* 2002;17:2495–9.

72 Legro RS, Strauss JF. Molecular progress in infertility: polycystic ovary syndrome. *Fertil Steril* 2002;78:569–76.

73 Glueck CJ, Streicher P, Wang P. Treatment of polycystic ovary syndrome with insulin-lowering agents. *Expert Opin Pharmacother* 2002;3:1177–89.

74 Bagis T, Gokcel A, Zeyneloglu HB *et al.* The effects of short-term medroxyprogesterone acetate and micronized progesterone on glucose metabolism and lipid profiles in patients with polycystic ovary syndrome: a prospective randomized study. *J Clin Endocrinol Metab* 2002;87:4536–40.

75 Pritts EA. Treatment of the infertile patient with polycystic ovarian syndrome. *Obstet Gynecol Surv* 2002;57:587–97.

76 Flier JS, Mantozoros C. Syndromes of insulin resistance and mutant insulin. In: DeGroot LJ, Jameson JL, editors. *Endocrinology* Vol. 1. W.B. Saunders Co.: Philadelphia, London, 2001; 799–807.

77 Van Malderem L, Magre J, Khallouf TE *et al.* Genotype–phenotype relationships in Berardinelli-Seip congenital lipodystrophy. *J Med Genet* 2002;39:722–33.

78 Petersen KF, Oral EA, Dufour S *et al.* Leptin reverses insulin resistance and hepatic steatosis in patients with severe lipodystrophy. *J Clin Invest* 2002;109:1345–50.

79 Fajans SS, Graeme IB, Polonsky KS. Molecular mechanisms and clinical pathophysiology of maturity-onset diabetes of the young. *N Engl J Med* 2001;345:971–80.

80 Velho G, Robert JJ. Maturity-onset diabetes of the young (MODY): genetic and clinical characteristics. *Horm Res* 2002;57 (Suppl 1):29–33.

81 Montagne CT, O'Rahilly S. The perils of portliness – causes and consequences of visceral adiposity. *Diabetes* 2000;49:883–8.

82 Havel PJ. Control of energy homeostasis and insulin action by adipocyte hormones: leptin, acylation stimulating protein, and adiponectin. *Curr Opin Lipidol* 2002;13:51–9.

83 McGarry JD. Dysregulation of fatty acid metabolism in the etiology of type 2 diabetes. *Diabetes* 2002;51:7–18.

84 Unger RH. Lipotoxic diseases. *Annu Rev Med* 2002;53:319–36.

85 Cooney GJ, Thompson AL, Furler SM *et al.* Muscle long-chain acyl CoA esters and insulin resistance. *Ann NY Acad Sci* 2002;967:196–207.

86 Kim JK, Gavrilova O, Chen Y *et al.* Mechanisms of insulin resistance in A-ZIP/17–1 fatless mice. *Biol Chem* 2000;276:8456–60.

87 Yamauchi T, Kamon J, Minokoshi Y *et al.* Adiponectin stimulates glucose utilization and fatty-acid oxidation by activating AMP-activated protein kinase. *Nature* In press.

88 Oral EA, Simha V, Ruiz E *et al.* Leptin-replacement therapy for lipodystrophy. *N Engl J Med* 2002;346:570–8.

89 Kelley DE, Goodpaster BH. Skeletal muscle triglyceride. An aspect of regional adiposity and insulin resistance. *Diabetes* 2001;24:933–41.

90 Houmard JA, Tanner CJ, Yu C *et al.* Effect of weight loss on insulin sensitivity and intramuscular long-chain fatty acyl-CoAs in morbidly obese subjects. *Diabetes* 2002;51:2959–63.

91 Song S. The role of increased liver triglyceride content: a culprit of diabetic hyperglycemia? *Diabetes Metab Res Rev* 2002;18:5–12.

92 Marchesini G, Brizi M, Bianchi G *et al.* Nonalcoholic fatty liver disease. A feature of the metabolic syndrome. *Diabetes* 2001;50:1844–50.

93 Boden G, Shulman GI. Free fatty acids in obesity and type 2 diabetes: defining their role in the development of insulin resistance and beta-cell dysfunction. *Eur J Clin Invest* 2002;32(Suppl. 3):14–23.

94 American Diabetes Association and National Institute of Diabetes, Digestive and Kidney Diseases. The prevention or delay of type 2 diabetes. *Diabetes Care* 2002;25:742–9.

95 Diabetes Prevention Program Research Group. Reduction in the incidence of type 2 diabetes with lifestyle intervention or metformin. *N Engl J Med* 2002;346:393–403.

96 Chiasson JL, Josse RG, Gomis R *et al.* for the STOP-NIDDM Trial Research Group. Acarbose for prevention of type 2 diabetes mellitus: the STOP-NIDDM randomised trial. *Lancet* 2002;359:2072–7.

97 Moller DE. New drug targets for type 2 diabetes and the metabolic syndrome. *Nature* 2001; 414:821–7.

3

Rationale and goals for glucose control in diabetes mellitus, and glucose monitoring

Ramachandiran Cooppan

INTRODUCTION

Diabetes mellitus is a chronic disease that results in major morbidity and mortality. As with any chronic illness, the goals of therapy are to alleviate the acute symptoms and complications, and then to focus on preventing the long-term consequences. While the initial goals can be reasonably achieved in most instances, the long-term complications can prove to be more of a challenge.

Type 1 disease is caused by autoimmune destruction of beta cells and type 2 diabetes is the result of alterations in insulin secretion and peripheral insulin resistance. Type 1 diabetes generally develops in younger individuals, while type 2 disease occurs in adults; however, the prevalence of type 2 diabetes mellitus is increasing among children and adolescents. The prevalence increased from 1% in the 15–24 year old group of Pima Indians in 1979 to 5% and has also emerged in the 10–15 year age group[1]. An increase has also been noted in African–American and Mexican–American youth. Similar trends have been seen in other parts of the world, such as Japan, Bangladesh, Libya and New Zealand[2]. In addition, many patients with type 2 diabetes already show evidence of complications at diagnosis[3].

Cardiovascular disease is the most important cause of death for patients with type 2 diabetes, with the risk starting to increase very early, during the stage of impaired glucose tolerance (IGT)[4]. These clinical issues therefore have important implications for glycemic control and the goals that we set for patients.

MICROVASCULAR DISEASE

A number of different mechanisms have been implicated in the pathogenesis of microvascular disease, this has been studied extensively in diabetic retinopathy and nephropathy. Chronic duration of the disease, metabolic abnormalities, including hyperglycemia, and genetic factors all play a role. There have been reports in the literature of patients who develop all the microvascular complications but who may not manifest overt clinical diabetes[5]. Abdella et al. reported on a 47-year-old man with IGT, who presented with nephrotic syndrome and renal failure, and had proliferative retinopathy on fundoscopy. These case reports serve to remind us that, while hyperglycemia is critical to the development of complications, milder degrees of glucose intolerance can also play a role via other mechanisms.

PATHOGENIC MECHANISMS FOR MICROVASCULAR DISEASE

The formation of advanced glycosylated end products

A high glucose concentration can lead to glycosylation of amino groups in proteins and the formation of advanced glycosylation end products (AGE). The production and deposition of these products are thought to contribute to the development of the long-term microvascular complications. AGEs bind to receptors and cause changes in signal transduction in macrophages or vascular endothelial cells. AGEs and oxidants have been implicated recently in the increased expression of vascular endothelial growth factor (VGEF), which can increase vascular permeability and cause retinal angiogenesis[6,7].

Increased aldose reductase activity

The aldose reductase pathway has been extensively studied because of the presence of this enzyme in the retina, kidney and nerves. The activity of the enzyme increases with hyperglycemia, and more glucose is converted to sorbitol. Sorbitol is slowly metabolized and has been postulated to lead to other metabolic changes that can cause neuropathy and retinopathy. This pathway has been most studied in relation to diabetic neuropathy[8].

Formation of excessive oxidants

Increases in oxidant formation are derived from many different sources, such as glucose auto-oxidation, protein glycation, and free radical formation. Oxidants can affect many cellular processes, including increases in oxidized low-density lipoprotein, cross-linked proteins and DNA. In addition, this increase in oxidants can lead to reduction of nitric oxide (NO), which can result in vasoconstriction and hypoxia. In one recent study of diabetic retinopathy, vitamin E was used in a dose-dependent manner (1000–2000 IU per day) and resulted in the normalization of the retinal blood flow changes in type 1 diabetic patients[9].

Alteration in the signal transduction pathway

Many changes occur in signal transduction with hyperglycemia, and the diacylglycerol, protein kinase C (DAG-PKC) activation pathway has been best studied. Hyperglycemia increases DAG and PKC actions through multiple intermediary substances, this can result in many cellular abnormalities. These include such changes as basement-membrane thickening, increased permeability, coagulation and contractibility abnormalities, as well as increased angiogenesis and cardiomyopathy. The use of a specific PKC beta isoform inhibitor, LY333531, has been studied and a delay in the hemodynamic changes seen in diabetic retinopathy, nephropathy and cardiovascular disease has been observed. The drug is now being studied clinically in patients with macular edema and neovascularization, to see whether visual loss can be prevented[10].

From the many theories that have been advanced to explain the pathogenesis of the microvascular complications of diabetes, it is evident that the one common abnormality in all theories is the presence of an elevated blood glucose level, which must be controlled optimally.

MACROVASCULAR DISEASE

Cardiovascular disease is the leading cause of mortality for people with diabetes. The majority of deaths are due to coronary heart disease, where the risk is 2–4 fold greater in patients, especially among women with diabetes, when compared with age-matched subjects without diabetes[11]. Gu et al. compared adults with diabetes with controls using the National Health and Nutrition Surveys (NHANES) database. Comparison of the first survey (1971–75) with the second (1982–84), showed that non-diabetic men had a 36.4% decline in age-adjusted heart disease mortality, compared with a 13.1% decline in diabetic men. In non-diabetic women the decline was 27%, but the rate increased 23% in women with diabetes[12].

Haffner and colleagues compared the mortality from coronary heart disease in type 2 diabetic patients and non-diabetics in Finland, and found a much higher risk, even among diabetics with no history of cardiac problems[13]. After the first cardiac event, 50% of patients with diabetes die within 1 year, and half die before they can reach a hospital[14]. This very high mortality suggests that a primary prevention strategy is needed to reduce the risk. The Scandanvian Simvastatin Survival Study (4S) and the Cholesterol and Recurrent Events (CARE)[15,16], are secondary prevention studies that showed a reduction in cardiovascular mortality in small numbers of patients with diabetes included in these studies. The Hypertension Optimal Treatment Trial (HOT) and the UK Prospective Diabetes Study (UKPDS)[17,18] also demonstrated a significant reduction in cardiovascular events, as well as in microvascular events (UKPDS), with blood pressure control.

In both type 1 and type 2 diabetes, accelerated macrovascular disease is a problem and the etiology is multifactorial, with hyperglycemia playing a significant role. In the type 2 patient there are multiple cardiovascular risk-factors that form part of the insulin resistance syndrome. There is considerable debate in the medical literature on the role of hyperglycemia as an independent risk factor for coronary heart disease. Balkau *et al.*, reviewed the mortality data from the Paris Prospective Study, and found that, in the upper levels of glucose distributions, the risk for death progressively increased with fasting and 2 h glucose levels[19]. A meta-regression analysis of 20 recent studies by Coutinho *et al.*[20] found that high fasting, 1 h, and 2 h glucose levels increased risk of cardiovascular events. The DECODE Study included over 25 000 patients, with a mean follow-up time of 7.3 years[21]. This study showed that a high blood glucose concentration 2 h after a glucose load was associated with increased risk of death, independent of fasting blood glucose levels. These studies do not imply a cause and effect relationship, but do suggest that, with increasing glucose levels, there may be worsening of the underlying risk factors for cardiovascular disease.

RESULTS OF STUDIES OF GLYCEMIC CONTROL AND MICROVASCULAR DISEASE

The ultimate proof that glycemic control is worthwhile has come from long-term randomized controlled trials (RCT). One systematic review and three long-term RCTs show the benefits of glucose control in both type 1 and type 2 diabetes. The systematic review, by Groeneveld *et al.*, looked at 16 small RCTs in type 1 diabetes that had a follow-up of 8–60 months[22]. The overall conclusion of these studies was that glycemic control was important in reducing microvascular complications.

The Diabetes Control and Complications Trial (DCCT)[23] study involved 1441 patients with type 1 diabetes who were randomized to either intensive glucose control or conventional treatment. While retinopathy was the main concern, renal, neurologic, cardiovascular and neuropsychological outcomes and adverse effects of the two treatments were also studied. The main results are summarized in Table 3.1. The benefits of strict glucose control in both primary prevention and secondary progression were clear, but it was noted that patients on the intensive treatment did have a three times greater increase in the number of severe hypoglycemic episodes. The hypoglycemia did not result in death or stroke, and the mortality did not differ in the two treatment cohorts. Despite the hypoglycemia difference, there was no clinically important changes in neuropsychological function between the groups. The patients appeared to adjust well to the demands of the intensive therapy program. Weight gain was a problem in the intensively treated group, with a mean gain of 4.6 kg at 5 years. There was no increase in the ketoacidosis

Table 3.1 Risk reduction (RR) in microvascular complications in the DCCT	
	RR (%)
Retinopathy	76
Severe diabetic retinopathy	61
Laser surgery	56
Microalb	43
Severe microalbuminuria	51
Albuminuria	56
Neuropathy	64

rates in either group. This benefit was achieved in the intensive treatment group with a mean blood glucose of 155 mg dL^{-1} and glycosylated hemoglobin (HbA1c) of ~7.2% with a normal average glucose being ~110 mg dL^{-1} and the HbA1c < 6.05%.

The DCCT results also demonstrated that there is no glycemic threshold for the development of long-term complications. A retrospective Joslin clinic study[24], and the prospective Stockholm Study[25], suggested that a threshold may exist for microalbuminuria around an HbA1c of 8–9%. However, the data from the DCCT indicate that, for every 10% reduction in HbA1c, there is a 39% reduction in the risk of retinopathy progression. The risk of developing microalbuminuria and neuropathy is also reduced. The magnitude of the risk reduction is greater at higher HbA1c levels and, at the same time as control improves the risk of hypoglycemia, increases with the lower HbA1c levels[6]. In a follow-up study of the DCCT, the Epidemiology of Diabetes Interventions and Complications (EDIC) study found that the benefits of intensive treatment persisted over the 4 years of follow-up[27].

Ohkubo and colleagues from Kumamoto, Japan, also demonstrated the benefits of intensive insulin therapy in a group of thin type 2 patients[28]. A total of 110 patients with type 2 diabetes were randomized to intensive treatment with multiple insulin injections (MIT) or conventional insulin therapy (CIT). After 6 years, the mean HbA1c was 7.1% in the intensive group and 9.4% in the control group. In the primary prevention cohort there was a 7.7% development of retinopathy in MIT group after 6 years, compared with 32% in the CIT group. In addition, in the secondary prevention cohort, in the MIT group, 19.2% had progression of retinopathy compared with 44% in the CIT group. Similar reductions in both the primary and secondary cohorts were found for nephropathy and neuropathy. The glycemic threshold to prevent the onset and progression of diabetic microangiopathy was an HbA1c < 6.5%, fasting blood glucose < 110 mg dL^{-1} and a 2 h postprandial blood glucose of < 180 mg dL^{-1}. Over the entire study period, six patients in the MIT group and four

patients in the CIT group had one or more mild hypoglycemic reactions, with no coma or seizures or need for assistance from another person.

The UKPDS led by Robert Turner is the largest type 2 diabetes study ever done[29]. This clinical study of 3867 newly diagnosed patients was designed to assess the effects of intensive treatment with four pharmacological monotherapies versus a diet-only control group, on cardiovascular and microvascular complications of type 2 diabetes. The goal of intensive treatment was a fasting plasma glucose of < 108 mg dL^{-1}, in the diet-treated group the aim was the best-achievable fasting glucose level, and oral drugs were added if there were hyperglycemic symptoms, or if the fasting plasma glucose was > 270 mg dL^{-1}. Over 10 years the HbA1c was 7.0% in the intensive group, compared with HbA1c 7.9% in the control group—an 11% reduction. These results are summarized in Table 3.2.

No glycemic threshold was found for any microvascular complication

The epidemiological analysis of the study also clearly demonstrated that there was a continuous association between the risk of cardiovascular complications and glycemia. In a second publication[30], the results from a subgroup of obese patients treated with metformin showed a 32% reduction in any diabetes-related endpoint, 42% reduction for diabetes-related death and 36% reduction for all cause mortality. In a substudy, 537 obese and normal weight subjects unable to maintain their glucose control on sulfonylurea were assigned to combination therapy. In this group there was an increased risk of diabetes-related death when compared with those treated with sulfonylurea alone. This observation also generated considerable discussion, but the American Diabetes Association has reviewed the study and its results and accepted the important role of all treatments for glucose control in reducing the incidence of microvascular complications[31].

Two other areas that demonstrate the importance of glucose control are pancreatic transplantation and pregnancy. A study by Fioretto

> **Table 3.2 UKPDS risk reduction for diabetes-related end-points during intensive therapy with sulfonylureas and insulin**
>
> | | Risk reduction[a] | P |
> |---|---|---|
> | Any diabetes-related end-point | 12% | 0.029 |
> | Myocardial infarction | 16% | 0.052 |
> | Microvascular disease | 25% | 0.0099 |
> | Retinopathy progression (at 12 years) | 21% | 0.015 |
> | Cataract extraction | 24% | 0.046 |
> | Microalbuminuria (at 12 years) | 33% | < 0.001 |
>
> [a]Compared with conventional therapy.

et al. looked at the effects of pancreas transplantation on diabetic nephropathy[32]. They performed renal biopsies before pancreas transplantation, and then 5 and 10 years afterwards, in eight patients with type 1 diabetes mellitus who had no uremia and mild to advanced diabetic nephropathy. All the patients had normal glycosylated hemoglobin values after transplantation, and albumin excretion dropped from 103 mg per day to 30 mg per day after 5 years. By 10 years, albumin excretion was down to 20 mg per day and the glomerular and tubular basement thickening, while not changed at 5 years, was also decreased significantly.

Poorly controlled diabetes during pregnancy increases congenital abnormalities and perinatal mortality. The American Diabetes Association and others have stressed meticulous glucose control not only during pregnancy but also in the preconception period. Gestational diabetes mellitus (GDM) complicates approximately 7% of all pregnancies and results in more than 200 000 cases annually[33]. It is associated with increased risk of fetal macrosomia, neonatal hypoglycemia, hyperbilirubinemia, hypocalcemia and polycythemia. The children of mothers with GDM are also at greater risk of childhood obesity and diabetes as young adults[34]. All women with diabetes should attempt to maintain blood glucose levels in the non-diabetic range. While treatment into the non-diabetic range is recommended, this must be achieved without significant increase in severe hypoglycemia. With these approaches there has been a reduction in fetal loss and congenital abnormality rates[35].

Macrovascular disease and glucose control

The issue of the direct benefit of glucose control has not yet been settled in a study where other risk factors are controlled and glucose control is the major outcome. The Veterans Affairs Cooperative Study on Glycemic Control and Complications in type 2 Diabetes (VA CSDM) was a feasibility trial of intensive insulin treatment in 153 adult men with type 2 diabetes[36]. The intensively treated patients had more hypoglycemia, required larger insulin doses, and had more statistically non-significant cardiovascular events. Interestingly, these events occurred in the group with HbA1c levels of 5.5–8%. The studies of glucose control and macrovascular outcome are summarized in Table 3.3.

The data from the table indicate that there is a cardiovascular benefit in lowering the blood glucose, in terms of a relative risk reduction (RRR) of 16–46%. But the problem with this observation is that the data comes for multiple sources and a specifically designed study is now needed to address this question.

Table 3.3 Glucose lowering in type 2 diabetes mellitus and cardiovascular disease risk

	Treatment	HbA1c change (%)	Outcome	Relative risk reduction (%)
UKPDS	Insulin/Su[a]	0.9	MI	16
UKPDS	Metformin	0.6	MI	39
Kumamoto	Insulin	2.3	CVD	46
VACSDM	Insulin/Su	2.2	CVD	−40
DIGAMI	Insulin	0.8	Death	29

[a]Su = Sulfonylurea.

GLUCOSE MONITORING

Self blood-glucose monitoring

In order to obtain blood glucose control and maintain it on a daily basis, it is essential for patients with diabetes to self-monitor blood glucose [self blood-glucose monitoring (SBGM)]. The data obtained from monitoring is used to assess the efficacy of the treatment program and the need for adjustments, to determine the frequency of hypoglycemia, as well as for reviewing medical nutrition therapy and the effects of exercise. A great deal of progress has been made in improving the accuracy and ease of use of glucose-monitoring equipment. In its position statement the American Diabetes Association made a number of recommendations[37]. It states that most patients with type 1 diabetes can only obtain blood glucose levels close to normal using SBGM with an associated increased risk of hypoglycemia under intensive therapies. Therefore, all insulin-treated patients and those on sulfonylureas and oral combination therapies need monitoring, to avoid asymptomatic hypoglycemia. The optimal frequency for testing is actually dictated by the needs and goals of the individual patient.

A recent report by Harris, using data from NHANES III, noted that the frequency of SBGM was more common as the HbA1c increased[38]. The report also noted that most patients treated with oral medications or diet rarely monitored their blood glucose. It was also noted that 39% of insulin treated, and 5–6% of oral agent or diet-controlled patients monitored themselves at least once daily.

In order to use SBGM properly, each patient should be taught by a diabetes nurse educator. This consultation can evaluate the correct testing technique, use of the monitor selected, and proper interpretation of the data. The use of newer oral drugs, rapid-acting insulin analogues and basal insulin also make it important to test more often because of the risk for severe hypoglycemia. Cox, in 1994, found that patients who recorded variable and frequent low blood glucose readings during routine SBGM were at higher risk of subsequent severe hypoglycemia[39].

HbA1c

The development of the HbA1c assay is one of the major advances in caring for patients with diabetes mellitus. Currently, most laboratories use the HbA1c measurement, however, this is not universal and the consensus statement by Marshall makes it apparent that standardization of the assay is an issue[40]. The report recommended that a DCCT-aligned HbA1c assay should be used, since this has the best data available on the relationship between control and complications.

Many different assay methods are available; they vary in the glycated components measured, interferences and the non-diabetic range. It is important for the clinician to know what the laboratory being used measures, and what the normal ranges are. The ADA position statement states that testing of the HbA1c should be performed routinely in all patients with diabetes, to document the level of their glycemic control. In general, the test should be repeated 3–4 times a year, but the actual frequency will vary depending on the individual patient and the goals set. Lytken Larsen *et al.* randomly assigned 240 matched patients with type 1 diabetes mellitus to either a three-monthly measurement of HbA1c, or blood glucose and urine testing to monitor treatment[41]. Treatment was modified based on the results of the tests and, after 1 year in the group having HbA1c measured, the mean HbA1c dropped from 10.1% to 9.5%. In the control group, the values were 10.0% and 10.1% respectively. As a result, the proportion of patients in poor control, defined as an HbA1c value > 10% decreased from 46% to 30%. Another interesting study by Chase *et al.* looked at the issue of severe hypoglycemic episodes in type 1 patients after the introduction of rapid acting lispro insulin in 1996[42]. They found additional reduction in the HbA1c levels, with no increase in the number of severe hypoglycemic episodes. While it is reasonable to measure the HbA1c three to four times a year in type 1 patients, the optimal frequency in type 2 diabetes is not clear, especially for stable patients who are diet treated. In the absence of definitive studies, stable patients should have their HbA1c measured twice a year, and those who are not in control or who are having therapy changes should probably be tested quarterly.

It is extremely important that patients and care-givers understand the basis for the test and how to use the information. It is better to individualize the approach rather than have fixed goals for all patients based on the studies discussed so far. The ability of the patient to participate in the treatment program is crucial for optimal control. Focusing only on the HbA1c levels, without addressing such issues as, the stresses of adolescence, puberty, the home environment, ageing, depression and economic issues, will create a counter-productive situation. This is especially important when setting goals in the elderly, where co-morbidities and many psychosocial and economic issues will determine the goals[43] (Table 3.4).

After many decades of questioning the role of glucose control in preventing long-term complications of diabetes mellitus, there is now data that indicate the benefits of good control. All patients cannot be controlled equally well, but all of them need to be improved. Any decrease in the HbA1c that can be obtained safely is important; the ideal being to keep the patients in the non-diabetic range. For the global epidemic of type 2 diabetes, it is

---

Table 3.4 Recommended targets for blood glucose

Preprandial plasma glucose	90–130 mg dL^{-1}	5.0–7.2 mmol/L
Peak postprandial plasma glucose	< 180 mg dL^{-1}	< 10.0 mmol/L
HbA1c (%)	< 7.0%[a]	
	< 6.5%[b]	

[a]American Diabetes Association[44].
[b]European Diabetes Policy Group 1999[45].

now apparent that the early treatment of patients with impaired glucose tolerance with lifestyle measures can have a major impact on progression to clinical disease. To improve diabetes care, and spread the message of glycemic control, will involve a major effort to educate both physicians and patients. Familiarity with the results of evidence-based trials and national standards of care will be essential. Close collaboration between the government and healthcare providers will also be required. There are major human and financial costs from the complications of diabetes and evidence that control matters

should inspire all involved in diabetes care to improve our efforts.

We need to balance our need to control glucose with the realities of daily life for our patients and the psychological stresses of living with a chronic disease. While the evidence is very persuasive for controlling diabetes mellitus to glycohemo-globin and fasting and postprandial goals, it is extremely important that the goals be set and adjusted for the individual patient. This situation should foster greater understanding of patients and their problems, and the need to continue to build long-term relationships with effective communications and support systems.

REFERENCES

1 Rosenbloom AL. The cause of the epidemic of type 2 diabetes in children. *Curr Opin Endocrinol Diabetes* 2000;7:191–6.

2 Rosenbloom AL, Joe JR, Young RS, Winter WE. The emerging epidemic of type 2 diabetes mellitus in youth. *Diabetes Care* 1999;22:345–54.

3 UK Prospective Diabetes Study group. Intensive blood-glucose control with sulfonylureas or insulin compared with conventional treatment and risk of complications in patients with type 2 diabetes. *Lancet* 1998;352:837–53.

4 Haffner SM, Stern MP, Hazuda P *et al.* Cardiovascular risk factors in confirmed predia-betic individuals. *N Engl J Med* 1990;263:2893–8.

5 Abdella N, Salman A, Moro M. Classical microangiopathic diabetic complications in the absence of overt diabetes mellitus. *Diabetes Res Clin Pract* 1990;8:283–6.

6 Aiello LP, Avery RL, Arrigg PG *et al.* Vascular endothelial growth factor in ocular fluid of patients with diabetic retinopathy and other retinal disorders. *N Engl J Med* 1994;331:1480–7.

7 Brownlee M, Cerami A, Vlassara H. Advanced glycosylation end products in tissue and the biochemical basis of diabetic complications. *N Engl J Med* 1988;318:1315–21.

8 Greene DA, Lattimer SA, Sima AAF. Patho-genesis and prevention of diabetic neuropathy. *Diabetes Metab Res Rev* 1988;4:201–21.

9 Bursell SE, Clermont AC, Aiello LP *et al.* High dose vitamin E supplementation normalizes retinal blood flow and creatinine clearance in patients with type 1 diabetes. *Diabetes Care* 1999;22:1245–51.

10 Bursell SE, King GL. Can protein kinase C inhibi-tion and vitamin E prevent the development of diabetic vascular complications? *Diabetes Res Clin Pract* 1999;45:169–82.

11 American Diabetes Association. Consensus Development Conference on the diagnosis of coronary heart disease in people with diabetes. *Diabetes Care* 1998;21:1551–9.

12 Gu K, Cowie CC, Harris MI. Diabetes and decline in heart disease mortality in US adults. *J Am Med Assoc* 1999;281:1291–7.

13 Haffner SM, Lehto S, Ronnemaa T *et al.* Mortality from coronary heart disease in subjects with type 2 diabetes and in nondiabetic subjects with and without prior myocardial infarction. *N Engl J Med* 1998;339:229–34.

14 Miettinen H, Lehto S, Salomaa V *et al.* Impact of diabetes on mortality after the first myocardial infarction. *Diabetes Care* 1998;21:69–75.

15 Pyorala K, Pedersen TR, Kjekshus J *et al.* Cholesterol lowering with simvastatin improves prognosis of diabetic patients with coronary heart disease: a subgroup analysis of the Scandinavian Simvastatin Survival Study (4S). *Diabetes Care* 1997;20:614–20.

16 Sacks FM, Pfeffer MA, Moye LA *et al.* The effects of pravastatin on coronary events after myocar-dial infarction in patients with average choles-terol levels. *N Engl J Med* 1996;335:1001–9.

17 Hansson L, Zanchetti A, Carruthers SG *et al.* The effects of intensive blood-pressure lowering and

low-dose aspirin in patients with hypertension: principal results of the Hypertension Optimal Treatment (HOT) randomized trial. *Lancet* 1998;351:1755–62.

18 Turner RC, Millins H, Neil HA *et al.* for the United Kingdom Prospective Diabetes Study Group. Risk factors for coronary disease in non-insulin dependent diabetes mellitus: United Kingdom Prospective Diabetes Study. *Br Med J* 1998;316:823–8.

19 Balkau B, Bertrais S, Ducimetiere P, Eschwege E. Is there a glycemic threshold for mortality risk? *Diabetes Care* 1999;22:696–9.

20 Coutinho M, Gerstein HC, Wang Y, Yusuf S. The relationship between glucose and incident cardiovascular events: a metaregression analysis of published data from 20 studies of 95,783 individuals followed for 12.4 years. *Diabetes Care* 1999;22:233–40.

21 The DECODE study group on behalf of the European Diabetes Epidemiology Group. Glucose tolerance and mortality: comparison of WHO and American Diabetes Association diagnostic criteria. *Lancet* 1999;354:617–25.

22 Groeneveld Y, Petri H, Hermans J, Springer MP. Relationship between blood glucose level and mortality in type 2 diabetes mellitus: a systematic review. *Diabetes Med* 1999;16:2–13.

23 The Diabetes Control and Complications Trial Research Group. The effect of intensive treatment of diabetes on the development and progression of long-term complications in insulin-dependent diabetes mellitus. *N Engl J Med* 1993;329:977–86.

24 Krolweski AS, Laffel LMB, Krolweski M *et al.* Glycosylated hemoglobin and the risk of microalbuminuria in patients with insulin dependent diabetes mellitus. *N Engl J Med* 1995;332:1251–5.

25 Reichard P. Are there any glycemic thresholds for the serious microvascular diabetic complications? *J Diabetes Complications* 1995;9:25–30.

26 The Diabetes Control and Complications Trial Research Group. The absence of a glycemic threshold for the development of long-term complications: The perspective of the diabetes control and complications trial. *Diabetes* 1996;45:1289–98.

27 The Diabetes Control and Complications Trial/Epidemiology of Diabetes Interventions and Complications Research Group. Retinopathy and nephropathy in patients with type 1 diabetes four years after a trial of intensive therapy. *N Engl J Med* 2000;342:381–9.

28 Ohkubo Y, Kishikawa H, Araki E *et al.* Intensive insulin therapy prevents the progression of diabetic microvascular complications in Japanese patients with non-insulin-dependent diabetes mellitus: a randomized prospective 6-year study. *Diabetes Res Clin Pract* 1995;28:103–17.

29 UK Prospective Diabetes Study (UKPDS) Group. Intensive blood-glucose control with sulfonylureas or insulin compared with conventional treatment and risk of complications in patients with type 2 diabetes (UKPDS 33). *Lancet* 1998;352:837–53.

30 UK Prospective Diabetes Study (UKPDS) Group. Effect of intensive blood glucose control with metformin on complications in overweight patients with type 2 diabetes (UKPDS 34). *Lancet* 1998;352:854–65.

31 American Diabetes Association. Implications of the United Kingdom Prospective Diabetes Study. *Diabetes Care* 1998;21:2180–4.

32 Fioretto P, Steffes MW, Sutherland DER *et al.* Reversal of lesions of diabetic nephropathy after pancreatic transplantation. *N Engl J Med* 1998;339:69–75.

33 American Diabetes Association. Gestational diabetes mellitus. *Diabetes Care* 2001;Suppl 1:S77–S79.

34 Pettit DJ, Baird HR, Aleck KA *et al.* Excessive obesity in offspring of Pima Indian women with diabetes during pregnancy. *N Engl J Med* 1983;308:242–5.

35 Canadian Diabetes Association. 1998 clinical practice guidelines for the management of diabetes in Canada. *Can Med Assoc J* 1998;159(Suppl 8):SS18–S19.

36 Abraira C, Colwell JA, Nuttall F *et al.* for the VA CSDM Group. Cardiovascular events and correlates in the Veterans Affairs Diabetes Feasibility Trial. *Arch Intern Med* 1997;157:181–8.

37 Tests of Glycemia in Diabetes. The American Diabetes Association. *Diabetes Care* 2001;24:S80–S82.

38 Harris M I. Frequency of blood glucose monitoring in relation to glycemic control in patients with type 2 diabetes. *Diabetes Care* 2001;24:979–82.

39 Cox DJ, Kovatchev BP, Julian DM *et al.* Frequency of severe hypoglycemia in insulin dependent diabetes mellitus can be predicted from self-blood monitoring blood glucose data. *J Clin Endocrinol Metab* 1994;79:1659–62.

40 Marshall SM, Barth JH. Standardization of HbAic measurements—a consensus statement. *Diabetic Med* 2000;17:5–6.

41 Lytken LM, Horder M, Mogensen EF. Effect of long-term monitoring of glycosylated hemoglobin levels in insulin-dependent diabetes mellitus. *N Engl J Med* 1990;323:1021–5.

42 Chase P, Lockspeiser T, Peery B *et al*. The impact of the diabetes control and complications trial and Humalog insulin on glycohemoglobin levels and severe hypoglycemia in type 1 diabetes. *Diabetes Care* 2001;24:430–4.

43 Cooppan R. Diabetes in the elderly: implications of the diabetes control and complications trial. *Compr Ther* 1996;22:286–90.

44 American Diabetes Association: clinical practice recommendations 2003. *Diabetes Care* 2003; 26(Suppl):S33–S50.

45 European Diabetes Policy Group. A desktop guide to Type 2 diabetes mellitus. *Diabetic Med* 1999;16:716–73.

4

The role of the diabetes educator in the management of diabetes mellitus

Carolé Mensing and Kathryn Mulcahy

INTRODUCTION

Diabetes self-management education (DSME) has long been revered as the cornerstone of care for all persons affected by diabetes. The diabetes educator provides this valuable service as an integral part of the healthcare delivery team. A large body of evidence supports the effectiveness of diabetes education[1] and, although there are variances in delivery methods, the educational process is universal. Since 1983, educators have focused on delivery of a formalized educational content. This content, as well as the process of DSME was most recently defined by the National Standards of DSME[2].

The overall combined goals of diabetes care and education continue to be: to optimize health and metabolic control, prevent or delay complications, and improve or optimize the patient's quality-of-life[3]. *Healthy People 2010* supports these goals and plans to increase the proportion of individuals with diabetes who receive formal diabetes education from 40 to 60%[4]. However, at present there continues to be significant knowledge and skill deficits in 50–80% of individuals with diabetes[5], and there are still under-served populations, i.e., only a small percentage of the people affected by diabetes attend educational events[6].

THE BROAD ROLE OF THE DIABETES EDUCATOR

The diabetes educator serves a pivotal role in the management of people with diabetes. The role is multidimensional, with boundaries for accountability that interface with both other members of the healthcare team, as well as internal and external customers[7]. For example, the general scope of practice of a diabetes educator in the USA (Table 4.1) has changing dimensions because of the multidisciplinary nature of the healthcare professionals who provide this service and the changing healthcare delivery system. Each professional who practices as a diabetes educator brings a unique

Table 4.1 Scope of practice

Scope and Standards of Diabetes Nursing (ANA, AADE), 1998. American Nurses Publishing.

The American Association of Diabetes Educators (AADE), 1999 Scope of Practice for Diabetes Educators and the Standards of Practice for Diabetes Educators. (Republished, TDE, vol. 28, No. 4, 2002)

American Dietetic Association Standards of Professional Practice for Dietetics Professionals, 1998.

American Diabetes Association Clinical Practice Recommendations 2002. *Diabetes Care* 2002;25 Suppl 1.

Report of the Task Force on the Delivery of Diabetes Self-Management Education and Medical Nutrition Therapy, Spectrum, Fall, 1998.

focus to the educational process. This phenomenon can have significant impact on the scope of practice for an individual educator, and is appropriate within the boundaries of each professional discipline. Diabetes educators are of diverse nature and bring varied skill-sets to the healthcare system. They frequently assume extended and complementary roles, such as in program, case or clinical management; as healthcare consultants; in public and professional education, or public health and wellness promotion; as well as researching diabetes management and education. The educator has a vital supportive role in the multidisciplinary team.

THE MULTIDISCIPLINARY TEAM

Over a decade or more ago, the multidisciplinary team began to be recognized as an effective and efficient method of care delivery and provider of the educational support demanded by diabetes. This team approach does not eliminate the primary practitioner or sole practitioner[8], but instead supports the variety of skills, timing, assistance and prerequisites brought by each of its members. The team brings a variety of services, interventions and assistance to fully integrate into a person's lifestyle as needed. Effective teams serve the population whether they be rural, inner city, small or large practice, special population needs, etc. They may have a patient-centered or population-based focus. More (team) effort is required[9].

The team is formed by a stepwise process:

- Ensure commitment of organizational leadership
- Gain support from care-providers
- Identify team members
- Identify the patient population
- Stratify the patient population
- Assess resources
- Develop a system for coordinated, continuous, quality care.

This process focuses on common goals, each member airing opinions and contributing to decisions about patient care and education. Efficient care delivery to all patients focuses on care delivery itself, mechanisms of identifying high-risk patients, cost-effective methods of education and treatment in the outpatient setting[9].

Team definition

Most teams work under the auspices of a physician. In the USA, much of the care is driven by standards of care and for insurance reimbursement. Traditional diabetes care is often symptom-focused, and managed according to acute presenting symptoms – this is the medical model. Care has now evolved into a patient-centered model, which is more appropriate than a provider-centered one.[10] Education by the multidisciplinary team is viewed as an ongoing strategy helping people to manage their diabetes with a continuous, proactive planned care.[10]

Numerous publications now support a chronic disease model for diabetes and there is evidence to support team care as an effective method of chronic disease management for diabetes[11]. The benefits of a team approach have been well-documented[12]:

"The role of the health care provider is to deliver appropriate treatment, including comprehensive medical care (prevention, detection, treatment of acute and chronic conditions related to diabetes) AND self-management education, including medical nutrition therapy, directed toward helping the person with diabetes make informed choices regarding self care."[13]

Team management

Team management is a coordinated multidisciplinary approach. It is crucial to share information to develop and implement a patient's care plan, and to evaluate success. The composition of the team will vary depending on the setting. Typically, a physician, or advanced practice provider, initiates direction and supervises medical care. A nurse or nutritionist participates in assessments, and other disciplines are utilized as available. A more comprehensive team (social worker, podiatrist, pharmacist, etc) may also be involved.

The team usually consists of three or four healthcare providers with complementary skills who are committed to one common goal or approach[10] and includes a physician or other primary-care provider, a nurse and a dietitian, at least one member is a Certified Diabetes Educator [(CDE) requires the passing of an exam administered by the National Certification Board for Diabetes Education][2]. The team is multidimensional, with accountability as defined by their individual discipline's scope of practice. A multidisciplinary team offers a variety of skills, experience that contributes to a common purpose[10].

Primary care physicians often provide the majority of diabetes care, augmented and enhanced by other healthcare professionals and community partners and services. In the USA, a primary care practitioner, advanced nurse practitioner, or physician assistant often take on the coordinating care role. Nurse practitioners have been shown to produce similar clinical outcomes to physicians in a primary care setting[14]. A primary care team consists of medical and educational managers. It is essential that a key individual coordinates the care effort between primary care providers, CDE and other healthcare providers.

The Diabetes Control and Complications Trial (DCCT) was a large clinical trial of people with type 1 diabetes mellitus, and included medicine, nursing, nutrition, education, and counseling[15,16]. The UK Prospective Diabetes Study (UKPDS), a clinical trial of people with type 2 diabetes, included teams of physicians, nurses, and dietitians[17]. O'Connor summarizes primary care setting progress towards the goal of better diabetes care[18]. These successful interventions utilize formal strategies to organize diabetes care (Table 4.2).

Not every team member needs to be involved with every patient, but will be guided by the assessed needs, selected by age grouping of the person (from pediatric to geriatric); special needs (language, literacy, learning abilities,

---

Table 4.2 Organizing diabetes care: strategies

1. Accurately *identifying* patients with diabetes
2. *Monitoring* one or more important clinical parameters, such as A1C or cholesterol levels
3. *Prioritizing* patients based on their clinical status and readiness to change
4. *Intensifying* care through active outreach or visit planning

---

family interactions, etc); level of information required (basic survival skills to advanced level); the intensity of management (meal planning to infusion pump); and availability. All these factors will influence the frequency of contact and amount of time allotted. Literature/publications can support both short- and long-term health outcomes; increasing patient and provider satisfaction, improving the quality-of-life, decreasing risk of complications and costs.

In each case, the team is needed to provide the ongoing care and education, glycemic management, health promotion, reduction of risks, telephone interventions, etc, which are guided by principles[11], clinical guidelines[3] and standards[2], as well as the 'process' of team education.

PROCESS OF TEAM EDUCATION

The 'gold standard', for education, is a coordinated team, often physician-led and nurse/dietitian supported. The role of the diabetes educator is recognized as an integral part of the instructional team. A 'diabetes educator' is defined as any qualified health professional, CDE or clinical diabetes specialist involved in the education process.

Some patients with complications require a more intense application of resources, increasing the cost per visit, amount of physician and allied health professional's time and variety of initiatives needed to improve healthcare[9]. This involves a move from recording simple vitals and giving a pamphlet, to complex patient education and counselling. Norris *et al.* suggest that behavior-change strategies were 'more effective' than a didactic approach, when combined with healthcare provider adjustments and reinforcement of educational messages[1].

In summary, the process of diabetes team management then is to individualize care and treatment, maximizing adherence. The diabetes educator and clinician roles emerge from this. The educator role convenes and coordinates the following team services: clinical, educational coordinating, consulting, and advocacy roles.

Educator role

All clinicians and educators need good clinical and educational backgrounds, and experiential expertise to fill certain requirements. Experience is needed in current clinical practice of diabetes care and management; and the principles of teaching–learning. These roles demand much flexibility, as the populations served and the settings (inpatient, outpatient, clinical, research) vary.

Diabetes educators offer support and a valuable service to the team, often fulfilling a role that it is difficult for a single physician to provide because of time and availability constraints. After initial instruction, educators provide continued personal and telephone or electronic contact for follow-through and assessment of progress. Many people require repeated instruction and teaching. Educators have the expertise, experience and, often, more scheduled time to assess, instruct and assist patients with the learning process, and working through the personal barriers to learning, such as language, reading levels, disabilities, etc. Scheduling of education, length and timing are often left to the educator, although new legislation promotes use of more group experience.

Instruction in the basics for survival and more advanced learning are common approaches. The revised standards identify 10 basic content areas to be delivered, educators are prepared to develop these as needed:

- Diabetes disease process
- Nutritional management
- Physical activity

- Medications
- Monitoring
- Complications
- Risk reduction
- Goal setting/problem solving
- Psychosocial adjustment
- Preconception care, pregnancy, gestational diabetes management

All members of the team are key players. Newer members of the clinical team are the CDE the clinical nurse specialist (CNS), advanced practice nurse (APN) and those with the advanced clinical role with the newest credentials: the Board Certified Advanced Diabetes Management (BC-ADM) certification. Each of these members has a strong basis in diabetes disease-specific practice, together with an expanded role. These are performed and guided by written procedures and policies, clinical practice guidelines and evidence-based research[21].

In conclusion, the educator role is an important part of the integration of clinical care into a more formal educational approach to diabetes. Patients must learn to be skilled and knowledgeable in diabetes self-care, able to access care, and facilitate ongoing decision-making related to their ongoing medical and self-care practices. They are at the center of their own team.

Clinician role

The clinical role of the diabetes educator is critical. Clinical background, including knowledge of the Clinical Practice Standards[3], facilitates recommendations for patient education and implementation of the treatment plan; it also fosters independence and access to the healthcare team. Clinical services (Table 4.3) provided often include objective analysis of current healthcare practices, preferences and knowledge base, and assisting the person with diabetes to achieve metabolic control, following the DCCT goal *Metabolic Control Matters*[15]. The person's understanding of their clinical status, acquisition of technical skills, communication with clinicians, and observation of physical and emotional challenges, etc are crucial to the development of a plan for care, guidance in achievement and educational planning.

Table 4.3 Clinician role
Self-care, family care assessment
Patient education skills
Communication, contact (acute/ongoing)
Review of clinical progress, problem-solving
Care trends, research, equipment, insurances team coordination
Care/case management

This clinician educator role may occur in the inpatient or outpatient setting, through referral from the same or a different clinical setting, and the service can be delivered in a variety of creative ways (person to person, electronically, via the mail service, etc). The clinical delivery alternatives also imply a modified team, which may include a variety of providers and specialists. Addressing risk reduction is a primary focus and the average patient will need hugely complex medical regimes, involving multiple antidiabetic, antihypertensive, and lipid-lowering agents to achieve target.

Management strategies consider[19]:

- Minimizing cost
- Minimizing weight gain
- Minimal injections (using a combination of pills, plus)
- Minimal circulating insulin (order of introduction of agents)
- Minimal patient effort (improve adherence, increase motivation, minimize effort)
- Hypoglycemia avoidance
- Postprandial targeting (better control achievement).

Family practice physicians appear to recognize and incorporate clinical and educational care into their diabetes-related visits. Chronic illness provides multiple opportunities for patient education over time and chronic illness visits can be used as 'teachable moments' to facilitate collaborative care[18]. Diabetes care requires distinctly different visits than an acute

care illness (probably also life style versus other chronic). A direct observational study found that 2.5 patient visits redo content and re-address physical needs, versus 2.1 visits for other chronic diseases, and 1.8 visits for acute care. More problems result in more visits. The amount of time spent on chronic topics, such as diet, advice, negotiation, assessment of compliance, exercise, etc, is more for advanced patients and less for patients undergoing procedures[18].

As the clinical role solidifies, educational programming and service development needs arise. The educator then assumes the role of coordinating these services, utilizing both business skills and quality management.

Coordinator role

Diabetes educators often find themselves faced with the challenge of starting a diabetes education program/service or they are hired to manage one. For many educators, with varying levels of clinical competence, starting, coordinating or managing a diabetes self-management program poses many challenges and the development of additional skills for diabetes educators has become as important as clinical skills. These skills include:

- Program development
- Strategic and business planning
- Marketing
- Financial management
- Human resource management
- Continuous quality improvement (CQI)
- Outcomes management.

The development of a strategic, marketing analysis plan, when starting a DSME program, will increase the potential for long-term success. Along with a thorough market analysis, the educator needs to conduct a financial analysis of the proposed service, and be prepared to present this to the sponsoring organization or community supporter. Budgeting is an important aspect of program development and will continue to be an important component of ongoing program management.

Table 4.4 Education standards

Canadian Diabetes Association: Diabetes Educator Section, Standards for Diabetes Education in Canada (2000). Education in Canada, 1995.

HCFA: Medicare Program; Expanded Coverage for Outpatient Diabetes Self-management Training and Diabetes Measurements. Federal Register: December 29, 2000 (USA).

International Consensus Standards of Practice for Diabetes Education. International Diabetes Federation Consultive Section on Education. 1997, Bakersville Press: UK.

National Standards for Diabetes Self-Management Education, Diabetes Care 2000;23 (USA).

Familiarity with the National Standards For Diabetes Self-Management Education, or other applicable standards (Table 4.4) is essential for coordinators in the early stage of starting a program. Standards define quality DSME that can be implemented in diverse settings and which will facilitate improvement in healthcare outcomes for people with diabetes. One example from the USA is comprised of ten evidence-based standards, which address structure, process and outcomes. The first national standard states that DSME must have documentation which describes its organizational structure, mission statement, and overall goals. It also states that quality must be an integral component of the program. There is strong scientific evidence in the business and healthcare literature which suggests that establishing a commitment to a strong organizational infrastructure which supports all of the above elements results in efficient and effective provision of services[22–25].

After the standards have been reviewed and 'homework' done, which includes community assessment, competitive analysis, target population and resource identification, a simple business plan is developed. It does not need to be complex, but serves as a guide for the leader and their team. According to the Joint Commission on Accreditation of Health Care Organizations (JCAHO), this type of documentation is important to both small and large organizations[26].

Once the target population, their needs, and the resources needed have been identified, a team will need to be formed. This 'core' clinical team usually consists of three or four healthcare professionals, with complementary skills, who are committed to a common goal and approach[27]. The diabetes educator may be the person who champions the case for diabetes education, but the organization's decision-makers must demonstrate their commitment to a multidisciplinary team, along with the resources and infrastructure that enables the team to function[10].

The diabetes education team will be the most important resource of the DSME. Without knowledgeable and competent diabetes educators, there will not be a program. The studies on diabetes education and diabetes care have rarely studied the characteristics of who actually provides the diabetes education, and what the outcome measures are of provider efficacy[28]. The studies have been clear that the provision of diabetes care and education always require a team. The national standards state that DSME must be provided by a multi-faceted educational instructional team, which may include a behaviorist, exercise physiologist, ophthalmologist, optometrist, pharmacist, physician, podiatrist, registered dietician, registered nurse, other professional, and para-professionals. They must be collectively qualified to teach all content areas, and must include, at a minimum, a registered dietician and registered nurse[13,29]. All instructors must be either a CDE or have recent didactic and experiential preparation in education and diabetes management. The research to date has shown that DSME is most effective when delivered by a multidisciplinary team with a comprehension plan of care[30–35]. If the program aims to become an ADA Education Recognized Program (ERP), the minimum team, as described in the national standards and adopted by the ADA ERP, must be in place[36].

Following the market survey, a mission statement and goals should be developed, before beginning to develop the team and program's services. There are several ways of approaching this. One common approach is to go back to the national standards and develop a curriculum based on Standard 7, which states that a written curriculum, with criteria for successful learning outcomes is required and the assessed needs of the individual will determine which content areas are delivered (Table 4.4). There are a number of curricula already developed, many of which meet standards and criteria.

The program services must be based on the selected curriculum, as well as on the needs of the target population. Demographics are analyzed for age, type of diabetes, payer mix (Medicare and some other insurers will mandate the delivery modality), and ethnic background. Clear descriptions of program services are important in order to market your program. There is still a widespread belief that 1:1 DSME is the best delivery modality, and that group teaching is a compromise made in response to economic pressure. However, there is data to support that group DSME is just as effective as individual education when utilized appropriately[37]. The dilemma becomes not whether to provide quality DSME programs in a group format, but whether diabetes educators have acquired the skills and strategies to provide effective educational, behavioral, and clinical interventions in a group format? The diabetes educator who has assumed a role as program coordinator, will need to be comfortable with applying change strategy not only for their patients but also for their staff. Quality management is also necessary to support the service.

Quality is a management philosophy that supports a continuous striving for service excellence and an unrelenting commitment to customer satisfaction. As individuals and organizations in healthcare began to attempt to define quality, hundreds of definitions came into existence. The definitions include terms such as quality assurance, quality assessment, total quality management, continuous quality improvement. The two models of quality activities most frequently cited have been the traditional structure, process, and outcome model of quality assurance, as described by Donebedian, and the industrial model of quality described by Deming, and Juran[37-41]. Quality is fundamentally a philosophy, and there is no one prescription for application. It is the concepts that need to be applied to the goal of striving for service excellence. There are a number of quality methodologies, with continuous quality improvement (CQI), being one of the most utilized. Two other frequently used methodologies are quality planning and quality measurement[40]. Understanding CQI is an important aspect for all diabetes educator, but especially for those who have assumed the coordinator role for program services. The steps in the CQI process are:

- Identify problem/opportunity
- Data collection
- Data analysis
- Identify alternative solutions
- Generate recommendations
- Implement recommendations
- Evaluate actions improvement.

Implementing a CQI program for DSME has now become one of the USA's national standards for DSME, and has been adopted by the ADA ERP[2,20]. In addition, the use and importance of measuring and formally reporting outcomes have risen. Outcome measurement is swiftly reviewed below.

Outcome measurement

Outcome measures have been defined as data that describe a patient's health status. Patient health outcomes have been measured for years, and their use has been increasing as researchers are beginning to see these outcomes as the best way to improve the performance of providing healthcare. Donebedian defines outcomes as "A measurable product and is the changed state or condition of an individual as a consequence of health care over time"[38] and an outcome is a change that occurs as a result of some intervention—it is not a single point in time[37]. The need to examine outcomes in healthcare and diabetes care has been reinforced by mandates from Healthcare Financing Administration (HCFA—

now renamed CMS, Centers for Medicaid and Medicare Services), Agency for Health Care Policy and Research (AHCPR), and accrediting bodies, such as the Joint Commission on Accreditation of Health Care Organizations (JCAHO), National Council on Quality Assurance (NCQA), and the American Diabetes Association Education and Provider Recognition programs.

Healthcare outcomes cross the healthcare continuum. They include educational, behavioral, clinical and long-term health status outcomes. Several outcome measurement instruments exist for assessing patient behavior, functional status, and QOL, for example: SF-36, PAID, and the Diabetes-Self-Management Assessment Report tool (D-SMART)[42–45]. Other outcomes that are important to different customers are: cost outcomes, such as cost effectiveness (ratio of costs of a program or process to the effects).

Evaluation, outcome measurement and reporting are critical to the future of DSME programs. The effectiveness of interventions must be documented in order to have a better understanding of which interventions are the most appropriate for a specific population. Diabetes education has long been held by many to be the cornerstone of effective diabetes care. Yet in 1997, when diabetes educators were asked by HCFA to provide specific evidence of what the attributes of effective education were, diabetes educators were left with little specificity. In 1999, in the USA at the AADE Research Summit, the question was asked: "Is diabetes education effective and what methods are the best?". The answer is: it depends on the following factors, what treatment, for what population, delivered by whom, under what set of conditions, for what outcome, and how did it come about[48]? Outcome measures associated with diabetes education programs include clinical (medical), educational (learning and behavioral), and psychosocial (QOL, coping, efficacy, etc)[49].

Through an extensive review of the literature and a process of expert consensus, the AADE Outcomes Task Force determined that health-related behaviors are the unique and measurable outcomes of effective diabetes education[48–53]. As the profession of diabetes education has

evolved, it has begun to shift focus from 'Did we deliver the right content' to 'Did the patient achieve the desired patient outcomes?' Research in diabetes education has not yet provided specificity in characteristics of 'best practice' in diabetes education. More detail is required about what steps in the process of diabetes education are important, including variables such as characteristics about the providers, population, delivery methodologies, and healthcare environment.

The process of assessing patient characteristics and determining what interventions are associated with the best outcomes is called clinical practice improvement (CPI)[54]. CPI is in many ways complementary to the CQI process as well as RCT, as it creates a permanent feedback loop aimed at all clinicians involved in the process of care delivery. It provides them with data about their daily practice, and the information necessary to understand and modify their interventions. The CPI framework is the basis for the AADE National Diabetes Education Outcomes System (NDEOS), which resulted from the work of the AADE Outcomes Task Force. Based on expert consensus, a comprehensive review of the literature, and a customer analysis of the AADE membership, the Outcomes Team determined that health-related behavior changes are the unique and measurable outcomes of diabetes education[46]. These behavior changes (which are compatible with the 10 DSME categories listed above) can be categorized in the following outcome areas:

- Physical activity (exercise)
- Food choices (eating)
- Medication administration
- Monitoring of blood glucose
- Problem solving for blood glucose: highs, lows, and sick days
- Risk-reduction activities
- Psychosocial adaptation.

Finding a definition of DSME that conveys your message in a clear and articulate way is important to the marketing of your program. One definition that has been used widely is the following: "Diabetes self-management education (including medical nutrition therapy[55]) is an interactive, collaborative, ongoing process involving the person with diabetes and the educator. It is a four-step process:

- Assess individual's education needs
- Identify individual's specific diabetes self-management goals
- Educate individual to achieve identified self-management goals
- Evaluate attainment of goals[49]."

Utilizing this information assists the diabetes education coordinator in developing and implementing a quality educational product. As the product expands, other educator roles may be identified and become appropriate, such as the coordinator of community education and case management.

Coordinator of professional, community education/consultant/advocate

Educators are often sought to provide professional and community intervention, together with prevention education, for a variety of groups ranging from other diabetes specialists to staff nurses, case managers, office nurses, pharmacists, primary care providers, and the general public. Each educator develops their skill sets based on their current practice environment and their personal areas of interest. Topics that they may be called on to present are diverse, and range from the core content areas in the National Standards, to clinical management, and less traditional areas, such as program development, quality management, and behavior change strategies. They may include support group and screening activities, school and camp programs, or work-site or faith-based presentations. The topic areas are as diverse and multidimensional as the role of the diabetes educator itself.

Coordinator of disease/case management

In recent years there has been an effort to identify new models of care for chronic diseases such as diabetes. The traditional model of acute care has been shown to inadequately address the needs of people with diabetes. A recent survey of patients who received their diabetes care from primary care providers, showed that they were receiving 64–74% of the ADA Provider Recognition Program recommended services[47]. The new models apply some recurring themes, such as systems approach, population based; preventive services, evidenced-based medicine; and outcomes management through IS solutions. These new models of care are often called disease and case management[48]. The diabetes educator has often been identified as a health professional with the requisite skill-set to coordinate such a model of care.

SUMMARY

Many physicians or health provider practices do not have access to a full comprehensive, multidisciplinary team, a diabetes educator in this expanded role, or this type of case and care management model. Contacting ADA or AADE can help identify educators in your local area. Regardless of practice setting, providers need to incorporate basic diabetes SM skills into routine office practice. A variety of materials and support supplies may be used to reinforce education. These may be obtained from ADA, AADE, CDC, etc. Reading level targeted material, larger print, graphics, models, sample products, audio, visual, and computer aids can all assist the learning process. A more balanced approach, especially for type 2 diabetes, emphasises risk reduction as well as glycemic control[56].

The appropriate allocation of the team educator role, as well as adequate teaching time, is necessary to facilitate the learning process. Skills demonstration, information repetition and situational problem solving are excellent tools for advancing the learning process. Content concepts should be limited, and specific behavioral instructions are better retained. General office staff reinforcement and encouragement help provide success.

Standards that include guidelines for curriculum, minimum professional expertise and training, advisory bodies, and systematic review of outcomes, are readily available to promote acceptable quality education nationwide for all people with diabetes. The voluntary recognition of ADA has created a template process. CMS has implemented accreditation for third party reimbursement, guided by these standards and the role of the educator.

As a result of the rapidly changing environment of healthcare financing and reimbursement, as well as the results of the DCCT and UKPDS, providers are faced with challenges of medical and educational care. Diabetes care and education has evolved into a highly specialized field with a focus on advanced practice, education and training requirements, and continuing to deliver care and education.

The diabetes educator is the 'gold standard' for maintaining the educational process, and the future holds the promise of easier implementation of therapies, together with the possibility that people with diabetes mellitus can live longer and better with education[57].

APPENDIX

Definitions

BC-ADM (Board-Certified Advanced Diabetes Management) – certified exam focused on advanced clinical management, requiring advanced degree for eligibility.

CDE-Certified Diabetes Educator – passing an exam administered by the National Certification Board for Diabetes Education. (AADE Scope of Practice, USA)

Clinical teaching – is communication, facilitates learning, provides structure, clients assume responsibility, to improve health, through changes in attitudes and behaviors[58–62]. The teaching role is generally accepted of all professionals. Process is: assess, analysis, planning, implementation, evaluation.

Diabetes education – a "planned series of events or experiences which include counseling, teaching of information, experiential skill building, discussions, problem solving, and assistance in reviewing ones life and determining if lifestyle changes necessary to support different, better health practices." The primary role of the educator is to educate the person with diabetes their family and support about diabetes self-management and related issues. (10 Curriculum)

Diabetes Clinical Specialist or advanced practitioner – professional with a masters degree and/ or certification in a specialty practice. They have training, expertise, autonomy and in many areas licensing with prescriptive ability. (ACCN/AADE)

Education – the interactive, collaborative, ongoing process involving the person with diabetes and the educator. (AADE Scope of Practice, USA)

Educator – healthcare professional who has mastered the core knowledge and skills (biological and social sciences; communication, counseling, education) and has current experience in the care of people with diabetes.

Goal – meet the academic, professional, experiential requirements to become a CDE. (AADE)

Patient education – expanding and evolving, now central to achieving adequate outcomes of care. Integrated throughout the care to individuals and groups, in all settings. Diagnostic–intervention–evaluation process model is used to practice patient education[62].

REFERENCES

1 Norris SL, Engelgau MM, Narayan KMV. Effectiveness of self-management teaching in type 2 diabetes: a systematic review of randomized trials. *Diabetes Care* 2001;24:561–87.

2 Mensing CR, Boucher J, Cypress M *et al*. National standards for diabetes self-management education. *Diabetes Care* 2000;23:682–9.

3 American Diabetes Association. Clinical practice recommendations 2002. *Diabetes Care* 2002; 25(Suppl 1).

4 United States Department of Health and Human Services PHS. *Healthy people 2010*. Washington DC: United States Department of Health and Human Services, 2000.

5 Clement S. Diabetes self-management education. *Diabetes Care* 1995;18:1204–14.

6 American Association of Diabetes Educators. *Executive summary of the diabetes educational and behavioral research summit 2001*. Chicago, IL: American Association of Diabetes Educators, 2001;6.

7   American Association of Diabetes Educators. The 1999 scope of practice for diabetes educators and the standards of practice for diabetes educators. In: *AADE 2000 Member Resource Guide.* Chicago, IL: American Association of Diabetes Educators, 2000.

8   American Association of Diabetes Educators. *Intensive diabetes management. The team approach.* Chicago, IL: American Association of Diabetes Educators, 1995.

9   Leichter SB, Cost and reimbursement as determinants of the quality of diabetes care: I. direct cost determinants. Cl diab 2001;19:142–4.

10 Etzwiler DD. Chronic care: a need in search of a system. *Diabetes Educ* 1997;23:569–73.

11 Center for Disease Control and Prevention. *Team care: comprehensive lifetime management for diabetes.* National Diabetes Education Program (NDEP-36). Atlanta, Georgia: US Department of Health and Human Services, 2001.

12 Lebovitz H. Therapy for diabetes mellitus and related disorders. In: Farkas-Hirsch R, editor. *The role of diabetes education in patient management.* 3rd edn. American Diabetes Association, 1998.

13 Franz MJ, Monk A, Barry B *et al.* Effectiveness of medical nutrition therapy provided by dieticians in the management of non-insulin-dependent diabetes mellitus: a randomized, controlled trial. *J Am Diet Assoc* 1995;95:1009–17.

14 Mundinger MO, Kane RL, Lenz ER *et al.* Primary care outcomes in patients treated by nurse practitioners or physicians: a randomized trial. *J Am Med Assoc* 2000;283:59–68.

15 Diabetes Control and Complications Trial Research Group. The effect of intensive treatment of diabetes on the development and progression of long-term complications in insulin dependent diabetes mellitus. *N Engl J Med* 1993;329:986–97.

16 National Institute of Diabetes and Digestive and Kidney diseases. *Metabolic control matters. Nationwide translation of the diabetes control and complications trial: analysis and recommendations.* NIH publication no. 94–3773. Bethesda, MD: US Department of Health and Human Services, 1994.

17 United Kingdom Prospective Diabetes Study Group. Intensive blood-glucose control with sulfonylureas or insulin compared with conventional treatment and risk of complications in patients with type 2 diabetes (UKPDS 33). *Lancet* 1998;352:837–53.

18 O'Connor PJ. Organizing diabetes care: identify, monitor, prioritize, intensify [editorial]. *Diabetes Care* 2001;24:1515 16.

19 Buse JB. Progressive use of medical therapies in type 2 diabetes. *Diabetes Spectrum* 2000;13:2000.

20 Yawn B, Zyzanski SJ, Goodwin MA *et al.* Is diabetes treated as an acute or chronic illness in a community family practice? *Diabetes Care* 2001;24:1390–6.

21 American Nurses Credentialing Center, www.Nursingworld.org/ancc/. Visited 13th March 2002.

22 American Association of Diabetes Educators, www.aadenet.org. Visited 13th March 2002.

23 Fox CH, Mahoney MC. Improving diabetes preventive care in a family practice residency program: a case study in continuous quality improvement. *Family Med* 1998;30:441–5.

24 Gilroth BE. Management of patient education in US hospitals: evolution of a concept. *Patient Educ Couns* 1990;15:101–11.

25 Heins JM, Nord WR, Cameron M. Establishing and sustaining state-of the art diabetes education programs: research and recommendations. *Diabetes Educ* 1992;18:501–8.

26 Mangan M. Diabetes self-management education programs in the Veterans Health Administration. *Diabetes Educ* 1997;23:87–695.

27 Joint Commission on Accreditation of Healthcare Organizations. *Framework for improving performance.* Oakbrook Terrace, IL: Joint Commission on Accreditation of Healthcare Organizations, 1994.

28 National Institute of Diabetes and Digestive and Kidney Diseases. *Metabolic control matters. Nationwide translation of diabetes control and complications trial: analysis and recommendations.* NIH publication no. 94–3773. Bethesda MD: US Department of Health and Human Services, 1994.

29 Young-Hyman D. Provider impact in diabetes education: what we know, what we would like to know, paradigms for asking. *Diabetes Educ* 1999;25(Suppl):34–42.

30 Aubert RE, Herman WH, Waters J *et al.* Nurse case management to improve glycemic control in diabetic patients in a health maintenance organization. *Ann Intern Med* 1998;129:605–12.

31 Abourizk NN, O'Conner PJ, Crabtree BF, Schnatz JD. An outpatient model of integrated diabetes treatment and education: functional, metabolic, and knowledge outcomes. *Diabetes Educ* 1994;20:416–21.

32 Etzweiler D. Chronic care: a need in search of a system. *Diabetes Educ* 1997;23:569–73.

33 Shamoon H, Vaccaro-Olko MJ. Diabetes education teams. Professional education in diabetes. In: *Proceedings of the DRTC Conference.* National Diabetes Information Clearinghouse and

National Institute of Diabetes and Digestive and Kidney Diseases, NIH, 1980.

34 Koproski J, Pretto Z, Poretsky L. Effects of an intervention by a diabetes team in hospitalized patients with diabetes. *Diabetes Care* 1997;20:1553–5.

35 Levetan CS, Salas JR, Wilets IF. Impact of endocrine and diabetes team consultation on hospital length of stay for patients with diabetes. *Am J Med* 1995;99:22–8.

36 American Diabetes Association, Education Recognition Program. Available at: http://www.diabetes.org. Visited June, 2000.

37 Rickheim PL, Weaver TW, Flader J. Assessment of group versus individual diabetes education: a randomized study. *Diabetes Care* 2002;25:269–74.

38 Donabedian A. *The definition of quality: a conceptual exploration.* Ann Arbor: Health Administration Press, 1980.

39 Deming WE. *Out of crisis.* Cambridge, MA: MIT-CAES; 1986.

40 Juran JM. *Juran's quality control handbook.* 4th edn. New York: McGraw-Hill, 1988.

41 Juran JM. *Reengineering processes for competitive advantage: business process quality management.* Wilton, CT: Juran Institute, 1994.

42 US Department of Health and Human Services, Agency for Health Care Policy and Research. Washington, DC: 1995. DHHS publication 95–0045.

43 Anderson RM, Fitzgerald JT, Wisdom K *et al.* A comparison of global versus disease-specific quality of life measures in patients with diabetes. *Diabetes Care* 1997;20:299–305.

44 Ware JEJ, Sherbourne CD. The MOS 36-item short-form health survey (SF-36): Conceptual framework and item changes. *Med Care* 1992;30:473–83.

45 Polonsky WH, Welch GM. Listening to our patient's concerns: understanding and addressing diabetes-specific emotional distress. *Diabetes Spectrum* 1997;9:8–11.

46 Peeples M, Mulcahy K, Tomky D, Weaver T. The conceptual framework on the National Diabetes Outcomes System (NDEOS). *Diabetes Educ* 2001;27:547–62.

47 Mulcahy KA, Peeples M, Tomky D *et al.* National diabetes education outcomes system: application to practice. *Diabetes Educ* 2000;26:957–64.

48 American Association of Diabetes Educators. Diabetes educational and behavioral research summit. *Diabetes Educ* 1999;25(Suppl).

49 American Diabetes Association. Task force. *Diabetes Spectrum* 1999;12:45.

50 Glasgow RE, Strycker LA. Preventive care practices for diabetes management in two primary care samples. *Am J Prev Med* 2000;19:9–14.

51 Peyrot M. Evaluation of patient education programs: how to do it and how to use it. *Diabetes Spectrum*1996;9:86–93.

52 Brown SA. Predicting metabolic control in diabetes: a pilot study using meta-analysis to estimate a linear model. *Nursing Res* 1994;43:362–8.

53 Glasgow R. Evaluating diabetes education. *Diabetes Care* 1992;15:1423–32.

54 McGlynn E. Choosing and evaluating clinical performance measures: The Joint Commission. 1998;24:470–9.

55 Franz MJ, Bantle JP, Beebe CA *et al.* Evidence-based nutrition principles and recommendations for the treatment and prevention of diabetes and related complications. *Diabetes Care* 2002;25:148–98.

56 Peyrot M, Rubin R. Modeling the effect of diabetes education on glycemic control. *Diabetes Ed* 1994;20:143–8.

57 Horn SD, Hopkins DSP. *Clinical practice improvement: a new technology for developing cost-effective quality care.* New York: Faulkner and Gray; 1994.

58 Pronk N, Goodman M, O'Connor PJ, Martinson B: Relationship between modifiable risks and short-term health care charges. *J Am Med Assoc* 1999;282:2235–39.

59 American Diabetes Association. *Annual review of diabetes.* American Diabetes Association, 2001.

60 Babcock D, Miller M. *Client education, theory and practice.* Mosby, 1994.

61 Pender NJ. *Health promotion in nursing practice.* Norwalk, CN; Appleton-Century Crofts, 1987.

62 Redman BK. *The practice of patient education.* 8th edn. Mosby, 1997.

5

Nutrition in the etiology and management of type 2 diabetes

Monika Toeller and Jim I Mann

INTRODUCTION

The prevalence of type 2 diabetes is increasing rapidly in many countries[1-3]. As there is currently no cure for diabetes, all measures that could contribute to prevention or treatment of the metabolic disturbances which precede or characterize the disease should be exploited. The important role of nutritional modifications in the prevention and treatment of type 2 diabetes is now well recognized[4-7].

Most persons with type 2 diabetes are overweight and/or insulin-resistant. Many of them also have dyslipidemia and hypertension, both of which are frequently present before type 2 diabetes is diagnosed. Nutritional intervention should therefore be started early enough to achieve the benefits that can be expected from medical nutritional treatment. This chapter describes the potential of nutritional measures to prevent or treat type 2 diabetes mellitus and its complications.

THE ROLE OF NUTRITION IN THE ETIOLOGY OF TYPE 2 DIABETES

Energy intake

There is now a considerable amount of evidence to suggest that rapid acculturation is associated with increased rates of type 2 diabetes[8]. Several characteristics of the Western way of life predispose to over-nutrition and obesity, which in turn increases the risk of developing insulin resistance and type 2 diabetes – particularly in individuals or populations with a genetic predisposition for diabetes. Physical inactivity and high intakes of energy-dense foods lead to an energy intake in excess of requirements[2,9].

An impressive decline in diabetes death rates in several places was reported during the First and Second World Wars. This trend was not found in places where there were no food shortages. On the other hand, the contribution of over-nutrition to risk of diabetes has also been demonstrated in many places. When food consumption per capita rose sharply in Japan, Taiwan and some Pacific Islands, there was also a sharp rise in the prevalence of type 2 diabetes[8].

A number of studies have demonstrated improvements in metabolic parameters among people with impaired glucose tolerance (IGT) after interventions aimed at reducing energy intake and increasing physical activity, suggesting that it may be possible to reduce the incidence of type 2 diabetes[10-13]. Indeed, some recent intervention studies have demonstrated the potential for weight loss to reduce the risk of progression from IGT to type 2 diabetes. The Finnish Diabetes Prevention Study included 522 overweight persons with IGT, randomized to a control group or to intensive lifestyle intervention. The cumulative incidence of type 2 diabetes after 4 years was 11% in the intervention group and 23% in the control group. The risk of type 2 diabetes was reduced by 58%, and this outcome was directly related to changes in lifestyle[14].

The Diabetes Prevention Programme in the USA included 3234 persons of diverse ethnic background with IGT[15]. Participants in the intensive lifestyle programme reduced their risk of developing type 2 diabetes by 58% over 3 years of follow-up, and the risk reduction was 71% among persons over the age of 60 years. Of interest is the finding that metformin, the pharmacological agent tested in this study, resulted in a risk reduction of 31%, which was less than the risk reduction observed for lifestyle intervention.

Excess body fat is perhaps the most important modifiable risk factor for the development of type 2 diabetes[8,12]. It is estimated that the risk of type 2 diabetes attributable to obesity is as great as 75%. However, it is important to emphasize that in intervention studies aimed at weight reduction there are major difficulties in disentangling the potential benefits of weight loss from the effects of altering intakes of individual foods and nutrients and increasing physical activity, all of which have the potential to reduce diabetes risk. Energy intake is difficult to assess adequately in large-scale epidemiological studies, even when the best presently available instruments are employed, and it has been demonstrated that overweight or obese persons underestimate their energy intake. Nevertheless, the consistency of beneficial effects shown in intervention studies in which body weight was reduced strengthens the recommendation that energy intake in excess of requirement and overweight should be avoided, particularly among those with a familial predisposition. Such advice probably offers the best hope of reducing the risk of developing resistance to the action of insulin, and progression to type 2 diabetes[6,11,16].

Carbohydrate and fibre

Many studies have examined the role of sucrose and sugars in the etiology of type 2 diabetes. A few have suggested a positive association, but the majority of studies have shown no association. Some have even suggested an inverse association between diabetes incidence and sucrose intake[8,11]. Poor assessment of dietary intake, inability to disentangle dietary and other confounding factors, as well as over-interpretation of data derived from observational studies characterize many of these studies. Despite the lack of direct evidence for the role of sugars in the etiology of type 2 diabetes, it is conceivable that excessive sucrose intake might predispose to obesity, and thus sucrose indirectly may be a predisposing factor for type 2 diabetes.

There is support for the suggestion that foods rich in slowly digested starch or high in fibre might be protective. Countries with high intakes of these foods have low rates of type 2 diabetes. In a cross-sectional study of normoglycemic men, intake of pectin was inversely associated with postprandial blood glucose levels, independent of total energy intake and body mass index (BMI)[5]. In the Health Professionals' Follow-up Study and the Nurses' Health Study, diets low in cereal fibre and with high glycemic loads were associated with an increased risk of type 2 diabetes after adjustment for other risk factors[10]. In the Iowa Women's Health Study the risk of self-reported diabetes was highest in the group with the lowest whole-grain intake. In contrast, a higher consumption of refined grains was associated with an increased risk of type 2 diabetes after adjustment for age and total energy intake. The ratio of whole grain to refined grain was related to a significantly lower risk of diabetes, suggesting a potential benefit for replacing refined grains with whole grains[17].

It is of interest that, in the studies quoted, cereal fibre appeared to contribute most to the protective effect; however, experimental studies have repeatedly demonstrated a more marked beneficial effect of soluble fibres than insoluble fibres on several measures of carbohydrate and lipid metabolism. Thus, fibre from fruit and vegetables might have been expected to have exerted a more marked protective effect than cereal fibre. Although further research is needed to investigate the effects of different types and sources of fibre, it seems to be prudent to encourage an increased consumption of total dietary fibre from different sources: whole grains, fruits, vegetables and legumes.

Types of fat

In the San Luis Valley Diabetes Study a high intake of fat was associated with an increased risk of IGT and type 2 diabetes. In the 1–3 year follow-up of this study, fat consumption predicted the progression to type 2 diabetes in persons with IGT[18]. A positive association has also been found between saturated fat and hyperglycemia or glucose intolerance in cross-sectional studies[5,18]. However, large cohort studies with diagnosed type 2 diabetes as an endpoint did not show an appreciable association with saturated fat intake[19]. Conversely, a high intake of vegetable fat was inversely associated with the risk of type 2 diabetes during 6 years of follow-up among participants in the Nurses' Health Study who were not obese[19]. With the exception of the San Luis Valley Diabetes Study, other epidemiological studies did not find a significant association between intakes of monounsaturated fat and risk of type 2 diabetes[18]. However, fats of a different nature are often highly correlated in the diets, and therefore confounding by one type of fat may have hindered the analysis for another type of fat. The relationship between nature of dietary fat and type 2 diabetes has been studied in persons with IGT and undiagnosed type 2 diabetes patients – who were reported to have higher proportions of saturated fatty acids in serum cholesterol esters than persons with normal glucose tolerance[20].

Perhaps the best evidence for the potentially deleterious effect of saturated fatty acids comes from the KANWU Study. In this study, replacing an appreciable proportion of dietary saturated fatty acids with monounsaturated fatty acids was associated with an increase in insulin sensitivity. It is also of interest to note that both in the Finnish Diabetes Prevention Study and in the US Diabetes Prevention Project, which showed a reduced risk of progression from IGT to type 2 diabetes, the dietary recommendations included advice to appreciably reduce saturated fatty acids. No studies are yet available to suggest conclusive associations between trans-fatty acids and the risk of type 2 diabetes.

The suggestion that n-3 polyunsaturated fatty acids may also play a role in the development of type 2 diabetes came from a prospective study of 175 elderly men and women who were habitual fish eaters. They were shown to have a 50% lower risk of developing glucose intolerance over a follow-up period of 4 years compared with persons who were not regular fish eaters[21].

It now appears that the effects of various fatty acids on the risk of type 2 diabetes are similar to their effects on lipoprotein-mediated risk of coronary heart disease[22–24]. According to the available data, modifying intake of dietary fats towards consuming less saturated fat and more unsaturated fats may reduce the risk of developing type 2 diabetes – in addition to reducing cardiovascular risk.

Other nutritional factors

There are no firm epidemiological data with regard to the role of dietary protein in the etiology of type 2 diabetes. Although vegetarians present with lower rates of type 2 diabetes compared with persons who eat meat, it is impossible to disentangle the association of animal protein with the risk of type 2 diabetes from other dietary factors, such as saturated fat and fibre intake[8]. The relationship between alcohol and other dietary variables similarly complicates attempts to evaluate a potential role for alcohol in the etiology of type 2 diabetes. In the Rancho Bernardo Study, increasing intakes of alcohol in obese men were associated with an increased risk of type 2 diabetes[25]. On the other hand, moderate alcohol intake has been shown to be associated with enhanced insulin sensitivity[26,27].

So far, no epidemiological studies have provided convincing support for the role of micronutrients in the etiology of type 2 diabetes. The suggestion that low birthweight infants, especially those who show rapid catch-up growth, are at increased risk of developing IGT and type 2 diabetes later in life is fairly consistent, but the possible relation of this phenomenon to maternal malnutrition needs further research.

Recent knowledge regarding the potential of nutritional factors in the prevention of type 2 diabetes can be summarized as follows:

- Structured programmes on lifestyle modification that emphasize a reduction in total energy and saturated fat intake, and encourage an increase in fibre consumption, together with increased physical activity and regular contact with the healthcare team, are the most promising approaches to reducing the risk of developing type 2 diabetes.
- Avoiding being overweight, and treating overweight and obesity are particularly important for those with a familial predisposition for type 2 diabetes.

MEDICAL NUTRITION TREATMENT IN THE MANAGEMENT OF TYPE 2 DIABETES

Goals of nutrition therapy for type 2 diabetes

Nutritional management aims to help optimize metabolic control and reduce risk factors for chronic complications of diabetes. This includes the achievement of blood glucose and glycosylated hemoglobin (HbA1c) levels as close to normal as is safely possible, and lipid and lipoprotein profiles, as well as blood pressure values, that may be expected to reduce the risk of macrovascular disease. Individual nutritional needs and the quality of life of the person with diabetes also have to be considered when defining nutritional objectives[6,7,11,16,28]. The nutritional recommendation for an individual patient should include practical advice regarding appropriate food choices and quantities. However, it should be stressed that nutritional recommendations for people with type 2 diabetes are similar to those aimed at the population as a whole for the promotion of good health and the prevention of metabolic disorders and vascular complications. Thus, the food for persons with diabetes should not differ appreciably from that recommended for other family members[6,29,30].

Energy restriction and body weight

Many individuals with type 2 diabetes are overweight. Insulin resistance increases with increasing

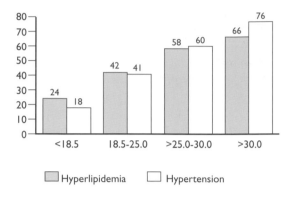

Figure 5.1 Prevalence of hyperlipidemia and hypertension (n%) by categories of BMI (kg m^{-2}) in a sample of 1988 persons with diabetes [930 male, 1058 female; mean age 57 ± 13 years; mean diabetes duration 8 (1–56) years].

body weight, and obesity may also aggravate hyperlipidemia and hypertension (Figure 5.1). Many short-term studies have demonstrated that weight loss, especially of intra-abdominal fat, in persons with type 2 diabetes is associated with decreased insulin resistance, improved glycemic control, reduced blood pressure and improvement of dyslipidemia[27,31] (Table 5.1). Thus, energy restriction and weight loss are important therapeutic objectives for obese individuals with type 2 diabetes[6,7]. However, long-term data are still missing to assess the extent to which metabolic improvements by means of weight loss can be maintained in people with type 2 diabetes. Long-term weight loss is often difficult to achieve, and it

Table 5.1 Nutritional factors and their possible impact on insulin resistance (↓ decrease, ↑ increase)

Total energy reduction	↓↓↓
Increased fibre intake	↓
Low glycemic index food	↓
Small amounts of alcohol	↓
Saturated fat intake	↑↑
Total fat	↑
Salt	↑

Table 5.2 Recommended nutrient intakes for persons with diabetes

Carbohydrate

45–60% total energy/day	Prefer foods rich in fibre and with low glycemic load (e.g. legumes, vegetables, fresh fruit, wholegrain bread, parboiled rice, pasta)
Sucrose/saccharose < 10% total energy/day	Beverages with high sucrose/glucose content are suitable to treat hypoglycemia
Non-nutritive sweeteners can be taken if desired	Consider ADI (accepted daily intake) levels

Total fat

25–35% total energy/day	
Saturated fatty acids plus trans-unsaturated fatty acids < 10% total energy/day	If LDL-cholesterol is elevated < 7% total energy/day
Polyunsaturated fatty acids up to 10% total energy/day	
Consider n-3–unsaturated fatty acids	e.g. in oily fish (at least 1–2 servings/ week), rapeseed
Monounsaturated fatty acids 10–20% total energy/day	oil, soybean oil, nuts, green leafy vegetables
Cholesterol < 300 mg/day	If LDL-cholesterol is elevated < 200 mg/day

Protein

10–20% total energy/day	0.8 g/kg of body weight in incipient or overt nephropathy

Alcohol

< 30 g/day for men; < 15 g/day for women	

---

has to be considered that genetic factors may play an important role in determining body weight. Environmental factors also often make losing weight difficult for those genetically predisposed to obesity. Nevertheless, the potential of structured weight loss programmes should be exploited in obese persons with type 2 diabetes to achieve the possible beneficial effects.

The UK Prospective Diabetes Study (UKPDS) reported that the initial glucose response in persons with type 2 diabetes was particularly related to the decreased energy intake. Once energy intake was increased, fasting glucose levels increased even when weight loss was maintained[32]. Prevention of weight regain seems to be an important target in those who lose weight, but evidently a long-term restricted energy intake is necessary to sustain the metabolic improvements.

Those who are overweight should be encouraged to reduce caloric intake so that their BMI moves towards the recommended range of 18.5–25 kg m^{-2}. Advice concerning the reduction of high fat and energy-dense foods will usually help to achieve a weight loss. If such measures do not result in a desired weight reduction, it may be necessary to offer specific weight reduction programmes, which also include increased physical activity and behaviour modification approaches[6,31]. The use of very low energy diets should be restricted to persons with a BMI > 35 kg m^{-2} (Reference 6).

Carbohydrate and type 2 diabetes

The recommended intake of carbohydrate for people with diabetes is 45–60% of total energy intake (Table 5.2). Provided that foods rich in fibre and with low glycemic index predominate, there are no known deleterious effects with this range of carbohydrate intake. When carbohydrate intakes are at the upper end of the proposed range, restriction of carbohydrate to around 45% of total energy and replacement of carbohydrate by monounsaturated fat may be tried for some patients with unsatisfactory glycemic control. However, there is concern that increased fat intake might promote weight gain and potentially contribute to insulin resistance. The advice for carbohydrate intake should therefore be individualized, based on nutrition assessment, metabolic results and treatment goals[6,7].

Vegetables, legumes, fresh fruit and whole-grain cereal-derived foods are the preferred sources of carbohydrate. They are rich in fibre, micronutrients and vitamins, and help to ensure the recommended intakes of other nutrients. However, many individuals with diabetes do not consume such foods on a regular basis (Figure 5.2).

A number of factors influence glycemic response to carbohydrate-containing foods, including the nature of the starch (amylose, amylopectin, resistant starch), the amount of dietary fibre and the type of sugar. Different carbohydrates have different glycemic responses and, clearly, the amount of carbohydrate is one important factor in postprandial

glucose levels. However, foods with a low glycemic index may confer benefits not only for postprandial glycemia in persons with type 2 diabetes, but also for their lipid profile[33–36]. Foods with a low glycemic index (e.g. legumes, pasta, parboiled rice, whole-grain breads, oats, certain raw fruits) should therefore be substituted when possible for those with a high glycemic index (e.g. mashed potatoes, white rice, white bread and rolls, sugary drinks).

People with diabetes should be encouraged to choose a variety of fibre-containing foods. It has been shown that increased fibre intake results in benefits for glycemic control, hyperinsulinemia and serum lipids[37–39]. A realistic goal in many individuals with type 2 diabetes might be to achieve a daily fibre intake of about 30 g. The available evidence from controlled clinical studies demonstrates that moderate intake of dietary sucrose in diets with an appreciable amount of fibre – with the sucrose displacing other fibre-depleted carbohydrate-containing food – does not worsen glycemic control in persons with diabetes[6,40,41]. Thus, sucrose and other added sugars may be included in moderation in the diets of people with type 2 diabetes, however, the bulk of dietary carbohydrate should be derived from foods with a low glycemic index and/or rich in fibre. It is of interest that low glycemic index foods and fibre-rich foods appear to have an effect independent of other attributes; many high fibre foods do indeed have a low glycemic index, and vice versa.

Fructose produces a reduction in postprandial glycemia when it replaces sucrose, however, this potential benefit is tempered by the fact that higher amounts of fructose may adversely effect plasma lipids by increasing triglycerides. But there is no reason to recommend that persons with diabetes avoid naturally occurring fructose, e.g. in fruits, vegetables and other foods. Adding fructose, sugar alcohols and other nutritive sweeteners, all of which are energy sources, does not have substantial advantage over added sucrose as a sweetener for people with diabetes and therefore should not to be encouraged[6,7]. Intake of food containing sugar alcohols, such as sorbitol, has been reported to cause diarrhoea. Furthermore, it is unlikely that sugar alcohols in

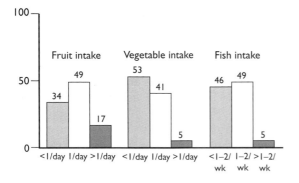

Figure 5.2 Frequency of fresh fruit, vegetable and fish intake (n%) in a sample of 1988 persons with diabetes [930 male, 1058 female; mean age 57 ± 13 years; mean diabetes duration 8 (1–56) years] in Germany in 2000.

the amounts likely to be ingested in foods or meals will contribute to a significant reduction in total energy or carbohydrate intake, although they are only partially absorbed from the small intestine.

Approved non-nutritive sweeteners may be used by people with diabetes to sweeten beverages, desserts, fruits, etc.[11,42]. The recommended acceptable daily intake (ADI), defined as the amount of a food additive that can be safely consumed on a daily basis over a person's lifetime without risk, should be considered when non-nutritive sweeteners are chosen. However, it is unknown whether the use of non-nutritive sweeteners improves glycemic control or assists in weight loss in persons with diabetes.

For individuals with type 2 diabetes treated with insulin, to avoid hypoglycemia and excessive postprandial hyperglycemia it is important that the timing and dose of insulin match the amount, type and time of carbohydrate-containing food intake. Individuals receiving intensive insulin therapy should adjust their premeal insulin dose based on the content and glycemic load of carbohydrate-containing snacks and meals. In persons with type 2 diabetes postprandial glucose responses to a variety of carbohydrates are similar if the amount of carbohydrate is constant[11]. Patients should therefore try to be consistent in day-to-day carbohydrate intake when they are treated with fixed daily insulin doses or with high doses of sulfonylurea, to avoid hypoglycemic episodes, as well as undesirably high postprandial blood glucose levels. Self-monitoring of blood glucose may be helpful in determining the most appropriate timing of food intake and optimal food choices for the individual patient. There are no general principles regarding the optimum frequency of snacks and meals. Individual preferences, the needs of different treatment regimes and total energy requirements are the main determinants of meal frequency and portion sizes[6].

Fat modification

The primary goal regarding dietary fat intake in individuals with type 2 diabetes is to decrease intake of saturated fatty acids. Compared with the non-diabetic population, persons with diabetes have an increased risk of cardiovascular disease and the intake of saturated fat is already undesirably high in most countries with a Western way of life. To assist in achieving optimal low-density lipoprotein (LDL)-cholesterol levels (< 100 mg dL^{-1}) it is recommended that the intake of saturated fatty acids plus trans-unsaturated fatty acids be limited to no more than 10% of total energy intake, and the amount of dietary cholesterol to < 300 mg/day[6,7,43]. In patients with elevated LDL-cholesterol, a further reduction of saturated fat to $< 7\%$, and of dietary cholesterol to < 200 mg/day, have been recommended for non-diabetics with dyslipidemia. Although specific studies in persons with diabetes are not available to conclusively demonstrate the effects of these limits, the goals for patients with diabetes remain the same as for other high-risk groups.

For those on weight-maintaining diets, the debate has focused on what is the best energy source alternative to saturated fat. Several studies now suggest that saturated fat could be replaced by carbohydrate food rich in fibre and/or by *cis*-mono-unsaturated fatty acids[6,7,44]. Diets high in *cis*-mono-unsaturated fatty acids, or low in fat and high in fibre-rich carbohydrate result in improvements in glycemia and lipid levels compared with diets high in saturated fat.

Controversial results have been reported from the few studies that evaluated the effects of polyunsaturated fat and glycemic control and serum lipid levels in persons with type 2 diabetes. It is currently recommended that intake should be $< 10\%$ of total energy, based upon the potential adverse consequences of increased lipid oxidation and reduced levels of high-density lipoprotein associated with high intakes[6,11].

N-3 polyunsaturated fat (omega-3 fatty acids) has the potential to reduce serum triglyceride levels, particularly in persons with hypertriglyceridemia, and to have beneficial effects on platelet aggregation and thrombogenicity[45]. Although studies of the effects of n-3 fatty acids in patients with diabetes have primarily used fish-oil supplements, there is evidence from the general population that foods containing n-3

Table 5.3 Dietary modifications for the prevention and treatment of diabetic nephropathy

When albumin excretion is raised (AER > 20 μg min⁻¹)

Avoid high protein intake, particularly high protein intake from animal sources

Restrict the consumption of meat to one serving per day (≈ 125 g)

Consume cheese only in small amounts

Two daily servings of milk or milk products are sufficient (e.g. one yoghurt and one glass of milk)

Large amounts of curd should not be consumed

Prefer consumption of protein from vegetable sources

When blood pressure is elevated (≥ 130/80 mmHg)

Reduce salt intake to target of < 6 g/day (particularly if salt sensitive)

Avoid added salt

Avoid obviously salted foods (particularly processed foods)

Prefer meals cooked directly from natural ingredients

When serum cholesterol is elevated (total cholesterol > 170 mg dL⁻¹ or LDL-cholesterol > 100 mg dL⁻¹)

Restrict intakes of saturated fat and trans-fatty acids (< 7% total energy) and dietary cholesterol intake (< 200 mg day⁻¹)

Substitute mono-unsaturated fat (*cis* configuration) for saturated fat

Increase intake of fibre

Choose meat with a lower fat content

Avoid processed meat as far as possible

Consume skimmed milk and fat-reduced milk products

Restrict the consumption of high-fat snacks (e.g. potato chips, chocolate, cakes and cookies)

Prefer use of vegetable oils, particularly oils rich in mono-unsaturated fat

Use fat and oils only in small quantities

Consume five portions of vegetables or fruits per day

Give preference to wholemeal or whole-grain cereals and cereal products

fatty acids have cardioprotective effects. Food sources of n-3 polyunsaturated fat include fatty fish and plant sources, such as rapeseed oil, soybean oil and nuts. The consumption of at least 1–2 helpings of fish each week will contribute to ensuring an adequate intake of n-3 fatty acids[6,11].

Trans-unsaturated fatty acids are produced during the hydrogenation of unsaturated fats and are found in many manufactured products, such as biscuits, cakes, confectionery, soups and some margarines. When studied independently of other fatty acids the effect of trans-fatty acids is similar to that of saturated fats in raising LDL-cholesterol. The intake of trans-fatty acids therefore should be minimized[7].

Dietary protein and diabetic nephropathy

A few studies suggest that persons with type 2 diabetes have an increased need for protein during moderate hyperglycemia, and an altered adaptive mechanism for protein-sparing during weight-loss, resulting in an increased protein requirement. However, in many countries the protein intake for persons with diabetes is relatively high and exceeds by far the recommended dietary allowance (RDA) of 0.8 g kg⁻¹ body weight for adults. On average, protein intake was 21% of daily energy in the UKPDS. In general, there seems to be little concern that persons with diabetes may develop a deficiency in protein intake[46]. The current recommendation for people with diabetes is that protein may provide 10–20% of total energy intake, and should not exceed this level (Table 5.3). In individuals with controlled type 2 diabetes, ingested protein does not increase glucose concentrations, although it is just as potent a stimulant of insulin secretion as carbohydrate[11].

An association between dietary protein intake and renal disease has been shown in a large-scale cross-sectional study of people with type 1 diabetes. Those with a protein intake above 20% of total energy intake had abnormal albumin excretion rates (AER > 20 µg min^{-1}), particularly when hypertension was present[46]. This suggests that a very high protein intake may have detrimental effects on renal function, and it may be prudent to avoid a protein intake > 20% of total daily energy intake.

Several studies have focused on reversing or retarding the progression of proteinuria, and preventing nephropathy. Only a few studies have evaluated nutritional modifications, particularly a reduction of protein intake in patients with type 2 diabetes. With small reductions in protein intake, to 0.8 g kg^{-1} body weight, albumin excretion rates were reduced in patients with microalbuminuria[47,48]. Whether substituting vegetable protein for protein from animal sources might result in beneficial effects has also been explored; however, there is still insufficient evidence to make firm recommendations regarding the source of dietary protein. The current recommendation advises a reduction of usually higher protein intake to 0.8 g kg^{-1} body weight per day in individuals with incipient diabetic nephropathy. This modification in protein intake means a major change in diet for many patients and, therefore, the education of the patient and family members should be assisted by a trained dietician whenever possible[11,46].

Alcohol

Precautions regarding alcohol intake that apply to the general population also apply to people with type 2 diabetes. If persons with diabetes choose to drink alcohol, intake should be no more than 15 g per day for adult women and 30 g

per day for adult men. This corresponds to approximately one or two drinks of wine or beer per day[6,11]. The cardioprotective effect of alcohol appears not to be determined by the type of the alcoholic beverages consumed. However, alcohol is an important energy source in overweight persons with type 2 diabetes, and alcohol consumption can be associated with raised blood pressure and hypertriglyceridemia. In individuals with diabetes, chronic intake of moderate amounts (5–15 g/day) of alcohol was associated with a decreased risk of coronary heart disease. However, conversely, a strong association between excessive habitual intake (> 30–60 g/day) of alcohol and raised blood pressure was found in both men and women[49].

Alcohol can have both hypoglycemic and hyperglycemic effects in people with diabetes, depending on the amount of alcohol acutely ingested. In studies where alcoholic beverages were consumed with food by people with diabetes, no acute effects were seen on blood glucose or insulin levels. Alcohol should therefore be consumed with food to reduce the risk of hypoglycemia and persons with diabetes are advised not to omit food when choosing to drink a moderate amount of alcoholic beverages[6,7].

Vitamins and minerals

Individuals with diabetes should be advised about the importance of acquiring daily vitamin and mineral requirements from natural food sources. Regular consumption of a variety of vegetables, fresh fruit (five or more servings of vegetables or fruits per day), legumes, low-fat milk, vegetable oils, nuts, whole-grain breads and oily fish should be encouraged to ensure that recommended intakes are met[11]. On the other hand, people with diabetes should be advised to restrict salt intake to under 6 g/day, particularly when elevated blood pressure is a problem.

Persons with diabetes may have increased oxidative stress, there has therefore been interest in recommending intake of antioxidant vitamins. However, placebo-controlled trials have failed to show a clear benefit from antioxidant supplementation and, in some cases, adverse effects

---

Table 5.4 Nutritional management as part of the continuing treatment and education process in persons with type 2 diabetes

Nutritional review and individual recommendations

At diagnosis

At each consultation if the patient is overweight or vascular risk factors are not well controlled

Every year as a routine

On the beginning of insulin therapy

On special request

Check

Is healthy eating a part of lifestyle?

Is energy intake appropriate for attaining or maintaining a desirable body weight (BMI < 25 kg m^{-2})?

Is alcohol intake moderate, or could it be exacerbating hypertension, hypertriglyceridemia or contributing to hypoglycemia?

Is money being spent unnecessarily on special diabetic food products?

Does the distribution of meals or snacks reflect the glucose-lowering medication?

Does raised blood pressure or abnormal albuminuria suggest a benefit from salt (< 6 g/day) or protein (0.8 g/kg/day) restriction?

Advise

Carbohydrate intake should be higher and fat intake lower than presently consumed in most countries – reducing saturated fats and/or trans-fats (e.g. in cream, chocolates, fast foods, high fat cheese, sausages, meat, spreads and fatty bakery)

The use of fresh fruit and vegetables (≥ 5 servings a day)

Consuming preferably whole-grain breads and cereals, parboiled rice, pasta, legumes

The use of vegetable oils (e.g. olive oil, rapeseed oil, soybean oil), nuts, seeds and oily fish

Sugar does not need to be excluded but should be limited (e.g. < 30–50 g/day)

Alcoholic beverages, if desired, should be consumed as part of the total caloric intake (no more than 1–2 small drinks/day)

Meals, snacks and food choices should match individual therapeutic needs, preferences and culture

---

have been suggested for beta-carotene supplements[11]. The role of folate supplementation in reducing cardiovascular events is still under further investigation. Vitamin and mineral supplementation in pharmacological dosages should be viewed as a therapeutic intervention, and recommended only in case of proven deficiencies[6]. There is no clear evidence of benefit from vitamin or mineral supplementation in people who do not have underlying deficiencies. Evaluation of the micronutrient status of a person with type 2 diabetes begins with a careful dietary history, as laboratory evaluation is often confounded by methodological problems. However, measurements of serum folate, vitamin B12, vitamin D, calcium, potassium, magnesium and iron concentrations may be clinically useful to define micronutrient deficiencies[11].

NUTRITIONAL ADVICE AND STRUCTURED TRAINING

Each patient with type 2 diabetes needs individual advice and structured training by his or her physician and other members of the healthcare team, to enable them to translate the principles of nutrition in type 2 diabetes into specific actions in daily life (Table 5.4). A balance must be achieved among the demands of metabolic control, risk factor management and the patient's well-being and safety. The therapeutic needs of an individual person will change with time and, therefore, continuing nutritional education must be provided[30,40]. To improve compliance, the main aspects of dietary advice given to a person with diabetes should also have a potential benefit for family members and should be acceptable to them.

A nutritional history should be taken at diagnosis, as well as at visits whenever the patient is not well controlled and it is thought that nutritional factors might have contributed to the unsatisfactory metabolic results. A nutritional review and individual nutritional recommendations should be provided at least once a year, or more often on special request[30].

Patients with incipient or overt diabetic nephropathy particularly need individual advice how to restrict protein intake without losing appetite and compliance to the proposed food intake[46]. Individual advice can be combined with structured group training. Since the clinical picture of diabetic nephropathy changes during the course of the disease, different priorities are required in the training programmes.

All steps in the nutritional management of a person with type 2 diabetes should be documented and the outcome evaluated by means of important markers, such as body weight, waist circumference, blood pressure, HbA1c, fasting and/or postprandial blood glucose (self-) monitoring, serum-lipids, albumin excretion rates and well-being or quality of life.

REFERENCES

1 American Diabetes Association. Type 2 diabetes in children and adolescents. Consensus statement. *Diabetes Care* 2000;23:381–9.

2 Seidell JC. Obesity, insulin resistance and diabetes – a world wide epidemic. *Br J Nutr* 2000;83 (Suppl 1):5S-8S.

3 Dunstan DN, Zimmet PZ, Welborn TA *et al.* The rising prevalence of diabetes and impaired glucose tolerance: the Australian Diabetes, Obesity, and Lifestyle Study. *Diabetes Care* 2002;25:829–34.

4 Hadden DR, Blair ALT, Wilson EZ *et al.* Natural history of diabetes presenting at age 40–69 years: a prospective study of the influence of intensive dietary therapy. *Q J Med* 1986;59:579–98.

5 Feskens EJ, Virtanen SM, Räsänen L *et al.* Dietary factors determining diabetes and impaired glucose tolerance: a 20–year follow-up of the Finnish and Dutch cohorts of the Seven Countries Study. *Diabetes Care* 1995;18:1104–12.

6 Mann J, Lean M, Toeller M *et al.* on behalf of the Diabetes and Nutrition Study Group (DNSG) of the European Association for the Study of Diabetes (EASD). Recommendations for the nutritional management of patients with diabetes mellitus. *Eur J Clin Nutr* 2000;54:353–5.

7 American Diabetes Association. Evidence-based nutrition principles and recommendations for the treatment and prevention of diabetes related complications. Position statement. *Diabetes Care* 2002;25:202–12.

8 Mann J, Toeller M. Type 2 diabetes: aetiology and environmental factors. In: Ekoe J-M, Zimmet P, Williams R, editors. *The epidemiology of diabetes mellitus*. Chichester, New York: John Wiley and Sons, 2001:133–40.

9 Turner RC, Millns H, Neil HA *et al.* Risk factors for coronary artery disease in non-insulin dependent diabetes mellitus: United Kingdom Prospective Diabetes Study (UKPDS: 23). *Br Med J* 1998;316:823–8.

10 Liu S, Manson JE, Stampfer MJ *et al.* A prospective study of whole-grain intake and risk of type 2 diabetes mellitus in US women. *Am J Publ Health* 2000;90:1409–15.

11 Franz MJ, Bantle JP, Beebe CA *et al.* Evidence-based nutrition principles and recommendations for the treatment and prevention of diabetes and related complications. Technical review. *Diabetes Care* 2002;25:148–98.

12 Hu FB, van Dam RM, Liu S. Diet and risk of type 2 diabetes: the role of types of fat and carbohydrate. *Diabetologia* 2002;44:805–17.

13 McAuley KA, Williams SM, Mann JI *et al.* Intensive lifestyle changes are necessary to improve insulin sensitivity: a randomized controlled trial. *Diabetes Care* 2002;25:445–52.

14 Tuomilehto J, Lindstrom J, Eriksson JG *et al.* Prevention of type 2 diabetes mellitus by changes in lifestyle among subjects with impaired glucose tolerance. *N Engl J Med* 2001;344:1343–50.

15 The Diabetes Prevention Program Research Group. The Diabetes Prevention Program: design and methods for a clinical trial in the prevention of type 2 diabetes. *Diabetes Care* 1999;22:623–31.

16 Ha TKK, Lean MEJ on behalf of the Diabetes and Nutrition Study Group (DNSG) of the European Association for the Study of Diabetes (EASD). Technical review: recommendations for the nutritional management of patients with diabetes mellitus. *Eur J Clin Nutr* 1998;52:467–81.

17 Jacobs DR, Meyer KA, Kushi LH, Folsom AR. Whole-grain intake may reduce the risk of ischemic heart disease death in postmenopausal women: the Iowa Women's Health Study. *Am J Clin Nutr* 1998;68:248–57.

18 Marshall JA, Hoag S, Shetterly S, Hamman RF. Dietary fat predicts conversion from impaired glucose tolerance to NIDDM. The San Luis Valley Diabetes Study. *Diabetes Care* 1994;17:50–6.

19 Colditz GA, Manson JE, Stampfer MJ *et al.* Diet and risk of clinical diabetes in women. *Am J Clin Nutr* 1992;55:1018–23.

20 Vessby B, Aro A, Skarfors E *et al.* The risk to develop NIDDM is related to the fatty acid composition of the serum cholesterol esters. *Diabetes* 1994;43:1353–7.

21 Feskens EJ, Bowles CH, Kromhout D. Inverse association between fish intake and risk of glucose tolerance in normoglycemic elderly men and women. *Diabetes Care* 1991;14:935–41.

22 Haffner SM. Management of dyslipidemia in adults with diabetes. Technical review. *Diabetes Care* 1998;21:160–78.

23 Svethey LP, Simons-Morton D, Vollmer WM *et al.* for the DASH Collaborative Research Group. Effects of dietary patterns of blood pressure: subgroup analysis of the Dietary Approaches to Stop Hypertension (DASH). Randomized clinical trial. *Arch Intern Med* 1999;159:285–93.

24 Adler A, Stevens RJ, Neil A *et al.* UKPDS 59: hyperglycaemia and other potentially modifiable risk factors for peripheral vascular disease in type 2 diabetes. *Diabetes Care* 2002;25:894–9.

25 Holbrook TL, Barrett-Connor E, Wingard DL. A prospective population-based study of alcohol use and non-insulin-dependent diabetes mellitus. *Am J Epidemiol* 1990;132:902–9.

26 Facchini F, Chen J, Reaven GM. Light to moderate alcohol intake is associated with enhanced insulin sensitivity. *Diabetes Care* 1994;17:115–19.

27 Riccardi G, Rivellese AA. Dietary treatment of the metabolic syndrome: the optimal diet. *Br J Nutr* 2000;83 (Suppl. 1):S143–S148.

28 Toeller M. Well-being in non-insulin-dependent diabetic patients – a long term follow-up. In: Lefèbvre PJ, Standl E, editors. *New aspects in diabetes.* Berlin, New York: Walter de Gruyter, 1992:127–43.

29 Coulston AM, Mandelbaum D, Reaven GM. Dietary management of nursing home residents with non-insulin-dependent diabetes mellitus. *Am J Clin Nutr* 1990;51:62–71.

30 European Diabetes Policy Group. A desktop guide to type 2 diabetes mellitus. *Diabetic Med* 1999;16:716–30.

31 Astrup A, Grunwald GK, Melanson EL *et al.* The role of low-fat diets in body weight control: a meta-analysis of ad libitum dietary intervention studies. *Int J Obes Relat Metab Disord* 2000; 24:1545–52.

32 UKPDS Group. UK Prospective Complications Study: response of fasting plasma glucose to diet therapy in newly presenting type 2 patients with diabetes. *Metabolism* 1990;39:905–12.

33 Frost G, Wilding J, Beecham J. Dietary advice based on the glycemic index improves dietary profile and metabolic control in type 2 diabetic patients. *Diabet Med* 1994;11:397–401.

34 Järvi AE, Karlström BK, Granfeldt YE *et al.* Improved glycemic control and lipid profile and normalized fibrinolytic activity on a low glycemic index diet in type 2 diabetes mellitus patients. *Diabetes Care* 1999;22:10–18.

35 Bouché C, Rizkalla SW, Luo J *et al.* Five-week, low-glycemic index diet decreases total fat mass and improves plasma lipid profile in moderately overweight nondiabetic men. *Diabetes Care* 2002;25:822–8.

36 Mann J, Hermansen K, Vessby B, Toeller M. Evidence-based nutritional recommendations for the treatment and prevention of diabetes and related complications. A European perspective [letter]. *Diabetes Care* 2002;25:1256–8.

37 Brown L, Rosner B, Willett WW, Sacks FM. Cholesterol lowering effects of dietary fiber: a meta-analysis. *Am J Clin Nutr* 1999;69:30–42.

38 Chandalia M, Garg A, Lutjohann D *et al.* Beneficial effects of high dietary fiber intake in patients with type 2 diabetes. *N Engl J Med* 2000;342:1392–8.

39 Jenkins DJA, Kendall CWC, Vuksan V *et al.* Soluble fiber intake at a dose approved by the US Food and Drug Administration for a claim of health benefits: serum lipid risk factors for cardiovascular disease assessed in a randomized controlled crossover trial. *Am J Clin Nutr* 2002;75:834–9.

40 Toeller M. Dietary programmes and the use of sweeteners in diabetes. In: Mogensen CE, Standl E, editors. *Concepts for the ideal diabetes clinic.* Berlin, New York: Walter de Gruyter, 1992:153–70

41 Nadeau J, Koski kg, Strychar I, Yale JF. Teaching subjects with type 2 diabetes how to incorporate sugar choices into their daily meal plan promotes dietary compliance and does not deteriorate metabolic profile. *Diabetes Care* 2001;24:222–7.

42 Toeller M. Diet and diabetes. *Diabetes Metab Rev* 1993;9:93–108.

43 Laitinen JH, Ahola IE, Sarkkinen ES *et al.* Impact of intensified dietary therapy on energy and nutrient intakes and fatty acid composition of serum lipids with recently diagnosed non-insulin dependent diabetes mellitus. *Am J Diet Assoc* 1993;93:276–83.

44 Garg A. High-monounsaturated fat diets for patients with diabetes mellitus: a meta-analysis. *Am J Clin Nutr* 1998;67:577S-582S.

45 Friedberg CE, Janssen MJEM, Heine RJ, Grobbee DE. Fish oil and glycemic control in diabetes: a meta-analysis. *Diabetes Care* 1999;21:494–500.

46 Toeller M, Buyken AE. Dietary modifications in patients with diabetic nephropathy. In: Hasslacher C, editor. *Diabetic nephropathy.* Chichester, New York: John Wiley & Sons, 2001:265–76.

47 Kasiske BL, Lakatua JDA, Ma JL, Louis TA. A metaanalysis of the effects of dietary protein restriction on the rate of decline in renal function. *Am J Kidney Dis* 1998;31:954–61.

48 Pijls LTJ, de Vries H, Donker AJM, van Eijk JTM. The effect of protein restriction on albuminuria in patients with type 2 diabetes mellitus: a randomized trial. *Nephrol Dialysis Transpl* 1999;14:1445–53.

49 Bell RA, Mayer-Davis EJ, Martin MA *et al.* Associations between alcohol consumption and insulin sensitivity and cardiovascular disease risk factors: the Insulin Resistance and Atherosclerosis Study. *Diabetes Care* 2000;53:1630–6.

6

Psychosocial issues and type 2 diabetes

Gary W Welch, Katie Weinger and Alan M Jacobson

INTRODUCTION

This chapter briefly discusses the social and cultural forces that are driving up both obesity and type 2 diabetes rates to epidemic levels in the USA. It also provides a review of the considerable psychological and social impacts on the individual living with type 2 diabetes and includes a discussion of current intervention approaches.

CULTURAL CHANGES AND THE RISE OF TYPE 2 DIABETES

Type 2 diabetes accounts for 90–95% of the 16 million diabetes cases in the USA[1]. The disease is nearing epidemic proportions due, in part, to our aging population, but mostly as a result of a sharp increase in the prevalence of obesity and its associated insulin resistance[2,3]. The Centers for Disease Control and Prevention reports that 56% of US adults are overweight or obese, up from 45% in 1991[3]. As many as 90% of those with type 2 diabetes are overweight or obese[4,5].

The three most important risk factors in the pathogenesis of this disease—sedentary lifestyle, poor dietary habits, and changes in body composition—are essentially modifiable risks, related to a set of profound social and cultural changes that have taken place recently in our society. Nestle and Jacobson[6] and others (e.g., Federation of American Societies for Experimental Biology, 1996[7]; Schumann, 2002[8]; Battle and Brownell[9]; Burros[10]; Bar-Or et al.[11]; US Department of Agriculture, 1997[12]; WHO, 2000[13]; *Tufts University Health & Nutrition Newsletter,*

2002[14]) have highlighted some of these social and cultural changes:

- The greater use of labor-saving devices and the automobile for transportation have reduced our habitual activity levels. More than 60% of American adults are not regularly physically active. In fact, 25% of all adults are not active at all.
- Greater access to mass-produced high-calorie foods that are relatively inexpensive and heavily advertised, with recent emphasis on larger portion sizes. There has been a rapid growth of the food industry and its use of sophisticated marketing and merchandising campaigns to stimulate food consumption, including fast foods, snacks, and drinks. For example, the McDonalds fast-food chain spends over a billion dollars a year on promotion of its products. The average US caloric intake is estimated to have risen from 1774 kcal day^{-1} in 1977–78 to 2002 kcal day^{-1} in 1994–96. Americans are eating more.
- The more hectic pace of modern life, longer working hours, and changes in family roles that reward convenience in terms of eating patterns, and limit time available for recreation and outside activities.

Reversing these recent cultural trends that impact eating and exercise habits will require a multifaceted public-health policy approach which should focus on the prevention of weight gain as early in life as possible as a key strategy[6,11]. Among adults, the Diabetes Prevention Program (DPP) study has shown that moderate exercise can help reduce the risk of developing type 2 diabetes in those who are most at risk[15]. By exercising moderately 30 min a day and losing 5–7% of body weight, high-risk study participants were able to reduce their odds of developing type 2 diabetes by 58%. Participants in the study had glucose intolerance at entry into the study and were at high risk for developing type 2 diabetes. The social and cultural causes of obesity and type 2 diabetes suggest that we need to make a dramatic shift from our current medical and behavioral models to a public health model involving prevention and public policy initiatives supported by medical and behavioral strategies. Indeed, current strivings for a medical cure of the multi-system defects inherent in type 2 diabetes involving the pancreas, liver, and peripheral tissues ignore the underlying social problems that are at the heart of the recent growth in obesity and type 2 diabetes rates.

THE PSYCHOLOGICAL AND SOCIAL IMPACT OF TYPE 2 DIABETES

The patient with type 2 diabetes must adjust to a demanding treatment regimen and the eventual onset of diabetes-related complications[16–20]. In this section we discuss some of these psychosocial issues and provide an update on treatment approaches in these areas. Most of the research on psychosocial issues in diabetes in the US has been carried out on Caucasians, principally in academic clinics and hospital diabetes centers, rather than in primary care settings, where most type 2 diabetes care is delivered. Despite these limitations, there is a sizeable body of research available that can help us understand the psychosocial impact of type 2 diabetes, and identify clinically useful interventions to manage patient problem-areas.

Type 2 diabetes is consistently described in clinical reports as demanding and complex from the patient's perspective[21–24]. Reflecting clinician time constraints, their training focus, institutional support, and reimbursement practices, most clinical interviews in diabetes practice focus largely on medical or educational aspects of type 2 diabetes, and concentrate little on psychosocial features that, for a subgroup of patients, should be at the forefront of priorities[25].

Psychosocial issues in type 2 diabetes have a significant influence on both patient outcomes and quality-of-life. High blood sugar levels, associated with poor blood sugar control, cause a range of medical complications (e.g., cardiovascular disease, retinopathy, neuropathy, nephropathy) that can impact many areas of the patients life, including ability to work, family functioning, quality-of-life, and sexual functioning[16,17,26]. As with other chronic medical conditions, the patient needs to carry out many daily treatment-related tasks if adequate blood glucose control is to be achieved. While a sound medical plan is important (e.g., a patient on oral agents who is under-medicated will find food and exercise regimens relatively ineffective), a good medical plan is a necessary but not sufficient condition to ensure good blood glucose control. Diet and exercise, blood glucose monitoring, timing and dosage of prescribed diabetes medications (insulin and/or oral agents), hypoglycemia management and prevention, foot care, sick day management, clinic visits, and various necessary medical screenings and education activities must all be successfully incorporated into life roles and any unexpected crises[25,27]. Changes to food habits can be particularly difficult to achieve and sustain. Also, diabetes regimen changes must be maintained by the individual patient within the context of helpful or unhelpful peer and social pressures, domestic and economic responsibilities, and distracting life events[28]. Self-care behavior change must be sustained over time to translate into improved blood glucose control and a reduction or slowing down of diabetes complications progression[29]. Type 2 diabetes typically emerges in middle adulthood, a period of life where lifestyle patterns and behaviors have become firmly established and may require greater effort to change. Also, during the pre-complications phase of type 2 diabetes, and even in the early phase of complications, the patient is often asymptomatic. Driving forces that might motivate a patient to seek medical care—unpleasant symptoms and awareness and fear of a serious illness—are therefore not present to provide a sufficient level of threat and motivation to make changes.

DIABETES-RELATED EMOTIONAL DISTRESS

It is common for patients to experience emotional distress from living with diabetes and the impact of its complications. The terms 'diabetes burnout'[24] and 'diabetes overwhelmus'[22] have been coined to capture this distress. The types of specific emotional problem faced by type 2 diabetes patients have been reported in several studies[30–32]. Approximately one-third reported "worry about the future and the possibility of diabetes complications" as a serious issue. Other areas endorsed as "serious" by approximately 15–20% of patients were:

- Guilt and anxiety at being off-track with treatment
- Scared about living with diabetes
- Not knowing if mood or feelings were related to diabetes
- Being constantly concerned about food and eating
- Feeling deprived around food
- Feeling depressed living with diabetes

The questionnaire used in these surveys is the Problem Areas In Diabetes (PAID) scale[30,33] (see Figure 6.1). This is a brief, one-page screening tool we recommend for busy diabetes clinicians. It can be given to patients routinely, to screen for overall high emotional distress related to living with type 1 or type 2 diabetes. A total score (overall emotional distress) is generated by simply adding the 0–4 values endorsed by the patient for each of the 20 questions in the PAID. This sum is then multiplied by 1.25 to provide a total score of 0–100. We recommend using a cut-off score of 50 to denote a high level emotional distress that warrants further professional attention. Individual questions scored as 'serious' (i.e., scored 4 on a scale of 0–4) identify individual areas a patient is finding difficult. These are specific 'hot spots' with which the patient is currently struggling emotionally. For patients scoring high on the total score or individual questions, the clinician might consider investing additional time exploring feelings and practical barriers to good diabetes self-care. It is rare in medical settings for patients to be asked even briefly about their illness-related feelings—despite the great value of this exercise to clinician for patients troubled with the emotional burden of diabetes[22,23].

A key task for the clinician is to give the patient a brief opportunity (i.e., a few minutes) to talk about how he or she feels about living with diabetes. The aim is to talk with the patient about feelings openly and in a safe way (supportive, non-judgmental). Good listening skills start with open questions, to stimulate the patient to talk about his or her feelings. For example, if a patient scores high on the PAID (above 50), the clinician may say:

> "It sounds as if you have been feeling overwhelmed with your diabetes care. Could you tell me a little more about how you have felt lately?"

Avoid closed questions at this point that simply require a 'yes' or 'no' response as these will close down conversation rather than opening it up, which is the goal. Avoid interrupting at this point, providing information, or showing personal reactions to what the patient has said. Some other suggestions: be aware of your own 'mental chatter' and try to simply listen to what the patient is saying when he or she talks. Be aware also of the patient's body language (tone of voice, facial expressions, use of hands and body posture, pauses and hesitations during difficult moments, etc). Maintain good eye contact and use small encouraging body signals (nod your head, say 'yes, go on', or 'hmm' to show you are staying with the patient's story). Then briefly summarize what you have heard from the patient both in terms of the specific emotions (e.g., guilt, anxiety, feeling alone, etc) and the reasons the patient gives for feeling that way. Check with the patient that what you have said is accurate:

> "If I've heard you correctly, you've felt ... because ... Does that sound accurate?"

Look for a response from the patient that might 'fine tune' your summary if needed. A patient who feels he or she has been heard by an empathic healthcare professional about the emotional distress of living with diabetes, even for a brief period, will feel less distressed and be

Instructions: *Which of the following diabetes issues are currently a problem for you?*
Circle the number that gives the best answer for you. Please provide an answer for each question.

	Not a problem ▼	Minor problem ▼	Moderate problem ▼	Somewhat serious problem ▼	Serious problem ▼
1 Not having clear and concrete goals for your diabetes care?	0	1	2	3	4
2 Feeling discouraged with your diabetes treatment plan?	0	1	2	3	4
3 Feeling scared when you think about living with diabetes?	0	1	2	3	4
4 Uncomfortable social situations related to your diabetes care (e.g. people telling you what to eat)?	0	1	2	3	4
5 Feelings of deprivation regarding food and meals?	0	1	2	3	4
6 Feeling depressed when you think about living with diabetes?	0	1	2	3	4
7 Not knowing if your mood or feelings are related to your diabetes?	0	1	2	3	4
8 Feeling overwhelmed by your diabetes?	0	1	2	3	4
9 Worrying about low blood sugar reactions?	0	1	2	3	4
10 Feeling angry when you think about living with diabetes?	0	1	2	3	4
11 Feeling constantly concerned about food and eating?	0	1	2	3	4
12 Worrying about the future and the possibility of serious complications?	0	1	2	3	4
13 Feelings of guilt or anxiety when you get off track with your diabetes management?	0	1	2	3	4
14 Not 'accepting' your diabetes?	0	1	2	3	4
15 Feeling unsatisfied with your diabetes physician?	0	1	2	3	4
16 Feeling that diabetes is taking up too much of your mental and physical energy every day?	0	1	2	3	4
17 Feeling alone with your diabetes?	0	1	2	3	4
18 Feeling that your friends and family are not supportive of your diabetes management efforts?	0	1	2	3	4
19 Coping with complications of diabetes?	0	1	2	3	4
20 Feeling 'burned out' by the constant effort needed to manage diabetes?	0	1	2	3	4

Figure 6.1 Problem areas in diabetes (PAID) questionnaire

more motivated to make any behavior changes that may be needed. Good listening enhances the therapeutic bond between patient and healthcare team member and can be used regularly to good effect in all areas of diabetes management. Referral can be made if appropriate to a diabetes nurse educator or other available member of the diabetes clinical team to tackle specific practical

issues arising from the emotional concerns identified by the patient (e.g., fear of complications, difficulties with the diet plan). The UK Prospective Diabetes Study (UKPDS)[29] has demonstrated the benefit of improved blood glucose control on progression of complications in type 2 diabetes. Screening for diabetes emotional distress and intervening where a high level of distress is present will support patient self-care efforts that, in turn, will contribute to improved blood glucose control[22].

STRESS AND BLOOD GLUCOSE CONTROL

Psychological stress has significant effects on the metabolism on individuals without diabetes by increasing counter-regulatory hormones, which could result in elevated blood sugars, among other impacts. In type 2 it is thought that stress can exert an effect on blood glucose control, either directly through these hormones or indirectly by disruption of the diabetes self-care regimen. Although the laboratory and clinical research to date does not appear to support a consistent stress–blood glucose response across all patients, there is evidence that a subgroup of individuals with diabetes are 'stress responders' but others are not[34]. Individuals with type 1 diabetes may have idiosyncratic responses to stress, with some showing increases in blood glucose levels and others decreases. However, for type 2 diabetes the effects of stress are more likely to result in increases in blood glucose, secondary to sympathetic activity[34,35].

Evidence from animal models also suggests a role for stress in the onset of type 2 diabetes[36]. Ineffective coping (e.g., avoidance, denial, detachment, anger) has been shown to be associated with poorer metabolic control in diabetes and adaptive coping (e.g., active problem solving and ability to obtain social support) with a stress-buffering role[37], highlighting the role of patient perceptions of stressful events. It is unclear whether relaxation training (e.g. biofeedback) produces glycemic benefits in type 2 diabetes[38]. Generally, there is a paucity of studies on stress in type 2 diabetes.

PSYCHIATRIC ILLNESSES

Patients with diabetes have elevated levels of psychiatric illnesses compared with the general population and similar to those found in other chronic illnesses. The most common psychiatric disorder in type 2 diabetes is major depression, while other significant disorders include anxiety disorders, alcohol and substance use disorders,

and eating disorders, principally binge-eating syndrome[20,39,40]. Lifetime prevalence of recent (i.e., within 6 months) psychiatric disorders among individuals with chronic illnesses, such as cancer, arthritis, and heart disease, has been found to be 40%, which is higher than for those without such illnesses[41]. A number of studies have been conducted recently to estimate psychiatric illnesses in type 2 diabetes. This chapter concentrates mostly on major depression as it is the most significant clinical problem seen in diabetes, but also discusses briefly anxiety disorders, alcohol abuse and dependence, and binge-eating disorder, which are commonly associated with obesity.

MAJOR DEPRESSION

The essential feature of major depression is depressed mood, or loss of interest in usual activities, which is experienced most of the day and nearly every day, for a period of at least 2 weeks. Accompanying these symptoms are appetite disturbance and weight change, sleep problems, either physical agitation or slowing down, decreased energy, feelings of worthlessness or excessive guilt, difficulty concentrating or thinking, and recurrent suicidal thoughts. Depression is present in 15–20% of patients with diabetes, regardless of diabetes type[42]. Several studies have found glycemic control significantly worse among depressed versus nondepressed diabetes patients[43–45]. The course of the illness is generally chronic; even after successful treatment it will reoccur in as many as 80% of diabetic patients and reoccur on an average of four episodes during a subsequent 5-year period[46]. Depression is recognized and treated in only one-third of cases. Depression also doubles the risk of type 2 diabetes onset, independent of its association with other risk factors[47,48]. Randomized controlled trials have shown both psychotherapy (i.e., cognitive behavioral therapy that targets negative thought patterns) and psychopharmacy [i.e., tricyclics and selective serotonin-reuptake inhibitors (SSRIs)] to have significant beneficial effects on both mood and glycemic control[49,50]. A recent meta-analysis of relevant studies demonstrated a significant and consistent association of diabetes complications and depressive symptoms[51]. Both diabetes complications and hyperglycemia are associated with diminished response to depression treatment and with an increased risk of recurrence. These findings suggest that optimal relief of depression in diabetes may require vigorous, simultaneous treatment of both the blood sugar control and psychiatric conditions.

There are a number of barriers that make detection of depression particularly challenging for the physician in the medical setting[52]. These include:

- Lack of time (most medical visits last 15 min or less)
- Somatization (patient presents the physical symptoms of depression such as fatigue, appetite change, or sleep disruption, but not the affective or cognitive symptoms)
- Stigmatization (which inhibits explicit questioning)
- Reimbursement problems (insurers may not allow physician billing for the management of psychiatric problems)
- Co-morbid medical conditions (camouflage depression by sharing somatic symptoms).

In the latter case, special attention should be paid to depressed mood, loss of interest in usual activities, guilt, difficulty concentrating, or suicidal thoughts the patient may also be experiencing, which suggest depression. If time constraints are a particular problem, a single question "Have you felt depressed or sad much of the time in the past year?" has been found to have a sensitivity of 85% and specificity of 66%[53].

ANXIETY

Although not well studied in diabetes, some research suggests anxiety disorders are more common in adults with type 2 diabetes than the general population[54–56] and anxiety symptoms are linked with poorer glycemic control[55]. Results parallel depression, in that women, African–Americans, and those with less education are more likely to report anxiety symptoms[20].

Formal anxiety disorders include panic disorder, which involves repeated episodes of intense fear that strikes often and without warning. Physical symptoms include chest pain, heart palpitations, shortness of breath, dizziness, abdominal distress, feelings of unreality, and fear of dying. Obsessive–compulsive disorder is characterized by repeated, unwanted thoughts or compulsive behaviors that seem impossible to stop or control. Phobias include two major types of phobias: social phobia and specific phobia. Social phobia involves the experience of an overwhelming and disabling fear of scrutiny, embarrassment, or humiliation in social situations, which leads to avoidance of many potentially pleasurable and meaningful activities. Specific phobias can produce extreme, disabling and irrational fear of something that poses little or no actual danger, the fear effectively leads to avoidance of these objects or situations and can cause people to limit their lives unnecessarily. Finally, generalized anxiety disorder (GAD) involves exaggerated, worrisome thoughts and tension about everyday routine life events and activities, lasting at least 6 months. Individuals with GAD always anticipate the worst, even though there is little reason to expect it and the fear is accompanied by physical symptoms, such as fatigue, trembling, muscle tension, headache or nausea.

Two clinically proven forms of psychotherapy used to treat anxiety disorders are behavioral therapy, including biofeedback, and cognitive-behavioral therapy. Cognitive-behavioral therapy teaches patients to understand and change negative thinking patterns, so the individual can react differently to the situations that cause them anxiety. In diabetes, behavioral interventions have reduced anxiety and improved glycemic control[57]. Psycopharmacological agents can be effective in the treatment of anxiety disorders and treatment with SSRIs is increasingly popular. Okada et al.[58] found reduced anxiety levels with fludiazepam, a benzodiazepine, in a study involving a small patient group, and glycemic control was improved in another study that focused on anxiety symptoms[59]. However, there is relatively little information on their use in type 2 diabetes[20]. Anxiety symptoms may be confused with the symptoms of low blood sugars among patients treated with sulfonylureas and insulin. Self-monitoring of blood glucose concentrations can help the anxious patient discriminate between hypoglycemia and anxiety[60]. When emotional and behavioral symptoms (e.g., persistent fears, worries, obsessions, compulsions) are predominant, as opposed to physical symptoms (e.g., palpitations and sweating), the diagnosis of anxiety disorder is more readily made[21].

ALCOHOL DEPENDENCY AND ABUSE

Alcohol-use disorders involve four problem areas:

- A strong need, or urge, to drink (craving)
- Not being able to stop drinking once drinking has begun (loss of control)
- Withdrawal symptoms, such as nausea, sweating, shakiness, and anxiety after stopping drinking (physical dependence)
- The need to drink greater amounts of alcohol to get 'high' (tolerance).

Alcohol dependence (alcoholism) refers to a repetitive pattern of excessive alcohol use with serious adverse consequences, often including lack of control, tolerance, and withdrawal. Alcohol abuse is a milder category that refers to continued drinking despite adverse consequences, in the absence of dependence[61]. Alcohol abuse and dependence disorders in the USA together have a lifetime prevalence of 18.2%[62]. As many as five out of six patients who meet diagnostic criteria for abuse or dependence go unrecognized in primary-care settings[63]. Although alcohol-use disorder rates in diabetes appear lower, when diabetes and alcohol-use disorders co-exist, they represent a considerable clinical challenge. Alcohol-induced fasting hypoglycemia can occur 6–36 h after alcohol intake in the context of low food-intake. Fasting depletes liver glycogen stores and alcohol impairs gluconeogenesis. Symptoms are neuroglycopenic and can include stupor and coma[64].

Chronic alcohol use can create medical and behavioral problems, including: blackouts, chronic abdominal pain, depression, liver dysfunction, hypertension, sexual dysfunction, sleep disorders, and work or interpersonal problems[65]. It can also affect nutritional status in type 2 diabetes, through direct changes to carbohydrate, lipid, and protein metabolism, but also indirectly by changing eating habits (e.g., meals become irregular or skipped). Chronic use can also promote hyperglycemia by the extra calories consumed and by enhancing insulin resistance and glucose intolerance[66]. Early detection is important and can be supported by use of the widely-used CAGE assessment[67]. After asking the patient whether or not they drink alcohol and if the answer is 'yes', then establishing the types, amounts, and frequency of drinking, the following four questions are presented to the patient:

- **C**: Have you ever felt you should CUT down on your drinking?
- **A**: Have people ANNOYED you by criticizing your drinking?
- **G**: Have you ever felt bad or GUILTY about your drinking?
- **E**: Have you ever had a drink first thing in the morning as an EYE OPENER?

CAGE can reveal problem areas that should be further explored. Individuals at risk include those with one or more positive CAGE responses. Alcohol dependence requiring referral is likely if the patient gives 3–4 positive responses for the past year[65]:

EATING DISORDERS

Although community prevalence rates of 1% for anorexia nervosa and 3% for bulimia nervosa can occur among young women, these disorders are not common in the older age group (over 40 years) where type 2 diabetes typically emerges. However, binge eating disorder (BED) is an eating disorder found among 70% of obese individuals, and 80% of type 2 diabetes patients are obese. The diabetes clinician will likely uncover BED if he or she is actively looking for it and asks questions about uncontrolled eating binges. BED is different from binge–purge syndrome (bulimia nervosa) as individuals with BED usually do not purge afterward by use of vomiting, laxative abuse, diuretic abuse, or insulin omission. In contrast to other eating disorders, where 90% or more of cases are female, one-third to one-fourth of all patients with BED are men. In the general population the prevalence of

BED is around 1–2%. Among mildly obese people in self-help or commercial weight-loss programs, 10–15% have BED. A recent survey found a BED prevalence of 25% in a consecutive series of type 2 diabetes patients attending a diabetes clinic at an academic medical center, but BED remains a neglected area of clinical research in type 2 diabetes. BED does not appear to be associated with poorer blood glucose control[40,68]. However, people with BED are typically extremely distressed by their binge eating. Most feel ashamed and try to hide their problem. Often they are so successful at this that close family members and friends don't know they binge eat. Several methods are being used to treat BED[69]. At this early stage of research we do not know which method or combination of methods is the most effective in controlling BED:

- Cognitive-behavioral therapy teaches patients techniques to monitor and change their eating habits, as well as to change the way they respond to difficult situations
- Interpersonal psychotherapy helps people examine their relationships with friends and family and to make changes in problem areas
- Treatment with antidepressants may be helpful for some individuals
- Self-help groups also may be a source of support.

SOCIAL SUPPORT

Social support can be defined as the availability of close family, friends, and other significant people in the individual's life that is provided through the individual's social network[70]. There is general agreement that there are several distinct types of social support[71,72]:

- Instrumental support (practical help)
- Informational (provision of information)
- Emotional (lending a good listening ear, showing understanding, helping talk over problems or make difficult decisions)
- Approval (giving verbal support).

Low perceived level of diabetes-related support has been related to a number of factors, including: lack of diabetes knowledge among individuals in the support network, resistance to making changes that would support improved patient self-care, the presence of serious interpersonal conflicts, and lack of specific requests for help from the individual with diabetes[24]. There is strong empirical support for the value of good social support to health and longevity. For example, a large study of men tracked for 4 years[73] showed higher cardiovascular disease, accident, and suicide-related deaths among those classified as socially isolated (i.e., not married, fewer than six friends or relatives, no membership in community groups). In diabetes, reviews have shown moderate positive correlations between social support and markers of self-care such as glycosylated hemoglobin (HbA1c)[27]. One study showed health-related quality-of-life is affected by the marital status of both type I and type 2 diabetic patients, with separated and divorced individuals generally experiencing lower levels of quality-of-life[26]. Weissberg-Benchell and Pichert[74] have provided some simple questions for the diabetes clinician interested in exploring social support:

- Who helps you care for your diabetes and how do they help?
- Are there things they do or say that make it harder for you to care for your diabetes?
- Who do you talk to for emotional support for having diabetes? Are they good listeners?

Social support is generally conceived of as a positive influence on health, although some support can be negative in type 2 diabetes if the patient fears being nagged or harassed about their self-care behaviors[75]. The 'diabetes police' is a term that has been coined to describe a pattern of behavior by family, friends, and others in the diabetes patient's social network where they monitor the patient's self-care behavior intrusively, and try to pressure the patient to improve self-care through persuasion, advice, criticism, and threats[24].

SEXUAL FUNCTIONING

Impaired sexual functioning is a well-recognized complication of type 2 diabetes in men and women. Men can develop erectile dysfunction (ED) 15 years earlier than men without diabetes[1], and 50–60% of men over 50 years have some type of problem with ED[1]. In women, type 2 diabetes has been shown to impact sexual desire, orgasmic capacity, lubrication, sexual satisfaction, sexual activity, and relationship with sexual partner[76]. More than 70% of male patients are thought to have organically based disease[77]. Interviews with patients should be undertaken with the sexual partner present, as relationship problems may be a primary or aggravating factor[78]. Performance anxieties and relationship problems have been identified as potential problem areas that may need sensitive investigation[77]. Sildenafil citrate (Viagra) has been reported to be well-tolerated and effective in improving erectile dysfunction in men with type 2 diabetes, even in patients with poor glycemic control and chronic complications[79]. The rate of adverse events, such as headache, flushing, dyspepsia, and dizziness, is similar to that for non-diabetic individuals[77].

COGNITIVE FUNCTIONING

Early research in cognitive functioning focused on type 2 diabetes as a theoretical model of accelerated aging (e.g., Kent[80]) but, more recently, there has been interest in potential changes in cognition that might make patient adherence to treatment more difficult[81]. Both chronically elevated high blood sugars and recurrent low blood sugar levels have the potential to independently contribute to cognitive dysfunction, for example through changes to the blood–brain barrier transport of glucose. A recent review on the cognitive impact of type 2 diabetes showed that verbal learning and memory skills are disrupted, but mainly for patients older than 60 years of age[82,83]. Other cognitive skills, such as attention, executive function, and psychomotor efficiency, were less affected. Although most research on cognition in diabetes has been conducted with type 1 patients, studies show that middle-aged type 2 individuals are apparently protected, insofar as researchers have only infrequently reported learning and memory impairments in that age group. It is likely that older adults have an increased risk of diabetes-associated memory dysfunction as a

consequence of a synergistic interaction between diabetes-related blood glucose changes and the structural and functional changes occurring in the central nervous system that are part of the normal aging process.

Multiple diabetes-related co-morbid conditions (i.e., hyperinsulinaemia, hypertension, hypercholesterolaemia) may individually and synergistically impact learning and memory skills (see review by Ryan and Geckle[83]). For example, hyperinsulinaemia may independently affect the central nervous system. Insulin levels usually rise with age, and are strong predictors of cognitive impairment in adults without diabetes. Data from the Framingham study showed that both hypertension and diabetes independently affect cognition generally, and memory skills in particular. Given their high rates in type 2 diabetes, it is notable that hypertension and hypercholesterolaemia interacts with hyperinsulinaemia to disrupt memory. Generally, there is evidence to support the view that verbal learning and memory skills are particularly vulnerable to disruption in type 2 diabetes compared with other cognitive skills as a result of diabetes and its co-morbidities.

While mild and severe hypoglycemia rates are lower in type 2 diabetes compared with type 1, due to residual insulin production in type 2, patients who use sulfonylureas or progress to insulin therapy can experience acute low blood sugars[84]. Such episodes cause both autonomic and neuroglycopenic changes. Neuroglycopenia appears to impact the cerebral cortex more than the deeper brain structures, in terms of cognitive functioning. Complex, attention-demanding and speed-dependent responses are most impaired, with accuracy often preserved at the expense of speed. Cognitive function does not recover fully until 40–90 min after blood glucose is returned to normal. Hypoglycemia also provokes changes in mood, including anxiety and depression, and increases fear of further hypoglycemia, which in turn can modify self-care behavior (e.g., over-treating with food) and thus blood sugar control[85].

In summary, there are a wide range of psychosocial issues that it is important to address in the clinical management of type 2 diabetes. For some patients, these issues are serious enough to warrant active treatment by the clinician, or referral to other healthcare professionals. This chapter briefly discussed some of these psychosocial issues and suggested practical, patient-centered strategies to aid the busy clinician. We should not lose sight of the fact that both obesity and type 2 diabetes are largely preventable diseases. As a society, we need to focus on the profound social and cultural changes that have recently occurred in our daily lifestyles which have reduced habitual activity and increased food intake. Practical preventive strategies at the societal and cultural level must be generated to reverse these trends. This may be the greatest challenge we face in tackling the current epidemic of type 2 diabetes.

REFERENCES

1 American Diabetes Association. *Medical management of Type 2 diabetes*. 4th edn. Alexandria, Va: American Diabetes Association, 1998.

2 Diabetes Research Working Group. *Congressional report on National Institutes of Health implementation of the recommendations of the Congressionally-directed Diabetes Research Working Group*. 1998.

3 Mokdad AH, Ford ES, Bowman BA *et al*. Diabetes trends in the U.S.: 1990–1998. *Diabetes Care* 2000;23:1278–83.

4 Cefalu W. *Practical guide to diabetes management*. New York: Medical Information Press, 1998.

5 Maggio C. The prevention and treatment of obesity: applications to Type 2 diabetes. *Diabetes Care* 1997;20:1162–744.

6 Nestle M, Jacobson MF. Halting the obesity epidemic: a public health policy approach. *Public Health Rep* 2000;115:12–24.

7 Federation of American Societies for Experimental Biology, Life Sciences Research Office. Executive Summary from the Third Report on Nutrition Monitoring in the United States. *J Nutr* 1996;126(7S):1907S–36S.

8 Schumann M. Megabrands: top brands hold the line in 2001. *Advertising Age* 2002; July 22:S1–S9. 200212. USDA. 1994–96 Continuing Survey of Food Intakes by Individuals [online article]. Available from: http://www.barc.usda.gov/bhnrc/foodsurvey/home.htm. Accessed 17 Oct 2002.

9 Battle EK, Brownell KD. Confronting a rising tide of eating disorders and obesity: treatment vs. prevention and policy. *Addict Behav* 1996;21:755–65.

10 Burros M. Losing count of calories as plates fill up. *New York Times*. April 2nd, 1997.

11 Bar-Or O, Foreyt J, Bouchard C *et al*. Physical activity, genetic, and nutritional considerations in childhood weight management. *Med Sch Sports Exerc* 1998;30:2–10.

12 Data tables: results from USDA's 1994–96 Continuing Survey of Food Intakes by Individuals and 1994–96 Diet and Health Knowledge Survey [online article], 1997. Available from: http:/:www.barc.usda.gov/bhnrc/foodsurvey/home.htm. Accessed 27 Oct 2002.

13 World Health Organization. *Obesity: preventing and managing a global epidemic. Report of a WHO Consultation* Geneva, 1999. WHO Technical Report Series 894. Geneva: WHO, 2000.

14 Special Report: Portion Distortion. *Tufts University Health & Nutrition Newsletter* 2002;18:4–5.

15 US Department of Health and Health Services. Diet and exercise dramatically delay type 2 diabetes. *Health Health Serv News* 2001: August 8th.

16 Bradley C (ed). *Handbook of psychology and diabetes: a guide to psychological measurement in diabetes research and practice*. London: Harwood Academic Publishers, 1994.

17 Rubin RR, Peyrot M. Quality of life and diabetes. *Diabetes Metab Res Rev* 1999;15:205–18.

18 Snoek FJ, Skinner CT. *Psychology in diabetes care*. New York: John Wiley & Sons, 2000.

19 Glasgow RE, Hiss RG, Anderson RM *et al*. Report of the health care delivery work group: behavioral research related to the establishment of a chronic disease model for diabetes care. *Diabetes Care* 2001;24:124–30.

20 Rubin RR, Peyrot M. Psychological issues and treatments for people with diabetes. *J Clin Psychol* 2001;57:457–78.

21 Jacobson AM. The psychological care of patients with insulin-dependent diabetes mellitus. *N Engl J Med* 1996;334:1249.

22 Rubin RR. Psychotherapy and counseling in diabetes mellitus. In: Snoek FJ, Skinner TC, editors. *Psychology in diabetes care*. New York: Wiley, 2000.

23 Anderson RM, Funnell M. The art of empowerment. In: Snoek FJ, Skinner TC, editors. *Psychology in diabetes care*. New York: Wiley, 2000.

24 Polonsky WH. *Diabetes burnout. What to do when*

you can't take it any more. Alexandria VA: American Diabetes Association, 2000.

25 Day JL. Diabetic patient education: determinants of success. *Diabetes Metab Res Rev* 2000;16:S70–S74.

26 Jacobson AM, deGroot M, Samson JA. The evaluation of two measures of quality of life in patients with type 1 and type 2 diabetes. *Diabetes Care* 1994;17:267–74.

27 Glasgow RE, Eakin EG. Medical office-based interterventions. In: Snoek FJ, Skinner TC, editors. *Psychology in diabetes care.* New York: Wiley, 2000.

28 Doherty Y, James PT, Roberts SH. Stage of change counselling. In: Snoek FJ, Skinner TC, editors. *Psychology in diabetes care.* New York: Wiley, 2000.

29 UK Prospective Diabetes Study Group. Intensive blood glucose control with sulfonylureas or insulin compared with conventional treatment and risk of complications with Type 2 diabetes (UKPDS). *Lancet* 1998;352:837–53.

30 Welch GW, Jacobson A, Polonsky W. The Problem Areas in Diabetes (PAID) scale. An examination of its clinical utility. *Diabetes Care* 1997;20:760–6.

31 Snoek FJ, Pouwer F, Welch GW, Polonsky WH. Diabetes-related emotional distress in Dutch and US diabetic patients. *Diabetes Care* 2000;23:1305–9.

32 Welch GW, de Groot M, Buckland GT, Chipkin S. Risk stratification of diabetes patients using diet barriers and self care motivation in an inner city hospital setting [Abstract]. *Diabetes* 1999;48(Suppl.1):1395.

33 Polonsky WH, Anderson BA, Lohrer PA *et al.* Assessment of diabetes-related emotional distress. *Diabetes Care* 1995;18:754–60.

34 Delamater AM, Cox DJ. Psychological stress, coping, and diabetes. *Diabetes Spectrum* 1994;7:46–49.

35 Surwit RS, Schneider MS. Role of stress in the etiology and treatment of diabetes mellitus. *Psychosom Med* 1993;55:380–93.

36 Surwit RS, Schneider MS, Feinglos MN. Stress and diabetes mellitus. *Diabetes Care* 1992;15:1413–22.

37 Peyrot MF, McMurry JF Jr. Stress buffering and glycemic control. The role of coping styles. *Diabetes Care* 1992;15:842–6.

38 Aikins JE, Kiolbasa TA, Sobel R. Psychological predictors of glycemic control with relaxation training in non-insulin dependent diabetes mellitus. *Psychother Psychosom* 1997;66:302–6.

39 Cohen, ST, Welch G, Jacobson AM *et al.* The association of lifetime psychiatric illness and increased retinopathy in patients with Type I diabetes mellitus. *Psychosomatics* 1997;38:98–108.

40 Crow K, Kendall D, Praus B, Thuras P. Binge eating and other psychopathology in patients with Type 2 diabetes mellitus. *Int J Eat Dis* 2001;30:22–226.

41 Wells KB, Golding JM, Burnam MA. Psychiatric disorder in a sample of the general population with and without chronic medical conditions. *Am J Psychiat* 1988;145:976–81.

42 Lustman PJ, Griffith LS, Clouse RE *et al.* Effects of nortriptyline on depression and glucose regulation in diabetes: results of a double-blind, placebo controlled trial. *Psychosom Med* 1997;59:241–50.

43 Mazze RS, Lucido D, Shamoon J. Psychological and social correlates of glycemic control. *Diabetes Care* 1984;7:360–6.

44 DeGroot M, Jacobson AM, Samson JA. Glycemic control and major depression in patients with type 1 and type 2 diabetes mellitus. *J Psychosom Res* 1999;46:425–35.

45 Lustman PJ, Griffith LS, Freedland KE, Clouse RE. The course of major depression in diabetes. *General Hospital Psychiatry* 1997;19:138–43.

46 Lustman PJ, Griffith LS, Freedland KE *et al.* Cognitive behavior therapy for depression in type 2 diabetes: a randomized controlled trial. *Ann Int Med* 1998;129:613–21.

47 Lustman PJ, Griffith LS, Clouse RE. Effects of nortriptyline on depression and glycemic control in diabetes: results of a double-blind, placebo-controlled trial. *Ann Intern Med* 1998;129:613–21.

48 Kawakami N, Takatsuka N, Shimizu H, Ishibashi H. Depressive symptoms and occurrence of type 2 diabetes among Japanese men. *Diabetes Care* 1999;22:1071–6.

49 Lustman PJ, Griffith LS, Clouse RE et al. Effects of nortriptyline on depression and glycemic control in diabetes: results of a double-blind, placebo-controlled trial. *Psychosom Med* 1997;59:241–50.

50 Lustman PJ, Griffith LS, Freedland KE, Clouse RE. Fluoxetine for depression in diabetes. *Diabetes Care* 2000;23:618–23.

51 De Groot M, Anderson R, Freedland KE *et al.* Association of depression and diabetes complications: a meta-analysis. *Psychosom Med* 2001;63:619–30.

52 Kroenke K. Discovering depression in medical patients: reasonable expectations. *Ann Intern Med* 1997;126:463–5.

53 Williams JW, Mulrow CD, Kroenke K *et al.* Case-finding for depression in primary care: a randomized trial. *Am J Med* 1999;106:36–43.

54 DeGroot M, Jacobson AM, Samson JA. Psychiatric illness in patients with type 1 and type 2 diabetes mellitus. *Psychosom Med* 1994;56:176A.

55 Peyrot M, Rubin RR. Levels and risks of depression and anxiety symptomatology among diabetic adults. *Diabetes Care* 1997;20:585–90.

56 Green L, Feher M, Catalan J. Fears and phobias in people with diabetes. *Diabetes Metab Res Rev* 2000;16:287–93.

57 Surwit RS, van Tilburg MA, Zucker N et al. Stress management improves long-term glycemic control in type 2 diabetes. *Diabetes Care* 2002;25:30–4.

58 Okada S, Ichiki K, Tanokuchi S et al. Effect of an anxiolytic on lipid profile in non-insulin-dependent diabetes mellitus. *J Int Med Res* 1994;22:338–42.

59 Lustman PJ, Griffith LS, Clouse RE et al. Effects of alprazolam on glucose regulation in diabetes. Results of double-blind, placebo-controlled trial. *Diabetes Care* 1995;18:1133–9.

60 Cox D, Gonder-Frederick L, Polonsky W et al. A multi-center evaluation of blood glucose awareness training-II. *Diabetes Care* 1995;18:523–8.

61 American Psychiatric Association. *Diagnostic and Statistical Manual of Mental Disorders*. 4th ed. Washington, DC: American Psychiatric Association, 1994.

62 Grant B, Harford TC, Dawson DA et al. Prevalence of DSM-IV alcohol abuse and dependence, United States 1992. *Alcohol Health Res World* 1994;18:18–27.

63 McQuade WH, Sheldon ML, Yanek LR et al. Detecting symptoms of alcohol abuse in primary care settings. *Arch Fam Med* 2000;9:814–21.

64 Avogaro A. Alcohol, glucose metabolism and diabetes. *Diabetes Metab Rev* 1993;9:129–46.

65 National Institute on Alcohol Abuse and Alcoholism. Eighth Special Report to the U.S. Congress on Alcohol and Health. Washington, DC: Secretary of Health and Human Services, 1993.

66 Emanuele NV, Swade TF, Emanuele MA. Consequences of alcohol use in diabetics. *Alcohol Health Research World* 1998;22:211–19.

67 Ewing JA. Detecting alcoholism. The CAGE questionnaire. *JAMA* 1984;252:1905–7.

68 Wing RR, Nowalk MP, Marcus MD et al. Subclinical eating disorders and glycemic control in adolescents with type I diabetes. *Diabetes Care* 1986;9:162–7.

69 Wolff GE, Clark MM. Changes in eating self-efficacy and body image following cognitive-behavioral group therapy for binge eating disorder. *Eat Behav* 2001;2:97–104.

70 Kaplan RM, Sallis JF, Patterson TC. *Health and human behaviour*. McGraw-Hill, 1993.

71 House JS. The nature of social support. In: House JS, ed. *Work stress and social support*. Reading, MA: Addison-Wesley, 1981: 13–40.

72 Lazarus RS, Fokman S. *Stress, appraisal, and coping*. New York: Springer Publishing Company, 1984.

73 Kawachi I, Colditz GA, Ascherio A et al. A prospective study of social networks in relation to total mortality and cardiovascular disease in men in the USA. *J Epidemiol Community Health* 1996;50:245–51.

74 Weissberg-Benchell J, Pichert G. Social support in diabetes. In: Anderson BJ, Rubin RR, eds. *Practical Psychology for Diabetes Clinicians*. 2nd ed. Alpharetta, GA: American Diabetes Association, 2002.

75 Boehm S, Schlenk EA, Funnell MM et al. Predictors of adherence to nutrition recommendations in people with non-insulin-dependent diabetes mellitus. *Diabetes Ed* 1997; 23:157–65.

76 Schreiner-Engel P, Vietorisz DA, Smith H. The differential impact of diabetes type on female sexuality. *J Psychosom Res* 1987;31:23–33.

77 Guay AT, Blonde L, Siegel RL, Orazem J. Safety and tolerability of sildenafil citrate for the treatment of erectile function in men with type 1 and type 2 diabetes. *Diabetes* 2000;49(Suppl 1):Abstract no. 363–P.

78 Veves A, Webster L, Chen TF, Payne S, Boulton AJ. Aetiopathogenesis and management of impotence in diabetic males: four years experience from a combined clinic. *Diabet Med* 1995;12:77–82.

79 Boulton AJ, Selam JL, Sweeney M, Ziegler D. Sildenafil citrate for the treatment of erectile dysfunction in men with type II diabetes. *Diabetologia* 2001;44:1296–1301.

80 Kent S. Is diabetes a form of accelerated aging? *Geriatrics* 1976;31:140–51.

81 Perlmuter LC, Hakami MK, Hodgson-Harrington C et al. Decreased cognitive function in aging non-insulin dependent diabetic patients. *Am J Med* 1984;77:1043–8.

82 Strachan M, Ewing F, Deary I, Frier B. Is Type II diabetes associated with an increased risk of cognitive dysfunction? *Diabetes Care* 1997;20:438–46.

83 Ryan CM, Geckle M. Why is learning and memory dysfunction in type 2 diabetes limited to older adults? *Diabetes Metab Res Rev* 2000;16:308–15.

84 Marcus AO. Safety of drugs commonly used to treat hypertension, dyslipidemia, and type 2 diabetes (the metabolic syndrome): part 1. *Diabetes Technol Ther* 2000;2:101–10.

85 Frier BM. Hypoglycaemia and cognitive function in diabetes. *Int J Clin Pract Suppl* 2001;123:30–7.

7

Oral hypoglycemic agents: sulfonylureas and meglitinides

Andreas F H Pfeiffer

INTRODUCTION

For many years sulfonylureas have been the mainstay of oral antidiabetic therapy based on their insulinotropic action on beta cells in the pancreatic Islets of Langerhans. Several alternative oral agents have now become available, broadening the spectrum of therapeutic alternatives. However, insulinotropic agents target one of the deficits that characterize diabetes mellitus type 2, namely a relative insufficiency of insulin secretion. Their therapeutic efficacy has been proven in several smaller trials, and in a large randomized prospective trial in type 2 diabetes—the UK Prospective Diabetes Study (UKPDS)—and was shown to be similar to the administration of insulin[1]. A recent study in the USA compared the glucose-lowering potential of insulin with sulfonylureas in a setting of treatment by family practitioners, and found similar potency for either treatment[2]. Insulin lowered the glycosylated hemoglobin (HbA1c) by 0.8% and the sulfonylurea by 1.1%, which is comparable to the outcome observed in the UKPDS.

A number of different insulinotropic agents have been developed, which differ in their insulinotropic potency, duration of action, routes of elimination and non-insulinotropic additional and side-effects[3]. Very recently, an additional group of insulinotropic agents acting on the sulfonylurea receptor has become avail-

able. These compounds are termed meglitinides, and presently consist of the benzoic acid derivative repaglinide and the tryptophane derivative nateglinide.

MECHANISM OF ACTION

Sulfonylureas and meglitinides (repaglinide and nateglinide) bind to a subunit of a potassium channel (K_{ATP}-channel) on beta cells named SUR1 (for sulfonylurea). SUR1 is a subunit of a potassium channel of the inward rectifier (IR) type, together with the channel-forming subunit named Kir6.2 (Reference 4). This channel is physiologically regulated by adenosine trisphosphate (ATP). ATP is generated by oxidative phosphorylation in the mitochondria and is derived from glucose metabolism. ATP closes the K_{ATP}-channel, which normally allows efflux of K^+ from the beta-cell, thereby generating the normal hyperpolarized membrane potential. Closure of the K_{ATP}-channel depolarizes the cell and activates voltage-driven Ca^{2+} channels. The ensuing influx of Ca^{2+} into the cell promotes fusion of insulin granules with the cell membrane, causing insulin release[5]. Sulfonylureas and the 'glinides', i.e. the meglitinides repaglinide and nateglinide, promote closure of the K_{ATP}-channel complex by binding to the SUR1–subunit. They can thereby enhance the effect of ATP, but also cause closure of the channels on their own. Sulfonylureas, therefore, cause an increase in basal insulin secretion and enhance glucose- or nutrient-induced insulin secretion. The degree to which basal and meal-stimulated insulin release is enhanced may differ between compounds.

THE INDICATION FOR SULFONYLUREA TREATMENT

Treatment goals for diabetes demand near normal glucose levels if possible in view of patient compliance and ability to follow therapeutic recommendations. This should be achieved with diet and exercise whenever possible. In the early phase of type 2 diabetes, insulin secretion typically is elevated[6], compared with healthy subjects, in an attempt to compensate for insulin resistance. Nevertheless, the chronically elevated levels of glucose, as occurs in manifest type 2 diabetes, indicate relative deficiency of insulin.

Insulinotropic agents are considered first-choice treatment in insulin-deficient patients who are not overweight, i.e. have a body mass index (BMI) < 25 kg m^{-2} (Reference 7). In overweight patients, metformin and alpha glucosidase inhibitors are recommended first-choice treatment and insulinotropic agents can be added where blood glucose control is insufficient. In obese patients with type 2 diabetes, sulfonylureas are considered second choice treatments since an increase in body weight of 2–4 kg was observed in most studies with either sulfonylureas or with insulin, but not with metformin. In obese patients, the use of sulfonylureas is indicated if hyperglycemia is not controlled by other agents, and many diabetologists will add a sulfonylurea to metformin.

EFFICACY

Sulfonylureas will decrease blood glucose on average by 30–60 mg dL^{-1} (1.5–3 mmol L^{-1}) and lower HbA1c by about 1.0–2.5%. The glucose-lowering potency of sulfonylureas is directly related to the initial glucose concentration at the onset of treatment, and is greater the higher the initial glucose concentration[2,6]. In the UKPDS, the starting HbA1c concentration was around 9% and was lowered to about 7% by diet during the run-in period. The HbA1c was lowered on average by 0.9% using chlorpropamide or glibenclamide (identical to glyburide in the US) compared with the diet group, and this difference persisted during the 10 years of the study in patients controlled by sulfonylureas[1]. Over this time, the mean HbA1c of all treatment groups increased by about 2%, reflecting the overall loss of beta-cell function. However, this increase in HbA1c was seen in all treatment groups and was not a consequence of sulfonylurea treatment, but rather was a consequence of the disease itself. Clearly, increased efforts are required to achieve good glucose control over time in patients with type 2 diabetes.

About 25% of the patients treated with sulfonylureas after diagnosis of type 2 diabetes will achieve a fasting plasma glucose < 140 mg dL^{-1}, which is still above the recommended ideal range of 80–120 mg dL^{-1}, but is often accepted as a satisfactory response[2,6]. A good response is predicted by a moderately elevated fasting blood glucose of 140–220 mg dL^{-1} before onset of treatment, and a high fasting plasma C-peptide and absence of markers of type 1 diabetes (GAD65 and/or IA2 antibodies). About 50–75% of newly diagnosed patients will require a second agent apart from life-style changes to achieve a blood glucose control of < 140 mg dL^{-1} or 7.8 mmol L, and thus are regarded as partial responders.

Patients with no or a poor response often have antibodies to GAD65 and belong to the group with 'latent autoimmune diabetes of adults' (LADA), which is a type 1 diabetes and represents about 10% of patients. Their age at onset of LADA is above 50 years and the BMI was around 23–25 kg m^{-2} in several studies, thus was lower than in type 2 diabetes where BMI of 27–30 kg m^{-2} are frequently reported. C-peptide in these patients is usually < 1 ng mL^{-1}, while this is elevated in type 2 diabetes.

Patients with a good initial response to sulfonylureas usually show a declining response over time, resulting in a failure rate of about 5% per year. Within 10 years of treatment the majority of patients with type 2 diabetes appear to develop an insufficient response to sulfonylureas, termed 'secondary failure'. Clinical causes may be an increased need of insulin due to weight gain, chronic inflammation, immobilization or dietary factors. However, a decline in beta-cell function has been observed in long-term studies, independent of the agents used for treatment, and represents a presently unmodifiable aspect of type 2 diabetes. The pathophysiology of this process is unknown. Early studies suggested that sulfonylureas may stress beta-cells by increased demand, possibly causing secondary beta cell failure. The UKPDS followed patients over about 9 years and documented that beta cell failure occurs independently of the type of treatment and was observed with metformin and with insulin to a similar degree as with sulfonylureas[1,8]. Beta-cell failure must apparently be regarded as an inherent aspect of the pathogenic process of type 2 diabetes and is not a consequence of particular treatments. However, since insulinotropic agents depend on beta-cell function, their failure causes loss of efficacy.

A possible cofactor causing a decline of beta-cell function may be seen in the chronic challenge of beta-cells by supranormal levels of glucose, termed glucose toxicity, which permanently activates the secretory signaling pathways, thereby leading to their desensitization. This includes the signaling pathway activated by K_{ATP}-channel inhibitors. The disturbances in lipid metabolism typical of type 2 diabetes with elevated free fatty acids provide another putatively toxic component, termed by analogy 'lipotoxicity'. However, these mechanisms remain speculative at present.

DRUG TYPES

Sulfonylureas were developed over 50 years ago and the first generation agents, such as tolbutamide, chlorpropamide and tolazamide, have a lower potency than the second generation agents (glipizide, glibenclamide/gliburide, gliclazide, glisoxepide)[4]. Potency correlates quite well with the affinity for the sulfonylurea

receptor, and second generation agents have a higher affinity for the sulfonylurea receptor. Glimepiride was proposed to possess some extrapancreatic effects and has therefore been termed a 'third generation' agent. However, with the development of a wide range of different sulfonylureas and meglitinides, the classification into different generations is more a marketing aspect than a meaningful characterization. The pharmacokinetic properties are summarized in Table 7.1.

The meglitinides differ structurally from the sulfonylureas and do not contain the sulfonylurea chemical motif. Repaglinide is a benzoic acid derivative, and nateglinide is derived from the amino acid tryptophane. Both compounds have substantially shorter duration of action than glibenclamide or glimepiride and have no active metabolites.

All these compounds bind to the sulfonylurea receptor and share the mechanism of action, i.e. all close the ATP-dependent potassium channel. The exact binding sites may differ somewhat, leading to complex displacement curves of radiolabeled glibenclamide[9], but the clinical significance of such rather subtle differences is unclear. Nateglinide has low affinity for the ATP-dependent potassium channel and, therefore, has rapid kinetics of association and dissociation, while repaglinide is intermediate between the high-affinity ligands glibenclamide or glimepiride and nateglinide.

DOSING SCHEDULE

With all compounds one should start treatment with the lowest effective dose and titrate upwards until sufficient control or a maximal dose is achieved. The drug dose can be increased every 1–2 weeks. The first generation compounds tolbutamide (500–2500 mg), tolazamide (100–1000 mg) and chlorpropamide (100–500 mg) required larger doses to be effective. Glipizide requires 5–20 mg, with 20 mg being the maximally effective dose, although doses of up to 40 mg have been approved. Glibenclamide (gliburide in the USA) can be given once daily, or in a divided dose of 1.75–10.5 mg for the micronized preparation, or up to 15 mg/day for

Table 7.1 Pharmacokinetic properties of sulfonylureas

Sulfonylurea	Enteral resorption	Bio-availability (%)	C max[a] (h)	T½[b] (h)	Plasma-protein-binding (%)	Placental passage
Tolbutamide	Fast	85–100	2–5	6–8	93–99	Yes
Chlorpropamide	Fast	> 90	2–4	35	> 87	Yes
Tolazamide	Slow	85–90	4–6	7	87–94	Yes
Glibenclamide (Gliburide)	Fast	> 95	1–3	8–10	99	Yes
Glibornurid	Fast	91–98	3–4	5–11	95–97	Yes
Glisoxepide	Fast	> 95	1	1.7	~ 93	Yes
Gliquidon	Fast	> 95	2–3	4–6	99	Yes
Glipizide	Fast	> 95	1–2	2.7–4	97–99	Yes
Gliclazide	Slow	95	4–8	♂, ♀ 11	85–97	Yes
Gliclazide MR	Fast	> 95	6	12–20	97	Yes
Glimepiride	Fast	> 95	2,5	5–8	99	Yes
Meglitinides						
Nateglinide	Fast	> 75%	1	1.5	97–99	
Repaglinide	Fast	> 90%	1	1.5	> 90	

[a] C max = maximum serum concentration.
[b] T½ = half-life.

the conventional, larger particle preparation. Glimepiride is given once daily in doses of 1–4 mg. Higher doses (8 mg) have been approved, but do not afford additional effects.

Gliquidon is administered once daily until a dose of 30 mg, higher doses, up to 120 mg, are given in a divided dose twice daily. The dose is also divided for patients with advanced renal impairment. Gliclazide was recently offered in a new once-daily formulation (MR) requiring lower doses of 30–120 mg, instead of 80–320 mg with the old twice daily formulation[10].

Dose per day	Onset of effect (min)	Max. effect (h)	Duration of effect (h)	Hepatic metabolism	Excretion by the kidney (%)	Other ways of excretion
0.5–2.0 g	60	2–5	12–18	80%, active metabolite too	> 75, < 1% unchanged	9% via feces
0.125–05 g			> 24	80%	> 95, 20% unchanged	Little via feces
0.125–05 g	100	6	6–12 (–16)	93%, five metabolites, three active	85	6% via feces
1.75–10.5	30	2–5	15–24	Complete, to inactive metabolites	50, almost 0% unchanged	50% via feces
12.5–75 mg				100%, six inactive metabolites	60–72, 0% unchanged	23–33% via feces
2–16 mg	30–45	1	5–10	50% inactive metabolites	70–80, 50% unchanged	15–25% via feces
15–120 mg	60–90	2–3		100% inactive metabolites	0–5	> 95% via feces
2.5–30 mg	30	1	8–10	> 9% inactive metabolites	64–87, 3–10% unchanged	15% via fcccs
40–320 mg		2	6	99%, seven inactive metabolites	60–70	10–20% via feces
30–120 mg	60–120	4–6	24	99% inactive metabolites	60–70	10–20% via feces
1–8 mg	30–60	2–6	24 h	100%, two metabolites	84	10% via feces
180–360 mg	15–30	30 min	3–4 h	Inactive metabolites	90	10% via feces
1.5–8 mg		30 min	3–4 h	Inactive metabolites	< 10%	90% via feces

Repaglinide and nateglinide are administered immediately before meals 2–4 times daily. Repaglinide is available in doses of 0.5–2 mg per meal and patients should be started with the lowest dose. Nateglinide is usually given in the dose of 120 mg/meal, although a 60 mg tablet is available[11–16].

EXTRAPANCREATIC EFFECTS OF SULFONYLUREAS AND MEGLITINIDES

Sulfonylureas cause a moderate improvement in the lipid profile due to improvement of lipid metabolism by increased levels of insulin and lowered levels of glucose, which is considered an indirect effect.

Large randomized trials, such as the UKPDS, usually showed a weight gain of 2–4 kg with longer-acting sulfonylureas, e.g. glibenclamide and chlorpropamide. This weight gain can be avoided by dietary advice if patients are compliant. Indeed, no weight gain was observed in smaller studies with glipizide, glimepride and the shorter-acting substances[17]. Weight gain is apparently related to the increase in insulin and its antilipolytic and trophic action on fat cells, and is probably enhanced by the addition of further agents inhibiting lipolysis, such as beta-blockers or the thiazolidinediones, which promote fat-cell differentiation and proliferation.

Glimepiride was shown to translocate glucose transporters to the cell membrane by a direct action in several experimental systems. In man, a modest effect on insulin sensitivity was shown in euglycemic clamps and insulin levels were slightly lower in glimepiride compared with glibenclamide treated patients[18]. A recent report compared glimepiride, glibenclamide and gliclazide in hyperinsulinemic euglycemic clamps and described an enhanced insulin action for glimepiride and somewhat less for glibenclamide compared with gliclazide[19]. However, the therapeutic benefit remains to be demonstrated.

Chlorpropamide has two unique effects: it can cause a flushing reaction after ingestion of alcohol, by inhibiting the metabolism of acetaldehyde, and it sometimes causes a syndrome of inappropriate anti-diuretic hormone (ADH) action (SIADH), by enhancing its effects. Chorpropamide is not now used in Europe and the USA.

Gliclazide was shown to have potent antioxidative actions in vitro and in vivo. Theoretically, this might be advantageous in patients with type 2 diabetes, but there are no studies with hard end-points that demonstrate this.

Some studies, such as the University Group Diabetes Study in 1976 (UGDP)[20], suggested that sulfonylureas are associated with a poor outcome after a myocardial infarction, but these studies have been heavily criticized[21], and do not correspond with current standards.

Theoretically, sulfonylureas might close ATP-dependent potassium channels possessing a SUR2a/b subunit, which are present on cardiomyocytes and coronary and arterial vessel smooth muscle cells, thereby preventing adaptive changes and relaxation of cardiomyocytes and vascular smooth muscle cells in response to hypoxia. This would occur by preventing smooth muscle cell hyperpolarization caused by potassium efflux, due to the closure of K_{ATP}-channels by the sulfonylurea, which might enlarge the infarct area. Although sulfonylureas bind the SUR1 on beta cells with much higher affinity than SUR2a/b, some activation appears possible. Glimepiride and nateglinide show much lower affinity for the cardiac SUR2b sulfonylurea receptor than for beta-cell SUR1 and are a safer choice in this respect. Most of the increased deaths after myocardial infarction in diabetes appear to be due to poor left ventricular function. There is no convincing evidence for negative effects of sulfonylureas from clinical trials. Moreover, the UKPDS has not provided evidence for an increased mortality of patients treated with glibenclamide or chlorpropamide, which would be expected to become apparent in such a large study. However, in conditions of hypoxia, such as after a myocardial infarction or during coronary interventions, negative effects have not been sufficiently studied. It therefore appears prudent to withdraw high affinity ligands of SUR2a/b in this condition[22].

SAFETY

Hypoglycemia is the major safety concern with sulfonylureas. Large studies have provided numbers for hypoglycemic episodes associated with some of the sulfonylureas used. The longer the duration of action and the more potent a compound, the higher the risk of hypoglycemia. Typically, elderly non-obese patients with type 2 diabetes who are given long-acting sulfonylureas and may miss a meal after having received the treatment are at highest risk. The presence of renal and/or hepatic insufficiency enhances the risk, due to impaired gluconeogenesis. In renal insufficiency, accumulation of compounds may occur due to decreased elimination.

There are few detailed studies about the use of sulfonylureas in renal impairment. Moderate reductions in creatinine clearance (up to 60 mL min⁻¹) require dose reductions, but allow the use of most sulfonylureas, whereas more severely compromised kidney function represents a contraindication. Gliquidone is almost completely eliminated in the feces after hepatic metabolism to inactive metabolites, and < 5% are eliminated via the kidney. This is therefore the safest agent to use for type 2 diabetes treatment in renal insufficiency[23,24].

The shorter-acting meglitinides may possess a lower risk of hypoglycemia simply because of the short duration of action and intake with meals, although not all studies have confirmed this assumption[13,25]. Observational studies have suggested that glimepiride is less frequently associated with severe hypoglycemia than glibenclamide, but this was not shown in prospective controlled trials.

A COMPARISON OF DIFFERENT SULFONYLUREAS AND MEGLITINIDES

Among sulfonylureas, no definitive advantages have been demonstrated for one compound compared with others in trials with hard endpoints. The potent long-acting sulfonylureas bear a higher risk of protracted hypoglycemias in elderly people who may miss meals, and in poorly controlled conditions. Shorter acting and less potent insulin releasers may be advantageous under these circumstances[13,25]. Specific advantages have been proposed for gliclazide, due to its antioxidant actions, and glimepiride, due to its insulin sensitizing effects, both of which are of unknown significance[26,27].

Meglitinides have been compared with glibenclamide and glipizide with regard to effects on average glucose- and meal-related insulin secretion. Indeed, repaglinide and nateglinide caused a more rapid increase in meal-related insulin secretion compared with glibenclamide, and achieved a more potent lowering of postprandial increases in glucose. Studies with nateglinide performed in patients with a fasting glucose slightly above 200 mg dL⁻¹ also showed that nateglinide was less potent in lowering fast-

ing plasma glucose. Used as a single agent, the therapeutic effect is relatively small and HbA1c was lowered by 0.6%. Thus, the drug appears most suitable for use in early diabetes. With more pronounced elevations of fasting glucose, combination with metformin was effective. This is, however, true for all combinations of sulfonylureas with metformin (see below). The faster-acting meglitinides may achieve better post-prandial control of blood glucose in combination with metformin or insulin sensitizers. It is unproven whether this difference of post-prandial glucose results in advantages for the patient with regard to the risk of macrovascular disease.

Increases in post-prandial glucose were shown to be associated with elevated risk of cardiovascular disease in impaired glucose tolerance (Lancet Decode 1999). This was not shown as well among patients with manifest type 2 diabetes. The extrapolation of studies in impaired glucose tolerance suggest that near normal control of glucose, both fasting and post-prandial, should decrease the cardiovascular risk associated with type 2 diabetes back to the normal range. Although this is plausible, and is expressed in the current treatment guidelines, it has not yet been proven in prospective trials. Such trials would have to overcome the difficulty that it is presently much harder to lower blood glucose into the normal range than to lower blood pressure or elevated cholesterol levels. However, the impact of clinical studies demonstrating a substantial advantage of normalizing—and not just lowering—blood glucose would be enormous and would change current treatment practices.

A reduction of post-prandial glucose levels, however, is most likely to be successful in a setting of normalized fasting glucose levels i.e. 80–120 mg dL⁻¹. Advantages of better control of post-prandial glucose are of unknown relevance with permanently elevated fasting glucose levels.

ORAL COMBINATION THERAPY

The combination of sulfonylureas with other non-insulinotropic agents results in additive effects and potently lowers blood glucose. The combination of metformin with sulfonylureas or meglitinides is frequently used, and additionally lowers HbA1c by 1–2%, depending on the dose of metformin added. A dose-related increase has been shown to occur to a ceiling of 2 g metformin added to the insulin releaser per day in two doses[28]. However, the mortality in the combination therapy group was increased compared with sulfonylurea monotherapy in the UKPDS[29]. This has been attributed to an exceptionally low mortality in the sulfonylurea monotherapy group. However, similar trends were observed in a population-based observational study, indicating an urgent need for further studies of this combination[30]. Similar improvements of blood glucose were reported for the combination of meglitinides with metformin[15] and for combinations of thiazolidinediones or α-glucosidase inhibitors and sulfonylureas. In all combinations, HbA1c was lowered by 1–2%, in addition to the effect of the insulinotropic agent.

Most patients will, in fact, require more than one agent to achieve treatment goals of HbA1c < 7%. The choice may be individualized, depending on body weight, compliance, kidney function and individual response to the treatment. The combination of insulinotropic agents with thiazolidinediones is highly effective in lowering blood glucose, but also additively increases body weight by 2–6 kg. The combination with α-glucosidase inhibitors was also shown to lower HbA1c by about 1%, but the lowering of fasting plasma glucose takes several weeks—for unknown reasons. This combination causes no additive weight gain.

Since all diabetes trials observed a positive relation between blood glucose and the occurrence of late complications, this approach is rational and well-justified, based on current evidence.

COMBINATION THERAPY WITH INSULIN

An effective approach for narrow control of blood glucose once other combinations fail or are unwanted for other reasons, is the use of evening administration of a long-acting insulin and an insulinotropic agent during the day. The evening dose of insulin should be titrated to achieve near normoglycemic blood glucose levels, while the insulinotropic agent improves post-prandial blood glucose control during the daytime[31]. Remarkably, a fair control may be achieved in some patients with type 2 diabetes, even when evening doses of 40 or more units of insulin are required. This scheme exploits the endogenous capacity for regulation of blood glucose still present with advanced type 2 diabetes, and may be tried before starting a multiple injection plan. However, this combination also is prone to cause substantial increases in body weight.

REFERENCES

1 UK Prospective Diabetes Study (UKPDS) Group. Intensive blood-glucose control with sulphonylureas or insulin compared with conventional treatment and risk of complications in patients with type 2 diabetes (UKPDS 33). *Lancet* 1998;352:837–53.

2 Hayward RA, Manning WG, Kaplan SH *et al.* Starting insulin therapy in patients with type 2 diabetes: effectiveness, complications, and resource utilization. *J Am Med Assoc* 1997;278:1663–9.

3 Schatz H, Mark M, Ammon H. Antidiabetika: Diabetes mellitus und Pharmakotherapie. Stutgart: Wissenschaftliche Verlagsgesellschaft mbH Stuttgart, 1986.

4 Hu S, Wang S, Fanelli B *et al.* Pancreatic beta-cell K(ATP) channel activity and membrane-binding studies with nateglinide: a comparison with sulfonylureas and repaglinide. *J Pharmacol Exp Ther* 2000;293:444–52.

5 Panten U, Schwanstecher M, Schwanstecher C. Sulfonylurea receptors and mechanism of sulfonylurea action. *Exp Clin Endocrinol Metab* 1996;104:1–9.

6 DeFronzo RA. Pharmacologic therapy for type 2 diabetes mellitus. *Ann Intern Med* 1999;131:281–303.

7 European Diabetes Policy Group 1999. A desktop guide to Type 2 diabetes mellitus. *Diabet Med* 1999;16:716–30.

8   United Kingdom Prospective Diabetes Study Group. United Kingdom Prospective Diabetes Study 24: a 6-year, randomized, controlled trial comparing sulfonylurea, insulin, and metformin therapy in patients with newly diagnosed type 2 diabetes that could not be controlled with diet therapy. *Ann Intern Med* 1998;128:165–75.

9   Fuhlendorff J, Rorsman P, Kofod H *et al.* Stimulation of insulin release by repaglinide and glibenclamide involves both common and distinct processes. *Diabetes* 1998;47:345-51.

10 Drouin P. Diamicron MR once daily is effective and well tolerated in type 2 diabetes: a randomized, double-blind, multi-national study. *J Diabetes Complications* 2000;14:185–91.

11 Moses RG, Gomis R, Frandsen KB *et al.* Flexible meal-related dosing with repaglinide facilitates glycemic control in therapy-naive type 2 diabetes. *Diabetes Care* 2001;24:11–15.

12 Owens DR, Luzio SD, Ismail I, Bayer T. Increased prandial insulin secretion after administration of a single preprandial oral dose of repaglinide in patients with type 2 diabetes. *Diabetes Care* 2000;23:518–23.

13 Landgraf R, Frank M, Bauer C, Dieken ML. Prandial glucose regulation with repaglinide: its clinical and lifestyle impact in a large cohort of patients with Type 2 diabetes. *Int J Obes Relat Metab Disord* 2000;24 (Suppl 3):S38–44.

14 Keilson L, Mather S, Walter YH *et al.* Synergistic effects of nateglinide and meal administration on insulin secretion in patients with type 2 diabetes mellitus. *J Clin Endocrinol Metab* 2000;85:1081–6.

15 Horton ES, Clinkingbeard C, Gatlin M *et al.* Nateglinide alone and in combination with metformin improves glycemic control by reducing mealtime glucose levels in type 2 diabetes. *Diabetes Care* 2000;23:1660–5.

16 Hollander PA, Schwartz SL, Gatlin MR *et al.* Importance of early insulin secretion: comparison of nateglinide and glyburide in previously diet-treated patients with type 2 diabetes. *Diabetes Care* 2001;24:983–8.

17 Simonson DC, Kourides IA, Feinglos M *et al.* Efficacy, safety, and dose–response characteristics of glipizide gastrointestinal therapeutic system on glycemic control and insulin secretion in NIDDM. Results of two multicenter, randomized, placebo-controlled clinical trials. The Glipizide Gastrointestinal Therapeutic System Study Group. *Diabetes Care* 1997;20:597–606.

18 Clark HE, Matthews DR. The effect of glimepiride on pancreatic beta-cell function under hyperglycaemic clamp and hyperinsulinaemic, euglycaemic clamp conditions in non-insulin-dependent diabetes mellitus. *Horm Metab Res* 1996;28:445–50.

19 Sato J, Ohsawa I, Oshida Y *et al.* Comparison of the effects of three sulfonylureas on *in vivo* insulin action. *Arzneimittelforschung* 2001;51:459–64.

20 Kilo C, Miller JP, Williamson JR. The crux of the UGDP. Spurious results and biologically inappropriate data analysis. *Diabetologia* 1980;18:179–85.

21 Genuth S. Exogenous insulin administration and cardiovascular risk in non-insulin-dependent and insulin-dependent diabetes mellitus. *Ann Intern Med* 1996;124(1 Pt 2):104–9.

22 Garrat K, Brady P, Hassinger N *et al.* Sulfonylurea drugs increase early mortality in patients with diabetes mellitus after direct angioplasty for acute myocardial infarction. *J Am Coll Cardiol* 1999;33:119–24.

23 Harrower AD. Pharmacokinetics of oral antihyperglycaemic agents in patients with renal insufficiency. *Clin Pharmacokinet* 1996;31:111–9.

24 Dedov II, Demidova I, Pisklakov SV, Antokhin EA. [Use of glurenorm in patients with non-insulin-dependent diabetes mellitus and liver diseases]. *Probl Endokrinol (Mosk)* 1993;39:6–8.

25 Landgraf R. Meglitinide analogues in the treatment of type 2 diabetes mellitus. *Drugs Aging* 2000;17:411–25.

26 Vallejo S, Angulo J, Peiro C *et al.* Prevention of endothelial dysfunction in streptozotocin-induced diabetic rats by gliclazide treatment. *J Diabetes Compl* 2000;14:224–33.

27 Elhadd TA, Newton RW, Jennings PE, Belch JJ. Antioxidant effects of gliclazide and soluble adhesion molecules in type 2 diabetes. *Diabetes Care* 1999;22:528–30.

28 Riddle M. Combining sulfonylureas and other oral agents. *Am J Med* 2000;108:15S–22S.

29 Effect of intensive blood-glucose control with metformin on complications in overweight patients with type 2 diabetes (UKPDS 34). UK Prospective Diabetes Study (UKPDS) Group. *Lancet* 1998;352:854–65.

30 Olsson J, Lindberg G, Gottsater M *et al.* Increased mortality in type 2 diabetic patients using sulfonylurea and metformin combination. *Diabetologia* 2000;43:558–60.

31 Riddle M. Combined therapy with a sulfonylurca plus evening insulin: safe, reliable and becoming routine. *Horm Metabol Res* 1996;28:430–3.

8

Metformin

Michael Stumvoll, Hans-Ulrich Häring and Stephan Matthaei

HISTORICAL ASPECTS AND INTRODUCTION

The glucose-lowering potential of the guanides was first described in medieval times, when extracts of *Galega officinalis* (goat's rue or French lilac) were used to treat diabetes in Europe[1]. In 1957, metformin—a dimethylated biguanide, and phenformin, a phenetylated biguanide, were introduced for the therapy of type 2 diabetes mellitus (Figure 8.1). However, because of the strong association with lactic acidosis, phenformin was withdrawn in the 1970s in most countries, including the USA[2]. In contrast, metformin continued to be used in Europe, Canada and many other countries, but was not approved by the US Food and Drug Administration until 1995[3].

There is now a large body of data documenting the clinical efficacy of metformin in the treatment of type 2 diabetes[4], and most of its clinical, pharmacological and basic cellular aspects have been addressed in several excellent reviews published over the past 20 years[5–12]. Recently, the UK Prospective Diabetes Study (UKPDS) showed that metformin is particularly effective in type 2 diabetic subjects with obesity, a condition commonly associated with insulin resistance[13]. Moreover, in essentially all clinical studies the improvement of hyperglycemia with metformin occurred in the presence of unaltered or reduced plasma insulin concentrations[14,15]. Taken collectively, these findings indicate the potential of metformin as an insulin-sensitizing drug, and forms the basis for metformin's current role in the treatment of type 2 diabetes[16] (Figure 8.2).

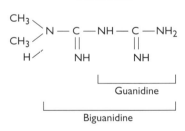

Figure 8.1 Chemical structure of biguanides.

CELLULAR MECHANISM OF ACTION

Despite almost 40 years of research, the precise cellular mechanism of metformin action is still not entirely understood. Several cellular mechanisms have been described, but a single unifying site of action, such as a receptor, an enzyme, or a transcription factor, has yet to be identified. Nevertheless, it is generally undisputed that metformin has no effect on the pancreatic beta

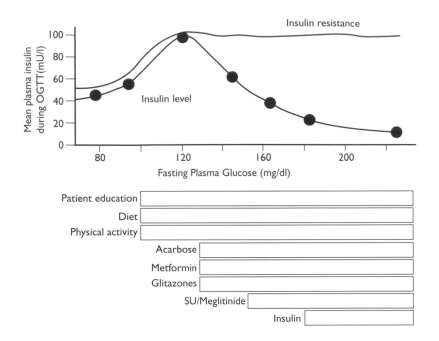

Figure 8.2 Starling's curve of the pancreas and rational treatment of type 2 diabetes mellitus. Starling's curve of the pancreas, as originally described by DeFronzo et al.[39], indicating the relationship of mean plasma insulin levels during an oral glucose tolerance test (OGTT) and fasting plasma glucose levels of subjects with normal glucose tolerance, impaired glucose tolerance, and type 2 diabetes. The therapeutic options should be selected according to the pathophysiological stage of the individual patient (modified from Reference 16). SU = sulfonylureas.

cell in stimulating insulin secretion[8]. Mild increases in glucose-stimulated insulin secretion after metformin treatment[17] are thought to be the result of reduced glucose toxicity on the beta cell, as a result of improved glycemic control[18].

Insulin binding and early insulin signalling events

A number of earlier studies demonstrated that *in vitro* or *in vivo* treatment with metformin improved the binding of insulin to its receptor on the surface of various cell types, such as human fibroblasts[19], human breast cells and lympho-cytes[20], rat adipocytes[21], mouse hepatocytes[22] and rat hepatoma cells[19]. In contrast, no effect was seen on adipocytes[23], monocytes[24] and erythro-cytes[25] from patients with type 2 diabetes. Insulin binding was also unaffected by metformin treat-ment in insulin-responsive cells, such as human[26] and rat adipocytes[27], and mouse[22] and rat[28,29] hepatocytes, suggesting that most of the cellular mechanism of action of metformin would be at the post-receptor level. One study of muscle in streptozotocin diabetic rats treated with metformin *in vivo* demonstrated a stimulatory effect on glycogen synthesis, which was accom-panied by increased autophosphorylation and

tyrosine kinase activity of the insulin receptor, but not by increased insulin binding[30]. Several more recent studies, however, have demon-strated a metabolic effect of metformin on insulin sensitive tissues in the absence of increased insulin binding[27,31–33], insulin receptor autophos-phorylation[27,32] or insulin receptor tyrosine kinase activity[27,31,32], substantiating the view that metformin stimulates, or potentiates, events distal of the insulin receptor.

Effect on glucose production

In vitro and animal data

In isolated rat hepatocytes, metformin increased insulin-suppression of gluconeogenesis[28,34]. In 24 h starved rodents, metformin inhibited conver-sion of ^{14}C pyruvate into plasma glucose[35] *in vivo*. In addition, in isolated kidney slices, metformin inhibited the conversion preferentially of lactate and pyruvate, less of alanine, but not of glutamate and oxaloacetate to glucose[35]. Metformin also decreased glucagon and dibuturyl cAMP-stimu-lated gluconeogenesis, suggesting that steps downstream of adenylate cyclase are inhibited[29]. It appears that metformin causes a decrease in intra-cellular ATP, which would inhibit gluconeogene-sis through stimulation of pyruvate kinase activity[36]. Alternatively, a primary inhibition of hepatic lactate uptake by metformin, demonstrated in rats *in vivo*, has also been suggested[37]. With respect to other insulin-dependent pathways in the liver (stimulation of glycogen and lipid synthesis), metformin has been shown to both potentiate insulin action and prevent insulin-induced insulin resistance in isolated rat hepatocytes[33]. Activation of AMP-activated protein kinase (AMPK) was shown to be required for metformin's inhibitory effect on hepatocyte glucose production[33A]. AMPK activation may in fact provide a unifying explanation for the pleiotropic metabolic effects of metformin, including those on skeleton muscle glucose uptake.

Effect on peripheral glucose metabolism

In vitro *data, glucose transport (Table 8.1)*
In vitro studies on isolated muscle from experi-

mentally diabetic rodents have shown that metformin stimulates glucose transport[51,52]. *In vitro* incubation with metformin increased insulin-stimulated, but not basal, glucose transport in muscle strips prepared from insulin-resistant healthy and diabetic subjects, while no effect was seen in strips from insulin-sensitive subjects[48,49]. In these studies, however, metformin concentrations (0.1 mM) 10 times higher than the therapeutic plasma concentration were used. The fact that stimulation of glucose transport was observed in the absence of an increase in insulin binding, or insulin receptor tyrosine kinase activity[32], suggests a post-receptor site of action.

In L6 myotubes and isolated rat adipocytes it was shown that the increase in glucose transport was due to an increase in glucose transporters in the plasma membrane[31,32,50], without an increase in mRNA levels or total cellular protein of GLUT

Table 8.1 *In vitro* studies—effect of metformin on insulin-mediated glucose metabolism

Effect	Cell/tissue type	Administration	Comment	Author
Glucose transport				
↑ I	Adipocytes humans	*In vitro*		Cigolini[26]
↑ I	Adipocytes, rat	*In vivo*	Hyperglycemia after injury	Frayn[47]
↑ I	Muscle strips, DM,N	*In vitro*	Effect only in insulin resistant subjects	Galuska[48,49]
↑ I	Adipocytes, rat	*In vitro/in vivo*	Stimulation of GLUT1 and GLUT4 translocation	Matthaei[31,32]
↑ I	L6 myotubes	*In vitro*	Stimulation of GLUT1 but not GLUT4 translocation	Hundal[50]
↑ I	Muscle, mouse	*In vivo*	Streptozotocin, no effect in non-diabetic animals	Bailey[51]
↑ I	Muscle, rat	*In vitro*	Alloxan diabetes, no effect in non-diabetic animals	Frayn[52]
↑ BI	Adipocytes, rat	*In vitro*	Prevention of GLUT4 down-regulation	Kozka[53]
↑ BI	Myotubes, humans	*In vitro*	Stronger effect with 25 mM versus 5 mM glucose	Sarabia[54]
NC	Adipocytes, DM	*In vitro*		Pedersen[23]
Glycogen synthesis				
↑ I	Muscle, mouse	*In vivo*	Streptozotocin diabetes	Bailey[51]
↑ I	Muscle, rat	*In vivo*	Streptozotocin diabetes	Rossetti[30]
Glucose oxidation				
↑ I	Muscle, mouse	*In vivo*	Streptozotocin diabetes	Bailey[51]
NC	Muscle, mouse	*In vitro*	Streptozotocin diabetes	Wilcock[85]

B = basal; I = insulin-stimulated; DM = patients with type 2 diabetes, N = normal subjects.

Table 8.2 Metabolic studies in humans with type 2 diabetes—effects of metformin

Author	N	Dose, duration (mg daily, wks)	FG (mg/dL)	FI (µU/ml)	Basal MCR	Insulin-stimulated MCR	Basal glucose production
Prager[42]	12, obese	1.7/4	244 → 160	–	–	↑	↓
Nosadini[25]	7, obese	2.55/4	156 → 113*	15 → 9*	NC	↑	↓
Jackson[43]	10, lean	2.0–2.5/12	172 → 103*	23 → 23	–	NC	↓
Hother-Nielsen[56]	9, obese	2.0–2.5/12	205 → 184*	50 → 43	↑	↑	–
Wu[57]	12, obese	2.5/> 12	~220 → ~180*	~13 → ~11	–	NC	–
DeFronzo[44]	14, lean/obese	2.5/12	207 → 158*	19 → 13*	NC	↑	↓
Riccio[59]	6, non-obese	1.7/4	~163 → ~143*	NC	–	↑	–
McIntyre[65]	12, obese	3/6	175 → 103*	14.9 → 15.7	↑	↑	NC
Johnson[45]	8, obese	2.55/12	149 → 122*	15.8 → 11.3	NC	↑	↓
Perriello[46]	21, lean/obese	1.0/acute	–	–	NC	NC	↓
Stumvoll[40]	10, obese	2.55/15	220 → 155*	12 → 10*	NC	–	↓
Cusi[41]	20, obese	2.55/16	196 → 152*	17 → 14	NC	NC	↓
Feny[134]	9, obese	1.7/3	148 → 119*	19 → 15	↑	–	NC
Abbasi[78]	11, lean/obese	2.5/12	224 → 175*	13 → 12	↑	–	NC

DM2 = type 2 diabetes; FDR = first degree relatives of patients with type 2 diabetes; FG = fasting glucose; FI = fasting insulin; MCR = metabolic clearance rate of glucose; ~ indicates values taken from a figure; * indicates significant change; NC = no change; PCO, women with polyocystic ovary syndrome.

1 and GLUT 4[31,32]. In rat adipocytes, the insulin-induced shift of GLUT 1 and 4 from the microsomal fraction to the plasma membrane was potentiated by metformin, suggesting an effect on insulin-stimulated glucose transporter translocation[32]. To fully account for the increase in insulin-stimulated glucose transport in this study, in addition, a stimulatory effect on the functional activity of glucose transporters was assumed. These data and the observations from the muscle strip experiments[48,49] suggest that, in muscle, metformin stimulates mechanisms shown to be defective in insulin resistant states and type 2 diabetes, such as translocation and functional activity of glucose transporters[54]. However, in human myotubes obtained from healthy, non-diabetic subjects, metformin also increased basal and insulin-stimulated glucose transport[54].

In vitro *data, glycogen synthesis (Table 8.2)*
In addition to the effects on glucose transport, there is some *in vitro* evidence for an effect of metformin on glycogen synthesis. In experimentally diabetic animals, metformin enhanced insulin-stimulated glycogen formation[30,47]. In *Xenopus* oocytes, incubation with metformin had no effect on basal glycogen synthesis, but potentiated insulin-stimulated glycogen synthesis[60]. Since this was accompanied by an increase in the amount of activated glycogen synthase, it was concluded that metformin facilitates some early regulatory steps in the insulin-signalling chain, leading to the activation of glycogen synthase. Moreover, the observation that metformin also increased glycogen synthesis in insulin-insensitive cells (human erythrocytes) demonstrates a direct, i.e. insulin-independent effect on this pathway[61].

MECHANISMS OF ACTION IN HUMANS

Glucose production

Accelerated endogenous glucose production is thought to be a key factor in the development of fasting hyperglycaemia in type 2 diabetes[38,39]. In patients with type 2 diabetes, metformin has been shown to inhibit endogenous glucose production in most[25,40,41–45] but not all studies (summarized in Reference 62) to various degrees (from a non-significant ~10% up to a significant ~30%, reviewed in Reference 62) (Figure 8.3). This could largely be accounted for by inhibition of gluconeogenesis[40,63], although an additional inhibitory effect of metformin on glycogen breakdown is likely[40,41]. The observation in many studies that, in the basal post-absorptive state, overall glucose disposal (metabolic plasma clearance rate of glucose) did not change while endogenous glucose production decreased[25,40,41,44–46], suggests that the improvement in glycemic control is largely attributable to the effect of metformin on glucose production.

Peripheral glucose metabolism

Most[25,42,44,45,59,64, 65], but not all studies[41,43,46,57] using the hyperinsulinemic–euglycemic clamp technique have shown a metformin-induced increase in insulin-stimulated glucose disposal in patients with type 2 diabetes varied from ~15% up to ~40% (reviewed in Reference 62) (Figure 8.4). Since muscle represents a major site of insulin-mediated glucose uptake[38,58], metformin must, either directly or via indirect mechanisms, have an insulin-like or insulin-

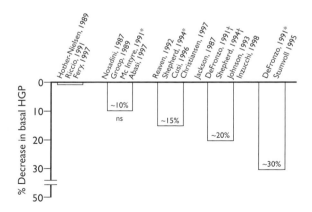

Figure 8.3 Summary of the effect of metformin on basal hepatic glucose production in type 2 diabetic patients (from Reference 62). HGP = hepatic glucose production.

sensitizing effect on this tissue. In humans, the increase in insulin-stimulated glucose disposal is mostly accounted for by non-oxidative pathways[45,59,66]. Non-oxidative glucose metabolism includes storage as glycogen, conversion to lactate and incorporation into triglycerides. No effect on lactate production was observed[40,41] and the implications for net triglyceride synthesis cannot be drawn. Nevertheless, it appears reasonable to propose that, in human muscle, glucose transport and, possibly as a consequence, glycogen synthesis, are the major targets of metformin action in the insulin-stimulated state. However, in the basal state, metformin had no effect on glucose clearance or whole body glucose oxidation, although the proportion of glucose turnover undergoing oxidation was increased[40]. Moreover, forearm glucose uptake in the post-absorptive state was not significantly altered[40].

Metabolic effects independent of improved glycemia

The interpretation of the above experiments is limited by the fact that treatment with metformin was always accompanied by improvement in glycemic control and sometimes also by reduction of body weight. It cannot be excluded therefore, that the effects on endogenous glucose production and glucose

disposal, at least in part, were secondary to reduced glucose toxicity[18] and/or weight loss[67], rather than resulting from the metformin *per se*. Only four studies have examined the metabolic actions of metformin in the absence of any changes in glycemic control or body weight.

In one study, 1 g of metformin was administered acutely to patients with type 2 diabetes and after 12 h no effect on insulin-stimulated glucose disposal was seen, while the excessive endogenous glucose production in the basal state was significantly reduced[46]. This suggests that, in patients with type 2 diabetes, improvement in insulin-stimulated glucose disposal is predominantly due to alleviation of glucose toxicity, while endogenous glucose production is immediately affected by metformin. In another study, lean, normal glucose-tolerant, insulin-resistant first-degree relatives of patients with type 2 diabetes acutely received 1 g of metformin and the exact opposite result was observed[66]. In subjects with impaired glucose tolerance (IGT) 6-week metformin treatment improved basal (HOMA) but not insulin-stimulated glucose disposal or glucose oxidation[68]. In this study, both fasting glucose and insulin decreased significantly. In android obese subjects with impaired glucose tolerance, increased insulin sensitivity (using an intravenous glucose tolerance test) was observed after only 2 days of metformin treatment (1700 mg day[−1])[69]. In obese women with the polycystic-ovary syndrome (PCOS) 6 months treatment with metformin also significantly improved insulin-stimulated glucose disposal[70,71]. In another study in obese women with PCOS the decrease in serum insulin levels was associated with an increased ovulatory response to clomiphene[72]. Glucose production was not assessed in the latter study. These apparent discrepancies could be explained by differences in the type of insulin resistance. In the highly selected group of lean, first-degree relatives and women with PCOS, mechanisms may contribute to insulin resistance that are different than those in normal-variety type 2 diabetes, where insulin resistance is predominantly the result of obesity and long-standing hyperglycaemia. Moreover, the reduction in

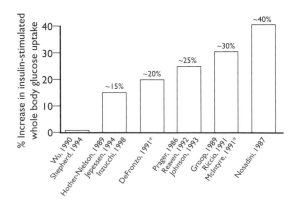

Figure 8.4 Summary of the effect of metformin on insulin-stimulated glucose disposal in type 2 diabetic patients (from Reference 62).

endogenous glucose production after metformin treatment may only be seen in subjects in whom it was increased to begin with, such as patients with type 2 diabetes. The latter is supported by observations showing that metformin alone does not cause hypoglycaemia, or lowers blood glucose in non-diabetic subjects[73,74]. The effect of metformin on endogenous glucose production in non-diabetic humans has not yet been studied.

Additional evidence of improved insulin action comes from studies combining insulin therapy and metformin. It was shown that requirements of exogenous insulin are reduced (by ~30%) by addition of metformin in obese patients with type 2 diabetes and in some patients with type 1 diabetes in whom glycemic control was unaltered[75–77].

OTHER MECHANISMS OF ACTION

It has been suggested that part of the antihyperglycemic effect of metformin is due to decreased release of free fatty acids (FFA) from adipose tissue and/or decreased lipid oxidation[46,78]. However, reduced FFA levels after metformin treatment have only been shown in some[44,57,78] but not all studies[40,41,67]. Moreover, *in vitro* studies have shown that metformin does not enhance the antilipolytic action of insulin on adipose tissue[79]. Only two studies have examined FFA turnover using isotope techniques and found either no difference[40] or a 17% reduction[59] after metformin treatment. In the latter study, the effect was only seen in the basal state, but not in the insulin-stimulated state, where FFA flux was largely suppressed. Thus, the metformin effect on peripheral glucose uptake may, at least in part, be mediated by suppression of FFA and lipid oxidation. In contrast, a causal relationship with endogenous glucose production is unlikely, since distinctly greater reductions in circulating FFA levels with acipimox failed to lower glucose production[80,81].

Evidence for other proposed mechanisms of metformin action is less convincing. Increased intestinal utilization of glucose has been suggested by animal studies[82–84]. More recently, *in vivo* treatment with metformin increased gene expression of the energy-dependent sodium-glucose co-transporter (SGLT1) in rat intestine[85]. However, such a mechanism has not been confirmed in humans[43].

Weight loss

Unlike other pharmacological therapies for type 2 diabetes (sulfonylureas, insulin) metformin treatment is not associated with weight gain. Consistently, clinical studies have shown either a small but significant decrease in body weight[44,86] or a significantly smaller increase in body weight compared to other forms of treatment[75]. One study has shown that weight loss during metformin treatment was largely accounted for by loss of adipose tissue[40]. This was explained by differential effects of metformin on adipose tissue and muscle. While metformin improves insulin sensitivity in muscle, it does not affect the antilipolytic action of insulin on adipose tissue[87]. The overall effect of metformin on body weight is attributed to a reduction in caloric intake[72,88], rather than an increase in energy expenditure[40,46,89]. Since reduction in body weight *per se* reduces insulin resistance, this may also represent a mechanism by which metformin improves insulin resistance.

To summarize, the partly divergent observations from the numerous metabolic studies regarding metformin's effect on muscle and liver (Tables 8.3 and 8.4) may reflect different mechanisms of metformin action in the basal versus the insulin-stimulated state. In the basal, post-absorptive state, the improvement of fasting hyperglycemia is mostly due to a decrease of the accelerated endogenous glucose production. This results from inhibition of both gluconeogenesis and glycogen breakdown. Direct or indirect effects on regulatory enzymes are likely to be involved. No data are available for suppression of glucose production during experimental hyperinsulinemia. However, the fact that reduction in basal glucose production occurs in the presence of lower or unaltered insulin levels suggests that glucose production in liver (and kidney[91,92]) is more sensitive to the restrictive action of insulin after treatment with metformin.

combination with sulfonylureas[86,120,121], troglitazone[122] and insulin, where a dose-sparing effect was consistently demonstrated[72–74,122–124]. Interestingly, among patients in whom sulfonylurea therapy has failed to obtain satisfactory glycemic control, the combination of bedtime NPH-insulin with metformin was advantageous compared with other combinations[124]. In contrast to insulin alone, insulin plus sulfonylurea or sulfonylurea alone, combining bedtime NPH-insulin with metformin gave a decrease in HBA1c without significant weight gain[123,124].

ADVERSE EFFECTS

While mild gastrointestinal disturbances are the most common side effects, lactic acidosis, though rare, is the most serious side effect of metformin treatment[126]. In 9875 patients one case of probable lactic acidosis was observed in 20 treatment months. The incidence of lactic acidosis is 10–20 times lower than with phenformin. This is explained by the hydroxylation of phenformin prior to renal excretion, a step which is genetically defective in 10% of Caucasians[126,127]. Metformin, in contrast, is excreted unmetabolized. In addition, in contrast to phenformin[128], metformin neither increases peripheral lactate production nor decreases lactate oxidation[40,41] making lactate accumulation unlikely. One study investigating individual cases of metformin-associated lactic acidosis showed that, in these patients, metformin should either have never been started, or should have been discontinued with the onset of acute illness[129]. Thus, strict adherence to the exclusion criteria of treatment (renal and hepatic disease, cardiac or respiratory insufficiency, severe infection, alcohol abuse, history of lactic acidosis, pregnancy, use of intravenous radiographic contrast) should minimize the risk of metformin-induced lactic acidosis.

GUIDELINES FOR THE CLINICAL USE OF METFORMIN

As recently reviewed[93], metformin or sulfonylurea therapy can be initiated when patients with NIDDM continue to have hyperglycemia despite diet and exercise. Metformin appears to be the drug of choice to start pharmacological treatment in insulin resistant and overweight/obese diabetic subjects[96,130]. However, since the antihyperglycemic effects of metformin are similar in lean and obese subjects, it can also be recommended as first-line treatment in the absence of obesity. It has been shown that the maximal antihyperglycemic effect of metformin is obtained using 2 g/day (Figure 8.5)[132]. Addition of metformin to sulfonylureas in patients with secondary sulfonylurea failure appears reasonable in view of their synergistic mechanisms of action, and has been shown to improve glycemic control. Furthermore, especially in overweight/obese patients, the addition of metformin to insulin has advantages over insulin alone[125,133]. Finally, metformin is not recommended for patients with type 1 diabetes, or in insulin-resistant states in the absence of overt type 2 diabetes. However,

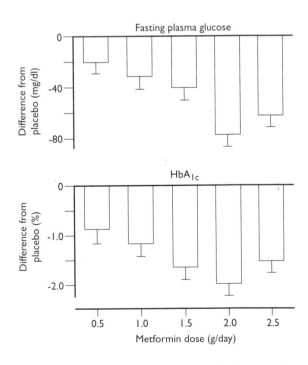

Figure 8.5 Effect of increasing metformin dose per day on fasting plasma glucose and HbA1c in type 2 diabetic patients (from Reference 132).

metformin is currently under investigation as an agent to prevent type 2 diabetes in subjects with impaired glucose tolerance as one of the three arms (versus diet and intensive life-style modification) of the Diabetes Prevention Program[131], but it has not yet been approved for use in subjects with impaired glucose tolerance.

REFERENCES

1 Bailey CJ, Day C. 1989 Traditional plant medicines as treatments for diabetes. *Diabetes Care* 1989;12:553–64.
2 Luft D, Schmulling R, Eggstein M. Lactic acidosis in biguanide-treated diabetics: a review of 330 cases. *Diabetologia* 1978;14:75–8.
3 Colwell J. Is it time to introduce metformin in the US? *Diabetes Care* 1993;16:653–5.
4 Johansen K. Efficacy of metformin in the treatment of NIDDM. *Diabetes Care* 1999;22:33–7.
5 Bailey CJ, Turner RC. Metformin. *N Engl J Med* 1996;334:574–9.
6 Dunn CJ, Peters DH. Metformin. A review of its pharmacological properties and therapeutic use in non-insulin-dependent diabetes mellitus. *Drugs* 1995;49:721–49.
7 Davidson MB, Peters AL. An overview of metformin in the treatment of type 2 diabetes mellitus. *Am J Med* 1997;102:99–110.
8 Bailey CJ. Biguanides and NIDDM. *Diabetes Care* 1992;15:755–72.
9 Klip A, Leiter L. Cellular mechanism of action of metformin. *Diabetes Care* 1990;13:696–704.
10 Bailey C. Metformin revisited: its actions and indications for use. *Diabetic Med* 1988;5:315–20.
11 Hermann L. Biguanides and sulfonylureas as combination therapy in NIDDM. *Diabetes Care* 1990;13:37–41.
12 Bailey C, Nattrass M. Treatment—metformin. *Baillieres Clin Endocrinol Metab* 1988;2:455–76.
13 UK Prospective Diabetes Study Group. Effect of intensive blood-glucose control with metformin on complications in overweight patients with type 2 diabetes (UKPDS 34). *Lancet* 1998;352:854–65.
14 DeFronzo RA, Goodman AM [The Multicenter Metformin Study Group]. Efficacy of metformin in patients with non-insulin-dependent diabetes mellitus. *N Engl J Med* 1995;333:541–9.
15 Hermann LS, Kjellström T, Nilsson-Ehle P. Effects of metformin and glibenclamide alone and in combination on serum lipids and lipoproteins in patients with non-insulin-dependent diabetes mellitus. *Diabet Metab* 1991;17:174–9.
16 Matthaei S, Stumvoll M, Kellerer M, Häring HU. Pathophysiology and pharmacological treatment of insulin resistance. *Endocrine Rev* 2000;21:585–618.
17 Ferner RE, Rawlins MD, Alberti KG. Impaired beta-cell responses improve when fasting blood glucose concentration is reduced in non-insulin-dependent diabetes. *Q J Med* 1988;66:137–46.
18 Yki-Järvinen H. Glucose toxicity. *Endocr Rev* 1992;13:415–31.
19 Goldfine ID, Iwamoto Y, Pezzino V *et al*. Effects of biguanides and sulfonylureas on insulin receptors in cultured cells. *Diabetes Care* 1984;7 (Suppl 1):54–8.
20 Pezzino V, Trischitta V, Purrello F, Vigneri R. Effect of metformin on insulin binding to receptors in cultured human lymphocytes and cancer cells. *Diabetologia* 1982;23:131–5.
21 Fantus I, Brosseau R. Mechanism of action of metformin: insulin receptor and postreceptor effects *in vitro* and *in vivo*. *J Clin Endocrinol Metab* 1986;63:898–905.
22 Lord JM, Atkins TW, Bailey CJ. Effect of metformin on hepatocyte insulin receptor binding in normal, streptozotocin diabetic and genetically obese diabetic (*ob/ob*) mice. *Diabetologia* 1983;25:108–13.
23 Pedersen O, Nielsen O, Bak J *et al*. The effects of metformin on adipocyte insulin action and metabolic control in obese subjects with type 2 diabetes. *Diabet Med* 1989;6:249–56.
24 Prager R, Schernthaner G. Insulin receptor binding to monocytes, insulin secretion, and glucose tolerance following metformin treatment: results of a double blind cross-over study in type II diabetics. *Diabetes* 1983;32:1083–6.
25 Nosadini R, Avogaro A, Trevisian R *et al*. Effect of metformin on insulin-stimulated glucose turnover and insulin binding to receptors in type II diabetes. *Diabetes Care* 1987;10:62–7.
26 Cigolini M, Bosello O, Zancanaro C *et al*. Influence of metformin on metabolic effects of insulin in human adipose tisssue *in vitro*. *Diabetes Metab* 1984;10:311–15.
27 Jacobs DB, Hayes GR, Truglia JA, Lockwood DH. Effects of metformin on insulin receptor tyrosine kinase activity in rat adipocytes. *Diabetologia* 1986;29:798–801.

28 Wollen N, Bailey CJ. Inhibition of hepatic gluco-neogenesis by metformin. Synergism with insulin. *Biochem Pharmacol* 1988;37:4353–8.

29 Alengrin F, Grossi G, Canivet B, Dolais-Kitabgi J. Inhibitory effects of metformin on insulin and glucagon action in rat hepatocytes involve post-receptor alterations. *Diabetes Metab* 1987;13:591–7.

30 Rossetti L, DeFronzo RA, Gherzi R *et al.* Effect of metformin treatment on insulin action in diabetic rats: *in vivo* and *in vitro* correlations. *Metabolism* 1990;39:425–35.

31 Matthaei S, Hamann A, Klein HH *et al.* Association of Metformin's effect to increase insulin-stimulated glucose transport with potentiation of insulin-induced translocation of glucose transporters from intracellular pool to plasma membrane in rat adipocytes. *Diabetes* 1991;40:850–7.

32 Matthaei S, Reibold JP, Hamann A *et al. In vivo* metformin treatment ameliorates insulin resistance: evidence for potentiation of insulin-induced translocation and increased functional activity of glucose transporters in obese (*fa/fa*) Zucker rat adipocytes. *Endocrinology* 1993;133:304–11.

33 Melin B, Cherqui G, Blivet M *et al.* Dual effect of metformin in cultured rat hepatocytes: potentiation of insulin action and prevention of insulin-induced resistance. *Metabolism* 1990;39:1089–95.

33A Zhou G, Myers R, Chen Y *et al.* Role of AMP-activated protein kinase in mechanism of metformin action. *J Clin Invest* 2001;108:1167–74.

34 Wollen N, Bailey CJ. Metformin potentiates the antigluconeogenic action of insulin. *Diabetes Metab* 1988;14:88–91.

35 Meyer F, Ipaktchi M, Clauser H. Specific inhibition of gluconeogenesis by biguanides. *Nature* 1967;213:203–4.

36 Argaud D, Roth H, Wiernsperger N, Leverve XM. Metformin decreases gluconeogenesis by enhancing the pyruvate kinase flux in isolated rat hepatocytes. *Eur J Biochem* 1993;213:1341–8.

37 Radziuk J, Zhang Z, Wiernsperger N, Pye S. Effects of metformin on lactate uptake and gluconeogenesis in the perfused rat liver. *Diabetes* 1997;46:1406–13.

38 Dinneen S, Gerich J, Rizza R. Carbohydrate metabolism in non-insulin-dependent diabetes mellitus. *N Engl J Med* 1992;327:707–13.

39 DeFronzo RA, Bonadonna RC, Ferrannini E. Pathogenesis of NIDDM. *Diabetes Care* 1992;15:318–68.

40 Stumvoll M, Nurjhan N, Perriello G *et al.* Metabolic effects of metformin in non-insulin-dependent diabetes mellitus. *N Engl J Med* 1995;333:550–4.

41 Cusi K, Consoli A, DeFronzo RA. Metabolic effects of metformin on glucose and lactate metabolism in noninsulin-dependent diabetes mellitus. *J Clin Endocrinol Metab* 1996;81:4059–67.

42 Prager R, Schernthaner G, Graf H. Effect of metformin on peripheral insulin sensitivity in non-insulin-dependent diabetes mellitus. *Diabetes Metab* 1986;12:346–50.

43 Jackson R, Hawa M, Jaspan J *et al.* Mechanism of metformin action in noninsulin-dependent diabetes. *Diabetes* 1987;36:632–40.

44 DeFronzo RA, Barzilai N, Simonson DC. Mechanism of metformin action in obese and lean noninsulin-dependent diabetic subjects. *J Clin Endocrinol Metab* 1991;73:1294–301.

45 Johnson AB, Webster JM, Sum C-F *et al.* The impact of metformin therapy on hepatic glucose production and skeletal muscle glycocgen synthase activity in overweight type II diabetic patients. *Metabolism* 1993;42:1217–22.

46 Perriello G, Misericordia P, Volpi E *et al.* Acute antihyperglycemic mechanisms of metformin in NIDDM. Evidence for suppression of lipid oxidation and hepatic glucose production. *Diabetes* 1994;43:920–8.

47 Frayn KN. Effects of metformin on insulin resistance after injury in the rat. *Diabetologia* 1976;12:53–60.

48 Galuska D, Zierath J, Thörne A *et al.* Metformin increases insulin-stimulated glucose transport in insulin-resistant human skeletal muscle. *Diabetes Metab* 1991;17:159–63.

49 Galuska D, Nolte LA, Zierath JR *et al.* Effect of metformin on insulin-stimulated glucose transport in isolated skeletal muscle obtained from patients with NIDDM. *Diabetologia* 1994;37: 826–32.

50 Hundal H, Ramlal T, Reyes R *et al.* Cellular mechanism of metformin action involves glucose transporter translocation from an intracellular pool to the plasma membrane in L6 muscle cells. *Endocrinology* 1992;131:1165–72.

51 Bailey CJ, Puah JA. Effect of metformin on glucose metabolism in mouse soleus muscle. *Diabetes Metab* 1986;12:212–18.

52 Frayn KN, Adnitt PI. Effects of metformin on glucose uptake by isolated diaphragm from normal and diabetic rats. *Biochem Pharmacol* 1972;21:3153–62.

53 Kozka IJ, Holman GD. Metformin blocks down regulation of cell surface GLUT4 caused by

chronic insulin treatment of rat adipocytes. *Diabetes* 1993;42:1159–65.

54 Sarabia V, Lam L, Burdett E *et al.* Glucose transport in human skeletal muscle cells in culture. Stimulation by insulin and metformin. *J Clin Invest* 1992;90:1386–95.

55 Garvey WT, Hueckstaedt TP, Matthaei S, Olefsky JM. Role of glucose transporters in the cellular insulin resistance of type II non-insulin dependent diabetes mellitus. *J Clin Invest* 1988;81:1528–36.

56 Hother-Nielsen O, Schmitz O, Andersen PH *et al.* Metformin improves peripheral but not hepatic insulin action in obese patients with type II diabetes. *Acta Endocrinol (Copenhagen)* 1989;120:257–65.

57 Wu M, Johnston P, Sheu W *et al.* Effect of metformin on carbohydrate and lipoprotein metabolism in NIDDM patients. *Diabetes Care* 1990;13:1–8.

58 DeFronzo RA. The triumvirate: B-cell, muscle, and liver: a collusion responsible for NIDDM. *Diabetes* 1988;37:667–87.

59 Riccio A, Del Prato S, Vigili de Kreutzenberg S, Tiengo A. Glucose and lipid metabolism in non-insulin dependent diabetes. Effect of metformin. *Diabetes Metab* 1991;17:180–4.

60 Detaille D, Wiernsperger N, Devos P. Potentiating effect of metformin on insulin-induced glucose uptake and glycogen metabolism with *Xenopus* oocytes. *Diabetologia* 1998;41:2–8.

61 Yoa RG, Rapin JR, Wiernsperger NF *et al.* Demonstration of defective glucose uptake and storage in erythrocytes from non-insulin dependent diabetic patients and effects of metformin. *Clin Exp Pharmacol Physiol* 1993;20:563–7.

62 Cusi K, DeFronzo RA. Metformin: a review of its metabolic effects. *Diabetes Rev* 1998;6:89–131.

63 Hundal RS, Krssak M, Dufour S *et al.* Mechanism by which metformin reduces glucose production in type 2 diabetes. *Diabetes* 2000;49:2063–9.

64 See ref. 56.

65 McIntyre HD, Ma A, Bird DM *et al.* Metformin increases insulin sensitivity and basal glucose clearance in type 2 diabetes mellitus. *Aust NZ J Med* 1991;21:714–19.

66 Widen E, Eriksson J, Groop L. Metformin normalizes nonoxidative glucose metabolism in insulin-resistant normoglycemic first-degree relatives of patients with NIDDM. *Diabetes* 1992;41:354–8.

67 Wing RR, Koeske R, Epstein LH *et al.* Long-term effects of modest weight loss in type II diabetic patients. *Arch Intern Med* 1987;147:1749–53.

68 Morel Y, Golay A, Pernegert T *et al.* Metformin treatment leads to an increase in basal, but not insulin-stimulated, glucose disposal in obese patients with impaired glucose tolerance. *Diabet Med* 1999;16: 650–5.

69 Scheen AJ, Letiexhe MR, Lefebvre PJ. 1995 Short administration of metformin improves insulin sensitivity in android obese subjects with impaired glucose tolerance. *Diabet Med* 12:985–9.

70 Diamanti Kandarakis E, Kouli C, Tsianateli T, Bergiele A. Therapeutic effects of metformin on insulin resistance and hyperandrogenism in polycystic ovary syndrome. *Eur J Endocrinol* 1998;138:269–74.

71 Moghetti P, Castello R, Negri C *et al.* Metformin effects on clinical features, endocrine and metabolic pofiles, and insulin sensitivity in polycystic ovary syndrome: a randomized, double-blind, placebo-controlled 6-month trial, followed by open, long-term clinical evaluation. *J Clin Endocrinol Metab* 2000;85:139–46.

72 Nestler JE, Jakubowicz DJ, Evans WS, Pasquali R. Effects of metformin on spontaneous and clomiphen-induced ovulation in the polycystic ovary syndrome. *N Engl J Med* 1998;338:1876–80.

73 Hermann L. Metformin: a review of its pharmacologic properties and therapeutic use. *Diabetes Metab* 1975;5:233–45.

74 McLelland J. Recovery from metformin overdose. *Diabet Med* 1985;2:410–11.

75 Mäkimattila S, Nikkilä K, Yki-Järvinen H. Causes of weight gain during insulin therapy with and without metformin in patients with Type II diabetes. *Diabetologia* 1999;42:406–12.

76 Giugliano D, Quatraro A, Consoli G *et al.* Metformin for obese, insulin-treated diabetic patients: improvement in glycaemic control and reduction of metabolic risk factors. *Eur J Clin Pharmacol* 1993;44:107–12.

77 Robinson AC, Johnston DG, Burke J *et al.* The effect of metformin on glycemic control and serum lipids in insulin-treated NIDDM patients with suboptimal metabolic control. *Diabetes Care* 1998;21:701–5.

78 Abbasi F, Carantoni M, Chen YD, Reaven GM. Further evidence for a central role of adipose tissue in the antihyperglycemic effect of metformin. *Diabetes Care* 1998;21:1301–5.

79 Cigolini M, Bosello O, Zancanaro C *et al.* Influence of metformin on metabolic effects of insulin in human adipose tisssue *in vitro*. *Diabetes Metab* 1984;10:311–15.

80 Puhakainen I, Yki-Järvinen H. Inhibition of lipolysis decreases lipid oxidation and gluconeogenesis from lactate but not fasting hyperglycemia or total hepatic glucose production. *Diabetes* 1993;42:1694–9.

81 Saloranta C, Taskinen M, Widen E *et al.* Metabolic consequences of sustained suppression of free fatty acids by acipimox in patients with NIDDM. *Diabetes* 1993;42:1559–1566.

82 Wilcock C, Bailey CJ. Sites of metformin-stimulated glucose metabolism. *Biochem Pharmacol* 1990;39:1831–4.

83 Penicaud L, Hitier Y, Ferre P, Girard J. Hypoglycaemic effect of metformin in genetically obese (*fa/fa*) rats results from an increased utilization of blood glucose by intestine. *Biochem J* 1989;262:881–5.

84 Bailey CJ, Mynett KJ, Page T. Importance of the intestine as a site of metformin-stimulated glucose utilization. *Br J Pharmacol* 1994;112:671–5.

85 Wilcock C, Bailey CJ. Accumulation of metformin by tissues of the normal and diabetic mouse. *Xenobiotica* 1994;24:49–57.

86 DeFronzo RA, Goodman AM [The Multicenter Metformin Study Group]. Efficacy of metformin in patients with non-insulin-dependent diabetes mellitus. *N Engl J Med* 1995;333:541–9.

87 Bellomo R, McGrath B, Boyce N. *In vivo* catecholamine extraction during continuous hemofiltration in inotrope-dependent patients. *ASAIO Transac* 1991;37:M324–M325.

88 Lee A, Morley JE. Metformin decreases food consumption and induces weight loss in subjects with obesity with type II non-insulin-dependent diabetes. *Obes Res* 1998;6:47–53.

89 Leslie P, Jung RT, Isles TE, Baty J. Energy expenditure in non-insulin dependent diabetic subjects on metformin or sulfonylurea therapy. *Clin Sci* 1987;73:41–5.

90 Nosadini R, Avogaro A, Trevisian R *et al.* Effect of metformin on insulin-stimulated glucose turnover and insulin binding to receptors in type II diabetes. *Diabetes Care* 1987;10:62–7.

91 Stumvoll M, Meyer C, Mitrakou A *et al.* Renal glucose production and utilization. New aspects in humans. *Diabetologia* 1997;40:749–57.

92 Meyer C, Stumvoll M, Nadkarni V *et al.* Abnormal renal and hepatic glucose metabolism in type 2 diabetes mellitus. *J Clin Invest* 1998;102:619–24.

93 Bailey CJ, Turner RC. Metformin. *N Engl J Med* 1996;334:574–9.

94 Dunn CJ, Peters DH. Metformin. A review of its pharmacological properties and therapeutic use in non-insulin-dependent diabetes mellitus. *Drugs* 1995;49:721–49.

95 Davidson MB, Peters AL. An overview of metformin in the treatment of type 2 diabetes mellitus. *Am J Med* 1997;102:99–110.

96 Johansen K. Efficacy of metformin in the treatment of NIDDM. *Diabetes Care* 1999;22:33–7.

97 UK Prospective Diabetes Study Group. Effect of intensive blood-glucose control with metformin on complications in overweight patients with type 2 diabetes (UKPDS 34). *Lancet* 1998;352:854–65.

98 Lalor BC, Bhatnagar D, Winocour PH *et al.* Placebo-controlled trial of the effects of guar gum and metformin on fasting blood glucose and serum lipids in obese, type 2 diabetic patients. *Diabet Med* 1990;7:242–5.

99 Teupe B, Bergis K. Prospective randomized two-years clinical study comparing additional metformin treatment with reducing diet in type 2 diabetes. *Diabetes Metab* 1991;17:213–7.

100 Dornan T, Heller S, Peck G, Tattersall R. Double-blind evaluation of efficacy and tolerability of metformin in NIDDM. *Diabetes Care* 1991;14:342–4.

101 Nagi D, Yudkin J. Effects of metformin on insulin resistance, risk factors for cardiovascular disease, and plasminogen activator inhibitor in NIDDM subjects. *Diabetes Care* 1993;16:621–9.

102 Tessari P, Biolo G, Bruttomesso D *et al.* Effects of metformin treatment on whole-body and splanchnic amino acid turnover in mild type 2 diabetes. *J Clin Endocrinol Metab* 1994;79:1553–60.

103 Grant PJ. The effects of high- and medium-dose metformin therapy on cardiovascular risk factors in patients with type II diabetes. *Diabetes Care* 1996;19:64–6.

104 Rains S, Wilson G, Richmond W, Elkeles R. The effect of glibenclamide and metformin on serum lipoproteins in type 2 diabetes. *Diabet Med* 1988;5:653–8.

105 Collier A, Watson HH, Patrick AW *et al.* Effect of glycaemic control, metformin and gliclazide on platelet density and aggregability in recently diagnosed type 2 (non-insulin-dependent) diabetic patients. *Diabetes Metab* 1989;15:420–5.

106 Josephkutty S, Potter JM. Comparison of tolbutamide and metformin in elderly diabetic patients. *Diabet Med* 1990;7:510–14.

107 Noury J, Nandeuil A. Comparative three-month study of the efficacies of metformin and gliclazide in the treatment of NIDD. *Diabetes Metab* 1991;17:209–12.

108 Boyd K, Rogers C, Boreham C *et al.* Insulin, gliben-clamide or metformin treatment for non insulin dependent diabetes: heterogenous responses of standard measures of insulin action and insulin secretion before and after differing hypoglycaemic therapy. *Diabetes Res* 1992;19:69–76.

109 Hermann LS, Kjellström T, Schersten B *et al.* Therapeutic comparison of metformin and sulfonylurea, alone and in various combinations. *Diabetes Care* 1994;17:1100–9.

110 Campbell IW, Menzies DG, Chalmers J *et al.* One year comparative trial of metformin and glipizide in type 2 diabetes mellitus. *Diabetes Metab* 1994;20:394–400.

111 Selby JV, Ettinger B, Swain BE, Brown JB. First 20 months' experience with use of metformin for type 2 diabetes in a large health maintenance organization. *Diabetes Care* 1999;22:38–44.

112 Reaven G, Johnston P, Hollenbeck C *et al.* Combined metformin-sulfonylurea treatment of patients with noninsulin-dependent diabetes in fair to poor glycemic control. *J Clin Endocrinol Metab* 1992;74:1020–26.

113 Giugliano D, De Rosa N, Di Maro G *et al.* Metformin improves glucose, lipid metabolism, and reduces blood pressure in hypertensive, obese women. *Diabetes Care* 1993;16:1387–90.

114 Landin K, Tengborn L, Smith U. Treating insulin resistance in hypertension with metformin reduces both blood pressure and metabolic risk factors. *J Intern Med* 1991;229:181–7.

115 Schneider J, Erren T, Zöfel P, Kaffarnik H. Metformin-induced changes in serum lipids, lipoproteins, and apoproteins in non-insulin-dependent diabetes mellitus. *Atherosclerosis* 1990;82:97–103.

116 Landin K, Tengborn L, Smith U. Metformin and metoprolol CR treatment in non-obese men. *J Intern Med* 1994;235:335–41.

117 Landin K, Tengborn L, Smith U. Effects of metformin and metoprolol CR on hormones and fibrinolytic variables during a hyperinsulinemic, euglycemic clamp in man. *Thromb Haemost* 1994;71:783–7.

118 Pentikainen PJ, Voutilainen E, Aro A *et al.* Cholesterol lowering effect of metformin in combined hyperlipidemia: placebo controlled double blind trial. *Ann Med* 1990;22:307–12.

119 Grant PJ, Stickland MH, Booth NA, Prentice CR. Metformin causes a reduction in basal and post-venous occlusion plasminogen activator inhibitor-1 in type 2 diabetic patients. *Diabet Med* 1991;8:361–5.

120 Gin H, Freyburger G, Boisseau M, Aubertin J. Study of the effect of metformin on platelet aggregation in insulin-dependent diabetics. *Diabetes Res Clin Pract* 1989;6:61–7.

121 Marena S, Tagliaferro V, Montegrosso G *et al.* Metabolic effects of metformin addition to chronic glibenclamide treatment in type 2 diabetes. *Diabetes Metab* 1994;20:15–19.

122 Groop L, Widen E. Treatment strategies for secondary sulfonylurea failure. Should we start insulin or add metformin? Is there a place for intermittent insulin therapy? *Diabetes Metab* 1991;17:218–23.

123 Hanuschak LN. Metformin useful in combination with exogenous insulin [letter]. *Diabetes Care* 1996;19:671–2.

124 Aviles-Santa A, Sinding J, Raskin P. Effects of metformin in patients with poorly controlled, insulin treated type 2 diabetes. *Ann Int Med* 1999;131:182–8.

125 Yki-Järvinen H, Ryysy L, Nikkilä K *et al.* Comparison of bedtime insulin regimens in patients with type 2 diabetes mellitus. *Ann Int Med* 1999;130:389–96.

126 Misbin RI, Green L, Stadel BV *et al.* Lactic acidosis in patients with diabetes treated with metformin. *N Engl J Med* 1998;338:265–6.

127 Oates NS, Shah RR, Idle JR, Smith RL. Influence of oxidation polymorphism on phenformin kinetics and dynamics. *Clin Pharmacol Ther* 1983;34:827–34.

128 Kreisberg R, Pennington L, Boshell B. Lactate turnover and gluconeogenesis in obesity: effect of phenformin. *Diabetes* 1970;19:64–9.

129 Lalau JD, Lacroix C, Compagnon P *et al.* Role of metformin accumulation in metformin-associated lactic acidosis. *Diabetes Care* 1995;18:779–84.

130 Nathan DM. Some answers, more questions, from UKPDS. *Lancet* 1999;352:832–3.

131 The Diabetes Prevention Program Diabetes Group. The Diabetes Prevention Program. Design and methods for a clinical trial in the prevention of type 2 diabetes. *Diabetes Care* 1999;22:623–34.

132 Garber A, Duncan T, Goodman A *et al.* Efficacy of metformin in type-II diabetes: results of a double-blind, placebo-controlled, dose-response trial. *Am J Med* 1997;102:491–7.

133 Buse J. Combining insulin and oral agents. *Am J Med* 2000;108 (Suppl 1):23–32.

134 Fery F, Plat L, Balasse EO. Effects of metformin on the pathways of glucose utilization after oral glucose in non-insulin-dependent diabetes mellitus patients. *Metabolism* 1997;46:227–33.

9

Alpha-glucosidase inhibitors (AGIs)

Markolf Hanefeld

INTRODUCTION

There is a strong role for impaired insulin secretion in the development and progression of type 2 diabetes, in particular due to a deficit in the early phase response to glucose load, as well as increasing insulin resistance[1,2]. It is believed that most subjects developing type 2 diabetes pass through a phase of impaired glucose tolerance (IGT). In this process—following the glucose toxicity theory—excessive postprandial hyperglycemia may act in a 'vicious circle', with harmful effects on both the insulin-producing beta-cells[3] and insulin sensitivity[4], leading to chronic hyperglycemia and progressive deterioration of diabetes, as shown in the UK Prospective Diabetes Study (UKPDS)[5].

There is increasing evidence that postprandial or 2 h post-challenge hyperglycemia is an independent risk factor for cardiovascular disease[6,7] and all-cause mortality[8,9]. Among other factors (Table 9.1), postprandial hyperglycemia strongly depends on the amount and of absorbed monosaccharides and velocity of absorption in the small intestine. Carbohydrates should account for $\geq 50\%$ of the daily supply of calories in type 2 diabetes. Monosaccharides play only a minor role as dietary carbohydrates since they consist mainly of complex carbohydrates, such as starch ($\sim 60\%$), and disaccharides, such as sucrose ($\sim 30\%$). Complex carbohydrates and disaccharides must be hydrolysed by intestinal and pancreatic enzymes before they can be transported through the mucosa of the bowel. Thus, any medication

Table 9.1 Determinants of postprandial glucose excursion

Fasting plasma glucose

(Early phase) insulin secretion

Hepatic gluconeogenesis

Insulin sensitivity of target tissues

Meal composition and quantity

Additives to meal (alcohol, spices, fibers)

Gastric emptying, intestinal digestion and
    absorption

Duration of the meal

Gut hormones (enteroinsular axis)

Medication affecting insulin sensitivity
    (beta-blockers, angiotensin converting-enzyme
    inhibitors etc.)

Physical activity

that delays breakdown of complex carbohydrates should decrease postprandial hyperglycemia and improve insulin sensitivity, as well as protecting the beta-cells of the pancreas.

Following the incretin concept[10], the digestion of carbohydrates in lower parts of the small intestine and colon may also have a stimulating effect on gastrointestinal hormones, such as glucagen-like peptide 1 (GLP_1)[11]. Alpha glucosidase inhibitors (AGIs—acarbose, miglitol, voglibose) are oral antidiabetics that specifically inhibit α-glucosidases in the brush border of the small intestine, these enzymes are essential for the release of glucose from more complex carbohydrates[12,13].

STRUCTURE AND MODE OF ACTION OF AGIs

The concept of alpha-glucosidase inhibition was developed by Puls *et al.*[14], as a method of controlling the release of glucose from starch and sucrose—the major carbohydrate components in western diet. Inhibition affects both degradation of complex carbohydrates and digestion of disaccharides. An appropriate agent (acarbose) of microbial origin (culture filtrates of actinoplanes) was first described in 1977 by Schmidt[12], and this inhibitor was introduced onto the market in 1990. Three AGIs are now in therapeutic use worldwide (Figure 9.1), and are frequently prescribed in Central and South Europe and Asia.

Acarbose is a pseudotetrasaccharide with a nitrogen bound between the first and second glucose unit. This modification of a natural tetrasaccharide is important for its high affinity for active centres of alpha-glucosidases of the brush border of the small intestine, and for its stability. 1-Desoxynojirimycin is the parent compound of other AGIs such as miglitol which, in contrast with acarbose, is a small molecule, similar to glucose. Voglibose is produced by reductive alkylation of valiolamine[15,16].

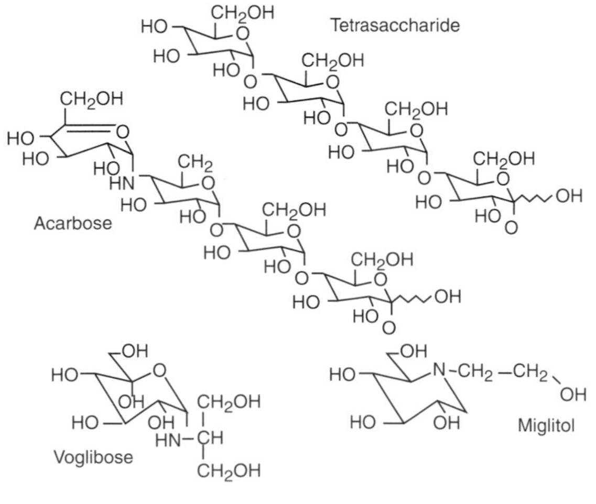

AGIs act as competitive inhibitors because of their high affinity for alpha-glucosidases, they block the enzymatic reaction particularly because of their nitrogen component. Thus, AGIs must be present at the site of enzymatic action at the same time as the carbohydrates. The effect on post-load glucose excursion and insulin after a starch-containing mixed meal is shown in Figure 9.2. In principle, all three AGIs act in the same way, by inhibiting alpha-glucosidase enzymes in the brush border of the upper part of the small intestine. There are, however, some differences with respect to the inhibitory efficiency on various alpha-glucosidases, which may be responsible for differences in the frequency of side-effects. Acarbose is most effective on glucoamylase, followed by sucrase, maltase and dextranase[14]. It also has a degree of inhibition of alpha-amylase, but has no effect on beta-glucosidases, such as lactase. Miglitol is a more potent inhibitor of disaccharide digesting enzymes, such as sucrase and maltase, than acarbose, and is also active on isomaltase but has no effect on alpha-amylase[17]. It also weakly interacts as a pseudomonosaccharide with the intestinal sodium-dependent glucose transporter, without having a clinically relevant effect on glucose absorption[18]. Voglibose is isolated from *Streptomyces* culture broths. It is a strong AGI with little effect on alpha-amylase.

PHARMACOLOGY OF AGIs

Acarbose is poorly absorbed (0.5–1.7%), and is degraded in the large intestine by bacterial enzymes into glucose, maltose and acarviosine. A non-absorbed fraction of 60–80% is excreted via feces (Table 9.2). About 35% of an oral dose appears as degradation products in the urine[15]; this may be clinically relevant in cases of impaired kidney function. Miglitol is rapidly absorbed and transported in the intestine in the same way as glucose. It is concentrated in the brush border of the small intestine. Miglitol is unchanged and excreted dose-dependently by the kidneys. Only 3–5% voglibose is absorbed, and it is almost completely excreted via the feces. After oral administration, about 90% unchanged drug remains. By extrapolation, the

Figure 9.1 Structures of AGIs in clinical use.

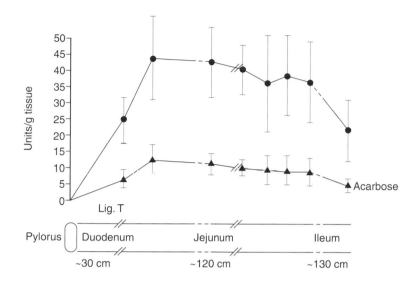

Figure 9.2 Mode of action of acarbose on postprandial glucose excursion.

most striking differences between AGIs in clinical use are with respect to absorption. Neither acarbose nor voglibose are absorbed in their active form, whereas miglitol is almost completely absorbed in the upper part of the small intestine, it has a long-lasting presence in

Table 9.2 Summary of pharmacological characteristics of AGIs in clinical use[15]

Drug	Acarbose	Miglitol	Voglibose
Extent of absorption	Low	High, dose dependent	Low, dose dependent
Unchanged drug	< 2%	> 96%	< 6%
Metabolites	< 35%	—	—
Bioavailability	< 2%	> 96%	< 6%
Clearance	Mainly renal by glomerular filtration	Mainly renal by glomerular filtration	Mainly renal
Protein binding	Low to high Species-dependent Saturable	Low	Low to high Species-dependent Saturable
Distribution	Extracellular Low tissue affinity	Extracellular Low tissue affinity	Low tissue affinity
Metabolism	Extrasystemic in the intestine	None	None
Excretion			
Faecal	> 65%	Low	Almost complete
Renal	< 35%	> 96%	< 5%
Biliary	< 5%	< 0.2%	—

Table 9.3 Dose–response of efficacy of acarbose[44] and miglitol[62] on plasma glucose (PG) and HbA1c after 24 weeks treatment

Change (%)	Fasting PG	1 h postprandial PG	2 h postprandial PG	HbA1c
Placebo	– 0.4	– 1.5	– 2.7	7.83
Acarbose (three times per day)				
25 mg	– 4.3	– 11.6	– 11.3	7.37
50 mg	– 11.8	– 15	15.5	7.08
100 mg	– 7.5	– 13	12.5	6.98
200 mg	– 15	– 19.4	22.5	6.79
Placebo	NA	NA	+ 3.6	+ 0.29
Miglitol				
25	NA	NA	– 8.4	– 0.08
50	NA	NA	– 17.7	– 0.18
100	NA	NA	– 28.9	– 0.60
				HbA1c initial
NA = not available				6.1–10.4%

an effect on fasting plasma glucose occurring after 8–12 weeks. In clinical practice, glucose monitoring should therefore include measurements 2 h after major meals. In a meta-analysis of 13 controlled clinical trials with acarbose[35], the mean reduction in fasting glucose was 24 mg ± 7.2 mg dL^{-1}, in postprandial glucose it was 54 mg ± 15.8 mg dL^{-1} and in HbA1c 0.90 ± 0.25%. The efficacy of therapeutic doses of miglitol is in the same range, with a somewhat higher effect on HbA1c at a dosage of 50 mg three times per day, versus the same dose of acarbose[45]. Fewer data are available for voglibose. Comparative studies with other oral antidiabetics show a weaker effect on HbA1c than for metformin[33], except for one study that showed a similar efficacy[46]. Except in one publication[47], a stronger effect of tolbutamide[48] and glibenclamide at 24–56 weeks follow-up has been consistently shown[35]. It is a consistent finding that metformin and the sulfonylureas were more effective on fasting blood glucose control, whereas the AGIs were superior in the control of postprandial hyperglycemia. No reliable data have been published comparing the new 'prandial' insulin-secretagogues repaglinide and nateglinide with AGIs in face-to-face investigations.

Combination therapy of AGIs with oral antidiabetics and insulin in type 2 diabetes

AGIs are frequently used as add-on therapy in patients insufficiently treated with sulfonylurea or metformin monotherapy. Less data exist on add-on therapy with AGIs as the first-line treatment. Recently, early combinations of oral antidiabetics with AGIs, to achieve perfect control of the glucotriad with lower dosage of the single drug and fewer side-effects, have been discussed. Co-administration of AGIs to patients treated with metformin has an effect complementary to the major action of metformin, reducing hepatic gluconeogenesis and improving peripheral glucose disposal. There is now evidence from long-term studies that the addition of acarbose[49] or miglitol[50] results in an average decrease of HbA1c of 0.8–0.9% in placebo-controlled long-term trials. The addition of metformin to patients on acarbose was particularly useful in fasting hyperglycemia[51].

Titration of metformin therapy should be started with a bed-time tablet, to optimize the effect on gluconeogenesis after midnight. Long-acting sulfonylureas, such as glibenclamide and glimepiride, are still in widespread use as first-line drugs. Addition of AGIs in subjects insufficiently treated with these insulin secretagogues has a synergistic effect to better control postprandial hyperglycemia. As consistently shown in controlled trials[48-51], an average reduction in HbA1c of 0.8–0.9% can be achieved with this combination. Long-term data so far available suggest that add-on therapy with AGIs may delay the chronic progression of beta-cell failure, by protecting them from postprandial glucose spikes[24,25]. Information comparing combination treatment of sulfonylurea plus metformin with the combination of either drugs with AGIs is scarce. Less favorable results are available on the combination of AGIs with insulin treatment in type 2 diabetes[52]. The only moderately successful option in this trial was the combination of day-time AGI with bed-time injection of a long-acting insulin.

AGIs AS ADJUNCT IN TYPE 1 DIABETES

AGIs have been used as adjunct in type 1 diabetic patients whose postprandial glucose excursions cannot be adequately controlled with an insulin regimen[53]. They reduce rapid rise in the early postprandial phase, and prevent spikes and troughs in the premeal phase[54]. This smoothing effect is beneficial to avoid hypoglycemic episodes and acute hunger attacks before meals, due to delayed gastric emptying. A reduction of 0.5% in HbA1c, by addition of acarbose, was shown in a 24-week placebo-controlled study, but no significant impact on frequency of hypoglycemic episodes was shown. In another study, nocturnal hypoglycemia was shown to be prevented when acarbose was given before dinner. Insulin dosage remained unchanged in the majority of cases. AGIs may therefore be helpful in brittle diabetes if best efforts to control postprandial glucose spikes by insulin regimen adjustment does not give an adequate control of postprandial glucose excursions. The same applies for excessive premeal hunger and nocturnal hypoglycemia.

SAFETY AND SIDE-EFFECTS

AGIs are the safest oral antidiabetics, but are associated with a rather high frequency of gastrointestinal side effects because they inhibit digestion of carbohydrates. With > 1 million patients having taken acarbose for > 1 year, no serious adverse event has been reported. As antihyperglycemic agents they carry no risk of causing hypoglycemia. When given in combination with oral insulin secretagogues, the frequency of hypoglycemic episodes was reduced[48] and there was no increase in hypoglycemias observed in insulin-treated patients[49]. A minor weight loss is observed in monotherapy with AGIs, and the weight gain caused by sulfonylureas is reduced if AGIs are added to the treatment regimen[48].

Gastrointestinal side-effects frequently noted by patients are meteorism, flatulence, diarrhoea (Table 9.4) or simple 'abdominal discomfort'. Gastrointestinal complaints exhibit strong inter-individual and regional differences, depending on nutrition habits, diet compliance and advice from medical staff. During the first weeks of treatment, and within the first 3 months, the enzyme content of the lower part of the small intestine increases and most of the carbohydrates reaching this part of the bowel can be digested here. This is indicated by a decrease in gastrointestinal side-effects to < 10% in long-term follow-up studies[25]. No malabsorption of carbohydrates is observed, together with

Table 9.4 Gastrointestinal and other side-effects, extrapolation from controlled and surveillance studies

Effect	Percentage
Meteorism	15–60
Flatulence	20–70
Diarrhea	5–16
Spasm and abdominal discomfort	3–4
Constipation	< 1
Headache	< 1
Nausea and vomiting	≈ 5

AGIs as add-on therapy, a further reduction of HbA1c of 0.4–0.54% was obtained. This combination may be useful in avoiding weight gain and gaining better control of postprandial hyperglycemia.

PRACTICALITIES

Efficacy, side-effects and compliance strongly depend on rational indications, education of patients on how to use the drug, and good dietary advice. Even with good clinical practice, a considerable variation in response and side-effects is seen. Side-effects depend, among other things, on the dose and time intervals for titration of optimal therapeutic dosage. It is essential to start with low doses of 25 mg of acarbose or miglitol twice a day, with a stepwise increase in 2–3 week intervals. A study in type 2 diabetes patients treated with sulfonylurea compared the tolerability of stepwise increase with an initial dose of 100 mg three times per day of acarbose[22]. The stepwise increase in dosage reduced specific side-effects from 70% to 31%. The maximum dosage for acarbose and miglitol is usually 100 mg three times per day. There are, however, controlled studies that show that 200 mg three times per day is more effective, but has a higher adverse event rate[44].

After 3–4 weeks gastrointestinal side-effects diminish to < 20% in almost all studies. In long-term studies, the great majority of discontinuation because of side-effects happens during the first 3 months. It is important to reinforce dietary advice before treatment and if side-effects occur. A high content of raffined carbohydrates, and a diet rich in fat and protein are causes of gastrointestinal discomfort. Patients should be made aware that side-effects are due to the mode of action, are mostly transient, and can be prevented by prudent diet. Table 9.6 summarizes some guidelines for patients to help overcome difficulties.

Patients should also take blood glucose levels twice a week at 1–2 h postprandial to see the benefit of treatment. With AGI treatment, fasting blood glucose levels in the first month of treatment is not indicative of therapy success.

USE OF AGIs IN PRIMARY PREVENTION OF TYPE 2 DIABETES

IGT is an accepted risk factor for both conversion to diabetes and cardiovascular disease. Prevalence of IGT in all nations with a westernized life-style is > 15% in subjects aged > 40 years. Primary prevention efforts with life-style modification are therefore of high priority. In terms of medical intervention in subjects with IGT, AGIs have been shown to improve insulin sensitivity and reduce proinsulin secretion[26–28]. In the STOP-NIDDM trial, a large placebo-controlled multinational study of 1429 subjects with IGT, acarbose reduced the annual incidence of diabetes by 36% in the intention to treat analysis[24]. This was associated with a significantly lower event-rate of cardiovascular co-morbidities. No serious adverse event associated with acarbose was observed during the 3.4 year follow-up.

CONTRAINDICATIONS

AGIs have very few contraindications: these are pregnancy and lactation period. They should not be given to patients with diverticulosis, large hernia, acute gastrointestinal diseases, colitis, inclusive and obstructive diseases of the bowel because of their adverse effects on gas production in the bowel, particularly in the colon. For acarbose, but not for miglitol, severe renal insufficiency (serum creatinine > 3.5 mg dL^{-1}) is a contraindication. Bile acid adsorbents, such as

---

Table 9.6 Advice to patients to overcome difficulties with AGIs

Start low, go slow

Prefer nutrients with complex carbohydrates (rice, pasta, full bread, vegetables, fruits)

Avoid refined carbohydrates (sugar, sweets)

Take only three meals

Avoid laxatives, such as sugar alcohols (sorbitol)

Control your postprandial blood glucose to experience the efficacy of treatment

In most cases gastrointestinal side-effect are transient

cholestyramine, antacid agents and digestive enzymes, may decrease the efficacy of these drugs. Clinical experience has shown that combination with the lipase inhibitor orlistat can exaggerate the gastrointestinal side-effects of both drugs, but no controlled data are available. Laxatives and sugar alcohols, such as sorbitol with its high osmotic activity, increase gastro-intestinal adverse reactions and should not be taken with AGI treatment.

REFERENCES

1 Haffner SM, Miettinen H, Gaskill SP, Stern MP. Decreased insulin action and insulin secretion predict the development of impaired tolerance. *Diabetologia* 1996;39:1201–7.

2 Tripathy D, Carlsson M, Almgren P *et al*. Insulin secretion and insulin sensitivity in relation to glucose tolerance. Lessons from the Bothnia study. *Diabetes* 2000;49:975–80.

3 Pratley RE, Weyer C. The role of impaired early insulin secretion in the pathogenesis of type II diabetes mellitus. *Diabetologia* 2001;44:929–45.

4 Gerich JE. Is insulin resistance the principal cause of type II diabetes? *Diabet Obes Metab* 1999;1:257–63.

5 UK Prospective Diabetes Study (UKPDS) Group. Intensive blood-glucose control with sulphony-lureas or insulin compared with conventional treatment and risk of complications in patients with type II diabetes (UKPDS 33). *Lancet* 1998;352:837–53.

6 Smidt N, Barzilay J, Shaffer D *et al*. Fasting and 2-hour post-challenge serum glucose measures and risk of incident cardiovascular events in the elderly. The Cardiovascular Health Study. *Arch Intern Med* 2002;162:209–16.

7 de Vegt F, Dekker JM, Ruhe HG *et al*. Hypergycaemia is associated with all cause and cardiovascular mortality in the Hoorn popula-tion: the Hoorn Study. *Diabetologia* 1999;42:926–31.

8 Hanefeld M, Schmechel H, Schwanebeck U, Lindner J [The DIS-Group]. Predictors of cor-onary heart disease and death in NIDDM: the Diabetes Intervention Study experience. *Diabetologia* 1997;40:123–4.

9 DECODE Study group on behalf of the European Diabetes Epidemiology Study Group. Glucose tolerance and mortality: comparison of WHO and American Diabetic Association diagnostic criteria. *Lancet* 1999;354:617–21.

10 Creutzfeldt W. The entero-insular axis in type 2 diabetes—incretins as therapeutic agent. *Exp Clin Endocrinol Diabetes* 2001;109(Suppl.2):288–303.

11 Göke B, Herrmann C, Göke R *et al*. Intestinal effects of alpha-glucosidase inhibitors: Absorption of nutrients and enterohormonal changes. *Eur J Clin Invest* 1994;24(Suppl.3):25–30.

12 Schmidt DD, Frommer W, Junge B *et al*. Alpha-glucosidase inhibitors. New complex oligosac-charides of microbial origin. *Naturwissenschaften* 1977;64:535–6.

13 Puls W, Keup U, Krause HP *et al*. Glucosidase inhibition. A new approach to the treatment of diabetes, obesity and hyperlipoproteinemia. *Naturwissenschaften* 1977;64:536–7.

14 Puls W. Pharmacology of glucosidase inhibitors *Oral Antidiabetics* 1996;119:497–525.

15 Krause HP, Ahr HJ. Pharmacokinetics and metabolism of glucosidase inhibitors. In: Kuhlmann J, Puls W, editors. *Handbook of experi-mental pharmacology*: *oral antidiabetics*. Vol. 119. Berlin: Springer, 1996: 541–5.

16 Taylor R, Bardolph E. Clinical evaluation of glucosidase inhibitors. *Oral Antidiabetics* 1996;119:633–46.

17 Junge B, Matzke M, Stoltefuss J. Chemistry and structure–activity relationships of glucosidase inhibitors. In: Kuhlmann J, Puls W, editors. *Handbook of experimental pharmacology*: *oral antidia-betics*. Vol. 119. Berlin: Springer, 1996: 541–5.

18 Joubert PH, Venter HL, Foukaridis GN. The effect of miglitol and acarbose after an oral glucose load: a novel hypoglycaemic mechanism. *Br J Clin Pharmacol* 1990;30:391–6.

19 Caspary WF. Sucrose malabsorption in men after ingestion of alpha-glucosidase hydrolase inhibitor. *Lancet* 1978;i:1231–3.

20 Holt RR, Atillasoy E, Lindenbaum J *et al*. Effects of acarbose on fecal nutrients, colonic pH, and short chain fatty acids and rectal proliferative indices. *Metabolism* 1996;45:1179–87.

21 Toeller M. Modulation of intestinal glucose absorption: postponement of glucose absorption by alpha-glucosidase inhibitors. In: Mogensen CE, Standl E, editors. *Pharmacology of diabetes 93–112*. Berlin: De Gruyter, 1991.

22 May C. Efficacy and tolerability of stepwise increasing dosage of acarbose in patients with non-insulin-dependent diabetes (NIDDM)

treated with sulfonylureas. *Diabetes Stoffwechsel* 1995;4:3–7.

23 Caspary WF, Lembke B, Creutzfeldt W. Inhibition of human intestinal alpha-glucoside hydrolase activity by acarbose and clinical consequences. In: Creutzfeldt W, editor. *Proceedings First International Symposium on Acarbose, Montreux, October 1981.* Amsterdam: Excerpta Medica, 27–37.

24 Chiasson JL, Josse RG, Gomis R *et al.* For the STOP-NIDDM trial research group. Acarbose can prevent the progression of impaired glucose tolerance to type 2 diabetes mellitus: the STOP-NIDDM trial. *Lancet.* 2002;359:2072–7.

25 Mertes G. Safety and efficacy of acarbose in the treatment of Type 2 Diabetes: data from 5-year surveillance study. *Diabetes Res Clin Pract* 2001;52:193–204.

26 Chiasson JL, Josse RG, Leiter LA *et al.* The effect of acarbose on insulin sensitivity in subjects with impaired glucose tolerance. *Diabetes Care* 1996;19:1190–3.

27 Laube H, Linn T, Heyen P. The effects of acarbose on insulin sensitivity and proinsulin in overweight subjects with impaired glucose tolerance. *Exp Clin Endocrinol Diabetes* 1998;106:231–3.

28 Shinozaki K, Suzuki M, Ikebuchi M *et al.* Improvement of insulin sensitivity and dyslipidemia with a new alpha-glucosidase inhibitor, voglibose, in non-diabetic hyperinsulinemic subjects. *Metabolism* 1996;45:731–7.

29 Schnack C , Prager RJF, Winkler J *et al.* Effect of 8 week α-glucosidase inhibition on metabolic control, C-peptide secretion, hepatic glucose output and peripheral insulin sensitivity in poorly controlled type 2 diabetic patients. *Diabetes Care* 1989;12:537–43.

30 Calle-Pascal A, Garcia-Honduvilla J, Martin Alvarez PJ *et al.* Influence of 16-week monotherapy with acarbose on cardiovascular risk factors in obese subjects with non-insulin-dependent diabetes mellitus: a controlled, double-blind comparison study with placebo. *Diabetes Metab* 1996;22:201–2.

31 Meneilly G, Ryan EA, Radziuk J *et al.* Effect of acarbose on insulin sensitivity in elderly patients with diabetes. *Diabetes Care* 2000;23:1162–7.

32 Hillebrand I, Boehme K, Frank G *et al.* Effects of the glycoside hydrolase inhibitor (BAY g 5421) on post-prandial blood glucose, serum insulin and triglycerides levels in man. In: Creutzfeldt, editor. *Frontiers of hormone research, the enteroinsular axis.* Basel: Karger, 1979;7:290–1.

33 Hanefeld M, Fischer S, Schulze J *et al.* Therapeutic potentials of acarbose as first-line drug in NIDDM insufficiently treated with diet alone. *Diabetes Care* 1991;14:732–7.

34 Hanefeld M, Haffner SM, Menschikowski M *et al.* Different effects of acarbose and glibenclamide on proinsulin and insulin profiles in people with type 2 diabetes. *Diabetes Res Clin Pract* 2002;55:221–7.

35 Leboritz HE. α-glucosidase inhibitors as agents in the treatment of diabetes. *Diabetes Rev* 1998;6:132–45.

36 Qualmann C, Nauck MA, Holst JJ *et al.* Glucagon-like peptide 1 (GLP-1) [17-36 amide] secretion in response to luminal sucrose from the upper and lower gut: a study using α-glucosidase inhibition (acarbose). *Scand J Gastroenterol* 1995;30:892–6.

37 Göke B, Fuder H, Wieckhorst G *et al.* Voglibose is an efficient alpha-glucosidase inhibitor and mobilize the endogenous GLP-1 reserve. *Digestion* 1995;56:493–501.

38 Göke B, Herrmann C, Göke R *et al.* Intestinal effects of alpha-glucosidase inhibitors: absorption of nutrients and enterohormonal changes. *Eur J Clin Invest* 1994;24(Suppl. 3):25–30.

39 Holman RR, Turner RC, Cull CA *et al.* A randomised double-blind trial of acarbose in type 2 diabetes shows improved glycemic control over 3 years (UK Prospective Diabetes Study 44). *Diabetes Care* 1999;22:960–4.

40 Wolever TMS, Chiasson JL, Josse RG *et al.* Small weight loss on long-term acarbose therapy with no change in dietary pattern or nutrient intake of individuals with non-insulin-dependent diabetes. *Int J Obes Relat Metab Disord* 1997;21:756–63.

41 Leonardt W, Hanefeld M, Fischer S *et al.* Beneficial effects on serum lipids in noninsulin-dependent diabetics by acarbose treatment. *Arzt Forschung* 1991;41:735–8.

42 Johnston PS, Feig PU, Coniff RF *et al.* Chronic treatment of African–American type 2 diabetes patients with type 2 diabetic patients with alpha-glucosidase inhibition. *Diabetes Care* 1998;21:416–21.

43 Coniff RF, Shapiro JA, Robbins D *et al.* Reduction in glycosylated hemoglobin and postprandial hyperglycemia by acarbose in patients with NIDDM: a placebo-controlled dose comparison study. *Diabetes Care* 1995;18:817–24.

44 Fischer S, Hanefeld M, Spengler M *et al.* European study on dose–response relationship of acarbose as a first-line drug in non-insulin-dependent diabetes mellitus: efficacy and safety of low and high doses. *Acta Diabetol* 1998;35:34–40.

45 Rybka J, Göke B, Sissmann J. European comparative study of 2 α-glucosidase inhibitors, miglitol and acarbose [abstract] *Diabetes* 1999;44(Suppl.1):101.

46 Hoffmann J, Spengler M. Efficacy of 24-week monotherapy with acarbose, metformin or placebo in dietary-treated NIDDM patients: the Essen II Study. *Am J Med* 1997;103:483–90.

47 Hoffmann J, Spengler M. Efficacy of 24-week monotherapy with acarbose, glibenclamide, or placebo in NIDDM patients. The Essen Study. *Diabetes Care* 1994;17:561–6.

48 Coniff RF, Shapiro JA, Seaton TB, Bray GA. Multicenter, placebo-controlled trial comparing acarbose with placebo, tolbutamide and tolbutamide-plus-acarbose in non-insulin-dependent diabetes mellitus. *Am J Med* 1998;98:443–51.

49 Chiasson JL, Josse RG, Hunt JA *et al.* The efficacy of acarbose in the treatment of patients with non-insulin-dependent diabetes mellitus: a multicenter controlled clinical trial. *Ann Intern Med* 1994;121:928–35.

50 Chiasson JL, Naditch L and the Miglitol Canadian University Investigator Group. The synergistic effect of miglitol plus metformin combination therapy in the treatment of type 2 diabetes. *Diabetes Care* 2001;24:989–94.

51 Hanefeld M, Bär K. Effizienz und Sicherheit der Kombinationsbehandlung von Typ-2-Diabetikern mit Acarbose und Metformin. *Diabetes Stoff* 1998;7:186–90.

52 Kelley DE, Schimel D, Bidot P *et al.* Efficacy and safety of acarbose in insulin-treated patients with type 2 diabetes. *Diabetes Care* 1998;21:2056–61.

53 Dimitriadis G, Hatziagellki E, Alexopoulos F. *et al.* Effects of α-glucosidase inhibition on meal glucose-tolerance and timing of insulin administration in patients with type I diabetes mellitus. *Diabetes Care* 1991;14:393–8.

54 Hollander P, Pi-Sunyer X, Coniff RF. Acarbose in the treatment of type 1 diabetes. *Diabetes Care* 1997;20:248–53.

55 Mertes G. Efficacy and safety of acarbose in the treatment of Type 2 diabetes: data from a 2-year surveillance study. *Diab Res Clin Pract* 1998;40:63–70.

56 Hollander PA. Safety profile of acarbose and alpha glucosidase inhibitor. *Drugs* 1992;44(Suppl. 3):47–53.

57 Gentile S, Turco S, Guarino G *et al.* Aminotransferase activity and acarbose treatment in patients with type-2 diabetes. *Diabetes Care* 1999;22:1217.

58 Ben-Am H, Krivo N, Nagachandran P *et al.* Interaction between digoxin and acarbose. *Diabetes Care* 1999;22:860–1.

59 Scheen AJ, Ferreira Alves de Megalheas AC, Salvatore T *et al.* Reduction of the acute bioavailability of metformin by the α-glucosidase inhibitor acarbose in normal man. *Eur J Clin Invest* 1994;24(Suppl. 3):50–4.

60 Hanefeld M, Fischer S, Julius U *et al.* and the DIS Group. Risk factors for myocardial infarction and death in newly detected NIDDM: the Diabetes Intervention Study, 11-year follow-up. *Diabetologia* 1996;39:1577–83.

61 Temelkova-Kurktschiev T, Köhler C, Henkel E *et al.* Post-challenge plasma glucose and glycemic spikes are more strongly associated with atherosclerosis than fasting glucose or HbA1c level. *Diabetes Care* 2000;23:1830–4.

62 Drent ML. Miglitol as single oral hypoglycemic agent in type 2 diabetes [Abstract]. *Diabetologia* 1994;37 (Suppl. 1):211.

10

Thiazolidinediones

Elise Hardy and Serge A Jabbour

INTRODUCTION

Thiazolidinediones are insulin-sensitizing agents used in the treatment of type 2 diabetes. These compounds have a thiazolidine-2-4-dione structure in common, and each has a distinct side chain (Figure 10.1). There are two of these agents currently on the market: pioglitazone (Actos), and rosiglitazone (Avandia), both of which were approved in the USA by the Food and Drug Administration (FDA) in 1999. Troglitazone (Rezulin), the first available thiazolidinedione, was withdrawn in March 2000 due to concerns about severe liver toxicity. This chapter reviews this class of agents and their role in the treatment of type 2 diabetes.

PHARMACOKINETICS AND METABOLISM

Pioglitazone

Pioglitazone is available in 15, 30, and 45 mg tablets. When administered after fasting, pioglitazone is measurable in the serum within 30 min[1]. Peak concentrations occur in 2 h. Administration of pioglitazone with food delays the time to peak concentration to 3–4 h, but does not diminish the extent of absorption. Pioglitazone alone has a half-life of 3–7 h; pioglitazone in combination with its active metabolites have a half-life of 16–24 h. Steady-state concentrations are reached within 7 days. Its volume of distribution is 0.63 L kg^{-1} and is > 99% protein-bound, principally to albumin. Pioglitazone is metabolized by hydroxylation, oxidation, and conjugation, into active and inactive metabolites. M-III, (active keto derivative), and M-IV, (active hydroxy derivative) are the principal metabolites in humans. Hepatic metabolism is extensive, and occurs via

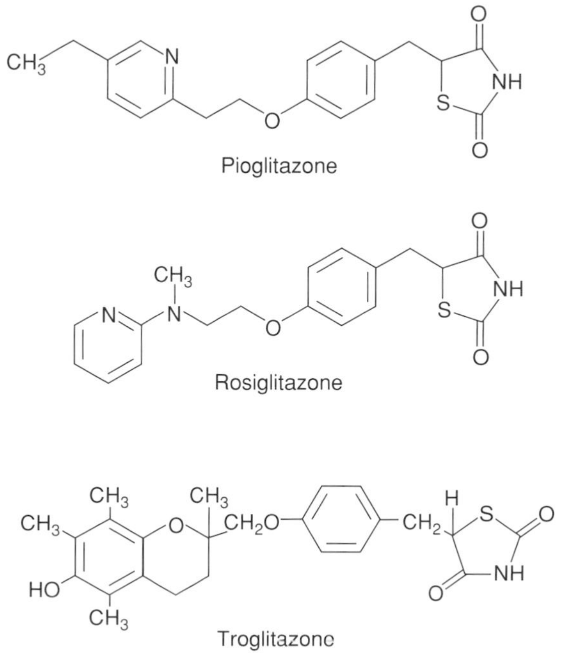

Figure 10.1 Structures of three thiazolidinediones.

assessed the effect of adding pioglitazone to stable therapy with metformin. Three hundred and twenty-eight subjects received pioglitazone 30 mg daily in combination with metformin or placebo. At 16 weeks, HbA1c was reduced by about 0.6% in the pioglitazone + metformin group compared with baseline. In contrast, HbA1c increased by almost 0.2% in the placebo + metformin group[20].

A 16-week trial compared the combination of insulin + pioglitazone with insulin alone. Five hundred and sixty-six patients with type 2 diabetes who were being treated with insulin received pioglitazone 15 mg or 30 mg once daily or placebo in addition to their pre-study insulin regimen. HbA1c was reduced by 0.73 and 1.0% in the 15 mg and 30 mg groups, respectively, compared with insulin + placebo[21].

Rosiglitazone

Rosiglitazone is effective as monotherapy in the treatment of type 2 diabetes (see Table 10.2). In a 26-week study of 959 patients with type 2 diabetes, rosiglitazone was given as 4 mg or 8 mg once a day, or 2 mg or 4 mg twice a day[22]. Drug-naïve patients showed the greatest reductions in HbA1c. The effect was dose-dependent, and the 4 mg twice daily dosing proved superior to the 8 mg once daily dosing (ΔHbA1c –0.8% and –1.1% compared to baseline, respectively). In patients who were not drug-naïve, the 4 mg twice daily dose was again the most effective, resulting in HbA1c decreases of –0.54% in patients who were previously treated with a single agent, and –0.43% in patients who were previously treated with multiple agents. In this study, fasting plasma glucose declined starting at the fourth week of therapy, and was maximally lowered at weeks 8–12. In another trial, rosiglitazone monotherapy in doses of 2 mg or 4 mg twice daily reduced HbA1c at 26 weeks by 1.1% or 1.5%, respectively, in patients with and without previous exposure to antihyperglycemic agents[23]. Both of these trials found that

Table 10.2 Summary of rosiglitazone trials

No. of patients	Duration of treatment	Additional medication	Change in HbA1c (%) compared with baseline					Reference
			PBO	4 mg QD	2 mg BID	8 mg QD	4 mg BID	
			Drug-naïve					
959	26 weeks	None	+0.35	–0.85	–0.89	–0.80	–1.11	22
			Prior oral monotherapy					
			+0.98	+0.14	+0.02	–0.26	–0.54	
			Prior oral combination therapy					
			—	—	—	—	–0.43	
493	26 weeks	None	+0.9	—	–0.3	—	–0.6	23
348	26 weeks	Metformin +PBO or +RSG	+0.45	–0.56	—	–0.78	—	25
319	26 weeks	Insulin +PBO or +RSG	+0.1	–0.6	—	–1.2	—	26

PBO = placebo, RSG = rosiglitazone.

HbA1c decreased initially at 8 weeks and achieved maximal effects at weeks 18–26.

Rosiglitazone has been studied in combination with sulfonylureas and metformin. In a trial of 574 patients with type 2 diabetes who were receiving therapy with a sulfonylurea, low-dose rosiglitazone or placebo were added to glibenclamide, gliclazide or glipizide. The maximum dose of rosiglitazone in this study was 2 mg twice daily, which resulted in the greatest decrease in HbA1c (–1.0% compared with placebo + sulfonylurea) at 26 weeks[24]. The combination of metformin and rosiglitazone was also found to be effective therapy in a study of 348 patients with type 2 diabetes. These patients discontinued all antihyperglycemic agents except for metformin, and were then randomized to receive placebo, rosiglitazone 4 mg once daily or 8 mg once daily. At week 26, HbA1c had decreased compared to baseline by 0.56% and 0.78% in the 4 mg and 8 mg groups, respectively, and increased by 0.45% in the placebo group[25].

In a recent trial, the addition of rosiglitazone to insulin therapy was evaluated in patients with type 2 diabetes. Patients who were taking insulin were randomized to receive placebo or rosiglitazone 4 mg or 8 mg once daily. HbA1c was reduced by a greater degree in the rosiglitazone groups at 26 weeks of therapy (–0.6% and –1.2% in the 4 mg and 8 mg groups, respectively, compared to baseline). The placebo group exhibited an average increase of 0.1% in HbA1c[26].

EFFECTS ON PANCREATIC INSULIN SECRETION

Thiazolidinediones consistently result in reduced plasma insulin levels, reflecting increased insulin sensitivity. Although these agents do not directly stimulate beta-cell insulin secretion, studies indicate that they restore normal insulin responsiveness in humans and animals with insulin resistance.

Accumulation of triglycerides in pancreatic islet cells may contribute to beta-cell dysfunction in insulin resistance[27]. In diabetic rats, troglitazone caused a 52% decrease in islet triglycerides, which correlated with improvements in insulin

responsiveness to glucose stimulation[27]. A study on obese rats demonstrated that rosiglitazone therapy resulted in the prevention or reduction of pathologic islet cell abnormalities, such as beta-cell hypertrophy[28].

Troglitazone has been shown to improve the ability of the beta-cell to respond to glucose in patients with impaired glucose tolerance[29], and to restore the pulsatile nature of insulin secretion by the beta-cell, which is impaired in patients with insulin resistance[30]. Rosiglitazone in combination with metformin has also been shown to improve beta-cell function to a greater extent than treatment with metformin alone[25].

LIPID EFFECTS

All three thiazolidinediones have been shown to increase high density lipoprotein (HDL) and modestly increase low-density lipoprotein (LDL) in patients with type 2 diabetes[1,3]. Pioglitazone and troglitazone also significantly decrease triglyceride levels[31].

In clinical trials, pioglitazone 45 mg raised HDL by 19.1% and LDL by 6.0% compared with baseline after 26 weeks of therapy[1]. Triglycerides fell by 9.3%. Pioglitazone was also reported to have dramatic effects on HDL in patients whose HDL levels fell into the lowest category. In a study of 408 patients with type 2 diabetes, pioglitazone 45 mg increased HDL by 31.6% after 26 weeks in patients who had HDL levels < 35 mg dL^{-1}. In contrast, HDL levels rose by 12.9% in patients who had baseline HDL levels > 45 mg dL^{-1} (Reference 32).

Compared with the baseline, rosiglitazone 8 mg raised LDL and HDL by up to 18.6% and 14.2% at 26 weeks and by 12.1% and 18.5% at 52 weeks, respectively. These results show that LDL levels remained stable, whereas HDL levels continued to rise over time. Triglyceride levels in rosiglitazone-treated patients were variable and usually not statistically different from placebo controls[3].

Small, dense LDL particles may be particularly atherogenic and are associated with type 2 diabetes[33]. Small studies have found that pioglitazone and rosiglitazone both increase the proportion of large, buoyant LDL particles, which may be less atherogenic[34,35]. The clinical significance of this effect is not yet clear.

Two small unblinded, non-randomized studies compared the effects of pioglitazone versus rosiglitazone on lipid values[36,37]. One study involving 144 patients with type 2 diabetes previously treated with troglitazone showed that conversion to pioglitazone or rosiglitazone resulted in equivalent effects on glycemic control. However, rosiglitazone increased triglyceride levels, whereas pioglitazone decreased these levels relative to previous treatment with troglitazone. Rosiglitazone also increased LDL slightly in contrast to pioglitazone, which decreased LDL. Neither agent had a dramatic effect on HDL after conversion from troglitazone[36]. In another small study comparing all three thiazolidinediones in patients with type 2 diabetes, pioglitazone again resulted in a decrease in triglycerides, whereas rosiglitazone increased these levels[37]. Further studies are required to confirm whether there is indeed a significant difference in the effects of these two medications on lipid profiles.

CARDIOVASCULAR EFFECTS

Atherosclerosis and vascular wall

PPARγ is expressed in human vascular smooth muscle cells (VSMCs)[38], endothelial cells[39], and macrophages[40]. It may directly regulate steps in the atherosclerotic process via its effects on these tissues. Table 10.3 lists the variety of effects attributed to PPARγ activation by thiazolidinediones. Most of these effects are anti-atherogenic. Interestingly, however, exposure to oxidized LDL induces PPARγ expression in monocytes and enables them to bind to and take up the oxidized LDL particles. In addition, PPARγ has been detected in high levels in the foam cells of atherosclerotic lesions[41,42]. *In vivo* studies thus far

---

Table 10.3 Effects of PPARγ activation by thiazolidinediones

Biological effect	Effect of PPARγ activation	Agent (tissue) studied	Reference
VSMC			
VSMC apoptosis	Stimulation	PIO (rat)	43
VSMC proliferation (insulin, bFGF, PDGF, EGF-dependent)	Inhibition	TRO/PIO (rat)	44,45
VSMC migration (PDGF-dependent)	Inhibition	TRO (human, rat)	38,44
Expression of Angiotensin II type 1 Receptor	Inhibition	TRO/PIO (rat)	46
Elaboration of matrix metalloproteinase 9	Inhibition	TRO (human)	38,47
Endothelial cells			
Expression of VCAM-1 and ICAM-1 adhesion molecules	Inhibition	TRO (human)	48
Monocytes/macrophages			
Macrophage apoptosis	Stimulation	RSG (human)	40
Elaboration of cytokines (TNFα, IL-1β, IL-6)	Inhibition	TRO (human)	49
Uptake of oxidized LDL	Stimulation	RSG (human)	41,42
CD 36 expression by macrophages	Stimulation	RSG (human)	41,42

bFGF = basic fibroblast growth factor ; PDGF = platelet-derived growth factor; EGF = epidermal growth factor; VCAM-1 = vascular cell adhesion molecule-1; ICAM-1 = intercellular adhesion molecule-1; PAI-1 = plasminogen activator inhibitor-1; TRO = troglitazone, PIO = pioglitazone, RSG = rosiglitazone.

show a benefit of treatment with thiazolidinediones on animal and human vasculature.

Troglitazone inhibited VSMC proliferation and migration, and reduced neointima/media area ratio by 62% relative to controls in balloon-injured rat aortas[44]. Rosiglitazone strongly inhibited atherosclerosis development in LDL-receptor-deficient mice, a finding that correlated with increased insulin sensitivity[50]. In another study, rosiglitazone decreased atherosclerotic lesion area by 60% compared with controls in mice with angiotensin II-accelerated atherosclerosis[51]. Pioglitazone has also been shown to markedly decrease neointimal cross-sectional areas relative to controls in air-injured rat carotid arteries[52].

In human studies, troglitazone and pioglitazone treatment resulted in a significant decrease in common carotid arterial intimal and medial complex thickness (IMT) (–0.080 mm, $n = 135$ and –0.084 mm, $n = 106$, respectively) after 3–6 months of treatment, as measured by carotid ultrasound. In contrast, control patients had a slight increase in IMT. There was not a significant correlation between this finding and HbA1c values[53,54]. Large randomized studies evaluating cardiovascular outcomes are necessary.

Cardiac structure and function

Thiazolidinediones were initially associated with increased cardiac weight in animal studies. However, human echocardiographic studies on rosiglitazone (4 mg twice daily) or pioglitazone (maximum 60 mg daily) for up to a year have shown no adverse effects on left ventricular mass or cardiac output[55,56].

BLOOD PRESSURE EFFECTS

Thiazolidinediones have been shown to lower blood pressure in animal and human studies. Mechanisms for the blood-pressure lowering effect have not been fully elucidated. An improvement in insulin resistance is likely responsible, at least in part.

PPARγ has been identified in vascular smooth muscle cells (VSMCs)[57]. Animal studies on VSMCs have shown that thiazolidinediones cause a decrease in intracellular calcium movement (troglitazone)[58,59], a blunted contractile response to calcium (pioglitazone)[60], an inhibition of endothelin-1 synthesis (troglitazone)[61], and possible stimulation of prostaglandin synthesis (troglitazone, not rosiglitazone)[62].

Rosiglitazone prevented the development of hypertension in insulin-resistant rats[63]. Pioglitazone was shown to lower blood pressure in rats to an extent that was not correlated with alterations in fasting insulin concentrations[60].

Troglitazone has been shown to reduce blood pressure in human studies among patients both with and without hypertension. In one study, troglitazone was shown to decrease blood pressure from 164/94 mmHg to 146/82 mmHg after 8 weeks of treatment in 18 patients with type 2 diabetes and hypertension. These effects were significantly correlated with a decrease in insulin resistance, as measured by plasma insulin levels[64]. Another study compared treatment with troglitazone and with glyburide in 22 patients with type 2 diabetes and normal blood pressure, at rest and during mental stress while taking an arithmetic test[65]. After 6 months of treatment, glucose was lowered equally in both groups. Systolic blood pressure was significantly decreased by troglitazone (–9 mmHg at rest and –11 mmHg during mental stress) but not glyburide. Peripheral vascular resistance was also decreased by troglitazone.

RENAL EFFECTS

PPARγ is expressed in the rat kidney, primarily in the collecting ducts[66]. Its presence in this location suggests that it may be involved in water and sodium retention[67]. It has also been detected in the mesangial cells of rats[68,69].

Plasminogen activator inhibitor-1 (PAI-1) indirectly inhibits the degradation of glomerular matrix, potentially leading to glomerulosclerosis. Treatment with troglitazone inhibited expression of PAI-1 in the rat glomerulus[69]. Treatment with troglitazone also caused decreased expression of alpha-smooth muscle actin, a marker of mesangial cell activation[68]. PPARγ may therefore be directly involved in the regulation of mesangial proliferation and glomerulosclerosis.

All three thiazolidinediones have been shown to delay the onset of proteinuria, or reduce established proteinuria in animals[28,68–70]. Troglitazone caused a reduction in urinary albumin excretion in rats, independent of its effect on blood glucose or blood pressure[69].

Improvement in renal function has also been observed in humans treated with thiazolidinediones. In patients with type 2 diabetes and microalbuminuria, troglitazone reduced urine albumin/creatinine ratio after 4 weeks of treatment, whereas metformin had no effect, despite superior improvement in glycemic control[71]. In a small randomized study, pioglitazone significantly reduced urinary albumin excretion from 142.8 to 48.4 µg min^{-1} after 3 months of treatment in patients with type 2 diabetes and microalbuminuria[72]. Those treated with glibenclamide or voglibose did not have a change in their urinary albumin excretion. Rosiglitazone also reduced albumin:creatinine ratio in patients with type 2 diabetes in a dose-dependent fashion[23]. Larger, longer-term studies are necessary to confirm the effects of thiazolidinediones on the delay and improvement of diabetic nephropathy.

EFFECTS ON DIABETIC RETINOPATHY

PPARγ is expressed in bovine retinal endothelial cells[73]. Troglitazone and rosiglitazone were studied in mice to determine their effects on retinal neovascularization. *In vitro*, thiazolidinediones inhibited the effects of vascular endothelial growth factor (VEGF) on migration and proliferation of retinal endothelial cells. *In vivo*, intravitreous injection of both agents inhibited development of retinal neovascularization. These results indicate that thiazolidinediones may be effective in the treatment of diabetic retinopathy pending further research in humans[73].

THIAZOLIDINEDIONES IN POLYCYSTIC OVARY SYNDROME

Polycystic ovary syndrome (PCOS) is characterized by menstrual irregularities, infertility, hyperandrogenism, obesity and insulin resistance.

Troglitazone has been studied in the treatment of this condition. In a recent trial involving 305 patients with PCOS, troglitazone resulted in significant improvement in several clinical parameters[74]. Ovulation occurred over 50% of the time in patients treated with the highest dose of troglitazone (600 mg) compared to 12% of the time with placebo. Thirteen pregnancies occurred on troglitazone compared with three on placebo, in spite of contraceptive counseling. Hirsutism and free testosterone levels significantly improved as well. In addition, there was a significant reduction in HbA1c and in circulating insulin levels on troglitazone therapy. These results point to an exciting new treatment option for PCOS; however, the newer thiazolidinediones have not yet been studied in this syndrome.

ADVERSE EFFECTS

The most commonly reported adverse events with both pioglitazone and rosiglitazone were upper respiratory tract infection and headache (see Table 10.4).

Hepatic effects

In combined North American clinical trials, troglitazone was associated with significant transaminase elevations (> 3 times the upper limit of normal) in about 2% of patients compared to 0.6% with placebo[75]. Troglitazone use led to liver failure and death in > 20 cases[76], resulting in its withdrawal from the market by the FDA in March 2000.

Unlike troglitazone, rosiglitazone and pioglitazone demonstrated no significant incidence of transaminase elevations in premarketing randomized clinical trials. Shortly after its approval by the FDA, two isolated reports of complex clinical cases suggesting a possible association between rosiglitazone and non-fatal hepatic toxicity were published[77–79]. However, to date the worldwide surveillance experience for both rosiglitazone and pioglitazone in millions of patients has shown convincingly that there is no 'signal' of hepatic damage, consistent with the clinical trial data. Nevertheless, given the thiazolidinedione structural similarity of piogli-

Table 10.4 Common adverse effects of therapy with pioglitazone and rosiglitazone[1,3]

Adverse effect	Rosiglitazone		Pioglitazone	
	Drug	Placebo	Drug	Placebo
URI	9.9	8.7	13.2	8.5
Headache	5.9	5.0	9.1	6.9
LFT abnormalities[a]	0.2	0.2	0.26	0.25
Edema	4.8	1.3	4.8	1.2
Anemia	1.9	0.7	1.0	0

[a]Defined as alanine aminotransferase (ALT) levels > 3 times the upper limit of normal. URI = upper respiratory tract infection, LFT = liver function test. Values expressed as percentages.

tazone and rosiglitazone to troglitazone, the FDA has maintained the requirement that clinical use of these drugs is accompanied by measurement of serum alanine aminotransferase (ALT) levels prior to initiation of therapy with either agent[1,3]. These drugs are not indicated in patients whose ALT levels exceed 2.5 times the upper limit of normal, or in patients who have clinical evidence of liver disease. If drug therapy is initiated, ALT should be checked every 2 months for the first year and periodically thereafter, or if symptoms of hepatotoxicity occur. If ALT levels exceed three times the upper limit of normal, the blood test should be repeated. If the abnormality persists, the drug should be discontinued immediately.

Hypoglycemia

In patients taking a sulfonylurea or insulin, the addition of pioglitazone or rosiglitazone may result in hypoglycemia, usually apparent beginning at 4 weeks of therapy. Under these circumstances, the sulfonylurea or insulin dose should be reduced and therapy with the thiazolidinedione continued.

Edema

Ankle edema occurred in about 5% of patients treated with rosiglitazone or pioglitazone. Edema was more frequent in insulin combination therapy with either drug (about 15% compared with 5.4–7% with insulin alone). Possible mechanisms include fluid retention and increased endothelial permeability[80]. In case reports, the edema has not been responsive to diuretics[81,82].

Anemia

Anemia was reported in 1% of patients treated with pioglitazone and 1.9% with rosiglitazone. In pioglitazone-treated patients, hemoglobin decreased by 2–3% within the first 4–12 weeks and remained stable thereafter[1]. Rosiglitazone also caused a decrease in hemoglobin of up to 1 g dL^{-1} (Reference 3). This effect is most likely related to hemodilution secondary to a slight increase in plasma volume[83]. Studies have shown that thiazolidinediones do not cause hemolysis, or affect red cell mass or erythropoiesis[83,84].

Weight gain

Pioglitazone and rosiglitazone are both associated with dose-dependent weight gain. The average weight gain was 0.5–3.5 kg in patients treated with either drug as monotherapy. When either drug was combined with insulin or a sulfonylurea, the weight gain was more dramatic. Mechanisms for weight gain with thiazolidinediones may include increased adipogenesis resulting from PPAR-γ activation, fluid retention, and increased appetite[85]. In a recent report, patients with a shorter duration of diabetes and higher body mass index (BMI) were significantly more likely to gain weight on pioglitazone therapy[86].

Cardiac effects

Patients with New York Heart Association Class III and IV cardiac status were excluded from clinical trials for both pioglitazone and rosiglitazone, and neither agent is indicated in this condition. Pulmonary edema unresponsive to diuretic therapy has been reported with troglitazone and rosiglitazone in patients who had a previous history of cardiomyopathy or congestive heart failure[82]. However, heart failure has also occurred in patients without a prior history of this condition. The rate of new onset or worsening heart failure is reported as 3% in rosiglitazone 8 mg in combination with insulin, compared with 1% on insulin alone[3]. These agents should be discontinued in patients who develop signs or symptoms of cardiac decompensation.

Ovulation

As discussed above, ovulation may be induced in previously anovulatory women treated with thiazolidinediones. Premenopausal women should be alerted to the possibility of becoming pregnant on these medications.

CONCLUSION

Thiazolidinediones are safe and effective therapy in most patients with type 2 diabetes. Preliminary reports indicate that these agents have many beneficial effects beyond mere glycemic control. In the future, long-term outcome studies evaluating heart disease and microvascular complications will offer more insight into the effects of therapy with these agents.

REFERENCES

1   *Prescribing information for pioglitazone.* Takeda Pharmaceuticals, 2000.
2   Aoyama E, Tsujiuchi H, Asahi S *et al. In vitro* studies on the metabolic pathways of pioglitazone [Abstract 418-P]. *Diabetes* 2001;50(Suppl 2):A105.
3   *Prescribing information for rosiglitazone.* Smith Kline Beecham Pharmaceuticals, 2001.
4   Freed MI, Allen A, Jorkasky DK, DiCicci RA. Systemic exposure to rosiglitazone is unaltered by food. *Eur J Clin Pharmacol* 1999;55:53–6.
5   Carey RA, Liu Y. Pioglitazone does not markedly alter oral contraceptive or hormone replacement therapy pharmacokinetics [abstract 405-P]. *Diabetes* 2000;49(Suppl 1):A100.
6   Inglis AML, Miller AK, Culkin KT *et al.* Freed MI. Rosiglitazone, a PPARγ agonist, does not alter the pharmacokinetics of oral contraceptives [abstract 0443]. *Diabetes* 2000;48(Suppl 1):A103.
7   Adams M, Montague CT, Prins JB *et al.* Activators of peroxisome proliferator-activated receptor gamma have depot-specific effects on human preadipocyte differentiation. *J Clin Invest* 1997; 100:3149–53.
8   Vidal-Puig AJ, Considine RV, Jimenez-Liñan M *et al.* Peroxisome proliferator-activated receptor gene expression in human tissues: effects of obesity, weight loss, and regulation by insulin and glucocorticoids. *J Clin Invest* 1997;99:2416–22.
9   Roden M, Price TB, Perseghin G *et al.* Mechanism of free fatty acid-induced insulin resistance in humans. *J Clin Invest* 1996;97:2859–65.
10 Oakes ND, Thalen PG, Jacinto SM, Ljung B. Thiazolidinediones increase plasma-adipose tissue FFA exchange capacity and enhance insulin-mediated control of systemic FFA availability. *Diabetes* 2001;50:1158–65.

11 Yonemitsu S, Nishimura H, Shintani M *et al.* Troglitazone induces GLUT4 translocation in L6 myotubes. *Diabetes* 2001;50:1093–101.

12 Sandouk T, Reda D, Hofmann C. The antidiabetic agent pioglitazone increases expression of glucose transporters in 3T3-F442A cells by increasing messenger ribonucleic acid transcript stability. *Endocrinology* 1993;133:352–9.

13 Iwata M, Haruta T, Usui I *et al.* Pioglitazone ameliorates tumor necrosis factor-alpha-induced insulin resistance by a mechanism independent of adipogenic activity of peroxisome proliferator-activated receptor-gamma. *Diabetes* 2001;50: 1083–92.

14 Inzucchi SE, Maggs DG, Spollett GR *et al.* Efficacy and metabolic effects of metformin and troglitazone in type II diabetes. *N Engl J Med* 1998;338:867–72.

15 Nolan JJ, Bernhard L, Beerdsen P *et al.* Improvement in glucose tolerance and insulin resistance in obese subjects treated with troglitazone. *N Engl J Med* 1994;331:1188–93.

16 Petersen KF, Krssak M, Inzucchi S *et al.* Mechanism of troglitazone action in type 2 diabetes. *Diabetes* 2000;49:827–31.

17 Maggs DG, Buchanan TA, Burant CF *et al.* Metabolic effects of troglitazone monotherapy in type 2 diabetes mellitus: a randomized, double-blind, placebo-controlled trial. *Ann Intern Med* 1998;128:176–85.

18 Aronoff S, Rosenblatt S, Braithwaite S *et al.* Pioglitazone hydrochloride improves glycemic control in the treatment of patients with type 2 diabetes. *Diabetes Care* 2000;23:1605–11.

19 Kipnes M S, Krosnick A, Rendell MS *et al.* Pioglitazone hydrochloride in combination with sulfonylurea therapy improves glycemic control in patients with type 2 diabetes mellitus: a randomized, placebo-controlled study. *Am J Med* 2001;111:10–17.

20 Einhorn D, Rendell M, Rosenzweig J *et al.* Pioglitazone hydrochloride in combination with metformin in the treatment of type 2 diabetes mellitus: a randomized, placebo-controlled study. *Clin Ther* 2000;22:1395–1409.

21 Rubin C, Egan J, Schneider R. Combination therapy with pioglitazone and insulin in patients with type 2 diabetes [abstract 0474]. *Diabetes* 1999;48(Suppl 1):A110.

22 Phillips LS, Grunberger G, Miller E *et al.* Once- and twice-daily dosing with rosiglitazone improves glycemic control in patients with type 2 diabetes. *Diabetes Care* 2001;24:308–15.

23 Lebovitz LE, Dole JF, Patwardhan R *et al.* Rosiglitazone monotherapy is effective in patients with type 2 diabetes. *J Clin Endocrinol Metab* 2001;86:280–8.

24 Wolffenbuttel BHR, Gomist R, Squatrito S *et al.* Addition of low-dose rosiglitazone to sulphony-lurea therapy improves glycaemic control in type 2 diabetic patients. *Diabet Med* 2000;17:40–7.

25 Fonseca V, Rosenstock J, Patwardhan R, Salzman A. Effect of Metformin and rosiglitazone combination therapy in patients with type 2 diabetes mellitus: a randomized controlled trial. *J Am Med Assoc* 2000;283:1695–1702.

26 Raskin P, Rendell M, Riddle MC *et al.* A randomized trial of rosiglitazone therapy in patients with inadequately controlled insulin-treated type 2 diabetes. *Diabetes Care* 2001;24:1226–32.

27 Shimabukuro M, Zhou YT, Lee Y, Unger RH. Troglitazone lowers islet fat and restores beta cell function of Zucker diabetic fatty rats. *J Biol Chem* 1998;273:3547–50.

28 Buckingham RE, Al-Barazanji KA, Toseland CD *et al.* Peroxisome proliferator-activated receptor-gamma agonist, rosiglitazone, protects against nephropathy and pancreatic islet abnormalities in Zucker fatty rats. *Diabetes* 1998:47:1326–34.

29 Cavaghan MK, Ehrmann DA, Byrne MM, Polonsky KS. Treatment with the oral antidiabetic agent troglitazone improves β cell responses to glucose in subjects with impaired glucose tolerance. *J Clin Invest* 1997;100:530–7.

30 Ehrmann DA, Schneider DJ, Sobel BE *et al.* Troglitazone improves defects in insulin action, insulin secretion, ovarian steroidogenesis, and fibrinolysis in women with polycystic ovary syndrome. *J Clin Endocrinol Metab* 1997;82: 2108–16.

31 Fonseca V, Valiquett TR, Huang SM *et al.* Troglitazone monotherapy improves glycemic control in patients with type 2 diabetes mellitus: a randomized, controlled study. *J Clin Endocrinol Metab* 1998;83:3169–76.

32 Prince MJ, Zagar AJ, Robertson KE. Effect of pioglitazone on HDL-C, a cardiovascular risk factor in type 2 diabetes [abstract 514-P]. *Diabetes* 2001;50(Suppl 2):A128.

33 Barakat HA, Carpenter JW, McLendon VD *et al.* Influence of obesity, impaired glucose tolerance, and NIDDM on LDL structure and composition. Possible link between hyperinsulinemia and atherosclerosis. *Diabetes* 1990;39:1527–33.

34 Ovalle F, Bell DSH. Differing effects of thiazolidinediones on LDL subfractions [abstract 1896-PO]. *Diabetes* 2001;50(Suppl 2):A453–4.

35 Winkler K, Friedrich I, Nauck M *et al.* Pioglitazone reduces dense LDL-particles in patients with type 2 diabetes [abstract 592-P]. *Diabetes* 2001;50(Suppl 2):A147.

36 Gegick CS, Altheimer MD. Comparison of effects of thiazolidinediones on cardiovascular risk factors: observations from a clinical practice. *Endocrinol Pract* 2001;7:162–9.

37 King AB. A comparison in a clinical setting of the efficacy and side effects of three thiazolidinediones. *Diabetes Care* 2000;23:557.

38 Marx N, Schonbeck U, Lazar MA *et al.* Peroxisome proliferator-activated receptor gamma activators inhibit gene expression and migration in human vascular smooth muscle cells. *Circ Res* 1998;83:1097–103.

39 Marx N, Bourcier T, Sukhova GK *et al.* PPARgamma activation in human endothelial cells increases plasminogen activator inhibitor type-1 expression: PPARgamma as a potential mediator in vascular disease. *Arterioscler Thromb Vasc Biol* 1999;19:546–51.

40 Chinetti G, Griglio S, Antonucci M *et al.* Activation of proliferator-activated receptors alpha and gamma induces apoptosis of human monocyte-derived macrophages. *J Biol Chem* 1998;273:25573–80.

41 Tontonoz P, Nagy L, Alvarez JGA *et al.* PPARγ Promotes monocyte/macrophage differentiation and uptake of oxidized LDL. *Cell* 1998;93:241–52.

42 Nagy L, Tontonoz P, Alvarez JGA *et al.* Oxidized LDL regulates macrophage gene expression through ligand activation of PPARγ. *Cell* 1998;93:229–40.

43 Aizawa Y, Kawabe J, Hasebe N *et al.* Pioglitazone enhances cytokine-induced apoptosis in vascular smooth muscle cells and reduces intimal hyperplasia. *Circulation* 2001;104:455–60.

44 Law RE, Meehan WP, Xi XP *et al.* Troglitazone inhibits vascular smooth muscle cell growth and intimal hyperplasia. *J Clin Invest* 1996;98:1897–905.

45 Dubey RK, Zhang HY, Reddy SR *et al.* Pioglitazone attenuates hypertension and inhibits growth of renal arteriolar smooth muscle in rats. *Am J Physiol* 1993;265:R726–32.

46 Takeda K, Ichiki T, Tokunou T *et al.* Peroxisome proliferator-activated receptor γ activators downregulate angiotensin II type 1 receptor in vascular smooth muscle cells. *Circulation* 2000;102:1834–9.

47 Marx N, Sukhova G, Murphy C *et al.* Macrophages in human atheroma contain PPARgamma: differentiation-dependent peroxisomal proliferator-activated receptor gamma (PPARgamma) expression and reduction of MMP-9 activity through PPARgamma activation in mononuclear phagocytes *in vitro*. *Am J Pathol* 1998;153:17–23.

48 Pasceri V, Wu HD, Willerson JT, Yeh ETH. Modulation of vascular inflammation *in vitro* and *in vivo* by peroxisome proliferator-activated receptor-[gamma] activators. *Circulation* 2000;101:235.

49 Jiang C, Ting AT, Seed B. PPAR-gamma agonists inhibit production of monocyte inflammatory cytokines. *Nature* 1998;391:82–6.

50 Li AC, Brown KK, Silvestre MJ *et al.* Peroxisome proliferator-activated receptor gamma ligands inhibit development of atherosclerosis in LDL receptor-deficient mice. *J Clin Invest* 2000;106:523–31.

51 Collins AR, Noh G, Hsueh WA, Law RE. PPARγ ligands attenuate angiotensin-II accelerated atherosclerosis in male low density receptor deficient (LDLR-/-) mice [abstract 292-PP]. *Diabetes* 2001;50(Suppl 2):A72–3.

52 Yoshimoto T, Naruse M, Shizume H *et al.* Vasculo-protective effects of insulin sensitizing agent pioglitazone in neointimal thickening and hypertensive vascular hypertrophy. *Atherosclerosis* 1999;145:333–40.

53 Minamikawa J, Tanaka S, Yamauchi M *et al.* Potent inhibitory effect of troglitazone on carotid arterial wall thickness in type 2 diabetes. *J Clin Endocrinol Metab* 1998;83:1818–20.

54 Koshiyama H, Shimono D, Kuwamura N *et al.* Inhibitory effect of pioglitazone on carotid arterial wall thickness in type 2 diabetes. *J Clin Endocrinol Metab* 2001;86:3452–6.

55 Schneider RL, Shaffer SJ. Long-term echocardiographic assessment in patients with type 2 diabetes mellitus treated with pioglitazone [abstract 504-P]. *Diabetes* 2000;49(Suppl 1):A124.

56 Sutton MSJ, Dole JF, Rappaport EB. Rosiglitazone does not adversely affect cardiac structure or function in patients with type 2 diabetes [abstract 0438]. *Diabetes* 1999;48(Suppl 1):A102.

57 Law RE, Goetze S, Xi XP *et al.* Expression and function of PPAR[gamma] in rat and human vascular smooth muscle cells. *Circulation* 2000;101:1311–8.

58 Song J, Walsh MF, Igwe R *et al.* Troglitazone reduces contraction by inhibition of vascular

smooth muscle cell Ca^{2+} currents and not endothelial nitric oxide production. *Diabetes* 1997;46:659–64.

59 Kawasaki J, Hirano K, Hirano M *et al.* Troglitazone inhibits the capacitative Ca^{2+} entry in endothelial cells. *Eur J Pharmacol* 1999;373: 111–20.

60 Buchanan TA, Meehan WP, Jeng YY *et al.* Blood pressure lowering by pioglitazone: evidence for a direct vascular effect. *J Clin Invest* 1995;96: 354–60.

61 Satoh H, Tsukamoto K, Hashimoto Y *et al.* Thiazolidinediones suppress endothelin-1 secretion from bovine vascular endothelial cells: a new possible role of PPARgamma on vascular endothelial function. *Biochem Biophys Res Commun* 1999;254:747–63.

62 Walker AB, Naderali EK, Chattington PD *et al.* Differential vasoactive effects of the insulin sensitizers rosiglitazone (BRL 49653) and troglitazone on human small arteries *in vitro. Diabetes* 1998;47:810–4.

63 Walker AB, Chattington PD, Buckingham RE, Williams G. The thiazolidinedione rosiglitazone (BRL-49653) lowers blood pressure and protects against impairment of endothelial function in Zucker fatty rats. *Diabetes* 1999;48:1448–53.

64 Ogihara T, Rakugi H, Ikegami H *et al.* Enhancement of insulin sensitivity by troglitazone lowers blood pressure in diabetic hypertensives. *Am J Hypertens* 1995;8:316–20.

65 Sung BH, Izzo JL, Dandona P, Wilson MF. Vasodilatory effects of troglitazone improve blood pressure at rest and during mental stress in type 2 diabetes mellitus. *Hypertension* 1999;34:83–8.

66 Yang T, Michele DE, Park J *et al.* Expression of peroxisomal proliferator-activated receptors and retinoid X receptors in the kidney. *Am J Physiol* 1999;277:F966–73.

67 Guan YF, Breyer MD. Peroxisome proliferator-activated receptors (PPARs): novel therapeutic targets in renal disease. *Kidney Int* 2001;60:14–30.

68 Asano T, Wakisaka M, Yoshinari M *et al.* Peroxisome proliferator-activated receptor gamma1 (PPARgamma1) expresses in rat mesangial cells and PPARgamma agonists modulate its differentiation. *Biochim Biophys Acta* 2000;1497: 148–54.

69 Nicholas SB, Kawano Y, Wakino S *et al.* Expression and function of peroxisome proliferator-activated receptor-gamma in mesangial cells. *Hypertension* 2001;37:722–7.

70 Yoshimoto T, Naruse M, Nishikawa M *et al.* Antihypertensive and vasculo- and renoprotective effects of pioglitazone in genetically obese diabetic rats. *Am J Physiol* 1997;272:E989–96.

71 Imano E, Kanda T, Nakatani Y *et al.* Effect of troglitazone on microalbuminuria in patients with incipient diabetic nephropathy. *Diabetes Care* 1998;21:2135–9.

72 Nakamura T, Ushiyama C, Shimada N *et al.* Comparative effects of pioglitazone, glibenclamide, and voglibose on urinary endothelin-1 and albumin excretion in diabetes patients. *J Diabetes Compl* 2000;14:250–4.

73 Murata T, Hata Y, Ishibashi T *et al.* Response of experimental retinal neovascularization to thiazolidinediones. *Arch Ophthalmol* 2001;119: 709–17.

74 Azziz R, Ehrmann D, Legro RS *et al.* Troglitazone improves ovulation and hirsutism in the polycystic ovary syndrome: a multicenter, double blind, placebo-controlled trial. *J Clin Endocrinol Metab* 2001;86:1626–32.

75 Watkins PB, Whitcomb RW. Hepatic dysfunction associated with troglitazone. *N Engl J Med* 1998;338:916–7.

76 Misbin, RI. Troglitazone-associated hepatic failure. *Am J Med* 1999;130:330.

77 Forman LM, Simmons DA, Diamond RH. Hepatic failure in a patient taking rosiglitazone. *Ann Intern Med* 2000;132:118–21.

78 Al-Salman J, Arjomand H, Kemp DG, Mittal M. Hepatocellular injury in a patient receiving rosiglitazone: a case report. *Ann Intern Med* 2000;132:121–4.

79 Ravinuthala RS, Nori U. Rosiglitazone toxicity. *Ann Intern Med* 2000;133:658.

80 Donnelly R, Gray S, Idris I. Rosiglitazone and ankle swelling: an acute dose-dependent effect on endothelial permeability [abstract 275-OR]. *Diabetes* 2001;50(Suppl 1):A68.

81 Gorson DM. Significant weight gain with rezulin therapy. *Arch Intern Med* 1999;159:99.

82 Thomas ML, Lloyd SJ. Pulmonary edema associated with rosiglitazone and troglitazone. *Ann Pharmacother* 2001;35:123–4.

83 Young MM, Squassante L, Wemer J *et al.* Troglitazone has no effect on red cell mass or other erythropoietic parameters. *Eur J Clin Pharmacol* 1999;55:101–4.

84 Dogterom P, Jonkman JHG, Vallance SE. Rosiglitazone: no effect on erythropoiesis or premature red cell destruction [abstract 0424]. *Diabetes* 1999;48(Suppl 1):A98.

85 Shimizu H, Tsuchiya T, Sato N, *et al.* Troglitazone reduces plasma leptin concentration but increases hunger in NIDDM patients. *Diabetes Care* 1998;21:1470–4.

86 King AB, Armstrong D. Characteristics of the patients who gain weight while on pioglitazone treatment [abstract 481-P]. *Diabetes* 2001;50(Suppl 1):A120.

11

Insulin treatment in type 2 diabetes

Julio Rosenstock and Kathleen Wyne

INTRODUCTION

Type 2 diabetes mellitus is clearly a progressive disease, with a relentless decline in insulin secretion[1]. The therapeutic armamentarium for the management of type 2 diabetes has been widely expanded with the introduction of new oral agents, but their blood glucose-lowering potency is limited[2]. Insulin therapy should no longer be viewed as a 'last resort', to be used after long-term oral agent combinations have failed, but rather as a therapeutic tool for earlier use in achieving glycemic targets. Simple strategies for starting insulin therapy, such as using evening basal insulin replacement in combination with oral agents, have been shown to be effective, and follow well the basal/bolus insulin concept[3]. Once patients on combination oral therapy are started on basal insulin replacement, a structured titration regimen may suffice to accomplish glycemic targets. The eventual need to intensify the regimen, with the addition of premeal short-acting insulin to address postprandial hyperglycemia, will depend on whether or not target HbA1c (glycosylated hemoglobin) levels are achieved and maintained.

Increased understanding of the natural history and progressive nature of type 2 diabetes mellitus, coupled with a growing awareness of the need for more effective treatment strategies and significant improvements in insulin therapy, merits a reassessment of the role of insulin in the treatment of type 2 diabetes.

RATIONALE FOR EARLY INSULIN REPLACEMENT IN TYPE 2 DIABETES

The initial defect: beta-cell dysfunction

Type 2 diabetes results from two fundamental pathogenic defects: impaired insulin secretion (or beta-cell dysfunction) and insulin resistance manifested by increased hepatic glucose production and reduced peripheral glucose uptake[4]. These defects are both genetically determined and influenced by environmental factors, such as physical inactivity and obesity[5]. Beta-cell ability to continue to secrete sufficient insulin in response to peripheral resistance has emerged as the pivotal point in determining whether or not a patient progresses towards type 2 diabetes mellitus[6]. Consequently, any assessment of insulin secretion must be interpreted as a function of insulin sensitivity[7].

Studies in a young and apparently healthy Caucasian population with normal glucose tolerance (NGT) demonstrated that beta-cell function varied quantitatively with differences in insulin sensitivity[8]. Analysis of first-degree relatives of patients with type 2 diabetes has shown that the relationship between insulin sensitivity and beta-cell function is reciprocal, in that changes in one directly affect the other – but not in a linear or logarithmic fashion (Figure 11.1).

The natural history of diabetes has been extensively studied in the Pima Indians of Arizona, among whom a high percentage of adults

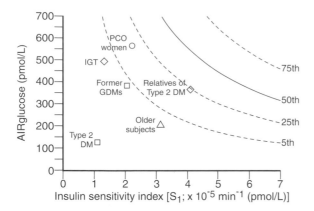

Figure 11.1 Percentile lines for the relationship between insulin sensitivity (SI) and the acute (first-phase) insulin response (AIRglucose): based on data from normal subjects with type 2 diabetes; healthy older subjects; women with a history of gestational diabetes (GDM); women with polycystic ovarian disease (PCO) and a family history of type 2 diabetes; subjects with impaired glucose tolerance (IGT); and subjects with a first-degree relative with type 2 diabetes. (Reprinted from Kahn et al. 2001[8], with permission.)

develop type 2 diabetes by age 40[9]. Further characterization of the beta-cell dysfunction has demonstrated that insulin-secretion defects are indeed present prior to progression to hyperglycemia, and can predict progression from NGT to impaired glucose tolerance (IGT), to diabetes[6,10]. A recent longitudinal study that monitored progression at yearly intervals in patients with initial NGT, found that transition from NGT to IGT was associated with an increase in body weight, a decline in insulin-stimulated glucose disposal, and a decline in the acute insulin secretory response to intravenous glucose (AIRglucose), but no change in endogenous glucose output[10]. Progression from IGT to diabetes was accompanied by a further increase in body weight, further decreases in insulin-stimulated glucose disposal and AIRglucose, and an increase in basal endogenous glucose output. Most notably, 31 of the 48 subjects who maintained NGT over this period also gained weight, but maintained normal beta-cell secretory capacity, with an increased AIRglucose to compensate for the decreasing insulin-stimulated glucose disposal. Thus, defects in insulin

secretion and insulin action occur early in the pathogenesis of diabetes, but the beta-cell secretory defect was the main determinant in progression towards type 2 diabetes. Similarly, studies in women who have a history of gestational diabetes show that progression to type 2 diabetes is correlated with the extent of impairment of insulin secretion[11].

The progressive nature of the insulin secretory defect was classically demonstrated by the UK Prospective Diabetes Study (UKPDS) in newly diagnosed patients with type 2 diabetes. Beta-cell function, as measured by the homeostasis model assessment method (HOMA), showed an inexorable decline over time, which explains why most patients with type 2 diabetes will eventually need insulin therapy if glycemic targets are to be achieved[1]. Although individuals in the UKPDS receiving sulfonylurea therapy demonstrated an early increase in beta-cell function, from 45% to 78% in Year 1 of the study (consistent with a secretagogue effect of the sulfonylurea agent), beta-cell function subsequently decreased along the same slope as that of the diet-treated group. This inevitable decline in beta-cell function also occurred in the metformin group, in which beta-cell function initially increased (similar to that in the sulfonylurea group) then declined from 66% to 38% by Year 6. It appears from the UKPDS that a significant loss of insulin secretory capacity, > 50%, is necessary for hyperglycemia to become overt.

Over time, insulin secretion declines, presumably accelerated by glucotoxicity and lipotoxicity[12–19]. Any therapeutic strategy that corrects hyperglycemia and reduces free fatty acid levels can potentially improve insulin action and increase insulin secretion[20]. It is conceivable that earlier intervention with a combination of agents that reduce insulin resistance and also promote insulin secretion may preserve beta-cell functional integrity and maintain a durable glycemic response but, eventually, supplemental insulin replacement will be needed to achieve near-normoglycemia. Insulin replacement may well be an option as part of the initial therapy in patients with type 2 diabetes, in an attempt to correct the pathogenic defects and effectively reach glycemic targets.

Indeed, short-term intensive insulin therapy in type 2 diabetes has been shown to improve insulin action by reversing glucotoxicity/lipotoxicity and, possibly, inducing 'beta-cell rest', which results in increased insulin secretion[21–25]. It is tempting to speculate, therefore, that much earlier insulin administration – perhaps from the outset of the disease – might be crucial for preserving beta-cell function. Preliminary support for this 'beta-cell rest' hypothesis is provided by a small study of newly diagnosed hyperglycemic type 2 diabetic patients, subjected to a period of 2 weeks of intensive insulin therapy resulting in near-normoglycemia[26]. Most of the patients subsequently sustained good glycemic control for long periods of time without pharmacologic intervention. These intriguing findings, albeit from small numbers of patients, suggest that insulin treatment in recently diagnosed type 2 diabetes might halt disease progression and permit long-term maintenance of nearly normal blood glucose levels, with better response to oral agents or to simpler long-term insulin supplementation.

Insulin therapy can improve insulin resistance

Insulin resistance, manifested by increased hepatic glucose production and reduced peripheral glucose disposal, is a major pathogenic defect in type 2 diabetes that correlates with obesity and hyperinsulinemia[27–29]. Consequently, concern has been raised that treatment with insulin may worsen insulin resistance. However, short-term intensive insulin therapy has been shown to decrease insulin resistance[21–23]. Peripheral insulin sensitivity has been assessed using the glucose-insulin clamp method, before and after restoration of near-normoglycemic control in type 2 diabetes patients on intensive insulin treatment. In each case, the treatment period was short (2–4 weeks) and a relatively high insulin dosage was required (>100 U daily). Figure 11.2 shows the tissue insulin sensitivity before and after treatment, expressed as a percentage of the mean value for insulin sensitivity of a non-diabetic control group that was matched in age, gender and weight to the diabetic subjects. The three

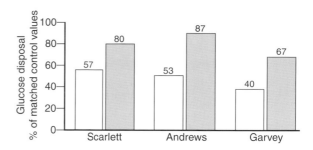

Figure 11.2 Improvement in insulin sensitivity, as measured by the glucose-insulin clamp technique, at baseline and after intensive insulin treatment[21–23]. Solid bars = after insulin; open bars = baseline.

studies showed remarkably similar results. Insulin sensitivity, compared with non-diabetic values, was increased by almost half with insulin treatment, indicating a marked reduction in insulin resistance. After treatment, insulin sensitivity improved toward the non-diabetic values, although some insulin resistance persisted, as would be expected. This improvement is presumably due to the resolution of the hyperglycemia and consequent reduced 'glucotoxicity'. Whether the improvement in insulin sensitivity persists when insulin treatment is continued for longer periods of time was not tested in these studies. However, these data show that – at least in the short term – successful insulin treatment reduces, rather than worsens, insulin resistance. Defronzo and colleagues showed that aggressive insulin therapy over 12 weeks, which resulted in near-normalization of HbA1c values (decreased from 10.1% to 6.6%), improved insulin resistance through improving insulin-stimulated glucose disposal; however this effect did not fully correct the inherent insulin resistance[25].

Insulin therapy and potential cardiovascular benefits

Insulin resistance and the consequent endogenous hyperinsulinemia are strongly associated with central obesity, hypertension and dyslipidemia, all factors that contribute substantially to cardiovascular (CV) risk and, in fact, characterize the metabolic syndrome [also called the insulin resistance syndrome (IRS)][29,30].

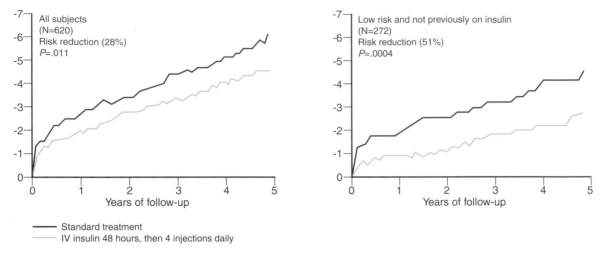

Figure 11.3 Mortality after MI reduced by insulin therapy in the DIGAMI study. Control (—), infusion (⋯⋯). (Reprinted from *BMJ* 1997;314:1512–15, with permission from the BMJ Publishing Group.)

Epidemiological studies in non-diabetic populations have shown an association between endogenous hyperinsulinemia and atherosclerosis[31], thus physicians have been concerned that initiating insulin therapy could be harmful and may accelerate coronary artery disease. However, the association of hyperinsulinemia and atherosclerosis is mainly an association between endogenous hyperproinsulinemia and atherosclerosis[32]. In fact, there is no evidence from animal or human studies that exogenous insulin administration causes accelerated atherosclerosis. The UKPDS actually was very reassuring in demonstrating that the insulin-treated patients, who presumably had exogenous hyperinsulinemia, showed no evidence at all of increased atherosclerotic-related events[33].

Furthermore, the 5-year Diabetes and Insulin-Glucose Infusion in Acute Myocardial Infarction (DIGAMI) trial showed that insulin infusion therapy during acute myocardial infarction (MI), followed by intensive multiple-dose insulin therapy, reduced the relative mortality risk by 28% compared with controls (conventional therapy) after an average follow-up of 3.4 years[34,35]. The subjects were randomized at the time of MI to either control (continued management according to the judgement of their physicians) or to intravenous infusion of insulin and glucose for 48 h,

followed by a four-injection regimen for as long as 5 years. The rationale underlying the study was the preliminary observations that, in animal experiments and small clinical studies, infarct size and outcome were improved by insulin-glucose-potassium infusion, which is thought to be related to suppression of otherwise elevated free fatty acid levels in plasma[36–43].

Figure 11.3 shows the cumulative total mortality rates in the whole population of 620 subjects randomized to the two treatments, as well as the rates for a predefined subgroup of subjects who were judged likely to survive the initial hospitalization and were not previously using insulin[35]. The whole population showed an 11% actual and a 28% relative risk reduction in mortality with intensive insulin treatment after 5 years, and the subgroup not previously using insulin showed a 15% actual and 51% relative risk reduction. Most of the benefit was apparent in the first month of treatment and, presumably, was partly due to immediate intravenous infusion of insulin; however, the survival curves tended to separate further over time, suggesting an ongoing benefit from intensive insulin treatment. This study suggests that insulin is an entirely appropriate treatment for type 2 diabetes patients with high cardiovascular risk, especially at the time of MI.

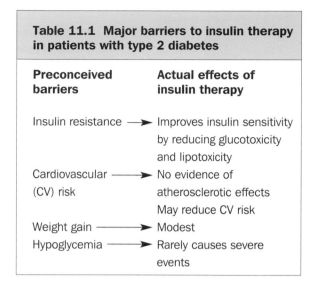

Table 11.1 Major barriers to insulin therapy in patients with type 2 diabetes

Preconceived barriers	Actual effects of insulin therapy
Insulin resistance ⟶	Improves insulin sensitivity by reducing glucotoxicity and lipotoxicity
Cardiovascular (CV) risk ⟶	No evidence of atherosclerotic effects May reduce CV risk
Weight gain ⟶	Modest
Hypoglycemia ⟶	Rarely causes severe events

BARRIERS TO INSULIN THERAPY (Table 11.1)

The major barriers for some physicians to the use of insulin in the treatment of type 2 diabetes are:

- The misconception that insulin therapy may increase the risk of cardiovascular disease (as reviewed above)
- Excessive concerns about weight gain or the potential risk of hypoglycemia
- The obvious inconvenience of having to instruct and persuade the patients to take injections.

Traditionally, insulin therapy has been considered a therapy of last resort in type 2 diabetes, due to these concerns and the lack of understanding that insulin deficiency is one of the initial defects that worsens with the progressive nature of the disease.

Insulin therapy and weight gain

Initiation of insulin therapy is typically associated with weight gain. The weight gain is most rapid in the first 3–6 months of therapy and is correlated with improvements in glycemic control. Some simple but partial explanation for the weight gain comes from patients typically maintaining the same prior dietary transgressions, but no longer having the caloric loss from glycosuria[44]. Most studies have shown no change

in basal metabolic rate (BMR) with improvement in glycemic control, perhaps due to the fact that the increase in BMR attributable to weight gain offsets the decrease in BMR attributable to improved glucose control[45–51]. BMR is typically higher in diabetic subjects than in non-diabetic subjects matched for body mass index (BMI). Bogardus and colleagues showed an improvement in resting metabolic rate after improving glucose control in obese Pima Indians with type 2 diabetes; the weight of the subjects was maintained constant from beginning to end of therapy by decreasing daily calorie intake[46]. Insulin therapy is also known to noticeably lower plasma non-esterified fatty acid concentrations, a change that is associated with a lowering of gluconeogenesis[52]. A decrease in non-esterified fatty acid concentrations may also lower heat production, by decreasing mitochondrial uncoupling, i.e. the ratio between heat and ATP production[53]. This emphasizes the importance of increasing daily activity and decreasing caloric intake to minimize weight gain. Of note, studies in obese patients with type 2 diabetes treated with insulin therapy have shown that, despite weight gain, cardiovascular risk factors, such as blood pressure, remained unchanged, and lipid patterns (triglycerides, lipoproteins) were generally improved[54–57]. These findings challenge the notion that insulin therapy negatively affects blood pressure and lipid profiles through weight gain. Importantly, as previously discussed, intensive insulin therapy has been shown to improve rather than worsen insulin sensitivity, by virtue of improving glycemic control, thus reducing and, to some degree, reversing the toxic effects of hyperglycemia (glucotoxicity).

In the UKPDS, patients in both the main study and the metformin substudy gained weight. In the main study, patients assigned to treatment with a sulfonylurea gained more weight than the conventional group, and those assigned insulin gained more weight than those on a sulfonylurea[33]. In the cohort followed for 10 years, those assigned to glyburide, compared with patients on conventional therapy, gained an excess of 1.7 kg and those on insulin gained an excess of 4.0 kg. In the metformin substudy, which included the more obese subjects in the trial (mean BMI ~31 kg m^{-2}), the changes of body weight were similar to those in the main study, except that the group randomized to metformin showed a weight gain that was similar to the conventionally treated group but lower than the groups treated with insulin or a sulfonylurea[58]. Indeed, combination insulin therapy with metformin is an effective strategy to potentiate the effectiveness of the insulin regimen while limiting weight gain (see below).

Insulin therapy and hypoglycemia

Hypoglycemia is the most important limiting factor for insulin adjustments to improve glycemic control. The risk of hypoglycemia depends on a number of factors, including age, weight, degree of insulin resistance, duration of disease, duration of insulin therapy, targeted degree of glycemic control, and history of hypoglycemic episodes. Additional causal factors in hypoglycemia include over-insulinization, dietary transgressions, strenuous unplanned exercise, excessive alcohol intake, and lack of awareness of hypoglycemia. The actual incidence of severe hypoglycemia in type 2 diabetes patients of < 2–3% per year, as shown by the UKPDS, is relatively very low[33,59]. Indeed, the UKPDS is the largest long-term treatment study using insulin for type 2 diabetes. Hypoglycemic episodes were monitored as a measure of outcome over 10 years of treatment. The groups treated with insulin from the start showed more hypoglycemia – as might be expected – with little difference between the non-obese and the obese groups, but most of the hypoglycemia was mild in severity. Severe hypoglycemic events occurred on average in only 2–3% of subjects in this group each year. This rate is certainly not trivial, but it is far less than the rate seen with intensive insulin treatment of type 1 diabetes in the Diabetes Control and Complications Trial (DCCT)[60].

It is conceivable that in patients with insulin resistance, exogenous insulin and the subsequent fall in glucose concentration into the normal range leads to a more physiologic endogenous insulin release from the beta-cells, which may contribute to decreased hypoglycemia[61]. However, most interventional insulin studies have failed to achieve target HbA1C levels, and it is possible that hypoglycemia would have become more common if patients had completely attained near-normoglycemia.

Limitations of insulin preparations

Over the years, multiple insulin preparations have been developed using recombinant DNA technology, resulting in major improvements in purity and production but still with significant limitations in pharmacokinetics and pharmacodynamics after subcutaneous injection[62,63]. A comparison of the kinetics of available insulins is given in Table 11.2.

Regular human insulin has a slow onset of action, with delayed peak concentrations requiring patients to administer their injection 20–40 min prior to a meal in an attempt to improve the mismatch with the postprandial hyperglycemic peaks[64]. This is inconvenient, infrequently achieved, and poses the risk of premeal hypoglycemia if the meal is inadvertently delayed. Furthermore, the duration of action of regular insulin is much longer than the normal endogenous insulin peak following meals, typically at least 6 h and up to 12 h when large doses are injected. This persistence of high insulin levels leads to a risk of hypoglycemia, which is often countered by between-meal snacks, which foster weight gain in type 2 diabetes patients.

Two short-acting insulin analogs, insulin lispro and insulin aspart, have absorption profiles that more closely match normal mealtime patterns[65–68]. Small alterations in their amino acid structure relative to human insulin reduce their tendency to aggregate into dimers or hexamers, thus speeding their absorption after subcutaneous injection. Lispro and aspart have very desirable action profiles at mealtimes; they have a rapid onset of action, 5–15 min, the peak of action occurs 1 h after injection, and the insulin effect practically vanishes 4–5 h after administration. Their quick onset of action matches normal mealtime peaks of plasma insulin better than does regular human insulin. Clinical studies, mostly in type 1 diabetes, have shown that these properties lead to less prominent peaks of glucose after meals and less late postprandial

Table 11.2 Pharmacokinetics of human insulin and analogs			
	Onset of action (h)	Peak (h)	Duration of action (h)
Human insulin			
Regular	0.5–1	2–4	6–10
NPH	2–4	4–8	12–16
Lente	2–4	4–8	12–16
Ultralente	4–6	Unpredictable	18–20
Insulin analog			
Lispro (Humalog)	5 min–15 min	1	4–5
Aspart (Novolog)	5 min–15 min	1	4–5
Glargine (Lantus)	1–2	Flat	~24

The time course of action of any insulin may vary between individuals, or at different times in the same individual. Consequently, table data should be considered only as general guidelines.

hypoglycemia[69–86]. However, rapid waning of the effects of mealtime lispro and aspart leads to greater dependency on adequate basal insulin levels between meals and overnight.

There has been a growing need for a long-acting 24 h basal insulin replacement that would mimic normal pancreatic basal insulin secretion to control hepatic glucose production in the postabsorptive state. Clinical use of insulin lispro or aspart has directed attention to the properties of extended-release human insulins, which have been used to provide basal insulin replacement.

The intermediate-acting insulins, neutral protamine Hagedorn (NPH) and lente, have gradual onset and the peak effect is usually at 4–8 h, with a total duration of 12–16 h. Human ultralente insulin is somewhat longer acting, but still usually falls short of a 24 h effect.

Human NPH, lente, and ultralente insulin all have mean durations of action of < 24 h, precluding them from providing adequate basal insulin replacement for many patients. All three, but especially NPH and lente, have pronounced peaks of action. Ultralente is thought to show a substantial day-to-day variation of action with erratic peaks. These limitations cause variations of glucose levels and unpredictable hypo-

glycemia, which are the leading factors limiting glycemic control at the present time. Indeed, the lack of reproducibility of glucose-lowering effects with conventional basal insulin preparations, including NPH and ultralente, has been a major limitation for most insulin regimens.

The first insulin analog with a prolonged duration of action to become available for clinical use is insulin glargine[63]. Insulin glargine results from two modifications of human insulin: a substitution of glycine at position A21 and the addition of two positive charges (two arginine molecules) at the C terminal of the B chain. Changes in amino-acid content shift the isoelectric point, reducing the aqueous solubility of insulin glargine at physiological pH and stabilizing the hexamer, delaying its dissociation into monomers. It is released gradually from the injection site and, because of the delay in absorption, its action is prolonged, allowing a relatively constant basal insulin supply. However, because insulin glargine is formulated as a clear acidic solution, it cannot be mixed with insulin formulated at a neutral pH, such as regular insulin. Studies have demonstrated no variation in absorption rates at various injection sites (e.g. arm, leg or abdomen)[87].

Glucose–insulin clamp studies have also compared the actions of insulin glargine with those of NPH and ultralente[88–90]. These studies have found that insulin glargine, compared with the other insulins, provides an essentially flat profile with a longer duration, about 24 h (Figure 11.4). Clinical trials have shown improvements in glycemic control similar to NPH, with a consistently lower frequency of nocturnal hypoglycemia[91–97]. Use of the flat or peakless insulin glargine profile now allows for a more vigorous titration regimen, and more patients can reach target HbA1c levels with considerably less risk of nocturnal hypoglycemia [98,99].

Insulin detemir (NN304) is another long-acting analog that is undergoing clinical trials[63]. The principle behind the longer duration of action is based on covalent acylation of the epsilon amino group of Lys B29. This modification promotes reversible binding of insulin to albumin, thereby delaying its resorption from subcutaneous tissue and, possibly because of size, reducing the rate of transendothelial transport[100]. The myristoyl fatty acid side-chain at the C terminus of the B-chain does not alter the aggregation properties of the molecule. NN304 has a slower disappearance rate from subcutaneous tissue, and a much flatter time-action

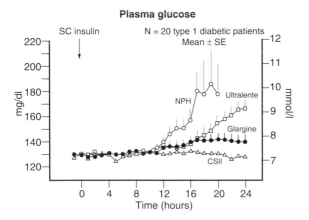

Figure 11.4 Insulin kinetics on duration of action during an isoglycemic 24-h clamp. Plasma glucose concentration after subcutaneous injection of glargine, NPH and ultralente, and after continuous subcutaneous infusion (CSII) of lispro. (©2000 American Diabetes Association. From *Diabetes*, vol. 49; 2000;2142–8. Reprinted with permission.)

profile than NPH[101]. In a 6-week crossover study, 73 patients with type 1 diabetes, who were given insulin detemir once daily before bedtime plus premeal soluble human insulin titrated to achieve equivalent glycemic control, required a two- to three-fold higher dose than those given NPH in the same way[102]. As a basal insulin, detemir has the potential disadvantage of having a shorter duration of action and thus may need to be given in a twice-daily regimen, which could limit its flexibility in the combined use with short-acting insulin analogs.

The mechanical barrier

Despite the improvements in insulin kinetics with the new insulin analogs, the need to mix and inject insulin remains a barrier to patients' acceptance and compliance. New pen-delivery devices are being created to make it easier for patients to carry their insulin with them and give injections in settings other than their homes[103,104]. Inhaled insulin preparations now under investigation are clearly very attractive, in that insulin is delivered in a non-invasive fashion, removing the ultimate barrier of insulin injections. Pharmacokinetic studies have shown rapid peaks of action for inhaled insulin, similar to lispro insulin but with slightly longer duration[105,106]. Time–action profiles of inhaled insulin compared with subcutaneous regular and lispro insulin were studied using a euglycemic glucose clamp[107]. After 120 min, subjects received 6 mg of inhaled insulin, 18 U of subcutaneous regular insulin or 18 U of subcutaneous insulin lispro. Inhaled insulin showed a faster onset of action than subcutaneous regular insulin and even insulin lispro, with early $t_{50\%}$ of 32, 48 and 40 min, respectively. The duration of action of inhaled insulin was intermediate between those of lispro and regular insulin (382, 309 and 413 min, respectively). The maximal metabolic action based on glucose infusion rates was comparable for the three groups.

The proof of concept for inhaled insulin, a dry powder aerosol delivery system of human insulin, was initially examined in an early Phase II study on 69 patients with type 2 diabetes. These patients were randomized to a 3-month treatment period of either continued oral agents alone (sulfonylurea and/or metformin), or in combination with one or two puffs of inhaled insulin before meals[108]. The inhaled insulin doses were titrated based on glucose testing four times daily. Patients continuing on oral agents alone showed little change in HbA1c at 12 weeks (–0.13%), while those receiving the inhaled insulin in addition to the oral agents exhibited a marked improvement in HbA1c (–2.28%). Full analysis of the Phase III studies in type 1 and type 2 diabetes, testing the efficacy and safety of inhaled insulin in different therapeutic scenarios, are awaited with great interest, as are long-term safety studies.

INSULIN REPLACEMENT STRATEGIES: THE BASAL/BOLUS CONCEPT

Insulin has been used therapeutically for more than 75 years and remains the most powerful anti-diabetes agent, with almost unlimited potential to lower plasma glucose levels. Ideally, insulin replacement therapy should be modelled with insulin preparations that can reproduce the physiologic patterns of insulin secretion in response to the 24 h postabsorptive and postprandial glucose profiles (Table 11.3). The basal/bolus insulin concept is a physiologically sound regimen that attempts to mimic the normal insulin patterns, to control glucose levels[64]. The role of basal insulin is to suppress hepatic glucose production, so that glucose levels remain constantly regulated overnight and during prolonged periods between meals[109]. Basal insulin meets about half of the patient's daily need for insulin, and basal insulin replacement may be sufficient when considerable endogenous insulin remains. Bolus insulin (10–20% of the total daily insulin requirements given at each meal) limits hyperglycemia after meals. Conceptually, each component of insulin replacement therapy should come from a different type of insulin, with a specific profile to fit the patient's needs.

The basal/bolus insulin concept has long been used in the management of patients with type 1 diabetes, but can also be applied to patients with type 2 diabetes. Since both fasting and postprandial glucose levels are abnormal in type 2 diabetes, and the underlying insulin deficiency typically progresses, most patients will need

> ## Table 11.3 The basal/bolus insulin concept
>
> **Basal insulin**
> - Nearly constant 24 h insulin levels
> - Suppresses hepatic glucose production between meals and overnight
> - Covers 50% of daily needs
>
> **Bolus insulin (mealtime)**
> - Immediate rise and sharp peak at 1 h
> - Limits postmeal hyperglycemia
> - Covers 10–20% of total daily insulin requirement at each meal
>
> Ideally, each component should be covered by a different insulin, with a specific profile.

both: initially basal insulin replacement and, eventually, mealtime insulin supplementation if glycemic targets are not achieved or cannot be maintained with basal insulin alone.

Starting insulin therapy with basal insulin

Rationale for early combination of oral agents plus basal insulin

It has been established that most patients with type 2 diabetes will eventually require insulin, 10–15 years after disease onset – but traditionally it is used as a 'last resort' after maximal combination therapy has failed. However, our improved understanding of the natural history of type 2 diabetes suggests that insulin therapy should be started sooner rather than later, and that insulin should be viewed as an essential therapeutic tool for achieving disease management goals at an early stage in the natural progression of the disease, rather than as a sign of failure on the part of physician or patient. Oral agents can be divided into two general categories: those augmenting the supply of insulin by increasing the secretion of insulin into the portal circulation, and those enhancing the effectiveness of insulin[2]. Injected insulin, in turn, increases insulin in the systemic circulation. The mechanisms of action for these classes of oral agents differ, they may therefore have complementary or additive effects and can help meet the individualized needs of patients.

The sulfonylureas and glitinides are oral agents that augment the supply of portal insulin[110–115]. They increase hepatic levels of endogenous insulin and enhance meal-mediated insulin release. Metformin and the thiazolidinediones are oral agents that enhance the effectiveness of insulin. Metformin improves insulin sensitivity at the liver and reduces hepatic glucose production[116–120]. The thiazolidinediones improve insulin action in peripheral tissues and enhance glucose uptake[121–125]. The α-glucosidase inhibitors have a different mechanism of action, decreasing postprandial glucose absorption by inhibiting digestion of complex carbohydrates and disaccharides, thereby retarding gastrointestinal glucose absorption[126,127].

Studies utilizing insulin therapy for patients with type 2 diabetes have been based on either the addition of insulin to oral therapy, or switching of the oral agents to insulin. Unfortunately, these studies usually enrol subjects who are 'failing' their oral agents, which occurs very late in the disease process.

The fundamental issue is which regimen will be the most cost-effective in achieving the target HbA1c of < 7%, with less hypoglycemia and fewer side effects, and with high acceptance by patients and physicians. Most importantly, and now under investigation, is whether starting with early insulin replacement strategies to achieve target glycemic control will prevent progression of the disease process and reduce the development of macrovascular complications.

Practical advantages of early combination oral agents plus insulin
Patients who no longer respond adequately to oral agents will benefit from combination therapy, which consists of maintaining use of oral antidiabetic agents together with supplemental insulin therapy (Table 11.4). The advantages of adding basal insulin to prior treatment with oral agents include the following:

- Only one insulin injection may be required each day, with no need for mixing different types of insulin

---

Table 11.4 Practical guidelines: combination therapy regimens

Average patient
- Early combination of insulin secretagogue and insulin sensitizer
- Most simple and cost-effective treatment:
  - Start low-dose, once-daily morning sulfonylurea and evening metformin
  - Eventually, full-dose sulfonylurea or glitinide in combination with increasing doses of metformin

For marked insulin resistance
- Combination of metformin + glitazone

If target HbA1c < 7% not achieved
- Try triple oral therapy
  or
- Add basal insulin while continuing oral therapy

- Titration can be accomplished in a slow, safe, simple fashion
- The use of insulin pens can enhance patient acceptance of the treatment
- Combination therapy eventually requires a lower total dose of insulin.

The result is an effective improvement in glycemic control with only limited weight gain. Adding insulin in the evening is a simple and effective strategy that can be regarded as 'bridge therapy'. It allows patients to overcome their initial resistance to start using insulin, facilitating long-term acceptance and compliance.

Sulfonylurea plus ultralente
One of the early studies that combined an oral agent with insulin was reported by the Oxford group in 1987[128]. Fifteen asymptomatic, sulfonylurea-treated type 2 diabetic patients were treated in a randomized crossover study of consecutive 8-week periods. The overnight mean basal plasma glucose level on sulfonylurea therapy was reduced to normal by adding ultralente insulin. Compared with ultralente insulin therapy alone, combining sulfonylurea with ultralente insulin therapy did not show a signif-

icant difference in glucose control, but it did significantly lower the required insulin dose for restoring fasting normoglycemia. The authors concluded that in type 2 diabetic patients who continue to have fasting hyperglycemia on maximal sulfonylurea therapy, the addition of a basal insulin supplement can easily result in normoglycemia.

Most notable is the recent report from the UKPDS emphasizing the importance of early initiation of insulin therapy in newly diagnosed patients with type 2 diabetes[59]. The Glucose Study 2 was introduced in the last eight UKPDS centers. This protocol differed from the main study in that insulin therapy was added immediately to treatment regimes of patients allocated to sulfonylurea therapy if maximal doses did not maintain fasting plasma glucose (FPG) levels ≤ 108 mg dL^{-1} (Figure 11.5). For those allocated to sulfonylurea, the modified UKPDS protocol used in the Glucose Study 2 meant that ultralente insulin was added if, on maximal sulfonylurea therapy (chlorpropamide 500 mg once daily, glipizide 20 mg twice daily), the mean of three successive FPG values increased to ≥ 108 mg dL^{-1}. Sulfonylurea therapy was continued unchanged; the starting dose of ultralente was based on body weight and administered once daily before the evening meal, then increased weekly or biweekly as necessary to maintain FPG ≤ 108 mg dL^{-1}. Human soluble insulin was added before meals if preprandial home blood glucose levels remained ≥ 126 mg dL^{-1}.

Median HBA1c over 6 years was significantly lower for those allocated to sulfonylurea + insulin (SI) [6.6% (6.0–7.6)] rather than insulin alone [7.1% (6.2–8.0), P = 0.0066]. The proportion of patients with HbA1c < 7% at 6 years was greater among patients taking SI compared with those taking insulin alone (47% versus 35%, P = 0.011) (Figure 11.6). The Glucose Study 2 shows that glycemic control can be significantly improved, with almost 50% of patients maintaining a HbA1c target of < 7% using insulin plus sulfonylurea therapy, and without promoting substantial increases in hypoglycemia or weight gain – despite the limitations of ultralente insulin.

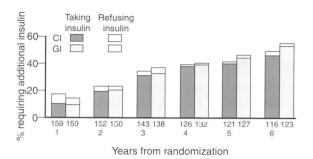

Figure 11.5 Proportions of patients (%) allocated to chlorpropamide (CI) or glipizide (GI) requiring early addition of insulin each year because FPG increased to ≥ 108 mg dL^{-1} (6.0 mmol L^{-1}) despite maximal sulfonylurea doses. Those requiring but refusing additional insulin are indicated separately. The number below each column is the number of patients per year. There were no significant differences between the chlorpropamide and glipizide groups at any time-point. (© 2002 American Diabetes Association. From *Diabetes Care* vol. 25, 2002;330–6. Reprinted with permission.)

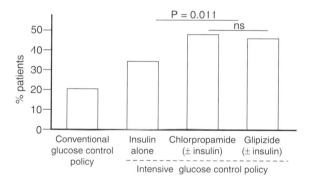

Figure 11.6 Proportion (%) of patients achieving HbA1c < 7% at 6 years. (© 2002 American Diabetes Association. From *Diabetes Care* vol. 25, 2002;330–6. Reprinted with permission.)

Sulfonylurea plus bedtime NPH

Combining a sulfonylurea with bedtime intermediate-acting insulin is an effective strategy for improving glucose control and overcoming secondary sulfonylurea failure. The rationale of combination therapy with sulfonylureas and insulin is based on the assumption that if bedtime insulin (BI) lowers the fasting glucose concentration to normal, then daytime sulfonylureas (DS)

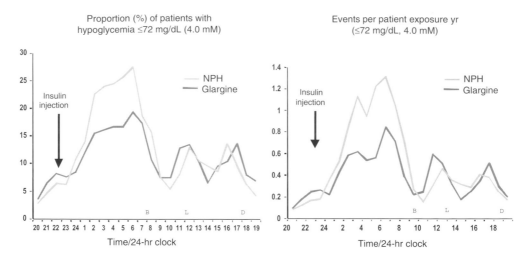

Figure 11.9 Treat to Target Study: hypoglycemia timing. B = breakfast; L = lunch; D = dinner. (Reprinted with permission from Rosenstock et al. 2002[99]).

substantial advantage for the insulin glargine – especially as this strategy has the potential to be applied to large populations of patients with type 2 diabetes managed by general physicians (Figure 11.9).

Starting insulin therapy with bolus insulin

The concept of initiating insulin therapy with bolus insulin has been demonstrated in patients with type 2 diabetes who were experiencing secondary oral agent failure to sulfonylurea (SU). Bastyr *et al.* added preprandial insulin lispro, or bedtime NPH or metformin to the sulfonylurea[134]. At the end of 12 weeks, HbA1c was significantly lower with all therapies and was even lower for the lispro plus SU group (7.6%) compared with either metformin combination or added bedtime NPH. Morning FBG was lowest with bedtime NPH, but the mean 2 h postprandial glucose after a test meal was lowest in the lispro plus SU group. The overall rate of hypoglycemia (episodes per 30 days) was low and showed no statistically significant difference between groups.

However, for patients starting insulin therapy, the need for multiple premeal injections makes the mealtime insulin supplementation strategy considerably more complex and less attractive than the once-daily evening dose of basal insulin. Perhaps in the future, when inhaled insulin becomes available, non-injectable premeal insulin replacement may become the first-line intervention, followed by basal insulin supplementation as required. Indeed, the efficacy of adding preprandial insulin, using an inhaled pulmonary delivery of dry powder insulin, to oral therapy was recently demonstrated in a 3-month Phase III clinical trial[135].

Patients with type 2 diabetes who did not maintain HbA1c < 8% on combination oral therapy (secretagogue plus metformin or a glitazone) were randomized to either inhaled insulin alone, continuing on the oral agents unchanged, or adding the inhaled insulin to the current doses of oral agents. The group receiving combination therapy oral agents plus inhaled insulin showed the largest decrease in HbA1c, 1.9%, with a decrease of 1.4% with inhaled insulin alone and 0.2% with continuing oral agents. Weight gain and hypoglycemia were comparable in the groups receiving insulin, with only one episode of severe hypoglycemia overall. While this study shows that adding prandial inhaled insulin results in a robust lowering of HbA1c, further long-term pulmonary safety studies will be required before this insulin can be made clinically available.

Starting therapy with basal/bolus

Traditionally, twice-daily mixtures of NPH and regular insulins have been widely used for type 2 diabetes for many years. However, most patients using this 'split-mixed' regimen rarely achieve reasonably good glycemic control by present standards, and often experience late morning or nocturnal hypoglycemia because of excessive levels of insulin at these times – as well as intermittent hyperglycemia due to insufficient insulin replacement.

Intensive insulin strategies using the twice daily split-mixed regimen are largely unsuccessful, except for the study by Henry *et al.* who studied a group of 14 patients with type 2 diabetes to determine whether tight glycemic control can be obtained using conventional insulin therapy in an outpatient setting by aggressively titrating insulin therapy[24]. Patients received conventional subcutaneous NPH and regular insulin before breakfast and supper for 6 months, with dose adjustments based on an algorithm built on frequent blood glucose measurements (4–6 times a day). The total dose of required exogenous insulin was 86 ± 13 U at 1 month, and 100 ± 24 U at 6 months. One month after initiating intensive insulin therapy, day-long glycemia had improved to within normal range and remained at this level through Month 6 of therapy. HbA1c, which was 7.7% at baseline, decreased to 5.1% at 6 months. This study underscores the importance of early insulin therapy, when the baseline HbA1c is only mildly elevated just above 7%, and insulin is aggressively titrated. These results are, however, hardly ever achieved when the split-mixed regimen, which fails to mimic the basal/bolus needs, is used in general practice and insufficient insulin is administered. Premixed 70/30 insulin is often used, but the insulin profiles do not come close to matching the normal endogenous secretory pattern to control fasting and postprandial hyperglycemia. In addition, the rigid premixed preparations have the significant limitation of having no flexibility for insulin adjustments according to the patient's blood glucose profile.

Multiple daily doses of short-acting insulin can be added when patients do not attain adequate control. Lindstrom and colleagues showed that this strategy may be effective in normalizing HbA1c, but was best accomplished with four injections of regular insulin per day[136]. They performed a randomized crossover study of 8 weeks of oral hypoglycemic agents followed by 8 weeks of two- or four-dose insulin regimens. Mean blood glucose and free-insulin profiles showed that patients taking the oral agents had higher blood glucose and lower postprandial insulin concentrations than those receiving insulin. When patients received the daily four-dose regimen of preprandial regular insulin and intermediate-acting NPH insulin at 10:00 pm, glycemic control improved. The mean HbA1c was 8.8% during treatment with oral therapy, compared with 5.6% on the intensive four-dose insulin regimen.

Perhaps the best evidence that near-normoglycemia is beneficial and feasible with multiple daily insulin injections in type 2 diabetes is the Kumamoto Study[137]. This 8-year study showed a sustained lowering of HbA1c levels and of microvascular complications in the patients treated with multiple injection therapy (short- and intermediate-acting insulin) with a goal of FBG < 140 mg dL^{-1}, 2 h postprandial < 200 mg dL^{-1}, an HbA1c < 7% and a mean amplitude of glycemic excursion < 100 mg dL^{-1}. No worsening of retinopathy or nephropathy was found in patients whose HbA1c, FBG and 2 h postprandial blood-glucose concentrations were below 6.5%, 110 mg dL^{-1}, and 180 mg dL^{-1}, respectively.

The longest study includes 15 patients who have been followed for 110 months while taking insulin after sulfonylurea failure[138]. While there was little difference in insulin dosage between the first weeks of insulin treatment and the 27-month examination, the dosage was increased by the 110-month examination from 51.3 ± 5.2 to 79.5 ± 10.8 U. Glycemic control was improved, with reduction of HbA1c from 8.9% during treatment with oral hypoglycemic agents to 7.3% at the 110-month examination. Body weight increased rapidly during the first 4–5 months, but after 12 months there was no significant change.

Adding oral agents to insulin therapy

Most of the studies reported on the combination of insulin plus oral sensitizers have been based on the addition of an oral agent, such as metformin or a glitazone, to patients already being treated with conventional insulin therapy. This is fundamentally a different issue from starting and then intensifying insulin replacement with strategies to achieve target glycemic control, as discussed extensively above. Nevertheless, the option of adding an insulin sensitizer, or even a secretagogue to patients who are already on insulin therapy should be considered if the HbA1c target is not achieved despite aggressive insulin replacement therapy.

Insulin plus Metformin

Several studies have used metformin as 'add-on' therapy to insulin, with significant improvements in HbA1c. The addition of metformin to pre-existing insulin therapy was first shown to have efficacy beyond that of continuing insulin alone in a study by Giugliano et al. in 1993[139]. Several studies have subsequently addressed this strategy, with decreases in HbA1c of 1–2.5%[140–143]. The largest HbA1c reduction was obtained with maximized intensive insulin therapy in 43 patients with type 2 diabetes who were randomized to added placebo or metformin[140]. The goal of this study was to maximally decrease HbA1c with intensive insulin adjustments, instead of the traditional goal of reducing insulin doses to demonstrate the sensitizer effect. HbA1c levels decreased by 2.5% in the metformin group, a significantly greater change than the decrease of 1.6% in the placebo group. Average final HbA1c levels were 6.5% in the metformin group and 7.6% in the placebo group. For patients who received placebo, the insulin dose increased 23 units, which is 29% more than the dose for patients who received metformin, whose insulin dose decreased slightly. The strategy of adding metformin to insulin can result in significant improvements in HbA1c, especially when the insulin dose is not decreased.

Insulin plus Thiazolidinediones

The clinical availability of the thiazolidinediones introduced the possibility of improving insulin sensitivity in muscle, liver and adipose tissue, thus potentiating the effects and reducing the doses of exogenous insulin. The first study to demonstrate the efficacy of this combination used troglitazone[144], which is now no longer available in the USA due to idiosyncratic hepatotoxicity. Subsequently, the addition of either pioglitazone or rosiglitazone to insulin in patients with poorly controlled type 2 diabetes (HbA1c ≥ 9%) showed a dose-related decrease in HbA1c of 1.2–1.3%, despite mild reductions in insulin dosages[145,146].

The addition of pioglitazone (15 or 30 mg daily) to pre-existing conventional insulin therapy for 16 weeks showed statistically significant decreases in HbA1c in 566 patients who were poorly controlled on conventional insulin alone[145]. Low-dose pioglitazone (15 mg) decreased HbA1c from 9.7% to 8.7%, and a medium dose (30 mg) decreased HbA1c from 9.8% to 8.6% while the insulin doses remained constant. Similarly, the addition of rosiglitazone (4 or 8 mg daily) to pre-existing insulin therapy for 26 weeks showed decreases in HbA1c in 209 patients who were poorly controlled[146]. Medium dose rosiglitazone (4 mg) decreased HbA1c from 9.1% to 8.5%, while high-dose treatment (8 mg) decreased HbA1c from 9.0% to 7.9%. Body weight increased by 2.3–3.7 kg during 16 weeks of treatment with pioglitazone, or 4.0–5.3 kg during the 26 weeks of treatment with rosiglitazone. The incidence of edema was comparable, 15.3% with pioglitazone and 14.7% with rosiglitazone.

Rosiglitazone has recently obtained FDA approval for use in combination therapy with insulin – pioglitazone had previously been granted this indication since its original FDA approval. Neither of these drugs, however, have yet obtained European approval for use in combination with insulin.

Safety issues remain a major concern, especially fluid retention and the potential risk of developing or worsening congestive heart failure (CHF) – particularly in high-risk patients with coronary disease with or without pre-existing CHF.

Further studies are ongoing to determine the long-term safety effects of the glitazones on fluid retention, and especially on the frequency and severity of CHF. When initiating these agents in any patient it is prudent to carefully evaluate the cardiovascular status, start at a very low dose and increase the dose very slowly (i.e. at 3–6- month intervals). In addition, long-term outcome studies are needed to confirm the potential cardiovascular beneficial effects that these drugs may have by improving insulin resistance. No studies are available on the potential benefits of adding glitazones to optimized intensive insulin therapy, in an attempt to further improve glycemic control to levels of HbA1c much lower than 7%.

PRACTICAL GUIDELINES FOR INSULIN REPLACEMENT THERAPY

For physicians managing patients with type 2 diabetes, practical guidelines for pharmacologic interventions are particularly important in view of the major changes there have been over the past 5 years in managing type 2 diabetes, and the growing movement toward starting aggressive pharmacotherapy earlier in the course of the disease. There has also been a paradigm shift that involves the increased use of flexible combination therapy, with lower doses of any of the insulin secretagogues plus an insulin sensitizer (metformin or glitazone) almost from the initiation of pharmacotherapy. This strategy is embraced by the community of diabetes experts, who view early insulin therapy to supplement oral treatment as an effective strategy in reaching a patient's glycemic target.

A practical approach to overcoming the complexity of MDI (multiple daily insulin injections) regimens – and perhaps the best and most acceptable way to initiate insulin therapy – is to start with evening basal insulin replacement for patients who are no longer responding to oral agents. Starting basal insulin replacement while maintaining the use of oral agents has considerable advantages:

- Only one daily injection may be required, without the need to mix different insulin preparations
- Titration can be accomplished in a slow, safe, and simple fashion

---

Table 11.5 Practical guidelines: starting basal insulin

- Continue oral agent(s) at same dosage (eventually reduce)
- Add single, evening basal insulin dose (~ 10 U):
  – Glargine (bedtime or anytime?)
  – NPH (bedtime)
- Adjust dose according to fasting blood glucose (FBG) monitoring
- Increase insulin dose weekly as needed:
  – Increase by 2 units if FBG > 100–120 mg dL^{-1}
  – Increase by 4 units if FBG > 121–140 mg dL^{-1}
  – Increase by 6 units if FBG > 141–180 mg dL^{-1}
  – Increase by 8 units if FBG > 180 mg dL^{-1}
- Do not increase insulin if FBG < 72 mg dL^{-1} or reduce insulin if evidence of hypoglycemia

---

- A lower total dose of insulin will eventually be required because of the synergy of effects from the oral combination therapy.

When insulin is combined with oral agents in asymptomatic patients with type 2 diabetes, it can be initiated as a simple regimen, with a low dose of 10 U of insulin glargine at bedtime (Table 11.5). Basal insulin glargine has the potential to facilitate and extend the use of the evening insulin strategy because of its long duration of action, peakless flat profile, more predictable response, and reduced risk of nocturnal hypoglycemia. Insulin glargine is typically given once - daily at bedtime but, based on its kinetics, it could theoretically be given at any time[147]. The patient can then increase the dose weekly according to fasting self-monitored blood glucose (SMBG) levels, based on an average of 2–3 consecutive days, as long as there is no evidence of nocturnal hypoglycemia, with no measurements ≤ 72 mg dL^{-1} (Table 11.5). Insulin adjustments with appropriate reductions will be required in instances of SMBG < 56 mg dL^{-1}, or with the occurrence of a severe hypoglycemic episode.

Whether all the oral agents should be continued once the insulin regimen has been optimized will depend on the individual patient response. The secretagogue may theoretically be stopped, but some patients may develop wide fluctuations in blood glucose levels suggesting the loss of endogenous insulin secretion and requiring resumption of the secretagogue, or the need for adding short-acting insulin analogs. Metformin should be continued to provide weight control as long as there is no evidence of renal impairment or CHF. A glitazone may be considered to reduce insulin resistance and potentially preserve beta-cell function, as long as there is no evidence of substantial weight gain and fluid retention.

Over time, the need to intensify insulin regimens arises in response to disease progression. The traditional way of supplying insulin, with a twice-daily, split-mixed insulin regimen, should be considered a strategy of the past. 'Premixed' insulin preparations, such as 70/30 or 75/25, do not provide enough flexibility and are seldom effective at reaching glycemic targets.

Clinical judgement should prevail to determine when to advance to a more intensive basal/bolus insulin regimen. Clearly, when the target fasting plasma glucose of 80–120 mg dL^{-1}

has been achieved and the HbA1c remains > 7%, further increments of the evening basal insulin glargine may be attempted, but this approach can result in an increased risk of hypoglycemia. At this point, therefore, adding a preprandial fast-acting insulin analog at the main meal or, eventually, at each meal will result in subsequent improvements in postprandial hyperglycemia and HbA1c levels. Postprandial hyperglycemia can be further improved if patients follow simple algorithms, based on self-monitoring of blood glucose levels to adjust and deliver sufficient premeal insulin doses, using insulin aspart or lispro independently from the basal insulin gargline with no mixing. This approach provides more flexibility and allows additional doses of supplemental insulin as needed to control postprandial hyperglycemia. In this fashion MDI regimens are progressively introduced as a further step toward intensifying insulin therapy to mimic normal physiology (Table 11.6). The use of effective and less troublesome injection devices, such as insulin pens, can facilitate the implementation of the new advances in insulin replacement therapy.

It is conceivable that this practical and simple strategy may have translational implications from clinical research studies into routine clinical practice and benefit large numbers of patients with type 2 diabetes who are followed by general practitioners. This structured regimen can realistically reach HbA1c targets in patients who have progressively intensified oral combination therapy by adding evening basal insulin glargine first and, eventually, premeal lispro, or aspart insulin, or inhaled insulin when available, to control fasting and postprandial glycemic levels.

FUTURE INSULIN REPLACEMENT THERAPIES

Traditionally, the approach to glucose-lowering therapy has been that most patients with type 2 diabetes require insulin – albeit used as a 'last resort' – after maximal combination therapy has failed, 10–15 years after disease onset. However, our improved understanding of the natural history of type 2 diabetes suggests that insulin therapy

---

Table 11.6 Practical guidelines: advancing to basal/bolus insulin

- Indicated when FBG in target range 80–120 mg dL^{-1} but:
  - HbA1c > 7% and/or
  - SBGM postprandial > 160–180 mg dL^{-1}
- Insulin options:
  - To glargine: add mealtime lispro or aspart
  - To bedtime NPH: add morning NPH and mealtime lispro or aspart
- Oral agent options:
  - Continue sulfonylurea for endogenous secretion?
  - Continue metformin for weight control?
  - Continue glitazone for glycemic stability?

should be started sooner, rather than later, and that insulin should be viewed as an essential therapeutic tool for achieving disease management goals at an earlier stage in the natural progression of the disease, rather than being a sign of failure on the part of the physician or the patient.

New strategies involving insulin analogs with improved pharmacokinetic properties – the new armamentarium of oral agents for type 2 diabetes – and future development in routes of insulin administration, will expand treatment options and combination regimens to facilitate the attainment of specific targeted glycemic levels in a safer and more effective manner. The prevention and retarding of the progression of microvascular and macrovascular complications are the ultimate objectives in the management of patients with type 2 diabetes.

REFERENCES

1 UK Prospective Diabetes Study Group. UK Prospective Diabetes Study 16. Overview of 6 years' therapy of type II diabetes: a progressive disease. *Diabetes* 1995;44:1249–58.

2 Inzucchi SE. Oral antihyperglycemic therapy for type 2 diabetes. *J Am Med Assoc* 2002;287:360–72.

3 Yki-Jarvinen H. Combination therapies with insulin in type 2 diabetes. *Diabetes Care* 2001;24:758–67.

4 DeFronzo RA Pharmacologic therapy for type 2 diabetes mellitus. *Ann Intern Med* 1999;131:281–303.

5 Stern MP, Gonzalez C, Mitchell BD *et al.* Genetic and environmental determination of type II diabetes in Mexico City and San Antonio. *Diabetes* 1992;41:484–92.

6 Weyer C, Bogardus C, Mott DM, Pratley RE. The natural history of insulin secretory dysfunction and insulin resistance in the pathogenesis of type 2 diabetes mellitus. *J Clin Invest* 1999;104:787–94.

7 Kahn SE, Prigeon RL, McCulloch DK *et al.* Quantification of the relationship between insulin sensitivity and B-cell function in human subjects. Evidence for a hyperbolic function. *Diabetes* 1993;42:1663–72.

8 Kahn SE, Prigeon RL, Schwartz RS *et al.* Obesity, body fat distribution, insulin sensitivity and islet β-cell function as explanations for metabolic diversity. *J Nutr* 2001;131:354S-60S.

9 Saad MF, Knowler WC, Pettitt DJ *et al.* The natural history of impaired glucose tolerance in the Pima Indians. *N Engl J Med* 1988;319:1500–6.

10 Bogardus C, Tataranni PA. Reduced early insulin secretion in the etiology of type 2 diabetes mellitus in Pima indians. *Diabetes* 2002;51:S262–S264.

11 Buchanan TA. Pancreatic B-cell defects in gestational diabetes: implications for the pathogenesis and prevention of type 2 diabetes. *J Clin Endocrinol Metab* 2001;86:989–93.

12 Bonner-Weir S, Trent DF, Honey RN *et al.* Responses of neonatal rat islets to streptozotocin: limited β-cell regeneration and hyperglycemia. *Diabetes* 1981;30:64–9.

13 Bonner-Weir S, Trent DF, Weir GC. Partial pancreatectomy in the rat and subsequent defect in glucose-induced insulin release. *J Clin Invest* 1983;71:1544–53.

14 Rossetti L, Shulman GI, Zawalich W *et al.* Effect of chronic hyperglycemia on *in vivo* insulin secretion in partially pancreatectomized rats. *J Clin Invest* 1987;80:1037–44.

15 Rossetti L, Smith D, Shulman GI *et al.* Correction of hyperglycemia with phlorizin normalizes tissue sensitivity to insulin in diabetic rats. *J Clin Invest* 1987;79:1510–15.

16 Leahy JL, Bonner-Weir S, Weir GC. Minimal chronic hyperglycemia is a critical determinant of impaired insulin secretion after an incomplete pancreatectomy. *J Clin Invest* 1988;81:1407–14.

17 Leahy JL, Weir GC. Evolution of abnormal insulin secretory responses during 48 h *in vivo* hyperglycemia. *Diabetes* 1988;37:217–22.

18 Leibowitz G, Yuli M, Donath MY *et al.* Beta-cell glucotoxicity in the *Psammomys obesus* model of type 2 diabetes. *Diabetes* 2001;50:S113–S117.

19 Unger RH. Lipotoxic diseases. *Ann Rev Med* 2002;53:319–336.

20 McGarry JD. Banting Lecture 2001: dysregulation of fatty acid metabolism in the etiology of type 2 diabetes. *Diabetes* 2002;51:7–18.

21 Scarlett JA, Gray RS, Griffin J *et al.* Insulin treatment reverses the insulin resistance of type II diabetes mellitus. *Diabetes Care* 1982;5:353–363.

22 Andrews WJ, Vasquez B, Nagulesparan M *et al.* Insulin therapy in obese, non-insulin-dependent diabetes induces improvements in insulin action and secretion that are maintained for two weeks after insulin withdrawal. *Diabetes* 1984;33:634–42.

23 Garvey WT, Olefsky JM, Griffin J *et al.* The effect

of insulin treatment on insulin secretion and insulin action in type II diabetes mellitus. *Diabetes* 1985;34:222–34.

24 Henry RR, Gumbiner B, Ditzler T *et al.* Intensive conventional insulin therapy for type II diabetes. *Diabetes Care* 1993;16:21–31.

25 Pratipanawatr T, Cusi K, Ngo P *et al.* Normalization of plasma glucose concentration by insulin therapy improves insulin-stimulated glycogen synthesis in type 2 diabetes. *Diabetes* 2002;51:462–8.

26 Ilkova H, Glaser B, Tunckale A *et al.* Induction of long-term glycemic control in newly diagnosed type 2 diabetic patients by transient intensive insulin treatment. *Diabetes Care* 1997;20:1353–6.

27 Carey DG, Jenkins AB, Campbell LB *et al.* Abdominal fat and insulin resistance in normal and overweight women: Direct measurements reveal a strong relationship in subjects at both low and high risk of NIDDM. *Diabetes* 1996;45:633–8.

28 Fujimoto WY. The importance of insulin resistance in the pathogenesis of type 2 diabetes mellitus. *Am J Med* 2000;108:9S-14S.

29 Reaven GM. Banting Lecture 1988. Role of insulin resistance in human disease. *Diabetes* 1988;37:1595–607.

30 Executive Summary of The Third Report of The National Cholesterol Education Program (NCEP) Expert Panel on Detection, Evaluation, and Treatment of High Blood Cholesterol in Adults (Adult Treatment Panel III). *J Am Med Assoc* 2001;285:2486–97.

31 Pyörälä K. Relationship of glucose tolerance and plasma insulin to the incidence of coronary heart disease: results from two population studies in Finland. *Diabetes Care* 1979;2:131–41.

32 Haffner SM, Hanley AJ. Do increased proinsulin concentrations explain the excess risk of coronary heart disease in diabetic and prediabetic subjects? *Circulation* 2002;105:2008–9.

33 UK Prospective Diabetes Study (UKPDS) Group. Intensive blood-glucose control with sulphonylureas or insulin compared with conventional treatment and risk of complications in patients with type 2 diabetes (UKPDS 33). *Lancet* 1998;352:837–53.

34 Malmberg K, Norhammar A, Wedel H, Ryden L. Glycometabolic state at admission: important risk marker of mortality in conventionally treated patients with diabetes mellitus and acute myocardial infarction: long-term results from the Diabetes and Insulin-Glucose Infusion in Acute Myocardial Infarction (DIGAMI) study. *Circulation* 1999;99:2626–32.

35 Malmberg K, Ryden L, Hamsten A *et al.* Effects of insulin treatment on cause-specific one-year mortality and morbidity in diabetic patients with acute myocardial infarction. DIGAMI Study Group. Diabetes Insulin-Glucose in Acute Myocardial Infarction. *Eur Heart J* 1996;17:1337–44.

36 Sodi-Pallares D, Testelli MR, Fischleder BL. Effects of an intravenous infusion of a potassium-glucose-insulin solution on the electrocardiographic signs of myocardial infarction. *Am J Cardiol* 1962;9:166–81.

37 Sodi-Pallares D, Bisteni A, Medrano G. The polarizing treatment of acute myocardial infarction. *Dis Chest* 1963;43:424–32.

38 Oliver MF, Kurien VA, Greenwood TW. Relation between serum-free-fatty acids and arrhythmias and death after acute myocardial infarction. *Lancet* 1968;1:710–14.

39 Rogers WJ, Stanley AW, Jr, Breinig JB *et al.* Reduction of hospital mortality rate of acute myocardial infarction with glucose-insulin-potassium infusion. *Am Heart J* 1976;92:441–54.

40 Rogers WJ, Segall PH, McDaniel HG *et al.* Prospective randomized trial of glucose-insulin-potassium in acute myocardial infarction. Effects on myocardial hemodynamics, substrates and rhythm. *Am J Cardiol* 1979;43:801–9.

41 Rackley CE, Russell RO, Jr, Rogers WJ *et al.* Clinical experience with glucose-insulin-potassium therapy in acute myocardial infarction. *Am Heart J* 1981;102:1038–49.

42 Oliver MF, Opie LH. Effects of glucose and fatty acids on myocardial ischaemia and arrhythmias. *Lancet* 1994;343:155–8.

43 Opie LH. Proof that glucose-insulin-potassium provides metabolic protection of ischaemic myocardium? *Lancet* 1999;353:768–9.

44 Welle S, Nair KS, Lockwood D. Effect of a sulfonylurea and insulin on energy expenditure in type II diabetes mellitus. *J Clin Endocrinol Metab* 1988;66:593–7.

45 Boden G, Ray TK, Smith RH, Owen OE. Carbohydrate oxidation and storage in obese non-insulin-dependent diabetic patients. Effects of improving glycemic control. *Diabetes* 1983;32:982–7.

46 Bogardus C, Taskinen M-R, Zawadzki J *et al.* Increased resting metabolic rates in obese subjects with non-insulin-dependent diabetes mellitus and the effect of sulfonylurea therapy. *Diabetes* 1986;35:1–5.

47 Franssila-Kallunki A, Group L. Factors associated with basal metabolic rate in patients with type 2

(non-insulin-dependent) diabetes mellitus. *Diabetologia* 1992;35:962–6.

48 Stumvoll M, Nurjhan N, Perriello G *et al.* Metabolic effects of metformin in non-insulin-dependent diabetes mellitus. *N Engl J Med* 1995; 333: 550–4.

49 Yki-Jarvinen H, Ryysy L, Kauppila M *et al.* Effect of obesity on the response to insulin therapy in noninsulin-dependent diabetes mellitus *J Clin Endocrinol Metabol* 1997;82:4037–43.

50 Lee A, Morley JE. Metformin decreases food consumption and induces weight loss in subjects with obesity with type II non-insulin-dependent diabetes. *Obes Res* 1998;6:47–53.

51 Makimattila S, Nikkila K, Yki-Jarvinen H. Causes of weight gain during insulin therapy with and without metformin in patients with Type II diabetes mellitus. *Diabetologia* 1999;42:406–12.

52 Yki-Jarvinen H, Helve E, Sane T *et al.* Insulin inhibition of overnight glucose production and gluconeogenesis from lactate in NIDDM. *Am J Physiol* 1989;256:E732–9.

53 Himms-Hagan J. Cellular thermogenesis. *Ann Rev Physiol* 1976;37:315–51.

54 Billingham MS, Milles JJ, Bailey CJ, Hall RA. Lipoprotein subfraction composition in non-insulin-dependent diabetes treated by diet, sulphonylurea, and insulin. *Metabolism* 1989;38:850–7.

55 Rivellese AA, Patti L, Romano G *et al.* Effect of insulin and sulfonylurea therapy, at the same level of blood glucose control, on low density lipoprotein subfractions in type 2 diabetic patients. *J Clin Endocrinol Metab* 2000;85:4188–92.

56 Cusi K, Cunningham GR, Comstock PJ. Safety and efficacy of normalizing fasting glucose with bedtime NPH insulin alone in NIDDM. *Diabetes Care* 1995;18:843–51.

57 Emanuele, N Azad N, Abraira C *et al.* Effect of intensive glycemic control on fibrinogen, lipids, and lipoproteins. Veterans Affairs Cooperative Study in type II diabetes mellitus *Arch Intern Med* 1998;158:2485–90.

58 UK Prospective Diabetes Study (UKPDS) Group. Effect of intensive blood-glucose control with metformin on complications in overweight patients with type 2 diabetes (UKPDS 34). *Lancet* 1998;352:854–65.

59 Wright A, Burden AC, Paisey RB *et al.* UK Prospective Diabetes Study Group. Sulfonylurea inadequacy: efficacy of addition of insulin over 6 years in patients with type 2 diabetes in the UK Prospective Diabetes Study (UKPDS 57). *Diabetes Care* 2002;25:330–6.

60 DCCT Research Group. The effect of intensive treatment of diabetes on the development and progression of long-term complications of insulin-dependent diabetes mellitus. *N Engl J Med* 1993;329:977–86.

61 Boyle PJ, Cryer PE. Growth hormone, cortisol, or both are involved in defense against, but are not critical to recovery from, hypoglycemia. *Am J Physiol* 1991;260:E395.

62 Bolli GB, Di Marchi RD, Park GD *et al.* Insulin analogues and their potential in the management of diabetes mellitus. *Diabetologia* 1999;42:1151–67.

63 Owens DR, Zinman B, Bolli GB. Insulins today and beyond. *Lancet* 2001;358:739–46.

64 Skyler JS. Diabetes mellitus, types I and II. In: Humes HD, editor. *Kelley's textbook of internal medicine* 4th edition. Philadelphia: Lippincott Williams & Wilkins, 2000.

65 Howey DC, Bowsher RR, Brunelle RL, Woodworth JR. [Lys(B28), Pro(B29)]-human insulin: a rapidly absorbed analogue of human insulin. *Diabetes* 1994;43:396–402.

66 Holleman F, Hoekstra JBL. Insulin lispro. *N Engl J Med* 1997;337:176–83.

67 Home P D, Barriocannal L, Lindholm A. Comparative pharmacokinetics of the novel rapid-acting insulin analogue, insulin aspart, in healthy volunteers. *Eur J Clin Pharmacol* 1999:55:199–203.

68 Gammeltoft S, Hansen, Dideriksen L *et al.* Insulin aspart: a novel rapid-acting human insulin analogue. *Expert Opin Invest Drugs* 1999;8: 1431–41.

69 Anderson JH Jr, Brumelle RL, Kovisto VA *et al.* Reduction of postprandial hyperglycaemia and frequency of hypoglycaemia in IDDM patients on insulin-analog treatment. *Diabetes* 1997;46: 265–70.

70 Raskin P, Riis A, Guthrie RA *et al.* Use of insulin aspart, a fast acting insulin analog, as the meal time insulin in the management of patients with type 1 diabetes. *Diabetes Care* 2000;23:583–8.

71 Tuominen JA, Karonen SL, Melamie *et al.* Exercise-induced hypoglycaemia in IDDM patients treated with a short-acting insulin analog. *Diabetologia* 1995;38:106–11.

72 Torlone E, Pampanelli S, Lalli C *et al.* Effects of short-acting insulin analog [Lys(B28), Pro(B29)] on postprandial blood glucose control in IDDM. *Diabetes Care* 1996;19:945–52.

73 Del Sindaco P, Ciofetta M, Lalli C *et al.* Use of the short-acting insulin analogue lispro in intensive treatment of type 1 diabetes mellitus: importance of appropriate replacement of basal insulin and time-interval injection-meal. *Diabet Med* 1998; 15:592–600.

74 Gale EAM. A randomized, controlled trial comparing insulin lispro with human soluble insulin in patients with type 1 diabetes on intensified insulin therapy. *Diabet Med* 2000;17:209–14.

75 Brunelle RL, Llewelyn J, Anderson JH *et al.* Meta-analysis of the effect of insulin lispro on severe hypoglycaemia patients with type 1 diabetes. *Diabet Care* 1998;21:1726–31.

76 Heinemann L. Hypoglycaemia and insulin analogues: is there a reduction in the incidence? *J Diabetes Complications* 1999;13:105–14.

77 Home PD, Lindholm A, Hylleberg B, Round P. Improved glycemic control with insulin aspart – a multicentre randomized double-blind cross-over trial in type 1 diabetes mellitus. *Diabetes Care* 1998;21:1904–9.

78 Home PD, Lindholm A, Riis A. Insulin aspart versus human insulin in the management of long-term blood glucose control in type 1 diabetes mellitus: a randomised controlled trial. *Diabet Med* 2000;17:762–70.

79 Heller SR, Amiel SA, Mansell P. Effect of the fast-acting insulin analog lispro on the risk of nocturnal hypoglycaemia during intensified insulin therapy. *Diabetes Care* 1999;22: 1607–11.

80 Lalli C, Ciofetta C, del Sindaco P *et al.* Long term intensive treatment of type 1 diabetes with the short-acting insulin analog Lispro in variable combination with NPH insulin at mealtime. *Diabetes Care* 1999;22:468–77.

81 Colombel A, Murat A, Krempf M *et al.* Improvement of blood glucose control in type 1 diabetic patients treated with lispro and multiple NPH injections. *Diabet Med* 1999;16:319–24.

82 Zinman B, Tildsley H, Chasson JL *et al.* Insulin lispro in CSII: results of a double-blind cross-over study. *Diabetes* 1997;46:440–3.

83 Melki V, Belicar P, Renard E *et al.* Improvement of HbA1c and blood glucose stability in IDDM patients treated with lispro insulin analog in external pumps. *Diabetes Care* 1998;21:977–85.

84 Renner R, Pfützner A, Trautmann M *et al.* Use of insulin lispro in continuous subcutaneous insulin infusion treatment: results of a multicenter trial. *Diabetes Care* 1999;22:784–8.

85 Garg SK, Carmain JA, Braddy KC *et al.* Pre-meal insulin analogue insulin lispro vs Humulin R insulin treatment in young diabetics with type 1 diabetes. *Diabet Med* 1996;13:47–52.

86 Mortensen HB, Lindholm A, Olsen BS, Hylleberg B. Rapid appearance and onset of action of insulin aspart in paediatric subjects with type 1 diabetes. *Eur J Pediatr* 2000;159:483–8.

87 Owens DR, Coates PA, Luzio SD *et al.* Pharmacokinetics of 125I-labeled insulin glargine (HOE901) in healthy men – comparison with NPH insulin and the influence of different subcutaneous injection sites. *Diabetes Care* 2000;23:813–19.

88 Lepore M, Pampanelli S, Fanelli CG *et al.* Pharmacokinetics of subcutaneous injection of long-acting human insulin analog glargine, NPH insulin, ultralente human insulin, and continuous subcutaneous infusion of insulin lispro. *Diabetes* 2000;49:2142–8.

89 Heinemann L, Linkeschova R, Rave K *et al.* Time-action profile of the long-acting insulin analog insulin glargine (HOE901) in comparison with those of NPH insulin and placebo. *Diabetes Care* 2000;23:644–9.

90 Scholtz HE, van Niekesk N, Mayer BH, Rosenkranz B. An assessment of the variability in the pharmacodynamics (glucose lowering effect) of HOE901 compared to NPH and ultralente human insulins using euglycaemic clamp technique. *Diabetologia* 1999;42(Suppl): A235.

91 Pieber TR, Eugene-Jolchine I, Derobert E. The European Study Group of HOE 901 in type 1 diabetes. Efficacy and safety of HOE 901 versus NPH insulin in patients with type 1 diabetes. *Diabetes Care* 2000;23:157–62.

92 Ratner RE, Hirsch IB, Neifing JL *et al.* Less hypoglycemia with insulin glargine in intensive insulin therapy for type 1 diabetes. *Diabetes Care* 2000;23:639–43.

93 Rosenstock J, Park G, Zimmerman J. Basal insulin glargine (HOE 901) versus NPH insulin in patients with type 1 diabetes on multiple daily insulin regimens. US insulin glargine (HOE 901) type 1 diabetes investigator group. *Diabetes Care* 2000;23:1137–42.

94 Raskin P, Klaff L, Bergenstall R *et al.* A 16–week comparison of the novel insulin analog insulin glargine (HOE901) and NPH human insulin used with insulin lispro in patients with type 1 diabetes. *Diabetes Care* 2000;23:1666–71.

95 Mohn A, Strang S, Wernicke-Panteu K *et al.* Nocturnal glucose control and free insulin levels in children with type 1 diabetes by use of the long-acting HOE901 as part of a three-injection regimen. *Diabetes Care* 2000;23:557–9.

96 Yki-Jarvinen H, Dressler A, Ziemen M. Less nocturnal hypoglycaemia and better post-dinner glucose control with bedtime insulin glargine compared with bedtime NPH insulin during insulin combination therapy in type 2 diabetes. HOE 901/3002 study group. *Diabetes Care* 2000;23:1130–6.

97 Rosenstock J, Schwartz SL, Clark CM Jr *et al.* Basal insulin therapy in type 2 diabetes: 28–week comparison of insulin glargine (HOE901) and NPH insulin. *Diabetes Care* 2001;24:631–6.

98 Riddle MC, Rosenstock J, HOE901/4002 Study Group. Treatment to target study: insulin glargine vs NPH insulin added to oral therapy of type 2 diabetes. Successful control with less nocturnal hypoglycemia. *Diabetes* 2002;51 (Suppl):A113.

99 Rosenstock J, Riddle MC, HOE901/4002 Study Group. Treatment to Target Study: timing and frequency of nocturnal hypoglycemia. The value of adding bedtime basal insulin glargine over NPH insulin in insulin-naïve patients with type 2 diabetes on oral agents. *Diabetes* 2002;51(Suppl): A482.

100 Markussen J, Havelund S, Kurtzhals P *et al.* Soluble, fatty acid acylated insulins bind to albumin and show protracted actions in pigs. *Diabetologia* 1996;39:281–8.

101 Heinemann L, Sinha K, Weyer C *et al.* Time-action profile of the soluble fatty acid acylated long acting insulin analogue NN304. *Diabet Med* 1999;16:332–8.

102 Hermansen K, Madsbad S, Perrild H *et al.* Comparison of the soluble basal insulin analog insulin determir with NPH insulin: a randomised, open, cross-over trial in type 1 diabetic subjects on basal-bolus therapy. *Diabetes Care* 2001;24:296–301.

103 D'Eliseo P, Blaauw J, Milicevic Z *et al.* Patient acceptability of a new 3.0 ml pre-filled insulin pen. *Curr Med Res Opin* 2000;16:125–33.

104 Gall MA, Mathiesen ER, Skott P *et al.* Effect of multiple insulin injections with a pen injector on metabolic control and general well-being in insulin-dependent diabetes mellitus. *Diabetes Res* 1989;11:97–101.

105 Bindra S, Rosenstock J, Cefalu WT. Inhaled insulin: a novel route for insulin delivery. *Expert Opin Investig Drug* 2002; 11:687–91.

106 JS Patton, Bukar J, Nagarajan S. Inhaled insulin. *Adv Drug Delivery Rev* 1999;35:235–47.

107 Heinemann L, Klappoth W, Rave K *et al.* Intra-individual variability of the metabolic effect of inhaled insulin together with an absorption enhancer *Diabetes Care* 2000;23:1343–7.

108 Weiss SR, Berger S, Cheng S *et al.* for the Phase II inhaled insulin study group. Adjunctive therapy with inhaled human insulin in type 2 diabetic patients failing oral agents: a multicenter Phase II trial. *Diabetes* 1999;48(Suppl):A12.

109 Cherrington, AD. Control of glucose production

110 Ashcroft FM, Gribble FM. ATP-sensitive K$^+$ channels and insulin secretion: their role in health and disease. *Diabetologia* 1999;42:903–19.

111 Zimmerman BR. Sulfonylureas. *Endocrinol Metab Clin North Am* 1997;26:511–21.

112 Doar JW, Thompson ME, Wilde CE, Sewell PF. Diet and oral antidiabetic drugs and plasma sugar and insulin levels in patients with maturity-onset diabetes mellitus. *Br Med J* 1976;1: 498–500.

113 Fuhlendorrf J, Rorsman P, Kofod H *et al.* Stimulation of insulin release by repaglinide and glibenclamide involves both common and distinct processes. *Diabetes* 1998;47:345–51.

114 Malaisse WJ. Stimulation of insulin release by non-sulfonylurea hypoglycemic agents: the meglitinide family. *Horm Metab Res* 1995;27:263–6.

115 Perfetti R, Ahmad A. Novel sulfonylurea and non-sulfonylurea drugs to promote the secretion of insulin. *Trends Endocrinol Metab* 2000;11: 218–23.

116 Musi N, Hirshman MF, Nygren J. Metformin increases AMP-activated protein kinase activity in skeletal muscle of subjects with type 2 diabetes. *Diabetes* 2002;51:2074–81.

117 Stumvoll M, Nurjhan N, Perriello G. Metabolic effects of metformin in non-insulin-dependent diabetes mellitus. *N Engl J Med* 1995;333:550–4.

118 Johansen K. Efficacy of metformin in the treatment of NIDDM: meta-analysis. *Diabetes Care* 1999;22:33–7.

119 Inzucchi SE, Maggs DG, Spollett GR. Efficacy and metabolic effects of metformin and troglitazone in type II diabetes mellitus. *N Engl J Med* 1998;338:867–72.

120 Kirpichnikov D, McFarlane SI, Sowers JR. Metformin: an update. *Ann Intern Med* 2002;137: 25–33.

121 Petersen KF, Krssak M, Inzucchi S *et al.* Mechanism of troglitazone action in type 2 diabetes. *Diabetes* 2000;49:827–31.

122 Mudaliar S, Henry RR. New oral therapies for type 2 diabetes mellitus: the glitazones or insulin sensitizers. *Annu Rev Med* 2001;52:239–57.

123 Frias JP, Yu JG, Kruszynska YT, Olefsky JM. Metabolic effects of troglitazone therapy in type 2 diabetic, obese, and lean normal subjects. *Diabetes Care* 2000;23:64–9.

124 Nolan JJ, Ludvik B, Beerdsen P *et al.* Improvement in glucose tolerance and insulin

in vivo by insulin and glucagon. In: Jefferson LS, Cherrington AD, editors. *Handbook of physiology.* Bethesda, MD: Am Physiol Soc, 2001:759–85.

resistance in obese subjects treated with troglitazone. *N Engl J Med* 1994;331:1188–93.

125 Maggs DG, Buchanan TA, Burant CF *et al.* Metabolic effects of troglitazone monotherapy in type 2 diabetes mellitus. *Ann Intern Med* 1998;128: 176–85.

126 Goke B, Herrmann-Rinke C. The evolving role of alpha-glucosidase inhibitors. *Diabetes Metab Res Rev* 1998;14 (Suppl):S31–S38.

127 Lebowitz HE. α-Glucosidase inhibitors as agents in the treatment of diabetes. *Diabetes Rev* 1998;6:132–45.

128 Holman RR, Steemson J, Turner RC. Sulphonylurea failure in type 2 diabetes: treatment with a basal insulin supplement. *Diabet Med* 1987;4:457–62.

129 Riddle MC, Hart JS, Bouma DJ *et al.* Efficacy of bedtime NPH insulin with daytime sulfonylurea for subpopulation of type II diabetic subjects. *Diabetes Care* 1989;12:623–9.

130 Gastaldelli A, Baldi S, Pettiti M *et al.* Influence of obesity and type 2 diabetes on gluconeogenesis and glucose output in humans: a quantitative study. *Diabetes* 2000;49:1367–73.

131 Shank ml, Del Prato S, DeFronzo A. Bedtime insulin/daytime glipizide: effective therapy for sulfonylurea failures in NIDDM. *Diabetes* 1995;44:165–72.

132 Riddle MC, Schneider J. Beginning insulin treatment of obese patients with evening 70/30 insulin plus glimepiride versus insulin alone. Glimepiride Combination Group. *Diabetes Care* 1998;21:1052–7.

133 Yki-Jarvinen H, Ryysy L, Nikkila K *et al.* Comparison of bedtime insulin regimens in patients with type 2 diabetes mellitus. A randomized, controlled trial. *Ann Intern Med* 1999;130:389–96.

134 Bastyr EJ, Stuart CA, Brodows RG *et al.* Therapy focused on lowering postprandial glucose, not fasting glucose, may be superior for lowering HbA1c. IOEZ Study Group. *Diabetes Care* 2000;23:1236–41.

135 Rosenstock J. Exubera Phase III Study Group. Mealtime rapid-acting inhaled insulin (Exubera) improves glycemic control in patients with type 2 diabetes failing oral agents: a 3–month, randomized, comparative trial. *Diabetes* 2002;51(Suppl. 2):A132.

136 Lindstrom TH, Arnqvist HJ, von Schenck HH. Effect of conventional and intensified insulin therapy on free-insulin profiles and glycemic control in NIDDM. *Diabetes Care* 1992;5:27–34.

137 Shichiri M, Kishikawa H, Ohkubo Y, Wake N. Long-term results of the Kumamoto Study on optimal diabetes control in type 2 diabetic patients. *Diabetes Care* 2000;23 (Suppl 2):B21–29.

138 Lindstrom T. Sustained improvement of glycemic control by insulin treatment after 9 years in patients with type 2 diabetes and secondary failure. *Diabetes Care* 1999;22:1373–4.

139 Giugliano D, Quatraro A, Consoli G *et al.* Metformin for obese, insulin-treated diabetic patients: improvement in glycemic control and reduction of metabolic risk factors. *Eur J Clin Pharmacol* 1993;44:107–12.

140 Aviles-Santa L, Sinding J, Raskin P. Effects of metformin in patients with poorly controlled, insulin-treated type 2 diabetes mellitus. A randomized, double-blind, placebo-controlled trial. *Ann Intern Med* 1999;131:182–8.

141 Bergenstal R, Johnson M, Whipple D *et al.* Advantages of adding metformin to multiple dose insulin therapy in type 2 diabetes. *Diabetes* 1998;47(Suppl. 1):abstract 347.

142 Relimpio F, Pumar A, Losada F *et al.* Adding metformin versus insulin dose increase in insulin-treated but poorly controlled type 2 diabetes mellitus: an open-label randomized trial. *Diabet Med* 1998;15:997–1002,

143 Robinson AC, Burke J, Robinson S *et al.* The effects of metformin on glycemic control and serum lipids in insulin-treated NIDDM patients with suboptimal metabolic control. *Diabetes Care* 1998;21:701–5.

144 Schwartz S, Raskin P, Fonseca V, Graveline JF. Effect of troglitazone in insulin treated patients with type II diabetes mellitus: Troglitazone and Exogenous Insulin Study Group. *N Engl J Med* 1998;338:861–6.

145 Rosenstock J, Einhorn D, Hershon K *et al.* Efficacy and safety of pioglitazone in type 2 diabetes: a randomized, placebo-controlled study in patients receiving stable insulin therapy. *Int J Clin Pract* 2002;56:251–7.

146 Raskin P, Rendell M, Riddle MC *et al.* [The Rosiglitazone Clinical Trials Study Group]. A randomized trial of rosiglitazone therapy in patients with inadequately controlled insulin-treated type 2 diabetes. *Diabetes Care* 2001;24:1226–32.

147 Hamann A, Matthaei S, Rosak C [The HOE901/4007 Study Group]. Once daily insulin glargine is effective and safe regardless of whether injected before breakfast or dinner, or at bedtime. *Diabetes* 2002;51(Suppl. 2):A53.

12

Combination therapy for treatment of type 2 diabetes

Anthony L McCall and Matthew C Riddle

INTRODUCTION

Combinations of oral antihyperglycemic agents together or with insulin are more appropriate for treatment of type 2 diabetes mellitus than for type 1 diabetes. This discussion concentrates on how to match the therapy of type 2 diabetes with the underlying pathophysiologic defects. While currently approved combinations are given most attention, therapeutic combinations that are not yet approved by the USA Food and Drug Administration (FDA) are also discussed to the extent that published data about them are available. Although the American Diabetes Association's optimal treatment goal [< 7% glycosylated hemoglobin (HbA1c)] is assumed as a therapeutic target, intensive insulin therapy, which in some cases is necessary to achieve this goal, is not discussed.

HISTORY OF COMBINATION THERAPY

Monotherapy

Since the development of sulfonylureas, pharmacotherapy for type 2 diabetes has commonly begun with one of these agents once dietary and lifestyle advice has proved insufficient to maintain glycemic control. Until the introduction of biguanides, patients were usually switched to once- or twice-daily insulin administration when secondary failure of sulfonylureas occurred. Sometimes insulin was combined with sulfonylureas, but for years there was little insight into how best to do this, nor clear demonstration of the value of this combination. After metformin came into use in some parts of the world, this agent was used as initial pharmacotherapy for many patients, especially those who were notably obese, until the time of secondary failure and initiation of insulin. In some cases, metformin and a sulfonylurea were used together to delay the need for insulin, but when insulin became necessary both oral agents were usually discontinued.

Delayed insulin use

An important aspect of this traditional approach to type 2 diabetes was that initiation of insulin therapy was often delayed until severe hyperglycemia occurred. One reason was the inconvenience of injecting insulin, which for many years involved use of glass syringes and needles that required sterilization before reuse, and the fact that insulins often caused inflammation and chronic tissue changes at the sites of injection. In addition, type 2 diabetes was often considered a mild disorder[1], for which insulin was not necessary or appropriate. This erroneous concept has since been rejected because of evidence of the severe microvascular and macrovascular complications of this form of diabetes, and better insulins and devices for delivering it have made treatment much less burdensome. However, many physicians now still use insulin only as a last resort.

Persisting reluctance to begin insulin seems related to several factors, including concern that insulin therapy causes hyperinsulinemia, weight gain, and hypoglycemia and, for these reasons, may lead to poor clinical outcomes. Poor outcomes are assured for any therapy if its use is delayed until the condition is far advanced. In the case of insulin, poor outcomes of patients with type 2 diabetes seem more likely due to delay of treatment than because insulin has any intrinsic toxicity. With this in mind, this chapter proposes a simple strategy for initiating insulin therapy for type 2 diabetes, using the principles of combination therapy.

The UKPDS and the progression of therapy

The United Kingdom Prospective Diabetes Study (UKPDS) was a landmark trial that examined the ability of several medications for treatment of type 2 diabetes and its related abnormalities to limit chronic complications. The main part of the UKPDS was a monotherapy trial of glycemic control. In this 'glucose control' study[2], sulfonylurea and insulin monotherapy were assessed for their ability to reduce complications, using an intensive treatment policy in comparison with a conventional policy based on dietary advice. Glycemic control achieved over a 10-year period, as estimated by median HbA1c, was 7% for the intensive policy group and 7.9% for the conventional policy group. The improvement of glycemic control reflected by this 0.9% difference of HbA1c resulted in a reduction of about 25% in microvascular endpoints, such as retinopathy, and a trend toward fewer rather than more cardiovascular events.

In a smaller substudy including patients who were more overweight, and also testing the effects of metformin, a lesser reduction of HbA1c occurred (about 0.6%), resulting in a trend for microvascular benefits and a significant benefit in some macrovascular endpoints, such as death and myocardial infarction[3]. These results provided convincing evidence of the benefit of good glycemic control with currently available monotherapies, and largely laid to rest the fear that treatment with either insulin or sulfonylureas increases cardiovascular mortality.

Progressive insulin secretory defect

An important physiological analysis performed by the UKPDS investigators estimated insulin secretion using a homeostasis (HOMA) model[4]. Fasting insulin and glucose levels were measured initially and repeated yearly over a 6-year period to determine by a mathematical model the natural history of beta-cell function. As shown in Figure 12.1 and, in more detail, in Figure 12.2, beta-cell function in the group assigned to diet treatment was initially reduced and then inexorably deteriorated. The groups taking sulfonylureas or metformin showed similar patterns of beta-cell function. That is, function was reduced at the outset and, after an immediate improvement associated with the onset of pharmacotherapy, deteriorated at the same rate as for the diet-treated group. Apparently, sulfonylureas did not accelerate the loss of beta-cell function, and metformin did not protect against it, as had been proposed. Thus, the UKPDS gave another important message, that type 2 diabetes is a progressive disorder, mainly because of declining insulin secretion over time.

It is hoped that current or future therapies, such as thiazolidinediones or gut peptide analogues, may ameliorate this progressive insulin secretory dysfunction. However, rigorous evidence that any therapy has this benefit is still lacking, despite some promising preliminary results.

Progressive attenuation of the response to monotherapy

Presumably linked to the gradual loss of insulin secretory function is a decline in the effectiveness of any monotherapy[5]. Figure 12.3 shows a gradual upward climb of HbA1c for patients using either conventional or intensive policy in the UKPDS. The deterioration of metabolic control was not prevented by any monotherapeutic regimen, including injected insulin, although the insulin regimen was not consistently advanced to intensive insulin therapy.

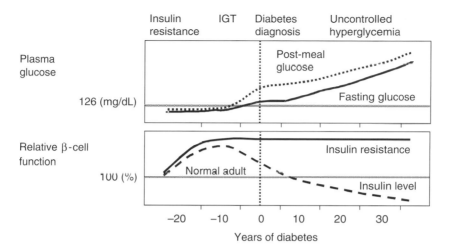

Figure 12.1 Progressive course of type 2 diabetes. This composite figure illustrates the principal pathophysiological defects in type 2 diabetes mellitus. The solid line (bottom panel) shows that insulin resistance starts well before the onset of hyperglycemia and the diagnosis of diabetes. The dashed line in the bottom panel shows that the onset of diabetes is caused by failure of the compensatory hyperinsulinemia that characterizes the metabolic syndrome of insulin resistance, the precursor to diabetes or impaired glucose tolerance (IGT). In the top panel, the dotted line shows that post-meal glucose levels rise as insulin deficiency progresses and that only later does fasting glycemia deteriorate (solid line). (Reproduced with permission from the publisher, from: Mudaliar SRD, Edelman SV, Intensive Insulin Therapy for Patients with Type 2 Diabetes Mellitus. In: LeRoith D, Taylor SI, Olefsky JM eds. *Diabetes Mellitus.* Philadelphia: Lippincott Williams & Williams, 2000.)

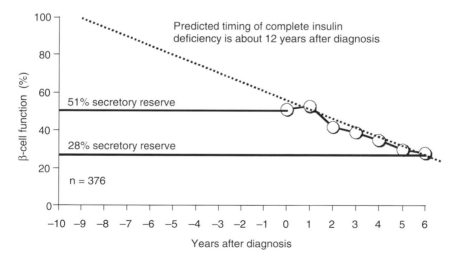

Figure 12.2 β-cell function on diet for 6 years. Based upon a homeostasis model (HOMA), residual maximal insulin secretory reserve is depicted at the time of diagnosis and yearly for 6 years in subjects receiving diet only in the UKPDS. This figure illustrates that nearly half of insulin secretion is lost at diagnosis. It also shows the progressive loss of insulin secretory reserve, which predicts essentially complete insulin deficiency in about a dozen years if further loss were linear. (Adapted with permission from The American Diabetes Association, from ref. 4. © 1995 American Diabetes Association.)

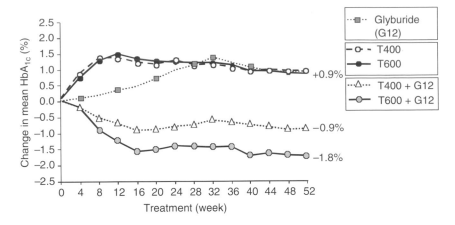

Figure 12.5 The greater therapeutic efficacy of combination oral agent therapy with an insulin secretagogue and an insulin sensitizer, in this instance the latter is the now discontinued drug troglitazone. As was shown for glyburide and metformin in Figure 12.4, this figure shows that either by continuation of glyburide at 12 mg doses (G12; maximal dosing) or substitution of troglitazone, no significant glycemic improvement occurs as measured by HgA1c change from baseline. By contrast, combination therapy is superior and reveals the dose-dependent benefit of the thiazolidinedione insulin sensitizer. (Reproduced with permission from The American Diabetes Association, from ref. 12. © 1998 American Diabetes Association.)

achieving equal or better glycemic control. This principle has been tested directly for the combination of glyburide and metformin[13].

Combinations of oral agents may seem more complex than monotherapy, but in some cases their convenience can be enhanced. Combining a single dose of a long-acting sulfonylurea, such as glimepiride or extended-release glipizide, with one or two tablets of metformin, may have equal or more benefit than three or four tablets of metformin alone. A metformin–glyburide combination pill (Glucovance), has recently been introduced and may signal a trend for the future. Convenient formulations of two agents in a single pill with dual actions may appeal to many patients and practitioners. While separate titration of agents may be desirable for many patients, for others a case can be made for combination preparations. This tactic may prove especially attractive for patients who must take not only two or more agents for glycemic control, but also many other medications for blood pressure, lipid abnormalities, heart disease, and other problems.

Avoiding insulin

A final aspect of convenience of combined oral agent therapy deserves comment, the convenience of avoiding insulin treatment. As mentioned above, many patients and physicians prefer not to use insulin if it can be avoided. Use of insulin may be frightening and may appear to be a punishment for poor lifestyle choices, and brings the risk of hypoglycemia. It remains to be seen whether combinations of three or even four oral agents will prove equally or better tolerated, and will lead to equal or better outcomes than earlier introduction of insulin.

Insulin and oral agents

The combination of insulin and oral agents can offer convenience for patients as well, by minimizing the number of injections of insulin required. While dosage of insulin may not be important to clinicians, patients taking insulin often perceive lower doses to be an advantage. More importantly, minimizing the number of injections and the size of an individual injection reduces the discomfort and inconvenience of multiple or large injections. This advantage is most evident for patients who are very insulin-resistant and therefore require > 100 units at a time, making a single injection not feasible if insulin is used as monotherapy

Non-glycemic effects of combination therapy

A final rationale for combination therapy relates to proven or potential benefits other than those resulting from better glycemic control. This concept has been most emphasized for metformin and the thiazolidinediones. Both of these classes of agents have potential non-glycemic effects that may reduce cardiovascular risk. In the UKPDS, metformin use by obese patients reduced cardiovascular events, such as myocardial infarction, relative to the rate seen with diet alone. Statistically significant benefits of this kind were lacking with insulin or sulfonylurea treatment[2,3]. This additional effect of metformin may have been related to the lack of weight-gain in the group using it in the UKPDS, which contrasted to the consistent gain in the groups assigned to sulfonylureas or insulin. Similarly, the thiazolidinediones may have various nonglycemic effects, among them reducing markers for procoagulant and inflammatory states, and normalizing endothelium-dependent vasorelaxation and smooth muscle migration. Some studies have found lipid and blood pressure benefits as well. Randomized clinical trials testing of whether these apparently protective physiologic effects will result in improved clinical outcomes are underway.

TACTICS FOR ACHIEVING CONTROL WITH COMBINATION THERAPY

Addressing dual defects with dual therapies

Both insulin deficiency and insulin resistance are present in most patients with diabetes. As a result, most patients will need treatment of both

physiologic abnormalities and, therefore, combination pharmacotherapy.

Secretagogues and insulin-assisting agents

Insulin secretagogues that are currently available include several sulfonylureas and the fast-acting, short-duration meglitinides. Insulin-assisting agents that are available include the biguanide metformin and the thiazolidinediones, rosiglitazone and pioglitazone. Not included in either of these groups are the alpha-glucosidase inhibitors acarbose, miglitol and voglibose. Conceptually, they do not neatly address a known physiologic defect of diabetes as do the other classes of agents. By delaying carbohydrate absorption from the small intestine, through inhibition of the breakdown of disaccharides and polysaccharides, they reduce the amount of insulin required to combat meal-related hyperglycemia. Thus, they may be considered another type of insulin-assisting agent. The most widely used forms of oral combination therapy for diabetes pair an insulin secretagogue with an insulin-assisting agent.

Combining insulin and insulin-assisting agents

Later in the course of type 2 diabetes, when insulin deficiency is more marked, oral therapy alone fails to maintain control and insulin therapy is needed. Continuation of previously used oral agents while starting insulin is a form of combination therapy that has become more common recently. This tactic allows insulin to be started with a simple regimen and titrated gradually, giving the patient time to learn the new procedures and gain confidence with insulin therapy. It also avoids the temporary loss of glycemic control that may occur when oral agents are discontinued and the dosage of insulin required is being established. Later, as a more complex insulin regimen becomes necessary, the benefit of ongoing oral-insulin combination therapy is less obvious, but use of insulin-assisting agents may continue to improve the results of treatment.

ORAL AGENT COMBINATION THERAPY

Secretagogues with biguanides

This combination has become very widely used in clinical practice and, for this reason, requires few comments. The first published data on oral agent combination in the US were for glyburide and metformin, as illustrated in Figure 12.4[11]. Drug dosing in this study (20 mg of glyburide and up to 2550 mg of metformin daily) was probably supramaximal for both the sulfonylurea and the metformin. Sulfonylureas have hyperbolic dose–response curves. Thus, doses for most patients need not exceed one-half of the approved maximal dose because this conveys most of the long-term glycemic benefit. Although metformin has been used for decades, only recently has an excellent dose–response study been published[14]. This study showed that maximal glucose lowering occurred at 2 g per day, suggesting the most appropriate full dosage regimen should be 1000 mg twice a day.

It is likely that similar benefit can be gained with combined use of other sulfonylureas or insulin secretagogues with metformin[15], although there is little published information. These authors tend to favor use of once a day sulfonylureas, such as glimepiride and extended release glipizide, in combination with metformin, because of their convenient once-daily dosing and reduced risk of hypoglycemia in comparison with glyburide.

Secretagogues with thiazolidinediones

Just as combining insulin secretagogues with insulin-assisting agents works well with metformin as the insulin-assisting agent, so too combinations of thiazolidinediones and secretagogues are effective. The large trial shown in Figure 12.5 found that adding troglitazone could restore glycemic control in patients with secondary failure of glyburide[12]. The study compared continued glyburide at maximal dosage with troglitazone alone in doses of 200, 400 and 600 mg, and to the combination of the two agents. The patients studied had fasting glucose between 140 and 300 mg dL^{-1}

(7.8–16.7 mmol L^{-1}) and C-peptide ≥ 0.5 nmol L^{-1} (1.5 ng m L^{-1}). It is perhaps important for the response to the thiazolidinedione in this study that the subjects were very obese, with mean body mass index (BMI) of 31–34 kg m^{-2} in the several subgroups, and had very poor glycemic control at baseline, with mean HbA1c 9.4–9.7%. The glycemic benefit of combination therapy in this study was substantial, with the highest dose of troglitazone plus glyburide lowering fasting serum glucose on average 79 mg dL^{-1} (4.4 mM) and lowering HbA1c 2.79% compared to glyburide alone. Thiazolidinediones have a relatively linear dose–response curve within the recommended dose range. This means that if ≥ 2% reduction of HbA1c is needed, maximally approved doses will usually be required to approach the glycemic target. Side effects, such as edema or weight gain may limit their use in a few patients.

Presumably, maximum doses of other thiazolidinediones will yield similar improvements to those demonstrated by troglitazone combined with sulfonylureas. In the case of rosiglitazone[16], evidence for this comes from a study in which 574 patients were randomized to continue sulfonylureas, or add submaximal doses of rosiglitazone (1 or 2 mg twice daily, compared to the maximal approved 4 mg twice daily dosage) for 26 weeks in a placebo-controlled trial. The higher dose of rosiglitazone reduced HbA1c by 1.0% and fasting plasma glucose by 44 mg dL^{-1} (2.44 mmol L^{-1}), while the lower dose reduced HbA1c by 0.6% and glucose by 24 mg dL^{-1} (1.35 mmol L^{-1}). Likewise, in a study of similar size[17], pioglitazone was given at less than the 45 mg maximal dosage (15 and 30 mg), and reduced HbA1c and fasting plasma glucose by 0.9% and 39 mg dL^{-1} (2.17 mmol L^{-1}) and 1.3% and 58 mg dL^{-1} (3.2 mmol L^{-1}) in a randomized comparison with placebo. Although studies directly comparing the effects of these agents have not been performed, these findings suggest they have roughly similar therapeutic power when combined at full dosage with sulfonylureas.

Short-acting secretagogues, such as repaglinide, can also be used in combination with thiazolidinediones. In a 22-week randomized study[18] of troglitazone (up to 600 mg) and repaglinide (up to 4 mg preprandially), combination therapy reduced HbA1c by 1.7% and fasting serum glucose by 80 mg dL^{-1} in comparison to monotherapy with repaglinide alone (0.8% and 43 mg dL^{-1}) or troglitazone (0.4% and 46 mg dL^{-1}).

Secretagogues with alpha-glucosidase inhibitors

Although alpha-glucosidase inhibitors are commonly used in Europe and Japan, they are less often used in the USA. Addition of an alpha-glucosidase inhibitor to an insulin secretagogue may reduce HbA1c by 0.5–1%. For example, in a 28-week trial of acarbose added to diet or sulfonylurea-treated subjects with inadequate control, the mean HbA1c reduction was 0.66% compared with placebo[19]. Much of this effect was due to reduction of postprandial hyperglycemia. The mean 1 h PPG level declined by 41 mg dL^{-1} (2.3 mmol L^{-1}) when acarbose was added.

Combinations of insulin-assisting agents

Insulin resistance may occur at multiple sites and several kinds of assisting agents exist, combinations can therefore be used. The glycemic effect is generally less robust than that seen in studies of combined secretagogue and sensitizer therapy. In one study[20], 3 months of treatment with metformin reduced fasting and postprandial plasma glucose levels by 20% (58 mg dL^{-1} or 3.2 mmol L^{-1}) and 25% (87 mg dL^{-1} or 4.8 mmol L^{-1}). The same duration of troglitazone treatment exerted similar monotherapeutic benefit, with a reduction in fasting and postprandial plasma glucose of 20% (54 mg dL^{-1} or 2.9 mmol L^{-1}) and 25% (83 mg dL^{-1} or 4.6 mmol L^{-1}). The combination of these therapies resulted in a further reduction of fasting and postprandial glucose of 18% (41 mg dL^{-1} or 2.3 mmol L^{-1}) and 21% (54 mg dL^{-1} or 3.0 mmol L^{-1}) and a reduction of mean HbA1c of 1.2%. Another study showed that addition of 30 mg of pioglitazone to metformin reduced HbA1c by 0.83 over 16 weeks, with further improvement in an open label extension of the trial that permitted higher doses of pioglitazone[21]. A third study showed that addition of full-dose (8 mg) rosiglitazone to metformin led to 1.2% reduction of HbA1c over 26 weeks[22]. These studies suggest that combining a thiazolidinedione with metformin is useful for some patients, especially those who are very obese and have marked insulin resistance with significant endogenous insulin remaining.

Combinations of three oral agents

Relatively few reports of triple oral agent therapy exist. A retrospective study[23] examined the addition of troglitazone 600 mg daily for patients inadequately controlled on metformin and the sulfonylurea glimepiride. In this study, significant declines in HbA1c occurred at 2 and 6 months (1.6 and 2.5%). In another small, non-randomized, prospective study[24] of patients offered troglitazone 400 mg for 3 months in addition to metformin and a sulfonylurea, about 62% of the patients achieved ≥ 1% decline and of these 68% reached the minimal HbA1c goal of 8%. Increasing the dose to 600 mg and extending the observation to 6 months did little to improve glycemia further. The only randomized placebo controlled trial[25] of triple agent oral therapy that has been published found that adding 400 mg of troglitazone for 6 month to patients with poor glycemic control (HbA1c 9.7%), already on a sulfonylurea and metformin, resulted in a mean 1.4% reduction of HbA1c. While this was far superior to placebo, only 43% of patients in this trial reached the minimally acceptable glycemic target of < 8% HbA1c.

The question should be raised whether use of triple oral agent therapy makes sense from a cost-effectiveness standpoint when compared with injected insulin, the main therapeutic alternative, but no comparative trials have been completed. The studies described above provide support for trying a thiazolidinedione for a few months in patients who are not successful with metformin plus a secretagogue, have HbA1c levels that are < 9%, and for whom using insulin is in any way problematic.

COMBINATION INSULIN AND ORAL AGENT THERAPY: TRANSITION TO INSULIN

Insulin with insulin secretagogues

Insulin therapy is needed for most patients with type 2 diabetes eventually. An evening insulin strategy is a simple way to begin insulin therapy that will achieve glycemic goals and is easily understood by patients. The rationale for evening insulin has previously been reviewed[26–28]. In brief, an evening injection of intermediate or long-acting insulin addresses a fundamental need in management of type 2 diabetes, by suppressing overnight endogenous glucose production and thereby preventing hyperglycemia prior to the first meal of the day. This approach is useful for most patients with type 2 diabetes, with the notable exception of patients taking morning glucocorticoid therapy. There are several versions of this strategy, using, respectively, intermediate-acting insulin at bedtime, intermediate and quick-acting insulin at dinnertime, or insulin glargine at bedtime. Most of the evidence for these regimens comes from trials of insulin combined with a sulfonylurea alone or with metformin, with the oral agents continued while the insulin dosage is gradually increased until control is reestablished.

NPH at bedtime

Addition of an injection of NPH insulin within an hour of bedtime is usually able to restore adequate glycemic control for patients who are no longer well-controlled with one or more oral agents alone. This tactic may be best employed in leaner patients (BMI ≤ 29), who seem to need short-acting insulin at suppertime less often. A multicenter trial has shown bedtime NPH insulin plus daytime oral agents achieves as good glycemic control as insulin taken in the morning with oral agents, or mixed intermediate and regular insulin twice daily without oral agents, however, there is less weight gain[29]. Other trials show better glycemic control with bedtime NPH plus a sulfonylurea than with a single injection of insulin alone[30–31]. Evening NPH insulin also reduces free fatty acids (FFA)

to a greater degree than use of daytime insulin[32]. Patients can begin with a low dose of NPH insulin, usually about 10 units. They are instructed to self titrate the dose up by 2–4 units every 3–7 days based upon the stability of their fasting glycemic response. Stable patients may titrate more quickly, based upon the pattern of response, but there is little reason to hurry because glucose control will steadily improve at any rate of titration so long as the oral agents are continued. The insulin dosage required is frequently in the range of 30–50 units daily, or about 0.4–0.5 units per kilogram of body weight. The target for fasting glucose should be individualized and adjusted when hypoglycemia occurs, but often can be the recommended 90–130 mg dL^{-1} (5–7.2 mmol L^{-1}) value in plasma-referenced home glucose-monitoring systems. Patients need to wake at a reasonably consistent time and eat breakfast consistently. Oral agents are continued, although sulfonylureas are usually given only with the first meal of the day.

A randomized trial has examined the choice of daytime therapy accompanying bedtime NPH insulin[33]. This study compared four different regimens in a prospective 1-year randomized controlled trial. The four regimens included bedtime insulin combined with

- Morning insulin
- Glyburide alone
- Metformin alone
- Glyburide combined with metformin.

The least weight gain occurred when metformin was the only oral agent, and hypoglycemia was a limiting factor when glyburide was used.

Premixed insulin with the evening meal

A second form of evening insulin that appears to work best for more obese patients (BMI ≥ 30) is the combination of morning sulfonylureas and suppertime mixed insulin, the latter commonly offered as 70/30 (70% NPH with 30% Regular) insulin. In a multicenter study using the long-acting sulfonylurea glimepiride[34], illustrated in Figure 12.6, patients achieved a more

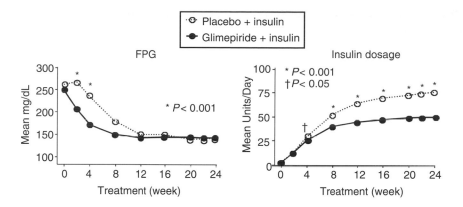

Figure 12.6 A transition strategy of adding insulin for obese patients failing oral agents using morning secretagogue plus a suppertime mixed insulin preparation (70/30 insulin combining NPH and Regular insulin). The titration of insulin dosing based upon the fasting glucose achieves more rapid control with combination therapy and does so at lower insulin doses. (Reproduced with permission from The American Diabetes Association, from ref. 34. © 1998 American Diabetes Association.)

rapid restoration of glycemic control with self-titration of 70/30 insulin while continuing the oral agent, rather than with insulin alone. Insulin was started at 10 units and titrated weekly, seeking fasting plasma glucose equivalent to 140 mg dL^{-1} (7.8 mmol L^{-1}, plasma-referenced). Nearly all subjects using the combination regimen reached the titration target rapidly, but 15% of the subjects in the placebo plus insulin group dropped out, mainly due to hyperglycemia during the transition to insulin. The mean HbA1c declined from almost 10% to 7.6% for subjects completing the trial in both groups. The mean dose in the insulin alone group was 78 units and, for the glimepiride plus insulin combination, was 49. More subjects on insulin alone needed doses higher than 100 units daily, and so had to take more than one injection. A smaller study with a more aggressive titration scheme found better glycemic control using 70/30 insulin with the evening meal plus glyburide once daily, than with evening insulin alone[35].

Insulin glargine at bedtime

A recently published study using insulin glargine[36] suggests this agent may offer another option for starting insulin with an evening injection. In this 1-year European study, 426 subjects were randomly assigned to either insulin glargine or NPH insulin at bedtime, while continuing previous oral therapy. The therapeutic target was a fasting blood glucose < 120 mg dL^{-1} (6.7 mmol L^{-1}), using a method that was probably not plasma-referenced. The insulin dosages used (23 units for glargine and 21 for NPH) and HbA1c values achieved (8.3 and 8.2%) were similar with the two insulins, but the rates of hypoglycemia were significantly less for the group using glargine (33% versus 51% for all symptomatic hypoglycemia), despite similar average insulin doses. Nocturnal hypoglycemia occurred in less than half as many subjects using glargine (13 versus 28%). Moreover, glucose control was better in the afternoon and evening with glargine, presumably because of its longer duration of action than NPH.

MULTIPLE INJECTIONS OF INSULIN AND INSULIN-ASSISTING AGENTS

Over time, glycemic control will eventually no longer be maintained by an evening injection of insulin plus oral agents, and additional doses of insulin will be needed. Physicians may choose to begin with more than one injection of insulin and not continue oral agents but, in some cases, this approach may not achieve the desired level of control. In either situation, a decision must be made on the possible value of using (or continuing to use) one or more oral agents along with multiple injections of insulin. Relatively little guidance on this point is provided by published studies.

Insulin and sulfonylureas

Several reviews have examined the evidence regarding the combination of a sulfonylurea with multiple injections of insulin[37–39]. The majority of studies show some benefit, presumably based on enhancement of remaining endogenous insulin secretion, but this is most apparent close to the time insulin becomes necessary. Little benefit may persist once little endogenous insulin remains, as evidenced by failure of a regimen including only one injection daily. In general, the authors discontinue secretagogues once more than one injection of insulin is necessary.

Insulin with metformin

A modest number of studies suggest better control is possible with this form of combination therapy than with insulin alone[38] and it is likely that enhancing the effectiveness of endogenous insulin is not the only benefit. Perhaps the most compelling evidence comes from a small 24-week, placebo-controlled study of the addition of metformin to insulin therapy that was aggressively intensified seeking optimal control[40]. Forty-three patients previously taking insulin, but with poor glycemic control, were randomized to receive either a placebo or metformin, while insulin therapy was optimized using two or more injections of NPH and Regular insulin. Metformin-treated patients achieved a 2.5% reduction of HbA1c (from 9.0 to 6.5%), while those taking insulin alone had a smaller 1.6% reduction (9.1 to 7.5%). With combination therapy, a slight reduction of insulin dosage occurred (96 to 92 units daily), but with insulin alone a greater dosage was used (102 to 125 units daily). Moreover, the patients taking insulin alone gained about 3 kg, while virtually no change of weight occurred during the impressive improvement of control with insulin–metformin combination therapy. Other studies have documented a similar weight-limiting effect of metformin during insulin treatment[33,39], and this may be of great importance, both for assisting glycemic control and minimizing cardiovascular risk.

Insulin with thiazolidinediones

The now discontinued drug troglitazone showed considerable benefit when added to insulin in a randomized, controlled trial[41]. Doses of 200 mg or 400 mg troglitazone were compared with placebo over 26 weeks in 350 patients taking > 30 units of insulin daily and having suboptimal glycemic control. Mean HbA1c was reduced 0.8 and 1.4% with the two doses of troglitazone, while fasting serum glucose was reduced 39 mg dL^{-1} (1.9 mmol L^{-1}) and 45 mg dL^{-1} (2.7 mmol L^{-1}). This occurred despite a reduction of 11% and 29% in insulin dose for the lower and higher troglitazone doses respectively. Troglitazone has been withdrawn from use due to serious liver toxicity.

Similar benefits for glucose control have been demonstrated for rosiglitazone, which is also now approved for use in combination with insulin. A recently published randomized, controlled trial[42] studied 319 subjects with suboptimal glycemic control (HbA1c > 7.5%) despite treatment with at least 30 units of insulin daily. After an 8-week period of insulin standardization, subjects were randomized to placebo, 4 mg, or 8 mg of rosiglitazone in addition to insulin. After a 26-week follow-up, the higher dose of rosiglitazone resulted in a 1.2% mean reduction of HbA1c (to 7.9%) and a 45 mg dL^{-1} (2.5 mmol L^{-1}) reduction of fasting glucose, despite a 12% mean reduction in insulin dose. As yet unpublished data with pioglitazone, which is approved for use with insulin in the US, suggests similar benefit with this thiazolidinedione as well.

One feature that distinguishes metformin from the thiazolidinediones is the weight gain associated with the latter class of drugs. Although this side effect is absent or not significant for most patients, occasionally marked weight-gain occurs. This is partly due to fluid retention, but increased adipose tissue mass commonly occurs as well. Clinically apparent peripheral edema is common, and there is much concern about the possibility of congestive heart failure in susceptible persons, especially when a thiazolidiendione is used together with insulin. The study of rosiglitazone described above is the only peer-reviewed publication on the combination of rosiglitazone or pioglitazone combined with insulin, and the data presented are reasonably reassuring[42]. The rates of congestive heart failure occurring during the trial, from which patients with severe heart disease were excluded, were 1%, 2%, and 2% in the three groups. There was no statistically significant difference between the placebo and rosiglitazone in this respect. Some patients using these agents, with (or without) insulin, have dramatic improvements of glycemic control, better information on the risk to benefit ratio is therefore urgently needed, including data on the hypothesis that these agents may have cardioprotective effects independent of improvement of glycemic control.

Alpha-glucosidase inhibitors with insulin

As with oral agent combination therapy with alpha-glucosidase inhibitors, a modest benefit on glucose-control may be seen when these drugs are combined with insulin[43]. However, perhaps because of the effectiveness of short-acting insulin in limiting postprandial hyperglycemia, this combination is not widely used. A point in favor of the combination, however, is the lack of weight-gain accompanying use of this class of oral agents.

Gut peptides and their analogs with insulin

In the future, it is likely that analogs of gut peptides which appear to have important physiologic roles in normal regulation of plasma glucose will also be used therapeutically. Amylin, a 37 amino acid peptide that is localized to the pancreatic islets and co-secreted with insulin, has effects on gastric emptying, glucagon secretion, and satiety that appear to be mediated in the brain[44]. Plasma levels of amylin are reduced (or lacking) in patients treated with insulin. Pramlintide is an analogue of amylin that is able to mimic its actions and has been tested in therapeutic trials in both type 1 and type 2 diabetes. In a 4-week trial in type 2 diabetes, pramlintide lowered fructosamine and HbA1c when used in doses of 30–60 µg injected three or four times daily[45]. While HbA1c was reduced only about 0.5%, this change is both statistically and potentially clinically significant in light of the study's short duration.

This agent may have other beneficial effects, notably weight-control, it may therefore prove useful as an adjunct to insulin therapy in the future. A little farther in the future lies the use of analogs of glucagon-like-peptide-1 (GLP-1), which is secreted by cells in the small intestine and has effects in some ways similar to those of amylin, but include the ability to enhance insulin secretion[46]. Analogs of GLP-1 may also prove to be excellent agents for use in combination with injected insulin.

SUMMARY

Combined oral agent therapy offers superior efficacy and an opportunity to minimize side effects. In selecting oral combinations, an important objective is minimizing the number of tablets needed and their cost, and this practical imperative is likely to lead to various formulations, including more than one agent in a single tablet. Combining oral agents may delay the need for insulin injections, but when insulin is needed it should be promptly started.

Continuing oral agents while starting a single evening injection of insulin is a simple and reliable way to make the transition to insulin therapy. Poor glycemic control with a single injection plus a secretagogue, an insulin-assisting agent, or both, may signal a decline of endogenous insulin and call for further daily injections. Similarly, poor glycemic control with two or more injections of insulin alone may call for addition of an insulin-assisting agent, such as metformin or a thiazolidinedione.

The glycemic and nonglycemic benefits, as well as risks, of combining insulin-assisting agents while intensifying insulin therapy must be better defined. It seems likely that such combinations will be necessary for most patients with type 2 diabetes to achieve the currently recommended glycemic target (< 7% HbA1c), and especially the more ambitious target that has been proposed recently (< 6.5% HbA1c) by some groups. Additional oral or injected agents, such as analogs of gastrointestinal hormones, including amylin and GLP-1, may soon become available and offer further options for combination therapy to achieve the glycemic targets of the future.

REFERENCES

1   Nathan DM, Singer DE, Godine JE, Perlmuter LC. Non-insulin-dependent diabetes in older patients. Complications and risk factors. *Am J Med* 1986;81:837–42.

2   United Kingdom Prospective Diabetes Study Group. Intensive blood–glucose control with sulphonylureas or insulin compared with conventional treatment and risk of complications in patients with type 2 diabetes (UKPDS 33). *Lancet* 1998;352:837–53.

3   United Kingdom Prospective Diabetes Study Group. Effect of intensive blood–glucose control with metformin on complications in overweight patients with type 2 diabetes (UKPDS 34). *Lancet* 1998;352:854–65.

4   UKPDS Study Group. Overview of 6 years' therapy of type II diabetes: a progressive disease (UKPDS 16). *Diabetes* 1995;44:1249–58.

5   Turner RC, Cull CA, Frighi V, Holman RR. Glycemic control with diet, sulfonylurea, metformin, or insulin in patients with type 2 diabetes mellitus: progressive requirement for multiple therapies (UKPDS 49). *J Am Med Assoc* 1999;281:2005–12.

6   Polonsky KS, Sturis J, Bell GI. Non-insulin-dependent diabetes mellitus: a genetically programmed failure of the beta cell to compensate for insulin resistance. *N Engl J Med* 1996;334:777–83.

7   Haffner SM, D'Agostino Jr. R, Mykkanen L *et al.* Insulin sensitivity in subjects with type 2 diabetes. Relationship to cardiovascular risk factors: the Insulin Resistance Atherosclerosis Study. *Diabetes Care* 1999;22:562–8.

8   Haffner SM, Stern MP, Hazuda HP *et al.* Cardiovascular risk factors in confirmed prediabetic individuals: does the clock for coronary heart disease start ticking before the onset of clinical diabetes? *J Am Med Assoc* 1990;263:2893–8.

9   Haffner SM, Lehto S, Ronnemaa T *et al.* Mortality from coronary heart disease in subjects with type 2 diabetes and in nondiabetic subjects with and without prior myocardial infarction. *N Engl J Med* 1998;339:229–34.

10   DeFronzo RA. Pharmacologic therapy for type 2 diabetes mellitus. *Ann Intern Med* 1999;131: 281–303 [Review].

11   DeFronzo RA, Goodman AM. Efficacy of metformin in patients with non-insulin-dependent diabetes mellitus. The Multicenter Metformin Study Group. *New Engl J Med* 1995;333:541–9.

12   Horton ES, Whitehouse F, Ghazzi MN *et al.* Troglitazone in combination with sulfonylurea restores glycemic control in patients with type 2 diabetes. The Troglitazone Study Group. *Diabetes Care* 1998;21:1462–9.

13   Hermann LS, Schersten B, Bitzen PO *et al.* Therapeutic comparison of metformin and sulfonylurea, alone and in various combinations. A double-blind controlled study. *Diabetes Care* 1994;17:1100–9.

14   Garber AJ, Duncan TG, Goodman AM *et al.* Efficacy of metformin in type II diabetes: results of a double-blind, placebo-controlled, dose-response trial. *Am J Med* 1997;103: 491–7.

15   Moses R, Slobodniuk R, Boyages S *et al.* Effect of repaglinide addition to metformin monotherapy on glycemic control in patients with type 2 diabetes. *Diabetes Care* 1999;22:119–24.

16   Wolffenbuttel BH, Gomis R, Squatrito S *et al.* Addition of low dose rosiglitazone to sulphonylurea therapy improves glycaemic control in Type 2 diabetic patients. *Diabet Med* 2000; 17:40–7.

17   Kipnes MS, Krosnick A, Rendell MS *et al.* Pioglitazone hydrochloride in combination with sulfonylurea therapy improves glycemic control in patients with type 2 diabetes mellitus: a randomized, placebo-controlled study. *Am J Med* 2001;111:10–17.

18   Raskin P, Jovanovic L, Berger S *et al.* Repaglinide troglitazone combination therapy: improved

glycemic control in type 2 diabetes. *Diabetes Care* 2000;23:979–83.

19 Buse J, Hart K, Minasi L. The PROTECT Study: final results of a large multicenter postmarketing study in patients with type 2 diabetes. Precose Resolution of Optimal Titration to Enhance Current Therapies. *Clin Ther* 1998;20: 257–69.

20 Inzucchi SE, Maggs DG, Spollett GR *et al.* Efficacy and metabolic effects of metformin and troglitazone in type II diabetes mellitus. *N Engl J Med* 1998;338:867–72.

21 Einhorn D, Rendell M, Rosenzweig J *et al.* Pioglitazone hydrochloride in combination with metformin in the treatment of type 2 diabetes mellitus: a randomized, placebo-controlled study. The Pioglitazone 027 Study Group. *Clin Ther* 2000;22:1395–1409.

22 Fonseca V, Rosenstock J, Patwardhan R, Salzman A. Effect of metformin and rosiglitazone combination therapy in patients with type 2 diabetes mellitus: a randomized controlled trial. *J Am Med Assoc* 2000;283:1695–1702.

23 Ovalle F, Bell DSH. Triple oral antidiabetic therapy in type 2 diabetes mellitus. *Endocr Pract* 1998;4:146–7.

24 Gavin LA, Barth J, Arnold D, Shaw R. Troglitazone add on therapy to a combination of sulfonylureas plus metformin achieved and sustained effective diabetes control. *Endocr Pract* 2000;6:305–10.

25 Yale J-F, Valiquett TR, Ghazzi MN *et al.* The effect of a thiazolidinedione drug, troglitazone, on glycemia in patients with type 2 diabetes mellitus poorly controlled with sulfonylurea and metformin. A multi-center, randomized, double-blind, placebo-controlled trial. *Ann Intern Med* 2001;134:737–45.

26 Riddle MC. Evening insulin strategy. *Diabetes Care* 1990;13:676–86.

27 Riddle MC. Combined insulin and sulfonylurea therapy for type 2 diabetes mellitus. *Diabetes Res Clin Pract* 1991;11:3–8.

28 Riddle MC. Combined therapy with a sulfonylurea plus evening insulin: safe, reliable, and becoming routine. *Hormone Metabol Res* 1996;28:430–3. [Review].

29 Yki-Järvinen H, Kauppila M, Kujansuu E *et al.* Comparison of insulin regimens in patients with non-insulin-dependent diabetes mellitus. *N Engl J Med* 1992;327:1426–33.

30 Riddle MC, Hart JS, Bouma DJ *et al.* Efficacy of bedtime NPH insulin with daytime sulfonylurea

for subpopulation of type II diabetic subjects. *Diabetes Care* 1989;12:623–9.

31 Shank ML, Del Prato S, DeFronzo RA. Bedtime insulin/daytime glipizide. Effective therapy for sulfonylurea failures in NIDDM. *Diabetes* 1995;44:165–72.

32 Taskinen MR, Sane T, Helve E *et al.* Bedtime insulin for suppression of overnight free-fatty acid, blood glucose, and glucose production in NIDDM. *Diabetes* 1989;38: 580–8.

33 Yki-Jarvinen H, Ryysy L, Nikkila K *et al.* Comparison of bedtime insulin regimens in patients with type 2 diabetes mellitus: A randomized, controlled trial. *Ann Intern Med* 1999;130:389–96.

34 Riddle MC, Schneider J. Beginning insulin treatment of obese patients with evening 70/30 insulin plus glimepiride versus insulin alone. Glimepiride Combination Group. *Diabetes Care* 1998;21:1052–7.

35 Riddle M, Hart J, Bingham P *et al.* Combined therapy for obese type 2 diabetes: suppertime mixed insulin with daytime sulfonylurea. *Am J Med Sci* 1992;303:151–6.

36 Yki-Jarvinen H, Dressler A, Ziemen M, HOE 901/300s Study Group. Less nocturnal hypoglycemia and better post-dinner glucose control with bedtime insulin glargine compared with bedtime NPH insulin during insulin combination therapy in type 2 diabetes. HOE 901/3002 Study Group. *Diabetes Care* 2000;23:1130–6.

37 Pugh JA, Wagner ML, Sawyer J *et al.* Is combination sulfonylurea and insulin therapy useful in NIDDM patients? A meta-analysis. *Diabetes Care* 1992;15:953–9.

38 Johnson JL, Wolf SL, Kabadi UM. Efficacy of insulin and sulfonylurea combination therapy in type II diabetes. A meta-analysis of the randomized placebo-controlled trials. *Arch Intern Med* 1996;156:259–64.

39 Yki-Jarvinen H. Combination therapies with insulin in Type 2 diabetes. *Diabetes Care* 2001;24:758–67.

40 Aviles-Santa L, Sinding J, Raskin P *et al.* Effects of metformin in patients with poorly controlled, insulin-treated type 2 diabetes mellitus. A randomized, double-blind, placebo-controlled trial. *Ann Intern Med* 2000;284:472–7.

41 Schwartz S, Raskin P, Fonseca V, Graveline JF. Effect of troglitazone in insulin-treated patients with type II diabetes mellitus. Troglitazone and Exogenous Insulin Study Group. *N Engl J Med* 1998;338:861–6.

42 Raskin P, Rendell M, Riddle MC *et al.* A randomized trial of rosiglitazone therapy in patients with inadequately controlled insulin-treated type 2 diabetes. *Diabetes Care* 2001;24:1226–32.

43 Hollander P, Pi-Sunyer X, Coniff RF. Acarbose in the treatment of type I diabetes. *Diabetes Care* 1997;20:248–53.

44 Young AA. Amylin's physiology and its role in diabetes. *Curr Opin Endocrinol Diabetes* 1997;4:282–90.

45 Thompson RG, Pearson L, Schoenfeld SL, Kolterman OG. *Diabetes Care* 1998;21:987–93.

46 Nauck MA. Glucagonlike peptide 1. *Curr Opin Endocrinol Diabetes* 1997;4:291–9.

13

Hypoglycemia in type 2 diabetes

Philip E Cryer

HYPOGLYCEMIA: THE LIMITING FACTOR

Comprehensive treatment, including glycemic control, makes a difference for people with diabetes. Glycemic control prevents or delays the microvascular complications—retinopathy, nephropathy and neuropathy—of both type 1 diabetes mellitus[1] and type 2 diabetes mellitus[2]; it may also reduce macrovascular events[1,2]. However, because of the imperfections of all current treatment regimens, iatrogenic hypoglycemia is the limiting factor in the glycemic management of diabetes[3–5]. Were it not for the potentially devastating effects of hypoglycemia on the brain—which requires a continuous supply of glucose from the circulation—diabetes would be rather easy to treat. Enough insulin, or any other effective drug, to lower plasma glucose concentrations to or below the normal range would eliminate the symptoms of hyperglycemia, prevent acute hyperglycemic complications (ketoacidosis, hypersmolar syndrome), almost assuredly prevent the long-term microvascular complications[1,2] and likely reduce atherosclerotic risk[6,7]. But the effects of hypoglycemia on the brain are real, and the glycemic management of diabetes is therefore complex.

The barrier of iatrogenic hypoglycemia precludes true glycemic control, i.e., euglycemia maintained continuously over time, in the vast majority of people with diabetes. Thus, compli-cations can develop or progress despite aggressive therapy. For example, in the Diabetes Control and Complications Trial (DCCT) in type 1 diabetes, retinopathy developed or progressed in 14% of the patients treated intensively (compared with 32% of those treated conventionally)[1]. Similarly, in the UK Prospective Diabetes Study (UKPDS) in type 2 diabetes, any microvascular endpoint was reached in 8% of the patients treated intensively (compared with 11% of those treated less intensively)[2].

The barrier of hypoglycemia may also explain why aggressive attempts at glycemic control have had little, if any, impact on the frequency of macrovascular events in people with diabetes[1,2]. It appears that the curve describing the relationship between mean glycemia (HbA1c) and macrovascular events, such as myocardial infarction, is shifted to the left (toward lower glycemia) compared with that between mean glycemia and microvascular complications[6] (Figure 13.1). Indeed, recent prospective epidemiological data, extending earlier studies based on fasting plasma glucose concentrations, indicate an increased risk of ischemic heart disease in individuals with HbA1c levels in the high normal range[7]. Because of the barrier of iatrogenic hypoglycemia it may simply not be practical to hold plasma glucose levels low enough over time to prevent atherosclerotic disease in a substantial proportion of people with diabetes using current treatment regimens.

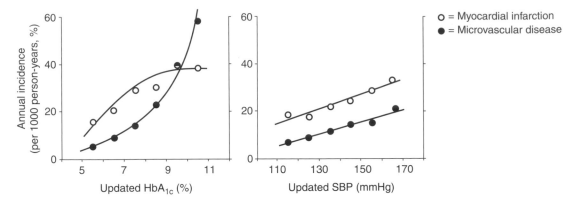

Figure 13.1 Relationship between updated systolic blood pressure (SBP), right, and updated HbA1c, left, and, the incidence of microvascular complications (closed symbols) and macrovascular, specifically myocardial infarction, complications (open symbols) of type 2 diabetes in the UKPDS. Drawn from data in Reference 6, with permission of BMJ Publishing Group.

The topic of hypoglycemia, including hypoglycemia in diabetes, has been reviewed in detail[4,5]. The focus in this chapter is on iatrogenic hypoglycemia in type 2 diabetes in the context of the larger body of knowledge concerning hypoglycemia in type 1 diabetes.

FREQUENCY OF HYPOGLYCEMIA

Hypoglycemia is a fact of life for people with established (i.e., C-peptide negative) type 1 diabetes[4,5]. Those attempting to achieve some degree of glycemic control suffer untold numbers of episodes of asymptomatic hypoglycemia; plasma glucose concentrations may be < 50 mg dL^{-1} (2.8 mmol L^{-1}) 10% of the time. They suffer an average of two episodes of symptomatic hypoglycemia per week—thousands of such episodes over a lifetime—and episodes of severe, at least temporarily disabling, hypoglycemia approximately once a year[1,8,9] (Table 13.1). Indeed, an estimated 2–4% of deaths of people with type 1 diabetes have been attributed to hypoglycemia.

Overall, the frequency of hypoglycemia is substantially lower in type 2 diabetes than in type 1 diabetes[12]. Event rates for severe iatrogenic hypoglycemia (requiring the assistance of another individual) during aggressive insulin therapy of type 1 and type 2 diabetes in several

series are summarized in Table 13.1. It appears that the rates are more than 10-fold lower in type 2 diabetes than in type 1 diabetes, even during aggressive therapy. The rates are undoubtedly even lower in patients with type 2 diabetes

Table 13.1 Severe hypoglycemia during intensive therapy of diabetes

	Episodes per 100 patient-years
Type 1 diabetes	
Edinburgh Series[8]	170
Stockholm Diabetes Intervention Study[9]	110
Diabetes Control and Complications Trial[1]	62
Type 2 diabetes	
Edinburgh Series[8]	73
VA Pump Study (MDI[a])[10]	10
VA Cooperative Study[11]	3
UKPDS[2]	?

[a]Multiple daily insulin injection group.

Table 13.2 Cumulative incidence of hypoglycemia in type 2 diabetes over 6 years in the UK PDS[13]

Therapy[a]	n	HbA1c (%)	Percent with hypoglycemia	
			Any	Major[b]
Diet	379	8.0	3.0	0.15
Sulfonylurea	922	7.1	45.0	3.3
Insulin	689	7.1	76.0	11.2[c]
Diet	297	8.2	2.8	0.4
Metformin	251	7.4	17.6	2.4

[a]Taking assigned medication.

[b]Requiring medical assistance or admission to hospital.

[c]Compared with severe hypoglycemia (that requiring the assistance of another individual) in 65% of type 1 diabetes over 6.5 years in the DCCT[1].

treated with oral hypoglycemic agents, although quantitative data from patients treated to near euglycemia are limited. Over 6 years in the UKPDS, major hypoglycemia (requiring medical assistance or hospitalization) was reported in 2.4% of type 2 diabetes patients treated with metformin, 3.3% of those treated with a sulfonylurea and 11.2% of those treated with insulin[13] (Table 13.2). In comparison, severe hypoglycemia (requiring the assistance of another individual) occurred in 65% of the patients with type 1 diabetes treated intensively (with insulin) over 6.5 years in the DCCT[1]. It should be recalled that, in contrast to median HbA1c levels of 7.2% in intensively treated type 1 diabetes throughout the DCCT[1], median HbA1c levels rose over time to ~8.1% in the intensively treated type 2 diabetes patients in the UKPDS[2]. Thus, the UKPDS data undoubtedly underestimate the frequency of iatrogenic hypoglycemia in patients with type 2 diabetes treated to glucose levels closer to the nondiabetic range.

The extent to which the frequency of iatrogenic hypoglycemia in type 2 diabetes is a function of the specific glucose-lowering drugs used to treat hyperglycemia or the stage of the disease is not entirely clear. The frequency of hypo-glycemia is highest in type 2 diabetes patients treated with insulin[13]. Among the sulfonylureas, hypoglycemia is more often reported in patients using long-acting agents, such as chlorpropamide or glyburide (glibenclamide), compared with those using a shorter-acting agent, such as glipizide[14,15]. The frequency of hypoglycemia in patients using rapid-acting insulin secretagogues—such as repaglinide and neteglinide—remains to be determined. In theory, monotherapy with a biguanide, a thiazolidinedione or an alpha-glucosidase inhibitor should not cause hypoglycemia; endogenous insulin secretion should decline appropriately as plasma glucose levels fall. Nonetheless, hypoglycemia, including major hypoglycemia, has been reported in patients treated with metformin[13] (Table 13.2). Thiazolidinediones increase the risk of hypoglycemia in patients treated with additional glucose-lowering agents, and alpha-glucosidase inhibitors preclude oral treatment of hypoglycemia with complex carbohydrates. The question arises whether the higher frequency of iatrogenic hypoglycemia in patients treated with insulin is the result of the greater glucose-lowering potency of that drug—given in sufficient doses—relative to that of the other drugs, and its pharmacokinetic imperfections. Alternatively, is it because patients who require treatment with insulin have advanced, insulin-deficient type 2 diabetes, with the associated compromised glucose counter-regulation discussed later in this chapter?

While estimates of hypoglycemic mortality rates in type 2 diabetes are not available, deaths caused by sulfonylurea-induced hypoglycemia have been well-documented[14]. The mortality of a given episode of severe sulfonylurea-induced hypoglycemia has been reported to be as high as 10%[14,15].

Hypoglycemia was found to become progressively more limiting to glycemic control over time in type 2 diabetes in the UKPDS[16]. The frequencies of severe hypoglycemia are similar in type 2 and type 1 diabetes matched for duration of insulin therapy[17]. Given progressive insulin deficiency in type 2 diabetes[2,13], these findings indicate that iatrogenic hypoglycemia becomes a progressively more frequent clinical problem, approaching that in type 1 diabetes, as patients approach the insulin deficient end of the spectrum of type 2 diabetes.

IMPACT OF HYPOGLYCEMIA

There is little published information about the clinical impact of hypoglycemia in type 2 diabetes. While it is reasonable to extrapolate from the experience in type 1 diabetes, there are obvious differences. As noted earlier, episodes of hypoglycemia become familiar events early in the course of type 1 diabetes. They are infrequent early in the course of type 2 diabetes, even during treatment with glucose-lowering medications, but become progressively more frequent as the patient approaches the insulin-deficient end of the spectrum of type 2 diabetes[16,17]. Furthermore, while type 2 diabetes occurs in all age groups, most affected people are middle-aged and older and, therefore, perhaps at higher risk of erratic food ingestion and even malnutrition, drug interactions, decreased drug metabolism and renal insufficiency, with reduced insulin clearance. They are also perhaps more susceptible to macrovascular events because of underlying cardiovascular disease.

Iatrogenic hypoglycemia causes both physical morbidity (and some mortality) and psychosocial morbidity[4]. The physical morbidity of an episode of hypoglycemia ranges from unpleasant symptoms, such as sweating, hunger, anxiety, palpitations and tremor, to neurological impairments, including behavioral changes, cognitive impairments, seizures and coma. Focal neurological deficits occur rarely. While seemingly complete neurological recovery is the rule following an episode of hypoglycemia, permanent neurological damage can occur. The extent to which the latter might be more frequent in older individuals with type 2 diabetes is unknown.

At the very least, an episode of hypoglycemia is a nuisance and a distraction; it can be embarrassing and lead to social ostracism. The psychological morbidity includes fear of hypoglycemia, guilt about that rational fear, high levels of anxiety and low levels of overall happiness[4]. Fear of hypoglycemia can be an impediment to glycemic control. Thus, hypoglycemia is often a psychological, as well as a pathophysiological, barrier to glycemic control. The performance of critical tasks, such as driving, is measurably impaired during hypoglycemia, as is judgement. Finally, the demands of the management of diabetes, including the prevention of both hyperglycemia and hypoglycemia, become progressively more intrusive over time in type 2 diabetes—albeit over a longer time-span than in type 1 diabetes.

PATHOPHYSIOLOGY OF GLUCOSE COUNTER-REGULATION

The prevention or correction of hypoglycemia normally involves both decrements in the secretion of insulin and increments in that of glucose counter-regulatory (plasma glucose-raising) hormones[4,5]. There are redundant glucose counter-regulatory factors, which exist in a hierarchy. Decrements in insulin are normally critically important in defence against falling plasma-glucose concentrations. This is the first defense against hypoglycemia. It occurs as glucose levels decline within the physiological range, and favors increased hepatic (and renal) glucose production (and decreased glucose utilization by tissues other than the brain). Among the glucose counter-regulatory hormones that are released as glucose levels fall just below the physiological range, increments in glucagon, which stimulates glycogenolysis and thus hepatic glucose production, play a primary role. Glucagon is the second defense against hypoglycemia. Albeit demonstrably involved, increments in epinephrine become critical only when glucagon is deficient. Epinephrine both stimulates hepatic (and renal) glucose production—both directly and by mobilizing gluconeogenic precursors—and limits glucose utilization by tissues such as muscle. Epinephrine is the third defense against hypoglycemia.

Insulin, glucagon and epinephrine therefore stand high in the hierarchy of redundant glucose counter-regulatory factors. Increments in cortisol and growth hormone are involved in defense against slowly developing hypoglycemia, but neither is critical to recovery from even prolonged hypoglycemia or to the prevention of hypoglycemia after an overnight fast. There is evidence that glucose autoregulation—hepatic glucose production as an inverse function of ambient glucose levels independent of hormonal, neural or other substrate glucoregulatory factors—is involved, albeit only during severe hypoglycemia. If other hormones, neurotransmitters, or substrates other than glucose (and nonesterified fatty acids that may mediate, at least in part, the actions of epinephrine) are involved, they play minor roles.

The key role of the normal virtual cessation of endogenous insulin secretion, and the rapid clearance of secreted insulin from the circulation, in the prevention or correction of hypoglycemia warrants emphasis. This is because of its relevance to the risk of hypoglycemia of the various glucose-lowering drugs used to treat type 2 diabetes.

Obviously, many factors in addition to the risk of iatrogenic hypoglycemia—such as efficacy, side effects, ease of adherence and cost—enter into the selection of a glucose-lowering agent for a given patient. However, to the extent the patient with type 2 diabetes has residual insulin secretion sufficient to achieve drug-facilitated euglycemia, monotherapy with a biguanide, a thiazolidinedione or an alpha-glucosidase inhibitor would seem preferable, since these drugs should allow endogenous insulin secretion to fall as plasma glucose levels fall. (Nonetheless, iatrogenic hypoglycemia has been reported in patients with type 2 diabetes treated with a biguanide (metformin)[13] as noted earlier.)

All insulin secretagogues, such as sulfonylureas and the rapid-acting insulin secretagogues, can produce absolute or relative insulin excess and, thus, hypoglycemia. An agent that would only enhance glucose-stimulated insulin secretion would be a preferable treatment. The extent to which the rapid-acting secretagogues will be found to have a lower risk of iatrogenic hypoglycemia during treatment to near euglycemia remains to be determined. Obviously, injected insulin can also produce absolute or relative insulin excess, largely because of the imperfectly regulated dosing and the flawed pharmacokinetics of injected insulin. Even with the shortest acting insulin preparations, such as lispro and aspart, the time-course of the glucose-lowering actions is much longer (hours) than those of normally secreted endogenous insulin (minutes).

Iatrogenic hypoglycemia is the result of the interplay of absolute or relative insulin excess and compromised glucose counter-regulation in established (C-peptide negative) type 1 diabetes[4,5]. As glucose levels decline, insulin levels do not decrease—they are simply a passive reflection of the absorption of exogenous insulin—and glucagon levels do not increase. The mechanism of the latter defect is not well understood, but it is tightly linked to, and possibly the result of, insulin deficiency. Thus the first and second defenses against hypoglycemia are lost in established type 1 diabetes. Further, the epinephrine response is typically attenuated, i.e., the glycemic threshold for the epinephrine response is shifted to lower plasma glucose concentrations. This reduction of the third defense is largely the result of recent antecedent iatrogenic hypoglycemia. The combination of absent glucagon and attenuated epinephrine responses causes the clinical syndrome of *defec-*

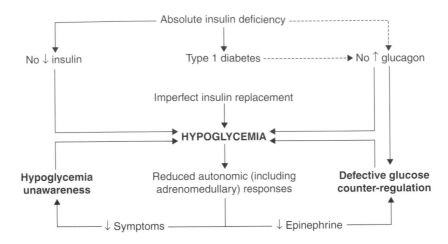

Figure 13.2 Schematic diagram of the concept of hypoglycemia-associated autonomic failure, and the pathogenesis of the syndromes of defective glucose counterregulation and hypoglycemia unawareness, in type 1 diabetes. Adapted with permission from: Cryer PE. Iatrogenic hypoglycemia as a cause of hypoglycemia-associated autonomic failure in IDDM: a vicious cycle. *Diabetes* 1992;41:255–60.

tive glucose counter-regulation, which is associated with a 25-fold or greater increased risk of severe iatrogenic hypoglycemia[18,19]. The reduced autonomic response (including the sympathetic neural norepinephrine and acetylcholine, as well as the adrenomedullary epinephrine response) causes the clinical syndrome of *hypoglycemia unawareness*—loss of the warning, largely neurogenic, symptoms of developing hypoglycemia, which, by compromising the behavioral defense (e.g., food ingestion), is also associated with a high frequency of severe iatrogenic hypoglycemia[20].

The concept of hypoglycemia-associated failure in type 1 diabetes[4,5,21,22] (Figure 13.2) posits that recent antecedent hypoglycemia causes both defective glucose counter-regulation (by reducing epinephrine responses in the setting of absent glucagon responses) and hypoglycemia unawareness (by reducing autonomic and thus neurogenic symptom responses). Perhaps the most compelling support for this concept is the finding, in three independent laboratories[22–24], that as little as 2–3 weeks of scrupulous avoidance of hypoglycemia reverses hypoglycemia unawareness and, at least in part, improves the epinephrine component of defective glucose counter-regulation in most affected patients.

The extent to which the concept of hypoglycemia-associated autonomic failure applies to type 2 diabetes remains to be defined. Glucose counter-regulatory defenses against developing hypoglycemia appear to be largely intact early in the course of type 2 diabetes. This likely explains the relatively low overall prevalence of iatrogenic hypoglycemia in type 2 diabetes, despite imperfect therapies. However, reduced hepatic (but not renal) glucose production responses to hypoglycemia—perhaps the result of reduced hepatic glycogen stores—have been observed in patients with relatively short duration type 2 diabetes, and intact glucagon and epinephrine responses (unpublished observation). Furthermore, patients with advanced type 2 diabetes selected for a relatively long-term requirement for treatment with insulin (in the absence of immunologic evidence of late onset type 1 diabetes) and shown to have reduced C-peptide levels, have been found to have virtually absent glucagon responses to hypoglycemia[25]. In addition, their epinephrine and symptomatic responses, among other responses, were shown to have shifted to lower plasma glucose concentrations following recent hypoglycemia[25]. Thus, hypoglycemia-associated autonomic failure may occur in advanced type 2 diabetes, and may

Table 13.3 Pathophysiology of glucose counter-regulation in type 1 and type 2 diabetes

Glucose		Insulin	Glucagon	Epinephrine
↓	Nondiabetic	↓	↑	↑
↓	T1DM	No ↓	No ↑	Attenuated ↑
	• Defective glucose counter-regulation			
	• Hypoglycemia unawareness			
↓	T2DM	↓-No ↓	↑-No ↑	↑-Attenuated ↑

Iatrogenic hypoglycemia is the result of the interplay of absolute or relative insulin excess and compromised glucose counter-regulation in type 1 diabetes and in advanced type 2 diabetes.

well explain the fact that iatrogenic hypoglycemia becomes progressively more limiting to glycemic control[16] as well as the high frequency of severe hypoglycemia[17] as patients approach the insulin deficient end of the spectrum of type 2 diabetes.

The pathophysiology of glucose counter-regulation in type 1 and type 2 diabetes is summarized in Table 13.3. While glucose counter-regulation is compromised early in the course of type 1 diabetes, defenses against falling glucose concentrations—decrements in insulin and increments in glucagon and epinephrine—are preserved early in the course of type 2 diabetes. However, these are progressively compromised over time as the patient approaches the insulin deficient end of the spectrum of type 2 diabetes. Thus, over time the risk of hypoglycemia in type 2 diabetes approaches that of type 1 diabetes[16,17].

RISK FACTORS FOR IATROGENIC HYPOGLYCEMIA

The conventional risk factors for iatrogenic hypoglycemia[4,5], conceptualized in type 1 diabetes but generally relevant to type 2 diabetes, are based on the premise that absolute or relative insulin excess—whether injected or secreted insulin—is the sole determinant of risk.

Absolute or relative insulin excess occurs when:

- Insulin, or insulin secretagogue or sensitizer, doses are excessive, ill-timed or of the wrong type.
- Exogenous glucose delivery is decreased, as following missed meals or snacks, or during an overnight fast.
- Endogenous glucose production is decreased, as following alcohol ingestion.
- Glucose utilization is increased, as during exercise.
- Sensitivity to insulin is increased, as during treatment with an insulin sensitizer, late after exercise, in the middle of the night, following weight loss, increased fitness or improved glycemic control.
- Insulin clearance is decreased, as in renal failure.

However, while they must be considered carefully, these conventional risk factors explain only a minority of episodes of severe iatrogenic hypoglycemia, at least in type 1 diabetes[26].

In type 1 diabetes and advanced type 2 diabetes, iatrogenic hypoglycemia is more appropriately viewed as the result of the interplay of insulin excess and compromised glucose counter-regulation, rather than absolute or relative insulin excess alone[4,5]. Risk factors related to compromised glucose counter-regulation that are well-established in type 1 diabetes[27], and are likely relevant to advanced type 2 diabetes, include:

- Insulin deficiency.
- A history of severe hypoglycemia, hypoglycemia unawareness, or both.
- Aggressive glycemic therapy *per se,* as evidenced by lower HbA1c levels, glycemic goals, or both.

These are clinical surrogates of compromised defenses against developing hypoglycemia. Absolute insulin deficiency indicates that insulin levels will not decrease and predicts accurately that glucagon levels will not increase as glucose levels fall. A history of severe hypoglycemia indicates, and hypoglycemia unawareness or even aggressive therapy *per se* implies, recent antecedent hypoglycemia which compromises the autonomic (including epinephrine) and neurogenic symptom responses to falling glucose levels by shifting the glycemic thresholds for these responses to lower plasma glucose concentrations.

An association between severe iatrogenic hypoglycemia, but not more moderate symptomatic hypoglycemia, and the angiotensin converting enzyme (ACE) DD genotype/high serum ACE activity phenotype has been reported in patients with type 1 diabetes[28]. However, that association was weak compared with the association between severe hypoglycemia and well-established risk factors, such as C-peptide negativity, hypoglycemia unawareness and lower HbA1c levels in the same study. A plausible mechanism is not apparent.

The risk factors for iatrogenic hypoglycemia are summarized in Table 13.4.

RISK FACTOR REDUCTION

Reducing the risk of iatrogenic hypoglycemia, while attempting to keep plasma glucose levels as close to normal as can be done safely, involves four steps[5,27].

First, the healthcare provider needs to address the issue of hypoglycemia in every contact with a patient undergoing drug treatment for diabetes. Is the patient having hypoglycemic episodes and, if so, is she or he aware of hypo-

Table 13.4 Risk factors for iatrogenic hypoglycemia

Absolute or relative insulin excess
1. Insulin, or insulin secretagogue or sensitizer, dose excessive, ill-timed, or of the wrong type
2. Decreased exogenous glucose delivery
   Missed meals or snacks, overnight fast
3. Decreased endogenous glucose production
   Alcohol
4. Increased glucose utilization
   Exercise
5. Increased sensitivity to insulin

Insulin sensitizer	Weight loss
Late after exercise	Improved fitness
Middle of the night	Glycemic control

6. Decreased insulin clearance
   Renal failure

Compromised glucose counter-regulation
1. Insulin deficiency
2. History of severe hypoglycemia, hypoglycemia unawareness, or both
3. Aggressive glycemic therapy *per se*
   Lower HbA1c
   Lower glycemic goals

glycemia? When do they occur? Are they severe? What is the temporal relation to drug administration, meals and snacks, alcohol use, and exercise? Are there low values in the self-monitoring of blood glucose (SMBG) log? Do family members think episodes that are not recognized by the patient are occurring? To what extent is the patient worried about actual or possible hypoglycemia? Hypoglycemia is more likely to be a problem in patients with type 1 diabetes, those with advanced type 2 diabetes and during aggressive glycemic therapy. Obviously, it can occur in other circumstances.

If hypoglycemia is a problem, as is often the case, the next step is to review the extent to which the principles of aggressive therapy—patient education and empowerment, frequent SMBG, flexible drug regimens, rational individualized glycemic goals, and ongoing professional guidance and support—are being applied.

The healthcare provider then needs to consider both the conventional risk factors for hypoglycemia—and adjust the drug regimen in relation to the meal and exercise plan appropriately—and the risk factors that imply compromised glucose counter-regulation. Given a history of severe hypoglycemia, a fundamental change in the treatment regimen is generally necessary; without this, the risk of recurrent severe hypoglycemia is high. With a history of hypoglycemia unawareness, a 2–3 week period of scrupulous avoidance of hypoglycemia is indicated; alleviation can be assessed by the return of awareness. While this has been accomplished with little or no compromise of glycemic control in personnel-intensive research settings[22-24], it may require some short-term compromise of glycemic control in the clinical setting. Given restoration of awareness, empirical approaches to improved glycemic control can then be tried.

TREATMENT OF HYPOGLYCEMIA

Obviously, prevention of iatrogenic hypoglycemia, as just discussed, is preferable to treatment of hypoglycemia. Episodes of asymptomatic hypoglycemia (detected by SMBG), and most episodes of mild to moderate symptomatic hypoglycemia, are effectively self-treated by ingestion of glucose tablets or carbohydrate in the form of juices, soft drinks, milk, crackers, candy or a meal[4,5]. However, the glycemic response to oral glucose is transient, typically < 2 h[29]. Therefore, ingestion of a snack or meal shortly after the plasma glucose concentration is raised is generally advisable.

Parenteral treatment is necessary when a hypoglycemic patient is unable or unwilling (because of neuroglycopenia) to take carbohydrate orally. While parenteral glucagon is often used, by family members, to treat hypoglycemia in type 1 diabetes, glucagon is less useful in type 2 diabetes because it stimulates insulin secretion as well as glycogenolysis. Thus, intravenous glucose is the preferable treatment for severe

iatrogenic hypoglycemia in type 2 diabetes. Because iatrogenic hypoglycemia, particularly that caused by a sulfonylurea, is often prolonged in type 2 diabetes, prolonged glucose infusion and frequent feedings are often required. It is critical that the absence of recurrent hypoglycemia is established unequivocally before the patient is discharged. This often requires hospitalization with prolonged medical supervision.

SUMMARY AND PERSPECTIVE

Iatrogenic hypoglycemia is the limiting factor in the glycemic management of diabetes, and a barrier to true glycemic control and its established microvascular and potential macrovascular long-term benefits. Severe hypoglycemia is less frequent overall in type 2 diabetes, compared with type 1 diabetes, even during aggressive glycemic therapy, because glucose counter-regulatory systems remain intact early in the course of type 2 diabetes. However, iatrogenic hypoglycemia becomes a progressively more frequent clinical problem, ultimately approaching that in type 1 diabetes, in advanced type 2 diabetes because of compromised glucose counter-regulation. The syndromes of defective glucose counter-regulation and hypoglycemia unawareness, and the concept of hypoglycemia-associated autonomic failure, in advanced type 2 diabetes are analogous to that which develops early in the course of type 1 diabetes. By practicing hypoglycemia risk reduction, i.e., addressing the issue, applying the principles of aggressive therapy, and considering both the conventional risk factors and those indicative of compromised glucose counter-regulation, healthcare providers should strive to reduce mean glycemia as much as can be accomplished safely. Clearly, given current treatment limitations, people with diabetes need more physiological approaches to glycemic control, tailored to their degree of insulin deficiency.

Hypoglycemia should not be used, by the provider or the patient, as an excuse for poor glycemic control, particularly in view of the growing array of glucose-lowering drugs that can be used to optimize therapy and achieve the best control possible in a given patient with type

2 diabetes. Nonetheless, better methods—such as those that would provide glucose-regulated insulin replacement—are clearly needed for people with type 2 diabetes, as well as for those with type 1 diabetes, if we are to achieve and maintain true euglycemia.

ACKNOWLEDGEMENTS

The author's work cited in this chapter was supported, in part, by US P.H.S. grants R37 DK27085, M01 RR00036, P60 DK20579 and T32 DK07120, and a fellowship award from the American Diabetes Association. The assistance of Ms Karen Muehlhauser in the preparation of this manuscript is gratefully acknowledged.

This chapter was written at approximately the same time as a review, entitled "Negotiating the Barrier of Hypoglycemia in Diabetes" was prepared, with Belinda P. Childs, for publication in *Diabetes Spectrum*. While not identical to that review, the organization and much of the phraseology of this chapter are similar. Therefore, permission has been obtained from the American Diabetes Association to reproduce that review here.

REFERENCES

1 The Diabetes Control and Complications Trial Research Group. The effect of intensive treatment of diabetes on the development and progression of long-term complications in insulin-dependent diabetes mellitus. *N Engl J Med* 1993;329:977–86.

2 The United Kingdom Prospective Diabetes Study Research Group. Intensive blood-glucose control with sulfonylureas or insulin compared with conventional treatment and risk of complications in patients with type 2 diabetes. *Lancet* 1998;352:837–53.

3 Cryer PE. Hypoglycemia: the limiting factor in the management of IDDM. *Diabetes* 1994;43:1378–89.

4 Cryer PE. *Hypoglycemia. Pathophysiology, diagnosis and treatment*. New York: Oxford University Press, 1997.

5 Cryer PE. Glucose homeostasis and hypoglycemia. In: Larsen PR, Kronenberg H, Melmed S, Polonsky K, eds. *Williams' textbook of endocrinology*. 10th edn. Philadelphia: Harcourt Health Sciences. In press.

6 Stratton IM, Adler AI, Neil AW *et al.* on behalf of the UK Prospective Diabetes Study Group. Association of glycaemia with macrovascular and microvascular complications of type 2 diabetes (UKPDS 35): prospective observational study. *BMJ* 2000;321:405–12.

7 Khaw K-T, Wareham N, Luben R *et al.* Glycated haemoglobin, diabetes, and mortality in men in Norfolk cohort of European Prospective Investigation of Cancer and Nutrition (EPIC-Norfolk). *BMJ* 2001;322:1–6.

8 MacLeod KM, Hepburn DA, Frier BM. Frequency and morbidity of severe hypoglycemia in insulin-treated diabetic patients. *Diabetic Med* 1993;10:238–45.

9 Reichard P, Berglund B, Britz A *et al.* Intensified conventional insulin treatment retards the microvascular complications of insulin-dependent diabetes mellitus (IDDM): the Stockholm Diabetes Intervention Study (SDIS) after 5 years. *J Intern Med* 1991;230:101–8.

10 Saudek CD, Duckworth WC, Giobbie-Hurder A *et al.* Implantable insulin pump vs. multiple-dose insulin for non-insulin dependent diabetes mellitus. A randomized clinical trial. *J Am Med Assoc* 1996;276:1249–58.

11 Abaira C, Colwell JA, Nuttall FQ *et al.* Veterans affairs cooperative study on glycemic control and complications in type II diabetes: results of the feasibility trial. *Diabetes Care* 1995;18:1113–23.

12 Gerich JE. Hypoglycaemia and counterregulation in type 2 diabetes. *Lancet* 2000;356:1946–7.

13 The United Kingdom Prospective Diabetes Study Research Group. Overview of 6 years of therapy of type II diabetes: a progressive disease. *Diabetes* 1995;44:1249–58.

14 Campbell IW. Hypoglycaemia and type 2 diabetes: sulphonylureas. In: Frier BM, Fisher BM, eds. *Hypoglycemia and diabetes. Clinical and physiological aspects*. London: Edward Arnold, 1993: 387–92.

15 Gerich JE. Oral hypoglycemic agents. *N Engl J Med* 1989;321:1231–45.

16 The United Kingdom Prospective Diabetes Study Research Group. A 6-year, randomized, controlled trial comparing sulfonylurea, insulin and metformin therapy in patients with newly diagnosed type 2 diabetes that could not be controlled with diet therapy. *Ann Intern Med* 1998;128:165–75.

17 Hepburn DA, MacLeod KM, Pell ACH *et al.* Frequency and symptoms of hypoglycemia experienced by patients with type 2 diabetes treated with insulin. *Diabetic Med* 1993;10:231–7.

18 White NH, Skor D, Cryer PE *et al.* Identification of type 1 diabetic patients at increased risk for hypoglycemia during intensive therapy. *N Engl J Med* 1983;308:485–91.

19 Bolli GB, De Feo P, De Cosmo S *et al.* A reliable and reproducible test for adequate glucose counterregulation in type 1 diabetes. *Diabetes* 1984; 33:732–7.

20 Gold AE, MacLeod KM, Frier BM. Frequency of severe hypoglycemia in patients with type 1 diabetes with impaired awareness of hypoglycemia. *Diabetes Care* 1994;17:697–703.

21 Dagogo-Jack SE, Craft S, Cryer PE. Hypoglycemia-associated autonomic failure in insulin dependent diabetes mellitus. *J Clin Invest* 1993;91:819–28.

22 Dagogo-Jack S, Rattarasarn C, Cryer PE. Reversal of hypoglycemia unawareness, but not defective glucose counterregulation, in IDDM. *Diabetes* 1994;43:1426–34.

23 Fanelli CG, Pampanelli S, Epifano L *et al.* Long-term recovery from unawareness, deficient counterregulation and lack of cognitive dysfunction during hypoglycemia following institution of rational intensive therapy in IDDM. *Diabetologia* 1994;37:1265–76.

24 Cranston I, Lomas J, Maran A *et al.* Restoration of hypoglycemia unawareness in patients with long duration insulin-dependent diabetes mellitus. *Lancet* 1994;344:283–7.

25 Segel SA, Paramore DS, Cryer PE. Hypoglycemia-associated autonomic failure in advanced type 2 diabetes. *Diabetes* 2002; 51:724–33.

26 The Diabetes Control and Complications Trial Research Group. Epidemiology of severe hypoglycemia in the Diabetes Control and Complications Trial. *Am J Med* 1991;90:450–9.

27 Cryer PE. Hypoglycemia risk reduction in type 1 diabetes. *Exp Clin Endocrinol Metab* 2001; 109:5412–23.

28 Pedersen-Bjergaard U, Agerholm-Larsen B, Pramming S *et al.* Activity of angiotensin converting enzyme and risk of severe hypoglycaemia in type 1 diabetes. *Lancet* 2001;357:1248–53.

29 Wiethop BV, Cryer PE. Alanine and terbutaline in the treatment of hypoglycemia in IDDM. *Diabetes Care* 1993;16:1131–6.

14

Metabolic emergencies in type 2 diabetes
Hyperosmolar non-ketotic hyperglycemia, ketoacidosis and lactic acidosis

Helen B Holt and Andrew J Krentz

HYPEROSMOLAR NON-KETOTIC HYPERGLYCEMIA

PATHOPHYSIOLOGY

Hyperosmolar non-ketotic hyperglycemia (HNKH), also known as hyperosmolar non-ketotic coma and hyperosmolar hyperglycemic state, is a medical emergency most frequently encountered in middle-aged or elderly subjects with type 2 diabetes[1–3]. There have been occasional reports of its occurrence in children. Biochemically, HNKH is characterized by a clinical and biochemical triad of:

* Marked hyperglycemia
* Profound dehydration
* Pre-renal uremia.

By convention, significant hyperketonemia, ketonuria and metabolic acidosis are absent (c.f. diabetic ketoacidosis, DKA), the arterial bicarbonate concentration usually being $> 15 \, \text{mmol} \, L^{-1}$. The syndrome of HNKH is considered to overlap with diabetic ketoacidosis[4]; patients presenting with features of both, i.e. plasma hyperosmolarity with a degree of ketoacidosis (and sometimes lactic acidosis—see below) are not uncommon. The distinction between these metabolic emergencies depends on arbitrary definitions.

Insulin deficiency—relative rather than absolute—permits the acceleration of hepatic glycogenolysis and gluconeogenesis[2]. The net result is an increase in hepatic glucose production and a slow, progressive rise in plasma glucose concentrations (Figure 14.1). Elevated circulating concentrations of counter-regulatory hormones antagonize the actions of insulin. Hyperglycemia is exacerbated by direct and indirect tissue actions of these hormones. Severe inter-current illnesses, e.g. sepsis, or acute myocardial infarction, are associated with marked elevations of counter-regulatory hormone concentrations. This, at least in part, explains the capacity of such conditions—to which patients with diabetes are more prone—to precipitate acute metabolic decompensation.

In addition to promoting further increases in hepatic glucose production, the high counter-regulatory hormone (glucagon, cortisol, catecholamines and growth hormone) levels, in concert with activation of the sympatho–adrenal system, reduce insulin-mediated glucose transport into skeletal muscle. As progressive hyperglycemia develops, the renal threshold for re-absorption of glucose (approximately $10 \, \text{mmol} \, L^{-1}$, but often higher in the elderly) is exceeded, resulting in increased renal losses of glucose; this provides some temporary protection against even greater degrees of hyperglycemia. However, the osmotic diuresis that accompanies the glycosuria ultimately leads to profound dehydration, as water moves from cells down an osmotic gradient only to be lost in the urine. The contraction of intra-vascular volume causes a fall in renal perfusion—particularly if oral fluid intake is insufficient to keep pace with polyuria. Consequently, the renal excretion of glucose declines, thereby exacerbating hyperglycemia. Renal losses of electrolytes (sodium, potassium, phosphate and magne-sium) accompany the osmotic diuresis. Dehydration and systemic hypotension also stimulate the secretion of the aforementioned catabolic hormones.

The absence of significant ketosis in the presence of a major decompensation in glucose metabolism remains incompletely explained. Direct suppression of lipolysis by the hyperosmolar state[4,5] has been postulated (this would counter the expected acceleration of lipolysis,

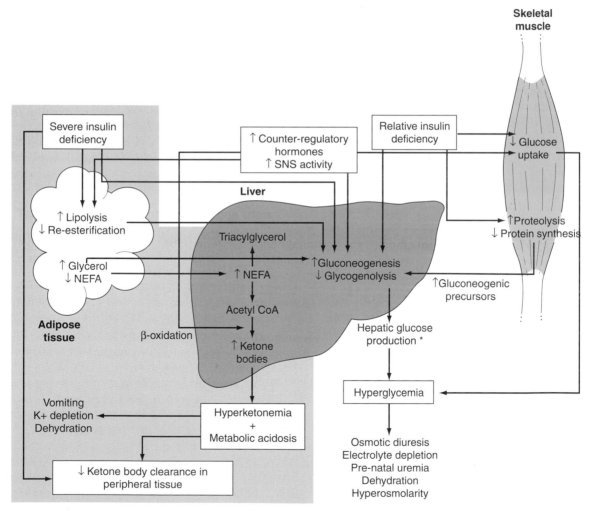

NEFA = Non-esterified fatty acids

□ = Denotes consequences of severe insulin deficiency on fat and ketone body metabolism

SNS = Sympathetic nervous system

* Renal gluconeogenesis also contributes to hyperglycemia

Figure 14.1 Pathogenesis of HNKH and DKA

resulting from decreased activation of hormone-sensitive lipase secondary to insulin deficiency and counter-regulatory hormone excess). It has also been suggested that the catabolic hormone response is generally less pronounced than that typically observed in DKA[6]. However, comparative studies—subject to the aforementioned caveats concerning definitions—have shown that peripheral blood concentrations of counter-regulatory hormones and insulin in patients with HNKH are similar to those observed in patients presenting with DKA[7]. By contrast, reports of peripheral blood C-peptide concentrations that are several-fold higher in patients with HNKH than in patients with DKA indicate some preservation of endogenous insulin secretion. This is to be anticipated in patients with type 2 diabetes, even though insulin secretion may be acutely inhibited by catecholamines via alpha-adrenergic stimulation in HNKH. Residual beta-cell function is likely to be relevant to the absence of ketosis in HNKH for two main reasons.

- First, in contrast to insulin-mediated glucose transport in skeletal muscle, hydrolysis of triaclyglycerol within adipocytes is readily inhibited at plasma insulin concentrations within the low-physiological range (there being a five- to ten-fold difference in insulin levels required for maximal effects on these processes). Insulin also promotes re-esterification of non-esterified fatty acids (NEFA) to triaclyglycerol. Although counter-regulatory hormones and sympatho–adrenal activation will shift this dose–response relationship to the right (i.e. higher insulin concentrations being necessary to suppress lipolysis), endogenous insulin will counter their lipolytic actions.
- Second, the fate of NEFA within the liver is subject to regulation by the portal insulin-to-glucagon ratio. Thus, higher portal insulin concentrations in patients with HNKH may protect against diversion of NEFA into the mitochondrial beta-oxidation pathway (see below, DKAs). Under these circumstances, intrahepatic re-esterification of NEFA to triacylglycerol will be favored.

INCIDENCE AND MORTALITY

The syndrome of HNKH is relatively uncommon, accounting for less than 1% of all primary diabetes-related hospital admissions[3,7]. However, HNKH is associated with a high case-fatality rate. A recent American Diabetes Association (ADA) Technical Review reported an average of mortality rate, based on reports in the literature, of approximately 15%[7]. Although the syndrome most commonly affects patients with known type 2 diabetes, previously undiagnosed cases account for approximately 25% of cases of HNKH in some series[8,9].

An association with ethnicity has emerged in some reports. In a series of hyperglycemic emergencies in adults from the multi-ethnic population of Birmingham, UK, patients from the minority African–Caribbean community were over-represented among patients presenting with HNKH, accounting for 26% of episodes. However, African–Caribbean patients comprised only 3% of those presenting with DKA, Caucasians accounting for the majority[8]. In contrast, in a series of black African patients presenting during a 12 month period in Johannesburg, severe DKA was more than twice as common as HNKH[10].

Outcomes for patients with HNKH tend to be worse for individuals of advanced age or with serious co-morbidity[9,11]. A high incidence of complications has long been recognized, particularly thrombo-embolic events resulting from a hypercoaguable state[2]. In a recent series of patients with HNKH who had a mean age of 75 years, the overall mortality rate was 17%[12]. The most frequent cause of death (31%) was septic shock. Mortality was higher for patients in whom cardiovascular disease was considered to be a precipitating factor for the metabolic decompensation. Other factors associated with a higher mortality rate included older age, relative hypotension on admission, hyponatremia, acidosis, and high plasma urea concentrations. In this particular series, thrombo-embolic events accounted for only three of 130 deaths[12]. While not all published series have reported associations between co-morbid and precipitating factors on mortality, the adverse effect of advanced age is well-recognized[13].

CLINICAL FEATURES

Symptoms of intense thirst, polyuria and gradual clouding of consciousness over preceding days are typical. Vomiting is characteristically absent, and the symptoms may develop insidiously over several weeks. Many patients are in a moribund state by the time they are admitted to hospital.

Severe dehydration with arterial hypotension (postural or, with greater degrees of dehydration, supine) is common. Mental status on admission is often impaired, with stupor and coma with more severe degrees of hyperosmolarity. Reversible focal neurological signs and motor seizures may occur[14]. However, since patients with type 2 diabetes are at increased risk of stroke, CT imaging should be considered if there are concerns about an acute intra-cranial vascular event. Kussmaul respiration (air hunger), frequently seen in DKA, is not a feature of the HNKH syndrome due to the absence of significant ketoacidosis. Signs of sepsis may be evident; serious co-morbidity is common.

PRECIPITATING FACTORS

The HNKH syndrome has many precipitating causes, which may co-exist in some patients. Respiratory and urinary tract infections are among the commonest precipitating illnesses, but many other conditions, such as myocardial infarction, pulmonary embolism and acute pancreatitis, are well-recognized. Certain anti-hypertensive drugs that have diabetogenic properties, including high-dose diuretics and beta-blockers, have been implicated in some reports[15,16]; diuretics may also exacerbate dehydration and potassium depletion. Other drugs linked causally to HNKH include phenytoin, cimetidine and chlorpromazine. Corticosteroids have potent effects on carbohydrate and lipid metabolism that, at high doses, will readily precipitate HNKH in predisposed individuals.

Non-compliance with insulin therapy, often in association with illicit drug use or excessive alcohol consumption, was found to be an important factor for hyperglycemic emergencies in urban African–American patients (a high percentage of whom actually presented with DKA), who tend to have higher admission rates than their Caucasian counterparts[17].

DIAGNOSIS

The HNKH state should be considered for any adult patient presenting with unexplained impairment of consciousness, acute focal neurological signs, dehydration or shock[8]. An erroneous preliminary diagnosis of stroke may be reached, particularly if the patient arrives in a comatose state with focal neurology. Urinalysis typically reveals heavy glycosuria and a 'negative' or 'trace' ketone reaction to a nitroprusside-based test. The diagnosis of HNKH is readily confirmed by a markedly raised plasma glucose concentration on fingerstick testing. Venous blood should be sent immediately to the clinical chemistry laboratory to confirm the degree of hyperglycemia. A significant elevation in blood urea nitrogen (BUN) is common, together with a raised hematocrit, and a mild leukocytosis. Plasma electrolytes must be measured and cultures of blood and urine taken, even in the absence of overt infection.

When plasma osmolality exceeds about 340 mosmol L^{-1}, some depression of consciousness is generally present[18]. Although there is considerable variation between individuals[19], alternative causes of an impaired level of consciousness should be considered in patients whose osmolality is less marked. Plasma osmolality can be measured directly in the laboratory (by freezing-point depression), or can be estimated approximately at the bedside from the formula:

Plasma osmolality = $2 \times$ (plasma Na^+ + plasma K^+) + plasma glucose + plasma urea (mosmol L^{-1}) (where Na^+, K^+, glucose and urea are in mmol L^{-1})

Normal ~285–295 mosmol kg^{-1}. The values for Na^+ and K^+ are doubled to allow for their associated Cl^- anions. Urea readily crosses the cell membrane, this molecule contributes relatively little to plasma tonicity.

Although total body sodium is usually low (as a consequence of the osmotic diuresis), plasma sodium concentration at presentation can be low, normal or high, depending on the concomitant water deficit. Dehydration is usually severe in the HNKH syndrome, with an average deficit in adults of 8–12 L of water.

Hyperglycemia may falsely depress the plasma sodium concentration (see below). The reciprocal relationship between plasma glucose and sodium is reportedly non-linear[20]. Hypertriglyceridemia may also result in apparent hyponatremia (although this caveat is avoided by the use of modern ion-specific electrodes); plasma should be examined for turbidity. Arterial plasma bicarbonate is generally > 15 mmol L[-1], although a degree of lactic acidemia may result from impaired renal excretion of H[+] ions, together with hypotension-induced under-perfusion of tissues.

Plasma potassium concentrations do not reliably reflect total body stores of this cation. Urinary losses of 400–700 mmol are not uncommon[4]. Thus, hyperkalemia at presentation may mislead the unwary clinician. Severe dehydration or hypotension may occasionally cause acute renal failure; oliguria, despite adequate rehydration, is an ominous sign. Many patients with type 2 diabetes of long duration have renal impairment, due to diabetic nephropathy. Renal function may be impaired by use of drugs, such as non-steroid anti-inflammatory agents.

TREATMENT

The use of written guidelines can facilitate the delivery of safe and effective therapy for hyperglycemic emergencies. However, treatment guidelines do not replace the need for careful clinical evaluation and appropriate modification of therapy according to individual circumstances. The following section relates to treatment of HNKH in adults. The syndrome is rare in children[21], but the incidence of type 2 diabetes in this age group is increasing.

Successful management of HNKH depends on early recognition of the diagnosis, good general care of the unconscious patient, and prompt treatment of underlying causes. Early transfer to a high-dependency or intensive care unit is recommended. Meticulously updated charts, on which the clinical and biochemical status of the patient is recorded, should be used; close attention to fluid balance is an aspect of care that requires particular emphasis. Initial treatment comprises intravenous fluid, electrolyte and insulin therapy (Table 14.1)[22–24]. Of these, rehydration is the most important consideration during the initial stages of treatment. This improves the delivery of insulin to tissues and reduces the concentrations of counter-regulatory hormones.

Rehydration

The average water deficit is 10–15% of body weight, translating into a requirement for 8–12 L (Reference 1). This dehydration affects the intravascular, interstitial and intracellular compartments. Initial therapy—during the first 2–3 h—aims to rapidly correct part of the deficit, approximately 50% being replaced over the first 24 h. There has long been disagreement over the choice of crystalloid—isotonic versus hypotonic saline—for initial rehydration in patients with HNKH. It should be remembered that 'physiological' saline is hypotonic relative to the patient's plasma at this point. Based on the literature and clinical experience we advocate that a litre of isotonic saline (0.9% NaCl) should be given during the first hour of treatment (Table 14.1). Thereafter, the rate of saline infused should be adjusted according to the clinical status of the patient. In the absence of concerns about cardiovascular or renal function, 1 L h[-1] of saline for the first 2–3 h will rapidly expand the intravascular fluid compartment. The infusion rate should be adjusted thereafter, according to the state of fluid balance, taking continuing polyuria into consideration.

If corrected plasma sodium rises > 150 mmol L[-1] then 1–2 L of hypotonic saline (0.45% NaCl) may be given over the next 2 h, with 0.9% saline being recommended according to hydration status. A rise in plasma sodium concentration is frequently observed during treatment, as blood glucose falls and water moves back into the intracellular compartment. The rise in sodium may also be partially explained by the aforementioned reciprocal relationship with blood glucose. When plasma glucose, measured hourly using a fingerstick and reflectance meter, has fallen to 10–15 mmol L[-1], isotonic glucose (5% dextrose) should be substituted (at a rate of approx. 250 mL h[-1] with added

Table 14.1 Guide to initial treatment of hyperosmolar non-ketotic hyperglycemia and DKA

Fluids and electrolytes

Volumes

1 L h^{-1} × 2–3, thereafter adjusted according to the degree of hydration and taking continuing polyuria into account

Caution in patients with known renal disease or cardiovascular insufficiency, in whom over-zealous hydration may result in fluid overload, or cardiac decompensation

Fluids

Isotonic ('normal') saline (150 mmol L^{-1}) for the majority of patients

Hypotonic ('half-normal') saline (75 mmol L^{-1}) if serum sodium exceeds 150 mmol L^{-1} (no more than 1–2 L; consider 5% dextrose with increased insulin if marked hypernatremia)

5% dextrose 1L 4–6 h^{-1} when blood glucose has fallen to 15 mmol L^{-1} (normal saline may be required in addition, according to electrolytes)

Potassium

No potassium in first litre of fluid unless initial plasma potassium < 3.5 mmol L^{-1}

Thereafter, add dosages shown below to each litre of fluid:

If plasma K^{+}: < 4.0 mmol L^{-1}, add 40 mmol KCl (severe hypokalemia may require more aggressive KCl replacement); 3.5–5.5 mmol L^{-1}, add 20 mmol KCl; > 5.5 mmol L^{-1}, add no KCl

Insulin

Consider intramuscular bolus of soluble insulin (10–15 U) if any delay in starting intravenous insulin infusion

Continuous intravenous infusion: 5–10 U h^{-1} (average 6 U h^{-1} in adults) initially, until blood glucose has fallen to 10–15 mmol L^{-1}. If plasma glucose does not fall in the first hour consider doubling initial rate of insulin infusion. Thereafter, adjust rate (1–4 U h^{-1} typically, in the absence of severe infection) with dextrose infusion to maintain blood glucose at 5–10 mmol L^{-1} until patient is eating again.

Intramuscular injections: 20 U soluble insulin i.m. immediately, then 5–10 U h^{-1} i.m. until blood glucose has fallen to ~15 mmol L^{-1}. Thereafter, change to ~10 U 6 hourly by subcutaneous injection until patient is eating again. Intravenous insulin is the preferred route.

Other measures

Search for and treat precipitating cause (e.g., infection, myocardial infarction)

Hypotension usually responds to adequate fluid replacement with crystalloids

Central venous pressure monitoring in elderly patients, or if cardiac disease is present

In DKA, pass nasogastric tube if conscious level impaired, to avoid aspiration of gastric contents

Urinary catheter if conscious level impaired, or no urine passed within 4 h of start of therapy

Continuous ECG monitoring may warn of hyperkalemia or hypokalemia (potassium should be measured at 0, 2, and 6 h and more often if < 3.5 or > 5.5 mmol L^{-1})

Consider cranial CT to exclude other pathology (e.g., cerebral hemorrhage, venous sinus thrombosis) if level of consciousness remains impaired following correction of metabolic disturbance

Treat clinical thrombo-embolic complications with heparin

Bicarbonate therapy only in patients with severe DKA, i.e. arterial pH < 7.0 or severe hyperkalemia (usually responds to insulin and rehydration)

Meticulous clinical and biochemical recording, using a purpose-designed flow-chart

potassium chloride, as required) for saline. In the severely dehydrated patient, saline may be co-infused (via a Y-shaped connector) with dextrose, as necessary, at this point.

Insulin

Recent ADA recommendations advocate administration of insulin (soluble, unmodified) as an intravenous infusion at a rate of 0.1 U kg^{-1} h^{-1} (Reference 7). However, the clinical status of the patient will often preclude accurate measurement of body weight. In the series from Birmingham, UK an insulin infusion rate of 6 U h^{-1} proved safe and effective[8,23]. Hourly intra-muscular injections (5–10 U) are effective, but may be less reliable in patients with severe dehydration. Some authorities advocate an initial intravenous bolus, e.g. 0.15 U kg^{-1} (Reference 7). The short half-life of insulin in the circulation (approximately 4.5 min) necessitates a continuous infusion of insulin. A modest decline in blood glucose concentration will usually be observed with rehydration alone; apparent failures of response to insulin may reflect inadequate intravenous fluid replacement, this should be reviewed urgently if blood glucose fails to decline by 4–6 mmol L^{-1} each hour during the early stages of therapy. Major degrees of insulin resistance are unusual, and an insulin infusion rate of 6 Uh^{-1} will usually be sufficient to effectively surmount the antagonistic effects of counter-regulatory hormones and cytokines. However, severe infection can sometimes lead to significant degrees of acute relative insensitivity to insulin that demand higher rates of insulin with careful monitoring of response.

The insulin infusion should be continued at 6 U h^{-1} until blood glucose has reached 10–15 mmol L^{-1}. At this point—when intravenous dextrose usually replaces saline (see above)—the insulin infusion rate should be adjusted; typically, 1–4 U h^{-1} will be required to maintain blood glucose in the target range of 5–10 mmol L^{-1}. This will minimize any further osmotic renal losses of water and electrolytes, since the renal threshold for the re-absorption of glucose is not exceeded. Care should be taken to avoid hypoglycemia at this stage.

When oral fluids and nutrition are recommenced, subcutaneous insulin replaces the intravenous infusion. Subcutaneous insulin is conveniently delivered as twice-daily biphasic soluble + isophane preparations, the intravenous insulin infusion being discontinued 60 min after injection (less if a rapid-acting analogue is used). Alternatively, pre-meal doses of soluble insulin or a rapid-acting analogue can be given, with pre-bed isophane, lente or insulin glargine. The intravenous insulin infusion rate will provide some guidance to the total daily dose of subcutaneous insulin. Any residual infection at this stage may necessitate a temporary increase in insulin dose, requirements falling as the clinical state of the patient improves.

Following discharge from hospital, insulin treatment is often recommended for the first 2–3 months. Patients with HNKH generally secrete sufficient endogenous insulin to be successfully treated in the longer term with oral antidiabetic agents, or even diet alone. Pointers to successful withdrawal of insulin in these circumstances will be excellent glycemic control, or even recurrent hypoglycemia, with relatively small doses of insulin. However, it should be borne in mind that low insulin requirements do not necessarily reliably equate with insulin-independence. These caveats demand that the clinical and biochemical picture is carefully evaluated before a decision is made to withdraw insulin therapy—an error may have disastrous consequences. Some centers measure glucagon-stimulated C-peptide concentration to confirm adequate endogenous insulin secretion. Close supervision and self-monitoring of blood glucose should be undertaken in the first few days after withdrawal of insulin therapy. Precipitating factors for HNKH, e.g. corticosteroid therapy, must be carefully avoided in the future, as far as possible.

Electrolyte replacement

Plasma potassium concentrations fall with rehydration and insulin therapy[3]; avoidance of hypokalemia during therapy is an important goal and plasma potassium must be carefully monitored. No potassium is recommended in the first litre of fluid unless the plasma potassium is < 3.5 mmol L^{-1} at presentation. Thereafter, potassium chloride should be added to each litre of fluid, unless hyperkalemia (> 5.5 mmol L^{-1}) is present, in which case the level should be re-checked at 1–2 h intervals. If plasma potassium is < 4.0 mmol L^{-1}, add 40 mmol KCl (severe hypokalemia may require more aggressive KCl replacement). When plasma potassium is 3.5–5.5 mmol L^{-1}, 20 mmol KCl should be added to each litre. Considerable care should taken in patients with pre-existing renal impairment or oliguria. Electrocardiographic monitoring is often advocated, in order to provide an early warning of serious hyper- or hypo-kalemia. However, this should not replace measurement of plasma potassium concentrations.

Whole body phosphate depletion (approximately 3–7 mmol kg^{-1})[7] in HNKH results from renal losses, unless significant renal impairment is present. Plasma phosphate levels tend to fall during rehydration[4]. In the absence of data suggesting benefit, we do not recommend routine replacement of phosphate, but this should be considered if clinical features are suggestive of significant hypophosphatemia or a marked deficiency of phosphate (< 0.3 mmol L^{-1}) is identified on laboratory testing. Some authorities advocate treatment of lesser degrees of hypophosphatemia in the presence of hypoxia, anemia or cardiorespiratory compromise. Care must be taken to avoid hypocalcemia during intravenous phosphate replacement—tetany may result.

COMPLICATIONS

Rhabdomyolysis

Non-traumatic rhabdomyolysis in patients with greater degrees of hyperosmolarity may occasionally precipitate acute renal failure[25]. This complication has been associated with a poorer prognosis for patients with HNKH in some reports. The diagnosis is suggested by a greatly elevated serum creatinine kinase concentration (usually well in excess of 1000 IU L^{-1}) in the absence of alternative causes, such as myocardial infarction, stroke, or end-stage renal failure. The diagnosis is confirmed by the presence of myoglobinuria. Hemodialysis or hemofiltration may be required.

Thrombo-embolic complications

Despite the high frequency of thrombo-embolic complications in patients with HNKH, the role of routine anticoagulation is unclear. Anti-coagulation in an acutely sick patient carries risks of gastrointestinal hemorrhage—an occasional cause of death in HNKH. We advocate treatment of clinically overt thrombo-embolic events as they arise; this approach will lead to occasional failure to recognize the insidious development of serious thrombosis. However, the risk–benefit equation will differ between patients, and this presents a dilemma for the clinician. In the absence of controlled clinical trials, the value of prophylactic anticoagulation with low molecular heparin remains uncertain[26].

KETOACIDOSIS

INTRODUCTION

Ketoacidosis in patients with type 2 diabetes is uncommon, but is increasingly being recognized—particularly in certain ethnic groups. DKA may be precipitated by acute severe illness, e.g. major sepsis. Alcoholic ketoacidosis is recognized principally in non-diabetics, but may also occur in patients with type 2 diabetes.

DKA is a metabolic emergency that is associated with a significant mortality rate, albeit generally lower (~5%) than that reported for HNKH[7,8]. Usually a hallmark of type 1 diabetes, DKA may be precipitated by acute severe illness, e.g. major sepsis, in patients with type 2 diabetes. DKA is characterized by an elevation of counter-regulatory (catabolic) hormone levels (see above) in the presence of an absolute or, more commonly, a marked relative deficiency of insulin[27,28]. Although residual beta-cell function is protective against ketoacidosis[29], suppression of secretion of insulin during acute severe illness may occasionally precipitate DKA. This was previously regarded as being an uncommon event, but in African–Americans with newly diagnosed type 2 diabetes (often obese), DKA is being increasingly diagnosed[30,31]. Diagnostic difficulties may be encountered in patients from certain ethnic groups who present in DKA yet who can be successfully managed without exogenous insulin after recovery[32]. Attempts have been made to identify clinical, biochemical and immunological criteria that might predict successful withdrawal of insulin; however, these have proved to have limited value[33].

CLINICAL FEATURES

The cardinal features of DKA are increasing polyuria and polydipsia, weight loss, generalized weakness and hyperventilation followed by drowsiness and, eventually, coma. Symptoms can develop rapidly—over 1–2 days—and it is often the onset of vomiting that precipitates emergency admission to hospital. Vomiting exacerbates urinary losses of water and electrolytes (particularly potassium). Signs of dehydration, hypotension and tachycardia are prominent in severe diabetic ketoacidosis.

Table 14.2 Causes of coma or impaired consciousness in diabetic patients

HKNH
DKA
Hypoglycemia
Lactic acidosis
Stroke (more common in diabetic patients)
Post-ictal (including hypoglycemia and severe hyperglycemia)
Cerebral trauma (may follow hypoglycemia)
Ethanol intoxication (may induce or exacerbate hypoglycemia in diabetic patients)
Sedative drug overdose

Metabolic acidosis stimulates the medullary respiratory center, causing deep and sometimes rapid breathing (Kussmaul respiration). The odour of acetone may be detectable on the patient's breath (although many people are unable to detect acetone). Impaired consciousness is common, although coma occurs in only ~10% of patients. Coma at presentation is associated with a worse prognosis, and co-existing causes, such as intra-cranial hemorrhage, head injury or sedative drug intoxication, should always be considered (Table 14.2).

PATHOPHYSIOLOGY

Diabetic ketoacidosis

In DKA, profound insulin deficiency, in concert with catabolic hormone excess, promotes adipocyte lipolysis (Figure 14.1). These effects are mediated via the activity of hormone-sensitive lipase, an enzyme exquisitely sensitive to inhibition by insulin. Concurrently, intra-adipocyte re-esterification is impaired, again by deficiency of insulin. This combination of effects results in the release of large quantities of long-chain NEFA, the principal substrate for hepatic ketogenesis, into the circulation. Hepatic ketogenesis is directly enhanced by portal delivery of NEFA. In DKA, hepatic re-esterification is impaired (see above) and NEFA are preferentially partially oxidized to ketone bodies via the beta-oxidation pathway[34]. These events are summarized in Figure 14.1. Hyperglycemia causes an osmotic diuresis when the renal threshold for glucose is exceeded, leading to dehydration and secondary losses of electrolytes[35,36]. Ketonuria compounds the loss of water, although its effect is quantitatively smaller. Insulin deficiency and glucagon excess exacerbate the renal sodium depletion via effects on renal sodium reabsorption[37]. Metabolic acidosis leads to displacement of intracellular potassium by hydrogen ions, which are subsequently lost in vomit or urine. DKA usually presents as an anion gap acidosis (anion gap typically 25–35 mmol L^{-1}; see below) but a wide variety of acid–base disturbances have been reported[38].

Alcoholic ketoacidosis

A severe metabolic acidosis in the absence of hyperglycemia, or another obvious cause of acidosis, such as renal failure, raises the possibility of alcoholic ketoacidosis[39]. This condition, which tends to be under-diagnosed, occurs in alcoholics. A combination of reduced oral carbohydrate intake due to vomiting (usually a consequence of alcohol-induced acute gastritis, or acute pancreatitis) and progressive dehydration set in motion a chain of metabolic events that lead to a major metabolic disturbance. Sympatho–adrenal activation, resulting from dehydration and sudden withdrawal of alcohol, stimulate lipolysis and hence ketogenesis. Hepatic metabolism of alcohol leads to a more reduced hepatic mitochondrial redox state that may alter the plasma 3-hydroxybutyrate to acetoacetate ratio. Under these circumstances, nitroprusside-based tests may under-estimate the degree of ketonemia. A similar diagnostic difficulty may be encountered when significant lactic acidosis co-exists with ketoacidosis (see below)[40].

MANAGEMENT

Diabetic ketoacidosis

Delays in initiating therapy for DKA may be disastrous, and the diagnosis should be considered in any unconscious or hyperventilating patient. Treatment broadly follows the same principles as the management of HNKH (see above and Table 14.1), comprising rehydration with intravenous fluids, administration of insulin (suppression of lipolysis being a key objective) and careful replacement of electrolytes. The acidosis is quantified by measurement of capillary pH, PCO_2 and bicarbonate concentration. Arterial PO_2 should be measured in severely shocked patients in order to quantify hypoxia. Tests for sickle cell and glucose-6-phosphate dehydrogenase (G6PD)-deficiency may be indicated in some patients.

Few centers have routine access to measurements of ketone body concentrations. Blood ketone body (acetoacetate and 3-hydroxybutyrate) concentrations of > 5 mmol L^{-1} confirm the diagnosis. More often, biochemical confirmation is based on semi-quantitative methods. The diagnostic criteria used in our unit include a plasma bicarbonate concentration (capillary or arterial) ≤ 15 mmol L^{-1} with significant ketosis, e.g. urine Ketostix reaction ++, or plasma Ketostix $> ++$. Plasma potassium levels are usually normal or high at presentation, despite a considerable total body deficit as a result of acidosis, insulin deficiency and renal impairment[41]. Hypokalemia at presentation signifies a marked deficiency of body potassium. Total body phosphate deficiency is a characteristic feature of DKA, that may also be seen in HNKH (see above). Benefits of phosphate replacement on the prognosis of either condition have not been substantiated in clinical trials[42–44]. Insulin treatment must not be interrupted during the later stages of therapy since the restraint of lipolysis will be removed.

Alcoholic ketoacidosis

In the absence of significant hyperglycemia, treatment of alcoholic ketoacidosis includes rehydration with intravenous dextrose and electrolyte replacement. Concomitant hyperglycemia requires intravenous insulin, and should prompt careful assessment of the need for long-term insulin therapy.

CONTROVERSIES IN THE MANAGEMENT OF DKA

Bicarbonate therapy

The role of intravenous bicarbonate in the management of DKA continues to be debated[7,45,46]. In the absence of any evidence of clinical or metabolic benefits[46], we suggest that bicarbonate be reserved for patients with the most severe degrees of acidosis (pH < 7.0), in whom cardio-respiratory collapse appears imminent. Bicarbonate may also be useful if there is life-threatening hyperkalemia. Care must be taken to avoid extravasation during administration; extra potassium (20 mmol per 100 mmol bicarbonate) should be administered in order to avoid iatrogenic hypokalemia.

Cerebral edema

The pathogenesis and treatment of cerebral edema is another prominent controversy in the management of DKA[47]. However, this devastating complication is largely confined to pediatric practice.

LACTIC ACIDOSIS

INTRODUCTION

Lactic acidosis is a rare complication of biguanide therapy. Phenformin was withdrawn in many countries in the 1970s because of an unacceptable risk of lactic acidosis. The relationship between lactic acidosis and metformin is more controversial. Intravenous bicarbonate therapy remains the mainstay of severe drug-induced lactic acidosis. Patients with type 2 diabetes may also be predisposed to lactic acidosis resulting from tissue hypoxia.

LACTATE METABOLISM

Anerobic glycolysis results in the production of lactate and hydrogen (H^+) ions. This predominantly occurs in skeletal muscle, brain, erythrocytes and the renal medulla. The liver, kidneys and heart normally extract lactate, but may contribute to lactic acid accumulation under conditions of severe ischemia[48]. At physiological plasma pH, lactic acid (pK_a 3.8) is almost completely dissociated. Lactate produced by glycolysis may be oxidized completely to CO_2 and water in the tri-carboxylic acid cycle, which consumes an equimolar quantity of hydrogen ions:

$$\text{lactate}^- + 3O_2 + H^+ \rightarrow 3CO_2 + 3H_2O$$

Alternatively, lactate may enter the gluconeogenesis pathway in the liver and kidney, to form glucose (the Cori cycle), a process that also consumes hydrogen ions:

$$2\,\text{lactate}^- + 2\,H^+ \rightarrow \text{glucose}$$

LACTIC ACIDOSIS

Pathological elevations of plasma lactate concentrations accompanied by acidosis may result from over-production of lactate and hydrogen ions (e.g., with tissue hypoxia), delayed clearance (e.g., reduced hepatic lactate clearance in severe shock, impaired gluconeogenesis in severe acidosis), or a combination of these two processes. Normal fasting lactate concentrations (in whole blood) are approx. 0.4–1.2 mmol L^{-1} (Reference 49). Severe lactic acidosis is defined arbitrarily as a high anion gap metabolic acidosis, with a blood lactate concentration of > 5 mmol L^{-1}. The anion gap (normal: 10–15 mmol L^{-1}) is calculated from plasma concentrations of:

[sodium + potassium] – [chloride + bicarbonate]
(all in mmol L^{-1})

Other causes of anion gap acidosis include DKA (see above), chronic renal failure and drug toxicity (methanol, ethylene glycol, salicylates). Severe lactic acidosis is encountered in two main clinical settings that are of relevance to patients with type 2 diabetes[48].

Anerobic (type A) lactic acidosis

This occurs predominantly in states of severe tissue hypoxia, such as cardiogenic shock, in which anerobic metabolism produces lactic acid. In such situations, nicotinamide adenine dinucleotide (NAD^+) for glycolysis is regenerated by conversion of pyruvate to lactate (Figure 14.2)[50]. Patients with type 2 diabetes are at risk of hypoxic cardiovascular complications that may place them at risk of type A lactic acidosis. The presence of concomitant hypoxic conditions, e.g. heart failure, is conventionally regarded as a contra-indication to biguanide therapy[51]. Combinations of over-production and decreased extraction of lactate may be encountered in conditions such as severe sepsis or shock.

Aerobic (type B) lactic acidosis

This is much less common and is associated with several systemic diseases (including diabetes—

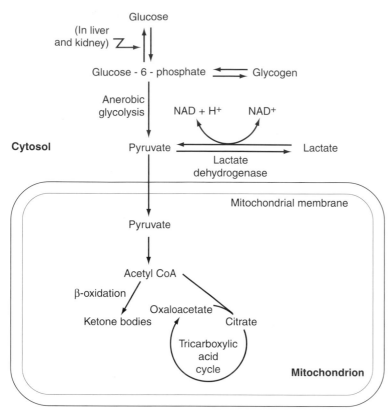

Figure 14.2 Lactate metabolism. Under anaerobic conditions, regeneration of NAD+ through lactate generation allows glycolysis to continue

NAD = Nicotinamide adenine dinucleotide

minor degrees of hyperlactatemia are common in DKA, for instance), certain drugs (notably biguanides), toxins and some inborn errors of metabolism. Tissue hypoxia is not an obvious feature of type B lactic acidosis, although hypotension and hypoxia may supervene as pre-terminal events.

LACTIC ACIDOSIS ASSOCIATED WITH DIABETES

Microvascular complications of diabetes, nephropathy being the most important, predispose to lactic acidosis in biguanide-treated patients[51,52]. Accumulation of metformin, which is excreted unchanged via the kidney, may increase the risk of lactic acidosis. However, the literature is inconsistent on the level of renal dysfunction that should prompt avoidance or withdrawal of metformin[51]; anecdotally, this is reflected by differing opinions among clinicians. Weighing risks and benefits for individual patients can be problematic. For example, many clinicians would avoid metformin in patients with advanced cardiovascular disease, yet this has to be balanced against evidence of vasoprotective actions in lower risk patients[53]. Similarly, should minor elevations of transaminase levels associated with hepatic steatosis (common in patients with type 2 diabetes) deter use of metformin in the light of preliminary evidence suggesting possible benefits[54]? To complicate matters further, the link between lactic acidosis, elevated plasma metformin concentrations and clinical outcomes has been challenged (see below). A list of cautions and contra-indications to metformin treatment, based on the literature and our current practice, is presented in Table 14.3.

Despite the high prevalence of macrovascular and microvascular complications, and consequent

Table 14.3 Cautions and contra-indications for metformin

Impaired renal function
Hepatic disease
   Acute or chronic hepatic dysfunction
Chronic alcoholism
Cardiovascular disease
   Cardiac failure
   Acute myocardial infarction
   Unstable coronary syndromes
   Severe peripheral arterial disease
Severe pulmonary disease
Other hypoxic conditions
   Severe sepsis
   Hemorrhagic shock
   Major trauma or surgery
Radiographic contrast media studies
   Withdraw metformin temporarily
Disseminated malignancy

Some of these cautions and contraindications are open to interpretation. Determining the balance of risks and benefits may be problematic in individual patients, particularly when only minor degrees of organ dysfunction are present.

risk of tissue hypoxia, severe lactic acidosis is rarely encountered in patients with type 2 diabetes[55]. However, lactic acidosis has a well-recognized association with biguanide therapy, especially with phenformin. Many patients treated with insulin or biguanides have asymptomatic daily fluctuations in blood lactate concentration, with levels reaching ~3 mmol L^{-1} (Reference 56). Increased delivery of lactate to the liver may explain why biguanides do not cause hypoglycemia when used as monotherapy (via the Cori cycle—see above). Metformin affects both production and clearance of lactate from the circulation. Anerobic glucose metabolism during metformin therapy generates lactate from splanchnic tissues, while hepatic lactate utilisation is reduced (secondary to inhibition of gluconeogenesis). Thus, lactate may accumulate in metformin-treated patients, a situation that could be rapidly accelerated if acute hypoxia supervenes.

BIGUANIDES AND LACTIC ACIDOSIS

The incidence of lactic acidosis among diabetic patients has declined considerably since the biguanide phenformin was withdrawn in many countries during the 1970s[52,56]. Lactic acidosis occurred 10–15 times more frequently during phenformin therapy than with metformin[52]. Phenformin (phenylethybiguanide) is a monosubstituted molecule with a lipophilic side-chain that binds with high affinity to the inner mitochondrial membrane[57]. In contrast to metformin, approximately 30% of an ingested dose of phenformin is metabolized in the liver to hydroxyphenyethyl biguanide. An inherited inability of some individuals to hydroxylate phenformin accounts for some of the higher risk of lactic acidosis than with metformin[58]. Lactic acidosis occurring in the course of phenformin treatment has a poor prognosis, with a 50% mortality rate[59].

Lactic acidosis complicating metformin therapy occurs much less commonly, most cases being reported among patients in whom biguanide therapy was contraindicated, for example by renal impairment[52]. Adverse experiences with phenformin have cast a lasting cloud over metformin. However, the nature of the relationship between metformin and lactic acidosis has been the subject of controversy. Lalau and colleagues have drawn attention to the paucity of evidence linking elevated metformin concentrations with lactic acidosis[60–62]. Accordingly, these authors propose that care should be taken to differentiate metformin-*associated* from metformin-*induced* lactic acidosis. More controversial still is their suggestion that metformin accumulation might actually improve the clinical outcomes for patients with lactic acidosis, via its aforementioned vasoprotective effects[60]. The clinical data on which this hypothesis is based seem open to alternative interpretations, and claims of benefit from metformin *per se* in this context must be regarded as speculative at present.

TREATMENT AND PROGNOSIS

Severe acute lactic acidosis generally has a poor prognosis that relates largely to the severity of underlying conditions. General intensive care is a crucial aspect of management. Despite considerable controversy surrounding the theoretical and clinical benefits of alkali therapy, intravenous bicarbonate remains the mainstay of supportive treatment for cases of severe type B lactic acidosis[63]. Massive doses of bicarbonate may be required to elevate arterial pH, and hemodialysis is often advocated to treat resulting sodium and water overload. Hemodialysis will also remove metformin, but conventional assumptions underpinning the role of dialysis in treating lactic acidosis attributed to metformin accumulation have been questioned[63,64]. The value of alternative approaches (e.g. using the pyruvate dehydrogenase stimulator dichloroacetate, Carbicarb) remain uncertain[64]. Accordingly, avoidance of circumstances that could precipitate lactic acidosis in vulnerable patients with type 2 diabetes continues to be an important consideration. Until more reliable evidence concerning risks and benefits of metformin becomes available, we advocate a cautious approach[53].

ACKNOWLEDGEMENTS

The support and encouragement of Drs M Nattrass and AD Wright is gratefully acknowledged. We also wish to thank Prof Sir KGMM Alberti for helpful comments.

REFERENCES

1 Arieff AI, Carroll HJ. Nonketotic hyperosmolar coma with hyperglycemia: clinical features, pathophysiology, renal function, acid-base balance, plasma-cerebrospinal fluid equilibria and the effects of therapy in 37 cases. *Medicine* 1972;51:73–94.

2 American Diabetes Association. Hyperglycemic crises in patients with diabetes mellitus. *Diabetes Care* 2001;24:154–61.

3 Delaney MF, Zisman A, Kettyle WM. Diabetic ketoacidosis and hyperglycemic hyperosmolar nonketotic syndrome. *Endocrinol Metab Clin North Am* 2000;29:683–705.

4 Cruz-Caudillo JC, Sabatini S. Diabetic hyperosmolar syndrome. *Nephron* 1995;69:201–10.

5 Gerich JE, Penhos JC, Gutman RA, Recant L. Effect of dehydration and hyperosmolarity on glucose, free fatty acid and glucose metabolism in the rat. *Diabetes* 1973;22:264–71.

6 Lindsey CA, Faloona GR, Unger RH. Plasma glucagon in nonketotic hyperosmolar coma. *J Am Med Assoc* 1974;229:1771–3.

7 Kitabchi AE, Umpierrez GE, Murphy MB *et al.* Management of hyperglycemic crises in patients with diabetes. *Diabetes Care* 2001;24:131–53.

8 Krentz AJ, Nattrass M. 1997. Acute metabolic complications of diabetes mellitus: diabetic ketoacidosis, hyperosmolar non-ketotic syndrome and lactic acidosis. In: Pickup JC, Williams G editors. *Textbook of Diabetes* 2nd edn. Oxford: Blackwell Science, 1997: 39.1–39.23.

9 Magee MF, Bhatt BA. Management of decompensated diabetes. Diabetic ketoacidosis and hyperglycemic hyperosmolar syndrome. *Crit Care Clin* 2001;17:75–106.

10 Zouvanis M, Pietersee AC, Seftel HC, Joffe BI. Clinical characteristics and outcome of hyperglycaemic emergencies in Johannesburg South Africans. *Diabetic Med* 1997;14:603–6.

11 McCurdy DK. Hyperosmolar hyperglycemic nonketotic diabetic coma. *Med Clin N Am* 1970;54:683–99.

12 Pinies JA, Cairo G, Gaztambide S, Vazquez JA. Course and prognosis of 132 patients with diabetic non-ketotic hyperosmolar state. *Diabet Metab* 1994;20:43–8.

13 Wachtel TJ. The diabetic hyperosmolar state. *Clin Geriatr Med* 1990;6:797–806.

14 Grant C, Warlow C. Focal epilepsy in diabetic non-ketotic hyperglycaemia. *Br Med J* 1985;290:1204–5.

15 Podolsky S, Pattavina CG. Hyperosmolar nonketotic diabetic coma: a complication of propranolol therapy. *Metabolism* 1973;22:685–93.

16 Fonseca V, Phear DN. Hyperosmolar non-ketotic diabetic syndrome precipitated by treatment with diuretics. *Br Med J* 1982;284:36–7.

17 Umpierrez GE, Kelly JP, Navarrete JE *et al.* Hyperglycemic crises in urban blacks. *Arch Intern Med* 1997;157:669–75.

18 Fulop M, Rosenblatt A, Kreitzer SM, Gerstenhaber B. Hyperosmolar nature of diabetic coma. *Diabetes* 1975;24:594–9.

19 Small M, Alzaid A, MacCuish AC. Diabetic hyperosmolar non-ketotic decompensation. *Q J Med* 1988;66:251–7.

20 Hillier TA, Abbott RD, Barrett EJ. Hyponatremia: evaluating the correction factor for hyperglycemia. *Am J Med* 1999;106:399–403

21 Gottshalk ME, Ros SP, Zeller WP. The emergency management of hyperglycemia-hyperosmolar nonketotic coma in the pediatric patient. *Pediatr Emerg Care* 1996;12:48–51.

22 Carroll P, Matz R. Uncontrolled diabetes mellitus in adults: experience in treating diabetic ketoacidosis and hyperosmolar nonketotic coma with low-dose insulin and a uniform treatment regimen. *Diabetes Care* 1983;6:579–85.

23 Wright AD, Walsh CH, Fitzgerald MG, Malins JM. Low-dose insulin treatment of hyperosmolar diabetic coma. *Postgrad Med J* 1981;57:556–9.

24 Keller U, Berger W, Ritz R, Truog P. Course and prognosis of 86 episodes of diabetic coma. A five year experience with a uniform schedule of treatment. *Diabetologia* 1975;11:93–100.

25 Lord GM, Scott J, Pusey CD *et al.* Diabetes and rhabdomyolysis. A rare complication of a common disease. *Br Med J* 1993;307:1126–8.

26 Rolfe M, Ephraim GG, Lincoln DC, Huddle KR. Hyperosmolar non-ketotic diabetic coma as a cause of emergency hyperglycaemic admission to Baragwanath Hospital. *S Afr Med J* 1995;85:173–6.

27 Chernick SS, Clark CM, Gardiner RJ, Scow RO. Role of lipolytic and glucocorticoid hormones in the development of diabetic ketosis. *Diabetes* 1972;21:946–54.

28 Schade DS, Eaton RP. Pathogenesis of diabetic ketoacidosis: a reappraisal. *Diabetes Care* 1979;2:296–306.

29 Madsbad S, Alberti KG, Binder C *et al.* Role of residual insulin secretion in protecting against ketoacidosis in insulin-dependent diabetes. *Br Med J* 1979;2:1257–9.

30 Umpierrez GE, Casals MM, Gebhart SP *et al.* Diabetic ketoacidosis in obese African–Americans. *Diabetes* 1995;44:790–5.

31 Musey VC, Lee JK, Crawford R *et al.* Diabetes in urban African–Americans. I. Cessation of insulin therapy is the major precipitating cause of diabetic ketoacidosis. *Diabetes Care* 1995; 18:483–9.

32 Balasubramanyam A, Zern JW, Hyman DJ, Pavlik V. New profiles of diabetic ketoacidosis: type 1 vs. type 2 diabetes and the effects of ethnicity. *Arch Intern Med* 1999;159:2317–22.

33 Yu EH, Guo H-R, Wu TJ. Factors associated with discontinuing insulin therapy after diabetic ketoacidosis in adult diabetic patients. *Diabet Med* 2001;18:895–9.

34 McGarry JD, Foster DW. Regulation of hepatic fatty acid oxidation and ketone body production. *Annu Rev Biochem* 1980;49:395–420.

35 Nabarro JDN, Spencer AG, Stowers JM. Metabolic studies in severe diabetic ketoacidosis. *Q J Med* 1952;21:225–48.

36 Podolsky S, Emerson KJ. Potassium depletion in diabetic ketoacidosis. *Diabetes* 1973;22:229.

37 DeFronzo RA, Sherwin RS, Dillingham M *et al.* Influence of basal insulin and glucagon secretion on potassium and sodium metabolism. Studies with somatostatin in normal dogs and in normal and diabetic human beings. *J Clin Invest* 1978;61:472–9.

38 Adrogue HJ, Wilson H, Boyd AE *et al.* Plasma acid-base patterns in diabetic ketoacidosis. *N Engl J Med* 1982;307:1603–10.

39 Thompson CJ, Johnston DG, Baylis PH, Anderson J. Alcoholic ketoacidosis: an under-diagnosed condition? *Br Med J* 1986;292:463–5.

40 Marliss EB, Ohman JL, Aoki TT, Kozak GP. Altered redox state obscuring ketoacidosis in diabetic patients with lactic acidosis. *N Engl J Med* 1970;283:978–80.

41 Beigelman PM. Potassium in severe diabetic ketoacidosis. *Am J Med* 1973;54:419–20.

42 Gibby OM, Veale KE, Hayes TM *et al.* Oxygen availability from the blood and the effect of phosphate replacement on erythrocyte 2,3-diphosphoglycerate and haemoglobin–oxygen affinity in diabetic ketoacidosis. *Diabetologia* 1978;15:381–5.

43 Wilson HK, Keuer SP, Lea AS *et al.* Phosphate therapy in diabetic ketoacidosis. *Arch Intern Med* 1982;142:517–20.

44 Fisher JN, Kitabchi AE. A randomized study of phosphate therapy in the treatment of diabetic ketoacidosis. *J Clin Endocrinol Metab* 1983;57:177–80.

45 Nattrass M, Hale PJ. Clinical aspects of diabetic ketoacidosis. In: Nattrass M, Santiago JV editors. *Recent advances in diabetes*. 1. Edinburgh: Churchill Livingstone, 1984: 231–8.

46 Hale PJ, Crase J, Nattrass M. Metabolic effects of bicarbonate in diabetic ketoacidosis. *Br Med J* 1984;289:1035–8.

47 Edge JA, Hawkins MM, Winter DL, Dunger DB. The risk and outcome of cerebral oedema developing during diabetic ketoacidosis. *Arch Dis Child* 2001;85:16–22.

48 Cohen RD, Iles RA. Lactic acidosis: diagnosis and treatment. *Clin Endocrinol Metab* 1980;9:513–41.

49 Foster KJ, Alberti KG, Hinks L *et al.* Blood intermediary metabolite and insulin concentrations after an overnight fast: reference ranges

for adults, and interrelations. *Clin Chem* 1978;24:1568–72.

50 Alberti KGMM, Nattrass M. Lactic acidosis. *Lancet* 1977;2:25–9.

51 Sulkin TV, Bosman D, Krentz AJ. Contra-indications to metformin therapy in patients with NIDDM. *Diabetes Care* 1997;20:925–8

52 Krentz AJ, Ferner RE, Bailey CJ. Comparative tolerability profiles of oral antidiabetic agents. *Drug Safety* 1994;11:223–41.

53 Howlett HCS, Bailey CJ. A risk-benefit assessment of metformin in type 2 diabetes. In: Krentz AJ, editor. *Drug treatment of type 2 diabetes.* Auckland: ADIS books, 2000: 61–76.

54 Marchesini G, Brizi M, Bianchi G *et al.* Metformin in non-alcoholic steatohepatitis. *Lancet* 2001;358:893–4.

55 Chan NN, Brain HPS, Feher MD. Metformin-associated lactic acidosis: a rare or very rare clinical entity? *Diabetic Med* 1999;16:273–81.

56 Nattrass M, Alberti KG. Biguanides. *Diabetologia* 1978;14:71–4.

57 Bailey CJ. Metformin—an update. *Gen Pharmacol* 1993;24:1299–1309.

58 Oates NS, Shah RR, Idle JR, Smith RL. Influence of oxidation polymorphism on phenformin kinetics and dynamics. *Clin Pharmacother* 1983;34:827–34.

59 Luft D, Schmulling RM, Eggstein M. Lactic acidosis in biguanide-treated diabetics: a review of 330 cases. *Diabetologia* 1978;14:75–87.

60 Lalau J-D, Race J-M. Lactic acidosis in metformin-treated patients. *Drug Safety* 1999;20:377–84.

61 Lalau J-D, Race J-M. Metformin and lactic acidosis in diabetic humans. *Diabetes Obes Metab* 2000;2:131–7.

62 Lalau J-D, Race J-M. Lactic acidosis in metformin therapy: searching for a link with metformin in reports of 'metformin-associated lactic acidosis'. *Diabetes Obes Metab* 2001;3:195–201.

63 Kreisberg RA. Pathogenesis and management of lactic acidosis. *Ann Rev Med* 1984;35:181–93.

64 Luft FC. Lactic acidosis update for critical care clinicians. *J Am Soc Nephrol* 2001;12(Suppl 17):S15–19.

15

Diabetic retinopathy and ocular complications

Brett Rosenblatt, Carl D Regillo and William E Benson

INTRODUCTION

Ophthalmic complications of type 2 diabetes mellitus include cataract, glaucoma and cranial nerve palsies, but diabetic retinopathy is by far the most frequent and potentially blinding complication. Nearly three decades ago it was estimated that diabetics are 20 times more likely to be blind than the general population[1]. Despite the great strides that have since been made in our understanding and management of diabetes, ocular complications continue to have a major impact on the well-being of patients with this disease. Results from several recent studies have made clear that, with tight metabolic control, vigilant screening and timely well-executed intervention, vision loss due to diabetes can be drastically reduced[2]. This chapter describes the ophthalmic complications associated with type 2 diabetes, with particular attention being given to their clinical characteristics and management.

EPIDEMIOLOGY

The prevalence of retinopathy increases with duration and severity of diabetes. Patients with type 2 diabetes are more likely to have signs of retinopathy at the time of diagnosis than those with type 1 diabetes. This difference is primarily a result of the frequent delay in diagnosis in older patients with more insidious onset of symptoms. However, over time, the prevalence of retinopathy increases at a slower rate in type 2 diabetics, who tend to have a more manageable disease, in contrast to the more difficult to control type 1 diabetics. The Wisconsin Epidemiologic Study of Diabetic Retinopathy (WESDR), a large population-based study, found a prevalence of retinopathy 10 years after diagnosis of 90% in type 1, compared with 60% in type 2 diabetes[3]. In the WESDR, type 2 diabetics requiring insulin had nearly twice the prevalence of retinopathy, in contrast to those who did not need insulin (70% versus 39%)[4].

The controversy regarding whether or not tight metabolic control prevents the development or progression of retinopathy has been settled by two large randomized studies. The first of these, the Diabetes Control and Complications Trial (DCCT), proved that tight glucose monitoring and control reduced diabetic complications, including retinopathy, in type 1 diabetes. The intensive-therapy group achieved a median glycosylated hemoglobin (HbA1c) of 7.2% (compared with 9.1% in the conventional group), and had a 65% risk reduction for clinically important progression of retinopathy at 10-year follow-up[5]. Results of the UK Prospective Diabetes Study (UKPDS) demonstrated that intensive treatment of hyperglycemia benefited type 2 diabetics as well. In the UKPDS over 5000 patients with recently diagnosed type 2 diabetes were randomly assigned to intensive or conventional treatment. Various hypoglycemic agents, including insulin, were used to maintain a fasting blood glucose level near 110 mg dL^{-1} in the intensive-treatment group, whereas diet alone was used in the conventional-treatment cohort. The intensive-treatment group achieved a median HbA1c of 7%, compared with the significantly higher 7.9% in the conventional-treatment group. Tighter control was associated with a 21% risk reduction for the progression of diabetic retinopathy at the 12-year follow-up (38% intensive group versus 48% conventional group)[6]. Physicians can now be assured that the current American Diabetes Association recommendation of aiming for a HbA1c of 7.0% is an indispensable aspect of diabetes management[7]. Despite the benefits that meticulous control of serum glucose provides, it may not prevent progression in diabetics with very advanced retinopathy[8].

The development and progression of retinopathy most certainly is influenced by many factors, including race, gender, hypertension and other vasculopathic systemic disorders. Epidemiologic studies have been unable to conclusively demonstrate a definitive association between these factors and retinopathy in patients with type 2 diabetes[9–15]. Pregnancy, however, has been shown to be a significant risk factor for development and progression of diabetic retinopathy. In women without retinopathy at the start of pregnancy, 10% will show mild retinal changes that resolve after delivery. However, in women with pre-existing retinopathy, up to 25% will progress to proliferative changes during pregnancy[16]. Those at greatest risk for severe visual deterioration are those who are rapidly brought under strict control[17]. Women should be encouraged to have their eyes examined and their glycemic control optimized prior to becoming pregnant.

CLINICAL FEATURES

Systemic complications of diabetes typically manifest clinically after permanent tissue damage has already occurred. Unlike the changes occurring in other organs, the microvascular alterations

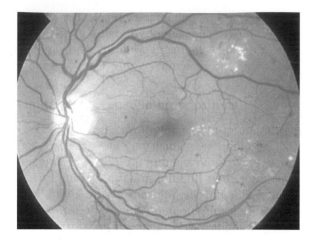

Figure 15.1 Diabetic retinopathy.

responsible for preventable vision loss can be observed directly through a dilated pupil (Figure 15.1). Clinicians caring for diabetics should be skilled at recognizing the signs and symptoms of diabetic retinopathy, not only because it minimizes visual sequelae, but also because the status of the retina reflects microvascular complications occurring elsewhere in the body.

Ophthalmologists classify diabetic retinopathy as non-proliferative diabetic retinopathy (NPDR) and proliferative diabetic retinopathy (PDR). The non-proliferative changes are also commonly referred to as background diabetic retinopathy. The ocular changes seen in eyes with NPDR all occur at the level of the retina, in contrast to PDR, which is characterized by the growth of blood vessels and fibrous tissue beyond the surface of the retina. The clinical features of diabetic retinopathy, including microaneurysms, cotton wool spots (CWS), retinal edema, exudates, venous abnormalities and neovascularization, are all secondary to compromised capillary endothelium, which leads to increased capillary permeability and fragility. Widespread small vessel damage leads to areas of ischemia, which can promote intraocular angiogenesis.

Numerous hypotheses explaining the microvascular complications of diabetes have been investigated, including the role of the polyol pathway, glycosylated end products, growth factors and oxidative stress[18–20]. Angiogenic factors, such as growth hormone (GH) and vascular endothelial growth factor (VEGF) are being evaluated for their mechanistic and potential therapeutic role in diabetic retinopathy. Increased concentrations, or over-expression of intraocular VEGF has been shown to lead to neovascularization, as well as increased permeability of retinal vasculature. Furthermore, inhibitors of VEGF have been shown to prevent ischemia-induced neovascularization in several animal models[21,22].

Protein kinase C (PKC) activation is required for VEGF to induce its effects on vascular endothelium. Orally ingested inhibitors of PKC, currently in clinical trials, have shown promise as an effective way of preventing many of the diabetes-induced vascular complications. Interest in the interaction between components of blood flow, including blood viscosity and red-cell deformability, has also increased recently. Blood viscosity, a potentially modifiable factor, has been shown in small studies to impact the progression and visual impact of diabetic retinopathy[23,24].

Non-proliferative diabetic retinopathy

Microaneurysms are the most common, and usually the first detectable, signs of retinopathy. These saccular out-pouching of capillaries appear as small discrete red dots within the retina, which tend to increase in number and size with progression of NPDR. Retinal hemorrhages, another early finding, result from ruptured microaneurysms, capillaries or venules. The morphology of retinal hemorrhages depend on how deep within the retina they lie. The deeper 'dot–blot' hemorrhages are round with distinct borders; whereas superficial nerve fiber layer hemorrhages assume a flame or splinter shape (Figure 15.2). These early, often subtle, manifestations of NPDR are important to recognize, because an increasing number of microaneurysms may indicate deterioration of retinopathy[25].

CWS are seen ophthalmoscopically as superficial white lesions with feathery margins (Figure 15.3). Although they are commonly called 'soft exudates', they result from ischemia,

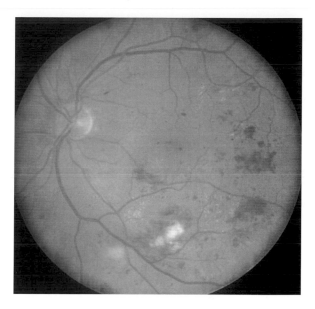

Figure 15.2 Non-proliferative retinopathy demonstrating retinal hemorrhages.

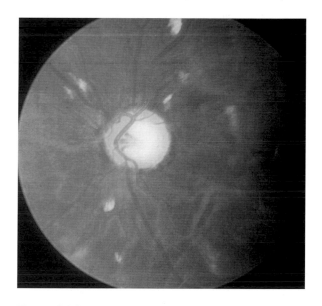

Figure 15.3 Numerous CWS.

not exudation. Local ischemia causes effective obstruction of axoplasmic flow in the normally transparent nerve fiber layer; the subsequent swelling of the nerve fibers gives CWS their characteristic white appearance. CWS are not specific for diabetes, and are commonly seen in association with hypertension, collagen-vascular disease, AIDS, carotid obstruction and cardiac valvular disease. The presence of even a single CWS deserves a systemic evaluation[26].

Hard exudates are extracellular deposits of lipid within the retina. They are sharply demarcated yellow 'waxy' lesions of varying size and configuration that, unlike CWS, have well-defined borders. This lipid derives from leaky vessels; hard exudates are therefore often associated with areas of retinal edema.

Macular edema, which is defined as thickening of the central retina, is the leading cause of legal blindness in diabetics[27]. Clinically significant macula edema (CSME) is edema or hard exudates that involve or threaten the part of the retina which subserves central vision (the fovea)[28]. This important sign is often difficult to visualize, because alterations of retinal thickness are subtle. It is best evaluated through the stereoscopic view provided by a contact lens and slit-lamp biomicroscope.

As NPDR advances, signs of retinal ischemia appear. These include increasing CWS, hemorrhages, venous irregularities and intraretinal microvascular abnormalities (IRMA). Venous beading (irregularly dilated venules) and IRMA (telangiectatic capillaries that shunt blood around areas of non-perfusion) often portend progression to proliferative changes. The Early Treatment Diabetic Retinopathy Study found that multiple retinal hemorrhages, venous beading, IRMA and widespread capillary nonperfusion were the clinical signs that best predicted progression to proliferative retinopathy. Eyes that had many of these features in excess have up to a 50% risk of progression to PDR after 1 year[29]. Although the macular edema, exudates, and capillary occlusions that occur in NPDR can occasionally cause legal blindness, affected patients usually maintain at least ambulatory vision. Proliferative diabetic retinopathy, on the other hand, is more likely to result in disabling, severe vision loss.

Proliferative diabetic retinopathy

Proliferative retinopathy is heralded by the growth of neovascular and fibrous tissue. The

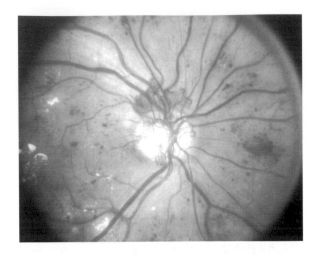

Figure 15.4 Neovascularization of the disc (NVD).

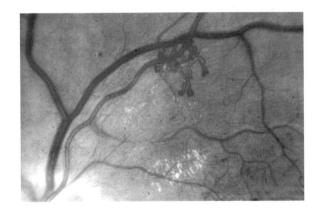

Figure 15.5 Neovascularization elsewhere (NVE).

overall prevalence of PDR in type 2 diabetics is 10%, but the rate is higher in those requiring insulin (14%) compared with those not requiring insulin (3%)[4]. Blood vessel growth from the optic nerve is termed neovascularization of the disc (NVD); whereas vessels arising from any other part of the retina is referred to as neovascularization elsewhere (NVE) (Figures 15.4 and 15.5). Neovascular tissue extends into the vitreous—the clear delicate connective tissue that fills the space bounded posteriorly by the retina and anteriorly by the lens. The complications of PDR are related to the propensity for new vessels to bleed (vitreous hemorrhage), as

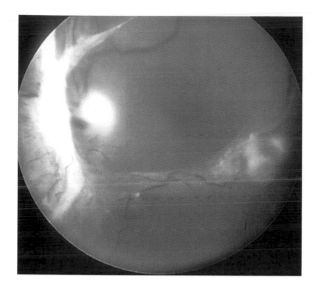

Figure 15.6 Tractional retinal detachment and vitreous hemorrhage.

well as the tendency of the vitreous body to shrink and pull the retina forward (traction retinal detachment) (Figure 15.6). Bleeding within the vitreous causes sudden painless loss of acuity.

The extent and location of the hemorrhage determine the magnitude of vision loss. Examining eyes with vitreous hemorrhage is difficult because blood in the vitreous obscures retinal details. When necessary, intraocular structures are assessed with ultrasonography. Tractional retinal detachments, the other major complication of PDR, appear as elevations of all or portions of the retina. Tractional retinal detachment occurs when fibrous tissue pulls on the retina, overwhelming the adhesive forces keeping it attached. Patients with detached retinas present with loss of vision corresponding to the part of the retina that has detached. For example, a superior retinal detachment will cause an inferior visual field defect because of the inverted topographic representation of the retina. Vision loss is often preceded by the sensation of flashing lights or floaters. If suspected, prompt referral to an ophthalmologist experienced in the repair of retinal detachments is critical.

MANAGEMENT

Non-proliferative diabetic retinopathy

Management of NPDR relies heavily on patient education, periodic screening and, when necessary, laser treatment. The American College of Physicians/American Academy of Ophthalmology has recommended a schedule for ophthalmic evaluation for patients with diabetes (Table 15.1). Periodic eye examinations enable ophthalmologists to identify patients who would benefit from prophylactic treatment, before serious complications develop. The potential sight-threatening sequelae associated with diabetic retinopathy and other ocular complications should be stressed to patients with diabetes; they should be made aware that regular eye exams are integral to their diabetes management. Patients, as well as all clinicians caring for diabetics, should be able to recognize the signs and symptoms of diabetic eye disease.

CSME, which can occur in non-proliferative or proliferative retinopathy, must be suspected in any patient with diabetes complaining of blurred vision. A delay in referral, or recognition of the signs or symptoms of macular edema, can diminish the success of intervention. Treatment of CSME with laser decreases the rate of moderately severe vision loss at 3 year follow-up from 30% in untreated to 15% in treated eyes[28]. Laser energy applied in a grid pattern to the area of retinal thickening facilitates the resorbtion of fluid, allowing the retina to resume its normal thickness and function. Focal laser treatment can also be used to close off the leaking vessels that are causing the edema. This requires precision; the exact location of leaking sources can only be identified by fluorescein angiography. This diagnostic study involves the intravenous injection of a fluorescent dye, which is captured on film or digital media as it passes through the retinal circulation. The proper management of diabetic macular edema relies heavily on the information provided by these detailed images of retinal vasculature (Figures 15.7 and 15.8).

Proliferative diabetic retinopathy

The goal of managing PDR is to prevent vitreous hemorrhage and retinal detachments. Pan-retinal

Table 15.1 Suggested follow-up and intervention for patients with diabetic retinopathy

Retinal abnormality	Follow-up	Action
None or minimal NPDR *None or rare microaneurysms*	Annually	Optimize control of serum glucose, hypertension, serum lipids, renal disease
Mild NPDR *Few scattered retinal hemorrhages and microaneurysms*	Every 6–12 months	Optimize control of serum glucose, hypertension, serum lipids, renal disease
Moderate NPDR *Moderate hemorrhages and microaneurysms; hard exudates or soft exudates may be present*	Every 6–12 months	Optimize control of serum glucose, hypertension, serum lipids, renal disease
Severe or very severe NPDR *Widespread retinal hemorrhages, venous abnormalities or IRMA*	Every 1–4 months	Consider early scatter laser treatment as retinopathy progresses
Macular edema *CSME if thickening or hard exudates threaten the fovea*	Every 2–4 months	Treat CSME with focal laser treatment Fluorescein angiogram necessary to locate leaking sources
Proliferative diabetic retinopathy (less than high risk) *Minimal neovascularization without bleeding*	Every 2–4 months	Consider early scatter laser treatment as retinopathy progresses
Proliferative diabetic retinopathy (high risk) *Extensive NVD, NVD with hemorrhage, extensive NVE with hemorrhage*	Every 1–4 months	Pan retinal photocoagulation is indicated More than 1500 laser burns, applied to peripheral retina in one or multiple sessions
Vitreous hemorrhage *Blood dispersed in the vitreous cavity, poor retinal view*	Every 1–3 months	Serial ultrasonography; Vitrectomy for persistent hemorrhage, for active retinopathy requiring laser (which is prohibited by hemorrhage) or for retinal detachment that threatens the macula
Traction retinal detachment *Elevation of part of the retina associated with fibrous tissue*	Every 1–3 months	Vitrectomy if threatening macula; otherwise careful observation

photocoagulation (PRP) involves the application of approximately 1500–2000, or more, laser burns to the peripheral retina, effectively ablating large areas of ischemic retina. It is believed that this, in turn, reduces the production of angiogenic substances, such as VEGF. In the Diabetic

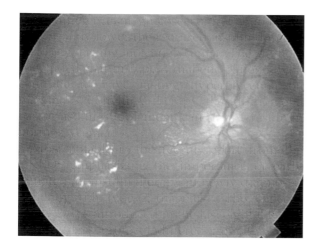

Figure 15.7 Macular edema with associated hard exudates.

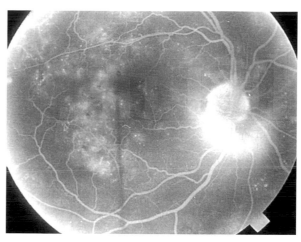

Figure 15.8 Fluorescein angiogram of same eye as in Figure 15.7, showing macular edema. Bright spots localize the focal areas of leakage.

Retinopathy Study (DRS) PRP reduced the rate of severe vision loss from 26% in observed eyes to 11% in treated eyes at 2 year follow-up, a 60% risk reduction[30].

PRP, although successful in promoting regression of the neovascularization in 72% of patients by 3 weeks, is associated with loss of peripheral vision and, occasionally, with other vision-compromising side effects[31]. PRP is typically reserved for patients with high-risk characteristics—eyes that have the most to gain from treatment (Figure 15.9).

The use of aspirin deserves special attention because its role in the management in diabetic retinopathy has been extensively debated. Many clinicians have been concerned that the antiplatelet effect of aspirin may promote intraocular bleeding. Others felt that the rheologic alterations induced by aspirin might decrease microvascular complications. However, evidence from a large randomized study revealed that aspirin has no clear beneficial or harmful effect on vision or progression of diabetic retinopathy. More importantly, this study found that those receiving aspirin had a 17% decreased risk of morbidity and death from cardiovascular disease[32]. Patients with diabetic retinopathy may take an aspirin daily unless otherwise contraindicated.

Vitrectomy, the surgical evacuation of the vitreous cavity, plays a vital role in the management of

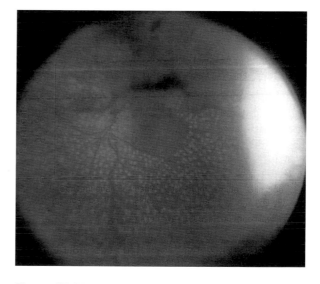

Figure 15.9 Wide-angle view of an eye following PRP.

severe complications of diabetic retinopathy. Removal of the vitreous limits the progression of neovascularization, because it eliminates the collagen fibrils that act as scaffolding upon which new blood vessels grow. Several studies have evaluated whether vitrectomy might improve the visual prognosis by reducing neovascularization and its concomitant complications. Two independent

in patients with type 2 diabetes. UKPDS 33. *Lancet* 1998;352:837–53.

7 American Diabetes Association. Standards of medical care for patients with diabetes mellitus. *Diabetes Care* 1998;21(Suppl):S23–S31.

8 Ramsay RC, Goetz FC, Sutherland DE *et al.* Progression of diabetic retinopathy after pancreas transplantation for insulin-dependent diabetes mellitus. *N Engl J Med* 1988;318:208–14.

9 Raab MF, Gagliano DA, Sweeney HE. Diabetic retinopathy in blacks. *Diabetes Care* 1990; 13:1202–6.

10 Arfken CL, Salicrup AE, Meuer SM *et al.* Retinopathy in African Americans and whites with insulin-dependent diabetes mellitus. *Arch Intern Med* 1994;154:2597–601.

11 Klein R, Klein BE, Moss SE. Is blood pressure a predictor of the incidence or progression of diabetic retinopathy? *Arch Intern Med* 1989; 149:2427.

12 Klein R, Klein BE. Epidemiology of proliferative diabetic retinopathy. *Diabetes Care* 1992;15:1875–91.

13 Klein R, Klein BE, Moss SE, Davis MD, DeMets DL. The Wisconsin epidemiologic study of diabetic retinopathy. II. Prevalence and risk of diabetic retinopathy when age is less than 30 years. *Arch Ophthalmol* 1984; 102:520–6.

14 Nelson RG, Wolfe JA, Horton MB *et al.* Proliferative retinopathy in NIDDM. *Diabetes* 1989;38:435.

15 Janka HU *et al.* Risk factors for progression of background retinopathy in long-standing IDDM. *Diabetes* 1989;38:460.

16 Klein BEK, Moss SE, Klein R. Effect of pregnancy on progression of diabetic retinopathy. *Diabetes Care* 1990;13:34–40.

17 Rosenn B, Miodovnik M, Kranias G *et al.* Progression of diabetic retinopathy in pregnancy: association with hypertension in pregnancy. *Am J Obstet Gynecol* 1992;166:1214–18.

18 Greene D, Sima A, Stevens M. Aldose reductase inhibitors: an approach to the treatment of diabetic nerve damage. *Diabetes Metab Rev* 1993;9:189–217.

19 Brownlee M. The pathologic implications of protein glycolation. *Clin Invest Med* 1995; 18:275–81.

20 Baynes J, Thorpe S. Role of oxidative stress in diabetic complications: a new perspective on an old paradigm. *Diabetes* 1999;48:1–9.

21 Williams J, Adamis A, Aiello L. Vascular endothelial growth factor in ocular neovascularization and proliferative diabetic retinopathy. *Diabetes Metab Rev* 1997;13:37–50.

22 Aiello L. Vascular endothelial growth factor: 20th century mechanisms, 21st-century therapies. *Invest Ophthalm Vis Sci* 1997;38:1647–52.

23 Fujisawa T, Ikegami H, Yamato E *et al.* Association of plasma fibrinogen level and blood pressure with diabetic retinopathy, and renal complications associated with proliferative diabetic retinopathy, in Type 2 diabetes mellitus. *Diabetic Med* 1999;16:522–6.

24 Widder RA, Brunner R, Walter P *et al.* Improvement of visual acuity in patients suffering from diabetic retinopathy after membrane differential filtration: a pilot study. *Transfus Sci* 1999;21:201–6.

25 Kohner EM, Sleightholm M. Does microaneurysm count reflect severity of early diabetic retinopathy? *Ophthalmology* 1986;93:586–9.

26 Brown GC, Brown MM, Hiller T *et al.* Cotton-wool spots. *Retina* 1985;5:206–14.

27 Patz A, Schatz H, Berkow JW *et al.* Macular edema: an overlooked complication of diabetic retinopathy. *Trans Am Acad Ophthalmol Otolaryngol* 1973;77:34–42.

28 Early Treatment Diabetic Retinopathy Study Research Group. Photocoagulation for diabetic macular edema: Early Treatment Diabetic Retinopathy Study Report no. 4. *Int Ophthal Clinics* 1987;27:265–72.

29 Early Treatment Diabetic Retinopathy Study Research Group. Fundus photographic risk factors for progression of diabetic retinopathy. Early Treatment Diabetic Retinopathy Study Report no. 12. *Ophthalmology* 1991;98:823–33.

30 Diabetic Retinopathy Study Group. Clinical applications of Diabetic Retinopathy Study (DRS) findings: Diabetic Retinopathy Study Report no. 8. *Ophthalmology* 1981;88:583–600.

31 Doft BH, Blankenship GW. Single versus multiple treatment sessions of argon laser panretinal photocoagulation for proliferative diabetic retinopathy. *Ophthalmology* 1982; 89:772.

32 Early Treatment Diabetic Retinopathy Study Research Group. Effects of aspirin treatment on diabetic retinopathy. Early Treatment Diabetic Retinopathy Study Report no. 8. *Ophthalmology* 1991;98:757–65.

33 Benson WE, Brown GC, Tasman W, McNamara JA. Complications of vitrectomy for non-clearing vitreous hemorrhage in diabetic patients. *Ophthalmic Surg* 1988;19:862–5.

34 Thompson JT, de Bustros S, Michels RG, Rice TA. Results and prognostic factors in vitrectomy for

diabetic vitreous hemorrhage. *Arch Ophthalmol* 1987;105:191–5.

35 Bernth-Peterson P, Bach E. Epidemiologic aspects of cataract surgery. III: Frequencies of diabetes and glaucoma in a cataract population. *Acta Ophthalmol* 1983;61:406–16.

36 Klein BEK, Klein R, Moss RE. Prevalence of cataracts in a population-based study of persons with diabetes mellitus. *Ophthalmology* 1985;92:1191.

37 Minckler D, Astorino A, Hamilton A. Cataract surgery in patients with diabetes. *Ophthalmology* 1998;105:949–50.

38 Krupsky S, Zalish M, Oliver M, Pollack A. Anterior segment complications in diabetic patients following extracapsular cataract extraction and posterior chamber intraocular lens implantation. *Ophthalmic Surg* 1991;22:526–30.

39 Straatsma BR, Pettit TH, Wheeler N, Miyamasu W. Diabetes mellitus and intraocular lens implantation. *Ophthalmology* 1983;90:336–43.

40 Hykin PG, Gregson RM, Stevens JD, Hamilton PA. Extracapsular cataract extraction in proliferative diabetic retinopathy. *Ophthalmology* 1993;100:394–9.

41 Benson WE, Brown GC, Tasman W. Diabetes and its ocular complications. Philadelphia: W B Saunders, 1988:27–34.

42 Tielsch JM, Katz J, Quigley HA, Javitt JC, Sommer A. Diabetes, intraocular pressure, and primary open-angle glaucoma in the Baltimore Eye Survey. *Ophthalmology* 1995;102:48–53.

43 Klein B, Klein R, Jensen S. Open-angle glaucoma and older-onset diabetes: the Beaver Dam Eye Study. *Ophthalmology* 1994;101:1173–7.

44 Little HL, Rosenthal AR, Dellaporta A, Jacobson DR. The effect of panretinal photocoagulation on rubeosis iridis. *Am J Ophthalmol* 1976;81:804.

45 Jacobson DR, Murphy RP, Rosenthal AR. The treatment of angle neovascularization with panretinal photocoagulation. *Ophthalmology* 1979;86:1270–5.

46 Regillo CD, Brown GC, Savino PJ *et al*. Diabetic papillopathy. Patient characteristics and fundus findings. *Arch Ophthalmol* 1995;113:889–95.

47 Watanabe K, Hagura R, Akanuma Y *et al*. Characteristics of cranial nerve palsies in diabetic patients. *Diabetes Res Clin Pract* 1990;10:19–27.

48 Burde RM. Neuro-ophthalmic associations and complications of diabetes mellitus. *Am J Ophthalmol* 1992;114:498–501.

49 Benson WE, Brown GC, Tasman W. Diabetes and its ocular complications. Philadelphia: W B Saunders, 1988:117–8.

16

Renal dysfunction and nephropathy in type 2 diabetes

Carl Erik Mogensen

INTRODUCTION

Nephropathy in type 2 diabetes has emerged as a serious clinical problem and is now more frequently seen than advanced renal disease in type 1 diabetes. In the 1970s, renal complications as a result of type 2 diabetes were rare, so this new development is surprising. Today, most patients in dialysis units have type 2 diabetics. We echo Eberhard Ritz's question: "Why and how did type 2 diabetes lose its 'renal innocence'?"[1].

There is probably not one single factor that is responsible for this new problem. In all likelihood there are now more frequent referrals of old severely ill patients with terminal renal failure. It is also clear that there is a dramatic increase in the prevalence of type 2 diabetes in the general population. This is partly due to the adoption of new 'less healthy' lifestyles. An even more important factor, however, is that survival of patients with type 2 diabetes is much better now, simply because of better treatment of hypertension and coronary heart disease, conditions that previously were quite common in these patients, and which could not be, or were not treated[1].

There is thus a change in life pattern of these patients—they often live long enough to develop renal disease, and even renal failure. The increase in number of patients is also a result of medical progress, where cardiovascular mortality to some extent has been replaced by end-stage renal disease (ESRD) as the terminal

fate of these patients. It should be noted that the strict classification of type 1 and type 2 diabetes may not be completely relevant, because there are many patients in whom classification is problematic; the pathogenesis and treatment strategy in both conditions is very similar. New studies suggest that the clinical course of renal disease is very much the same in the two types of diabetes[2-5].

Type 2 diabetes is a polygenic condition that acts in a complicated interplay of lifestyle and environment. Ironically, our improved living conditions, with more abundant food and less hard physical work, has 'created' new degenerative diseases, which are not due to physical burdens and hard work.

HISTORICAL ASPECTS

In the pre-insulin era, patients who developed complications related to diabetes would be type 2 diabetics, because type 1 patients would simply not survive long enough. As early as the 19th century, it was recognised that the urine of diabetic patients contained abnormal amounts of coagulable matter, probably proteins[6,7]. The French physician, Rayer[8] described the characteristic renal hypertrophy that was rediscovered only in the 1970s, and German physicians identified renal involvement in diabetes; when glucosuria would disappear due to a severe decrease in renal function, patients would quite often have heavy proteinuria and be edematous[1].

Pathologists were also aware of the typical diabetic kidney, and Arman Epstein lesions were identified because of lack of treatment[9]. Understanding of the disease was completely changed by observations by Kimmelstiel and Wilson in 1936, who found glomerular lesions in eight patients, all of whom were probably type 2 diabetic patients[10]. Kimmelstiel and Wilson clearly understood that the disease was due to diabetes. However, for many years renal complications were still considered to be rare in type 2 diabetes, and the clinical course was not considered malignant ('benign diabetes')[11].

In the last few years, there has been a change in treatment strategy, partly because of the UK Prospective Diabetes Study (UKPDS) study, which clearly negated the concept that glycemic treatment, especially with sulfonylurea agents, but also with metformin and even insulin, could be deleterious[12–15]. The opposite is true. In the US, it has been a prevalent concept that especially sulfonylureas could be harmful to patients with diabetes, due to the effect on cardiac function. This debate seems not to be completely closed, as some doctors from the FDA still argue that certain oral agents could be harmful to diabetics.

EVALUATION OF DIABETIC RENAL DISEASE AND CLASSIFICATION

It is now widely accepted that patients with type 1 diabetes exhibit a very characteristic evolution of renal changes (Table 16.1). Initially, there may be hyperfiltration and renal hypertrophy, but there is a normal albumin excretion rate, unless patients are badly controlled with respect to glycemia. Blood pressure is normal.

By contrast, patients with type 2 diabetes quite often have hypertension related to abnormalities of the metabolic syndrome and obesity[16]. They may also exhibit signs of loss of renal autoregulation, resulting in a high blood pressure being inflicted on the glomeruli[17]. In type 1 diabetes, there are usually no symptoms or laboratory signs in the next stage. However, there is an increasing thickening of the basement membrane and expansion of the mesangium. Glomeruli filtration rate (GFR) is quite often high because of glycemic dysregulation[18]. The

same may be the case in patients with type 2 diabetes, but there may also be renal changes due to long-standing hypertension, and therefore it is not uncommon that many patients show signs of microalbuminuria early on.

The typical stage seen in type 1 diabetes with incipient nephropathy is microalbuminuria, generally found after 5–15 years of diabetes (Table 16.2). The renal excretion of albumin is clearly elevated, and patients with type 1 diabetes start to exhibit elevated blood pressure, however, this quite often remains in the 'normal' range of blood pressure.

In type 2 diabetes, arterial hypertension is very common, and when a patient with microalbuminuria is followed for many years s/he is at an increased risk of overt renal disease and, importantly, cardiovascular mortality[19–21]. This observation was made in Europe many years ago and it has now been confirmed in a number of subsequent studies. Persistent microalbuminuria is a clear omnious sign of both renal involvement and cardiovascular disease, and perhaps also an indicator for treatment, as discussed later in this chapter.

The next stage is proteinuria, diagnosed by old-fashioned methods. If biopsies are performed, clear changes are found in type 1 diabetes. GFR starts to fall, and correlates to the blood pressure and glycemia, the rate of fall is about 10 mL min^{-1} year^{-1} [21]. Proteinuria gradually increases, correlated again to glycemia and perhaps dyslipidemia. High blood pressure is common in type 1, and even more so in type 2 diabetes. Two large trials have shown that the decline in GFR in type 2 diabetes is quite rapid, as was also documented in other studies. Thus, patients with proteinuria and type 2 diabetes have a very poor prognosis, not only due to renal disease and lurking ESRD, but also due to the increase in risk of cardiovascular mortality, that may soon be better controlled by new agents which control the risk elements[21,22]: beta-blockers controlling dysrhythmia, diuretics controlling fluid overload, angiotensin converting enzyme (ACE)-inhibition controlling increased pressure in the kidney and cardiac abnormalities, e.g. angiotensin receptor blockers (Table 16.3).

There has been some discussion about the significance of non-diabetic renal disease in diabetic patients. In the author's experience this

Table 16.1 Characteristics in the development of renal dysfunction and nephropathy in type 2 diabetes

Stage 1 Clinical diagnosis without pre-diagnostic diabetes	Normal serum creatinine and somewhat elevated GFR (but not to the same extent as in type 1 diabetes). Blood pressure may be elevated since essential hypertension may be related to the metabolic syndrome, and type 2 diabetes
Stage 2 'Silent stage'	After the diagnosis and treatment of hyperglycemia, abnormal albuminuria is usually not found. GFR may decrease slightly with better glycemic control. Blood pressure has a tendency to increase
Stage 3a	Microalbuminuria may be found at the clinical diagnosis due to the fact that diabetes has been undiagnosed for years
Stage 3b	Microalbuminuria typically develops from normoalbuminuria after some years with diabetes related to blood pressure elevation and glycemic control. Hypertension is quite common in such patients. GFR is still normal. In some studies a tendency to decrease in GFR has been found with high normoalbuminuria
Stage 4 Overt diabetic nephropathy	Proteinuria typically after 10–15 years with diabetes GFR declines variably related to metabolic control and blood pressure. The risk factors; hyperglycemia and especially hypertension even borderline should be aggressively treated. Blood pressure may be reduced to values as low as possible. Cardiovascular disease is common. On biopsy these patients typically have lesions but a few percentages do not show any changes initially. Retinopathy is quite often found, but not obligatory
Stage 5	Late stage, just before or with renal insufficiency

Table 16.2 Albumin excretion in microalbuminuria

Range short term collections	20–200 μg min^{-1}
24 h urines	30–300 mg 24 h^{-1}
Albumin creatinine ratio (morning or spot urine)	Men: 2.5–25 mg mmol^{-1} creatinine Women: 3.5–35 mg mmol^{-1} creatinine

Table 16.3 Optimal blood pressure level in diabetic patients

Without nephropathy	< 135/85 mmHg
With nephropathy	< 130/80 mmHg
	< 125/75 mmHg

is quite rare, but selected studies in nephrology departments suggest that the problem may be more common, and it is now generally accepted that non-diabetic renal disease is much more common in diabetic patients than in the background population. It has taken many years to reach this view[23].

Understanding of diabetic renal disease has been distorted by the following hypotheses:

- It has been claimed that high blood pressure would be essential to maintain renal function—a prevailing concept in the USA for many years[24]
- It has also been alleged that hyperglycemia is not important in the genesis of diabetic renal disease—clearly an unsound and faulty statement
- It has also been claimed that genetic factors are decisive in determining renal disease—this has never been adequately substantiated[25].

The view that non-diabetic renal disease, like glomerulonephritis was important also disturbed the situation for some years[23,26].

It is now clear that normalizing or even 'subnormalizing' blood pressure is essential[27,28]. It is also clear that hyperglycemia is the main risk factor in the genesis of diabetic renal disease. Genetic factors have not been identified, and there is no reason to believe that they are decisive, although they may modulate the development. This is, however, not proven. The combined effects of high blood pressure and hyperglycemia are almost sufficient to explain the development of diabetic renal disease.

DIAGNOSTIC PROCEDURES

It is imperative to ensure the correct diagnosis of diabetic renal disease in patients with type 2 diabetes; fortunately, the procedures to do this are usually very simple. First it should be ensured that the patients actually have diabetes, based on the medical history, treatment, blood glucose measurements and glycosylated hemoglobin (HbA1c) levels. From this background, the diagnosis is usually certain. There may, of

course, be cases that are not so obvious, for example, where a patient who has diabetes but has become euglycemic by weight loss may still have renal lesions from diabetes. In this case, a biopsy may be needed, unless the medical history is known. In the presence of diabetes, it is often a good idea to examine the patient for other diabetic lesions, such as retinopathy. It is perhaps surprising, but retinopathy is not always found in type 2 diabetic patients with microalbuminuria, or even proteinuria[26].

Measurements of albuminuria are essential, and usually it is necessary to repeat the tests two or three times at intervals of some weeks or months[29,30]. An early morning urine test is usually used, and albumin creatinine ratio measured in this specimen; the test is very simple and reliable. If the test is positive, two more should be taken to be assure the degree of renal involvement. Steps should be taken to ensure that glycemic control is satisfactory, since there may be a fall in albuminuria levels with better glycemic control. There are several simple tests available for measuring albumin concentrations that are easy and reliable to use, such as nephelometry, radioimmuno assays, or dip-stick tests. All patients should be followed longitudinally in the outpatient clinic[31,32].

Some patients may already have signs of renal disease at the time of diagnosis, and possibly also of retinopathy[33]. This situation can arise as some patients may not have been aware of their diabetes, because symptoms can be mild, or even non-existent. Measurement or examination of urine sediment may be useful to differentiate from other renal diseases. It may be of value to perform renal sonography; usually in diabetes the kidney is of normal size, or larger than normal, at least in the absence of proteinuria. Regarding measurements of renal function it is usually sufficient to measure serum creatinine, although exact measurements of GFR may be warranted in some cases, e.g. determined as chromium–EDTA clearance, or creatinine clearance, but usually this is not needed in the clinical setting.

In rare situations renal biopsy may be indicated, particularly if the disease has developed very rapidly; in most cases, typical diabetic lesions are found[23]. In some situations the renal biopsy may not show specific diabetic abnormalities, which is not necessarily a sign of non-diabetic renal disease (minimal-change disease). Structural lesions could also be explained by hypertension[34,35]. Screening for urinary tract infection, which may be more common in diabetic patients due to cystopathy, is a very reasonable procedure. Quite often blood pressure is moderately elevated in these patients, so careful measurements of blood pressure is always warranted. This is sometimes related to sodium retention[36]. Careful clinical examination regarding edema is also important.

The conclusion is that in the daily life and follow-up of diabetic patients the diagnosis of diabetic renal disease is not difficult. Usually patients are followed longitudinally, and it is possible to observe the slow increase in albuminuria in these patients of 5–20% per year[37]. This increase is related to glycemic control and blood pressure; patients with high blood pressure and poor control often show a rapid rate of progression.

Measurements of serum lipid levels are also warranted, although this parameter is not decisive in determining treatment for these patients[38–41]. Some clinicians are more inclined to renal biopsies, but usually the treatment strategy is exactly the same and it is extremely rare that the treatment strategy is altered by the results of a biopsy. Steroid treatment may be needed in rare cases of nephrotic syndrome. Careful cardiovascular examination is also part of the general examination strategy because cardiovascular disease is so common in these patients, related to the microalbuminuria.

PREVENTION

It has been suggested that there may be a genetic background for the development of renal disease in type 2 diabetes[25], but this has not been clearly defined. There may be a higher risk in certain patients, and some patients may show a clustering of risk factors, but there are no genetic markers for hypertension, nor for adiposity. Risk factors/markers are indicated in Tables 16.4 and 16.5.

Table 16.4 Risk factors/markers for development of diabetic nephropathy in type 2 patients

	Type 2
Normoalbuminuria (above median)	+
Microalbuminuria	+
Sex	M > F
Familial clustering	+
Predisposition to arterial hypertension	+
Increased sodium/lithium counter transport	+/–
Ethnic conditions	+
Glycemic control	+
Prorenin	–
Smoking	?
Cholesterol	+
Presence of retinopathy	+
Protein intake	

+ = present; - = not present; ? = scanty, or no relevant information.

Table 16.5 Pathogenesis of diabetic nephropathy

Familial/genetic pathways
Metabolic pathways
    Glucose itself
    Non-enzymatic glycosylation
    Increased protein kinase C activity
    Abnormal polyol metabolism
    Biochemical abnormalities of extracellular matrix
Hemodynamic pathways
Cytokines and growth factors
Endothelial dysfunction

Both experimental and human studies (although intervention studies may not be so clear-cut) show that glucose toxicity is an important factor in the genesis of diabetic renal disease. This is perhaps not surprising[42], the mechanistic background for glucose toxicity is not completely clear but advanced glycation end-products may play an important role, along with the activation of the polyol pathway. Activation of protein kinase C and growth factors are of potential interest, but a detailed discussion of these pathogenetic factors is outside the scope of this chapter[26]. All studies show that the duration of diabetes is of importance but, as mentioned earlier, lesions may be present even at the clinical diagnosis of diabetes. The UKPDS study was important in this respect and, in particular, it verified the effectiveness of sulfonylurea agents, insulin and metformin. Combination therapy is quite often used and there is no reason to believe that any of these treatment strategies should be problematic. Unfortunately, the difference between the well-treated and the less-treated groups in the UKPDS was not dramatic; HbA1c levels 7.0 versus 7.9.

Besides optimal glycemic control, it is also clear that antihypertensive treatment is of top priority, as documented in the UKPDS, where both beta-blockers and ACE-inhibitors, together with other types of antihypertensive therapy, were effective in preventing albuminuria. The UKPDS showed that the lower the blood pressure, the better the outcome, and, therefore, the usual goals for antihypertensive treatment may be lower in diabetics; 140/90 in non-diabetics and 135/85 in diabetics. One should, however, be careful regarding patients who may be at risk for renal arteriostenosis. Careful follow-up in such patients is essential. Patients who are generally artherosclerotic should be followed even more carefully, particularly patients who are smokers[43].

TREATMENT STRATEGY

The first sign of diabetic renal disease in the clinical setting is the presence of microalbuminuria. The genesis of microalbuminuria is complex, being not only related to long-standing diabetes, but also to blood pressure elevation, which is also quite common in these patients. Loss of renal autoregulation may also be important, due to lesions in the vasculature of the kidney and the systemic blood pressure may therefore be transferred unhindered to glomeruli in these patients[17,44]. Optimal glycemic control is important in patients with microalbuminuria, just as during prevention of renal damage. However, antihypertensive treatment is a key feature in these patients, and blood pressure should probably be much lower in patients with microalbuminuria and overt renal disease, perhaps around 125/80. Several studies show that ACE-inhibitors or angiotensin-receptor blockers are effective in the treatment of these patients, but other agents may be used if the goal for antihypertensives is not reached[31,32,45–52].

According to the newly published candesartan and lisinopril microalbuminuria (CALM) study[53], it is possible to combine ACE-inhibitors with receptor blockers. Small doses of ACE-inhibitors are usually not sufficient, and monitoring of renal function by measuring serum creatinine and albuminuria is obviously imperative in these patients.

When inhibiting the renal angiotensin system is not adequate, diuretic treatment should be added, and is almost obligatory in patients with diabetes because of the tendency to sodium retention.

Beta-blockers also are useful, overriding hypoglycemic unawareness is extremely rare so the counter-indication for beta-blockers is not present in most patients. On the contrary, many patients need beta-blockers for cardiac protection against dysrhythmia and heart insufficiency. Combination therapy with calcium-channel blockers is also useful, but most physicians will not start treatment with these agents alone, and instead use them as supplementary therapy.

The goal in antihypertensive treatment is stable serum creatinine, a decline in albuminuria, and decline in blood pressure. There seems to be no lower limit for blood pressure, and if patients can manage a level of 120/75, this may be very useful in renal protection. So far there is no evidence of a 'J-shaped curve' in these patients.

There are few studies that have used low protein diets in diabetic patients. Studies so far

Table 16.6 RENAAL and IDNT trial comparison cohort baseline characteristics	
RENAAL	IDNT
Age: 60 ± 7.5 years	Age: 59 ± 8 years
sCr: 1.9 mg dL^{-1}	sCr: 1.7 mg dL^{-1}
BP: 152/82 ± 19/10 mmHg	BP: 156/85 ± 18/11 mmHg
HbA1c: 8.5 ± 1.6%	HbA1c: 8.1 ± 1.7%
UA/Cr 1867 ± 2701 mg g^{-1} (~ 3.9 g 24 h^{-1})	UPE: 4.2 ± 4.1 g 24 h^{-1}

performed are not positive in patients with type 2 diabetes[54,55]. A low protein diet may not be warranted, but rather it may be useful to use a low sodium diet, especially if the patient does not respond to ordinary therapy. In some cases, restriction of sodium may be useful in achieving the goal for antihypertensive treatment.

There is little evidence that treatment of dyslipidemia will protect renal function, and the few studies that do exist are somewhat conflicting. Obviously, treatment of hyperlipidemia is more important for the prevention of cardiac and vascular disease.

Cigarette smoking is also considered to be a risk factor, and patients should be given advice regarding smoking cessation[43]. Sodium restriction is important[36].

TREATMENT IN OVERT DIABETIC RENAL DISEASE

Treatment strategy is essentially the same throughout the course of diabetic renal disease, from incipient to overt[45]. Two studies, the Renaal and the Irbesartan (IDNT) studies, show that treatment with angiotensin-receptor blockers can postpone ESRD and help proteinuric patients with type 2 diabetes. Both studies showed that there is a considerable effect in these patients. However, prognosis unfortunately remains poor[56,57] (Tables 16.6, 16. 7 and 16.8).

The Renaal study[56] showed a significant effect on all pre-defined end-points considered together, namely ESRD, doubling of serum creatinine, and mortality. Mortality in itself was not significant, but mortality along with ESRD was

Table 16.7 RENAAL and IDNT trial comparison patient characteristics: race		
	RENAAL $n = 1513$	**IDNT** $n = 1715$
Race %		
Caucasian	49	73
Hispanic	18	5
Asian	17	4
Black	15	14
Other	1	4

positively effected by the treatment. This study may be a little more encouraging than the IDNT study[57] but, in principle, the two studies of similar design gave the same results. The IDNT study also included patients who were treated with a calcium-channel blocker. The angiotensive receptor blocker was more successful in preventing or postponing the course of renal disease. The Renaal study also showed a beneficial effect on hospitalization for cardiac insufficiency, which is indeed a noteworthy result.

Another study, the IRMA-II[58], showed a positive effect on patients with microalbuminuria regarding reduction in albuminuria, but not in preventing a fall in GFR. From a more theoretical point of view it may be more advantageous to treat the patient with microalbuminuria early on, perhaps even before the onset of microalbuminuria. There is evidence to suggest that renal disease in diabetes is a self-perpetuating

Table 16.8 RENAAL and IDNT trial results: comparison of primary endpoint and components

Composite and components	Losartan versus pbo RR%	Irbesartan versus pbo RR%	Irbesartan versus amlo RR%	Amlodipine versus pbo RR%
DsCr, ESRD, death	16 $p = 0.024$	20 $p = 0.024$	23 $p = 0.006$	−4 NS
Doubling of SCr	25 $p = 0.006$	33 $p = 0.003$	37 $p = 0.001$	−6 NS
ESRD	28 $p = 0.002$	23 NS	23 NS	0 NS
Death	NS	NS	NS	NS
ESRD or death	20 $p = 0.010$	?	?	?

RR = risk reduction; NS = not significant; pbo = placebo.

process, and with more advanced disease there may be less autoregulation and more transmission of systemic blood pressure to glomeruli[59].

It is clear that anti-lipidemic treatment could also be of importance to these patients although there is no clinical trial regarding renal endpoints. Obviously, cardiovascular disease is important and this may well be positively affected by a lipid-lowering agent, especially statins. Further studies are needed in this area.

ESRD AND TYPE 2 DIABETES

An increasing number of patients develop ESRD, and about 50% of patients in dialysis units in the USA suffer from diabetes, mainly type 2 diabetes. This is a dramatic development since the early 1970s when diabetic patients were rare, and very few were accepted. Those who were accepted had a poor prognosis—the prognosis is still poor, but is much better than previously[60].

SUMMARY

Hyperglycemia is an important contributor to complications, including nephropathy. In order to obtain the best possible glycemic control throughout the course of diabetes, it is important to diagnose renal disease early on by screening for microalbuminuria. Blood pressure elevation is also an important factor and normal-

izing blood pressure throughout the course of type 2 diabetes is, of course, essential.

Studies show that treatment with ACE-inhibitors can prevent the development of microalbuminuria. Many studies also show that microalbuminuria can be reduced by antihypertensive treatment, especially with ACE-inhibitors, but also with other agents. Usually agents that block the RAS are an essential part of the treatment process.

Effects on strong end-points in microalbuminuric patients are difficult to ascertain because of the long follow-up needed. However, the HOPE study suggested a positive effect in microalbuminuric diabetic patients on strong end-points. New studies using angiotensin-receptor blockers show a positive effect in patients with proteinuria and type 2 diabetes on the progression of renal disease. ACE-inhibitors seem to be important in preventing cardiovascular disease and mortality, and angiotensin-receptor blockers (ARBs) are important in preventing or postponing ESRD. There may thus be a theoretical case for using a combined blockade, or dual blockade of the renin–angiotensin system. There is also a good pathophysiological rationale for such a combination. Further studies are, however, needed.[61]

Patients with diabetic renal disease need effective antihypertensive treatment, as well as ACE-inhibition, with diuretic and beta-blocker treatment, as well as calcium blockers with prolonged action.

Dyslipidemia should be treated carefully, although there are no clinical studies that suggest whether the renal outcome is better with treatment with statins or other lipid-lowering agents. All general risk factors should be treated, and patients should be urged to quit smoking, lose weight, and have a low sodium diet. The role for protein reduction is less clear, and even weak in patients with other types of renal disease.

REFERENCES

1 Ritz E, Rychlik I, editors. *Nephropathy in type 2 diabetes*. Oxford Press: Oxford, 1999.

2 Ritz E, Stefanski A. Diabetic nephropathy in type 2 diabetes. *Am J Kidney Dis* 1996;27:167–94.

3 Biesenbach G, Janko O, Zazgornik J. Similar rate of progression in the predialysis phase in type 1 and type 2 diabetes mellitus. *Nephrol Dial Transplant* 1994;9:1097–102.

4 Ritz E, Orth SR. Nephropathy in patients with type 2 diabetes mellitus. *N Engl J Med* 1999;341: 1127–33.

5 Hasslacher C, Ritz E, Wahl P *et al*. Similar risks of nephropathy in patients with type 1 or type 2 diabetes mellitus. *Nephrol Dial Transplant* 1989;4:859–63.

6 Schmitz R. Über die prognostische Bedeutung und die Ätiologie der Albuminurie bei Diabetes. *Berlin Klin Wschr* 1891;28:373–7.

7 Fahr T. Über atypische Befunde aus den Kapiteln des Morbus Brightii nebst anhangsweisen Bemerkungen zur Hypertoniefrage. *Virchows Arch Path Anat* 1924;248:323.

8 Rayer P. *Traité des maladies des reins et des alterations de la sécrétion urinaire étudiées en elles-mêmes et dans leurs rapports avec les maladies des uretères de la vessie, de la prostate et de l'urètre*. Paris: Librairie de l'Académie Royale de Médecine, NB, 1839.

9 Ebstein W. Weiteres über Diabetes, insbesondere über die Complication desselben mit Typhus abdominalis. *Dtsch Arch Klin Med* 1882;30:1.

10 Kimmelstiel P, Wilson C. Intercapillary lesions in the glomeruli of the kidney. *Am J Pathol* 1936; 12:83–97.

11 Fabre J, Balant LP, Dayer PG *et al*. The kidney in maturity onset diabetes mellitus: a clinical study of 510 patients. *Kidney Int* 1982;27:167–94.

12 UK Prospective Diabetes Study Group. Intensive blood-glucose control with sulfonylureas or insulin compared with conventional treatment and risk of complications in type 2 diabetes (UKPDS33). *Lancet* 1998;352:837–53.

13 UK Prospective Diabetes Study Group. Tight blood pressure control and risk of macrovascular and microvascular complications in type 2 diabetes (UKPDS38). *Br Med J* 1998;317:703–12.

14 UK Prospective Diabetes Study Group. Efficacy of atenolol and captopril in reducing risk of macrovascular and microvascular complications in type 2 diabetes (UKPDS39). *Br Med J* 1998;317:713–20.

15 Gaster B, Hirsh IB. The effects of improved glycemic control on complications in NIDDM. *Arch Intern Med* 1998;158:134–40.

16 Gaede P, Vedel P, Parving HH *et al*. Intensified multifactorial intervention in patients with type 2 diabetes mellitus and microalbuminuria; the Steno type 2 randomized study. *Lancet* 1999;353: 617–22.

17 New JP, Marshall SM, Bilous RW. Renal autoregulation is normal in newly diagnosed normotensive NIDDM patients. *Diabetologia* 1998;41:206–11.

18 Vedel P, Obel J, Nielsen FS *et al*. Glomerular hyperfiltration in microalbuminuric NIDDM patients. *Diabetologia* 1996;39:1584–9.

19 Valmadrid CT, Klein R, Moss SE *et al*. The risk of cardiovascular disease mortality associated with microalbuminuria and gross proteinuria in persons with older-onset diabetes mellitus. *Arch Intern Med* 2000;160:1093–100.

20 Gall MA, Hougaard P, Borch-Johnsen K *et al*. Risk factors for the development of incipient and overt diabetic nephropathy in patients with non-insulin-dependent diabetes mellitus: prospective observational study. *Br Med J* 1997;314:783–8.

21 Mogensen CE. The kidney in diabetes: how to control renal and related cardiovascular complications. *Am J Kidney Dis* 2001;37:S2–S6.

22 Wang SL, Head J, Stevens L *et al*. Excess mortality and its relation to hypertension and proteinuria in diabetic patients. The WHO multinational study of vascular disease in diabetes. *Diabetes Care* 1996;19:305–12.

23 Olsen S, Mogensen CE. How often is NIDDM complicated with non-diabetic renal disease? An analysis of renal biopsies and the literature. *Diabetologia* 1996;39.1638–45.

24 Mogensen CE. Diabetic renal disease: the quest for normotension—and beyond. *Diabet Med* 1995;12:756–69.

25 Bain SC, Chowdhury TA. Genetics of diabetic nephropathy and microalbuminuria. *J R Soc Med* 2000;93:62–6.

26 Mogensen CE. Microalbuminuria, blood pressure and diabetic renal disease: origin and development of ideas. In: Mogensen CE, editor. *The kidney and hypertension in diabetes mellitus.* 5th edn. Boston, MA: Kluwer Academic Publishers, 2000: 655–706.

27 Weir MR. Diabetes and hypertension: how low should you go and with which drugs? *Am J Hypertens* 2001;14:17S–26S.

28 Adler AI, Stratton IM, Neil HAW *et al.* on behalf of the UK Prospective Diabetes Study Group. Association of systolic blood pressure with macrovascular and microvascular complications of type 2 diabetes (UKPDS 36): prospective observational study. *Br Med J* 2000;321:412–19.

29 Gerstein HC, Mann JFE Qilong Y. Albuminuria and risk of cardiovascular events, death, and heart failure in diabetic and non-diabetic individuals. *J Am Med Assoc* 2001;286:421–6.

30 Rachmani R, Levi Z, Lidar M *et al.* Considerations about the threshold value of microalbuminuria in patients with diabetes mellitus: lessons from an 8-year follow-up study of 599 patients. *Diabetes Res Clin Pract* 2000;49:187–94.

31 Ravid M, Lang R, Rachmani R *et al.* Long-term renoprotective effect of ACE inhibition in NIDDM: a 7-year follow-up study. *Arch Intern Med* 1996;156:286–9.

32 Ravid M, Brosh D, Levi Z *et al.* Use of enalapril to attenuate decline in renal function in normotensive, normoalbuminuric patients with type 2 diabetes mellitus. A randomized controlled trial. *Ann Intern Med* 1998;128:982–8.

33 Olivarius N de F, Andreasen AH, Keiding N, Mogensen CE. Epidemiology of renal involvement in newly-diagnosed middle-aged and elderly diabetic patients. Cross-sectional data from the population-based study "Diabetes Care in General Practice", Denmark. *Diabetologia* 1993;36:1007–16.

34 Ruggenenti P, Remuzzi G. Nephropathy of type 1 and type 2 diabetes: diverse pathophysiology, same treatment? *Nephrol Dial Transplant* 2000;15:1900–2.

35 Vestra MD, Saller A, Bortoloso E *et al.* Structural involvement in type 1 and type 2 diabetic nephropathy. *Diabetes Metab* 2000;26:8–14.

36 Dodson PM, Beevers M, Hallworth R. Sodium restriction and blood pressure in hypertensive type 2 diabetics: randomised blind controlled and crossover studies of moderate sodium restriction and sodium supplementation. *Br Med J* 1989;298:227–30.

37 Nielsen S, Schmitz A, Rehling M, Mogensen CE. The clinical course of renal function in NIDDM patients with normo- and microalbuminuria. *J Intern Med* 1997;241:133–41.

38 Lam KSL, Cheng IKP, Janus ED *et al.* Cholesterol lowering therapy may retard the progression of diabetic nephropathy. *Diabetologia* 1995;38:604–9.

39 Nielsen S, Schmitz O, Møller N *et al.* Renal function and insulin sensitivity during simvastatin treatment in type 2 (non-insulin-dependent) diabetic patients with microalbuminuria. *Diabetologia* 1993;36:1079–86.

40 Tonolo G, Ciccarese M, Brizzi P *et al.* Reduction of albumin excretion rate in normotensive microalbuminuric diabetic patients during long-term simvastatin treatment. *Diabetes Care* 1997;20:1891–5.

41 Hommel E, Andersen P, Gall MA *et al.* Plasma lipoproteins and renal function during simvastatin treatment in nephropathy. *Diabetologia* 1992;35:447–51.

42 Pirart J. Diabetes mellitus and its degenerative complications: a prospective study of 4,400 patients observed between 1947 and 1973. *Diabetes Care* 1978;1:168–88.

43 Orth SR, Ritz E, Schrier RW. The renal risks of smoking. *Kidney Int* 1997;51:1669–77.

44 Christensen PK, Hansen HP, Parving HH. Impaired autoregulation of GFR in hypertensive non-insulin dependent diabetic patients. *Kidney Int* 1997;52:1369–74.

45 Mogensen CE. Intervention strategies for microalbuminuria: The role of angiotensin II antagonists, including dual blockade with ACE-I and a receptor blocker. *J R AAS* 2000;1:63.

46 Cooper M, McNally PG, Boner G. Antihypertensive treatment in NIDDM, with special reference to abnormal albuminuria. In: Mogensen CE, editor. *The kidney and hypertension in diabetes mellitus.* 5th edn. Boston, MA: Kluwer Academic Publishers, 2000: 441–60.

47 De Pablos PL, Martin FJM. Effects of losartan and diltiazem on blood pressure, insulin sensitivity, lipid profile and microalbuminuria in hypertensive type 2 diabetic patients. *Clin Drug Invest* 1998;16:361–70.

48 Esmatjes E, Flores L, Inigo P *et al.* Effect of losar-

tan on TGF-β1 and urinary albumin excretion in patients with type 2 diabetes mellitus and microalbuminuria. *Nephrol Dial Transplant* 2001;16:90–3.

49 Lozano JV, Llisterri JL, Aznar J *et al.* Losartan reduces microalbuminuria in hypertensive microalbuminuric type 2 diabetics. *Nephrol Dial Transplant* 2001;16:85–9.

50 Lacourcière Y, Bélanger A, Godin C *et al.* Long-term comparison of losartan and enalapril on kidney function in hypertensive type 2 diabetics with early nephropathy. *Kidney Int* 2000;58:762–9.

51 Foggensteiner L, Mulroy S, Firth J. Managment of diabetic nephropathy. *J R Soc Med* 2001;94:210–17.

52 Mann JFE, Gerstein HC, Pogue J *et al.* for the HOPE investigators. Renal insufficiency as a predictor of cardiovascular outcomes and the impact of ramipril: the HOPE randomized trial. *Ann Intern Med* 2001;134:629–36.

53 Mogensen CE, Neldam S, Tikkannen I *et al.* for the CALM Study Group: randomised controlled trial of dual blockade of the renin-angiotensin system in hypertensive, microalbuminuric, non-insulin dependent diabetes: the candesartan and lisinopril microalbuminuria (CALM) study. *Br Med J*, 2000;321:1440–4.

54 Hermansen K. Diet, blood pressure and hypertension. *Br J Nutr* 2000;83:S113–119.

55 Pijls LTJ, de Vries H, Donker AJ *et al.* The effect of protein restriction on albuminuria in patients with type 2 diabetes mellitus: a randomised trial. *Nephrol Dial Tranpl* 1999;14:1445–53.

56 Brenner BM, Cooper ME, de Zeeuw D *et al.* for the Reduction of End-points in NIDDM with the Angiotensin II Antagonist Losartan (RENAAL) Study Investigators. Effects of losartan on renal and cardiovascular outcomes in patients with type 2 diabetes and nephropathy. *N Engl J Med* 2001;395:861–9.

57 Lewis EJ *et al.* IDNT. Irbesartan type II Diabetic Nephropathy Trial. *N Engl J Med* 2001;345:851–60.

58 Parving HH, Lehnert H, Bröchner-Mortensen J *et al.* The effect of Irbesartan on the development of diabetic nephropathy in patients with type 2 diabetes *N Engl J Med* 2001;345:870–8.

59 Parving HH, Hovind P, Rossing K, Andersen S. Evolving strategies for renoprotection: diabetic nephropy. *Nephrol Hypertens* 2001;10:515–22.

60 Bergrem H, Leivestad T. Diabetic nephropathy and end-stage renal failure: The Norwegian story. *Adv Ren Replace Ther* 2001;8:4–12.

61 Hilgers KF, Mann JF. ACE inhibitors versus AT(1) receptor antagonists in patients with chronic renal disease. *J Am Soc Nephrol* 2002;13:1100–8.

one of the most common causes for hospital admission and lower limb amputations among diabetic patients[8].

Neuropathic symptoms are present in 15–20% of diabetic patients, 7.5% of whom experience chronic neuropathic pain[9]. Pain associated with diabetic neuropathy exerts a substantial impact on the quality-of-life, particularly by causing considerable interference with sleep and enjoyment of life[10]. Despite this significant impact, a quarter of the diabetic patients and one-fifth of the non-diabetic subjects had no treatment for their pain in a survey dating from 1990[9]. Pain is a subjective symptom of major clinical importance as it is often this complaint that motivates patients to seek healthcare. People with diabetes experience more chronic pain than the non-diabetic population. It has been found that 25% of diabetic patients had chronic pain, compared with 15% of non-diabetic subjects[9]. This difference is largely attributable to pain associated with polyneuropathy.

CLINICAL MANIFESTATIONS

Distal symmetric polyneuropathy

The term 'hyperglycemic neuropathy' is used to describe sensory symptoms in poorly controlled diabetic patients that are rapidly reversible following institution of near-normoglycemia[3]. The most frequent form is DSP, commonly associated with autonomic involvement. Onset is insidious and, in the absence of intervention, the course is chronic and progressive. It seems that the longer axons to the lower limbs are more vulnerable to the nerve lesions induced by diabetes (length-related distribution). This notion is supported by the correlation found between the presence of DSP and height. It has also been suggested that DSP occurs primarily in the lower limbs because of the upright posture, with the microvessels being particularly vulnerable, because of impairment of the control mechanisms of vasoconstriction that would normally protect vessels from back pressure during standing[11].

DSP typically develops as a dying-back neuropathy, affecting the most distal extremities (toes) first. The neuropathic process then extends proximally up the limbs and later may also affect the anterior abdominal wall and then spread laterally around the trunk. Occasionally, the upper limbs are involved, with the fingertips being affected first (glove-and-stocking distribution). Variants, including painful small-fiber or pseudosyringomyelic syndromes and an atactic syndrome (diabetic pseudotabes), have been described. Small-fiber unmyelinated (C) and thinly myelinated (Aδ) fibers, as well as large-fiber myelinated (Aα, Aβ) neurons, are typically involved. However, it is as yet uncertain whether the various fiber damage develops following a regular sequence, with small fibers being affected first, followed by larger fibers, or whether the small-fiber or large-fiber involvement reflects either side of a continuous spectrum of fiber damage. However, there is evidence suggesting that small fiber neuropathy may occur early, often presenting with pain and hyperalgesia before sensory deficits or nerve conduction slowing can be detected[3]. The reduction or loss of small fiber-mediated sensation results in loss of pain sensation (heat pain, pinprick) and temperature perception to cold (Aδ) and warm (C) stimuli. Large fiber involvement leads to nerve conduction slowing, and reduction or loss of touch, pressure, two-point discrimination, and vibration sensation, which may lead to sensory ataxia (atactic gait) in severe cases. Sensory fiber involvement causes 'positive' symptoms, such as paresthesiae, dysesthesiae (hypersensitivity), and pain, as well as 'negative' symptoms, such as numbness.

Persistent or episodic pain that typically may worsen at night and improve during walking is localized predominantly in the feet. The pain is often described as a deep-seated aching, but there may be superimposed lancinating stabs, or it may have a burning thermal quality[12]. In a recent clinical survey of 105 patients with painful polyneuropathy, the following locations of pain were most frequent: 96% feet, 69% balls of feet, 67% toes, 54% dorsum of foot, 39% hands, 37% plantum of foot, 37% calves, and 32% heels. The pain was most often described by the patients as 'burning/hot', 'electric', 'sharp', 'achy', and 'tingling', was worse at night-time and when the patient was tired or stressed[10]. The average pain intensity was moderate, approximately 5.75/10 on a 0–10 scale, with the 'least' and 'most' pain being 3.6 and 6.9/10, respectively. Allodynia (pain due to a stimulus that does not normally cause pain, e.g. stroking) may occur. The symptoms may be accompanied by sensory loss, but patients with severe pain may have few clinical signs. Pain may persist over several years[13] causing considerable disability and impaired quality-of-life in some patients[10], whereas it remits partially or completely in others[14,15], despite further deterioration in small fiber function[15]. Pain remission tends to be associated with sudden metabolic change, short duration of pain or diabetes, preceding weight loss, and less severe sensory loss[14,15].

Compared with the sensory deficits, motor involvement is usually less prominent, and restricted to the distal lower limbs, resulting in muscle atrophy and weakness at the toes and foot. Ankle reflexes are frequently reduced or absent. At the foot level, the loss of the protective sensation (painless feet), motor dysfunction, and reduced sweat production due to autonomic involvement, result in a markedly increased risk of callus and foot ulcers. Thus, the neuropathic patient is a patient at high-risk of developing severe and potentially life-threatening foot complications, such as ulceration, osteoarthropathy (Charcot foot), and osteomyelitis, as well as medial arterial calcification and neuropathic edema.

DSP is the major contributory factor for diabetic foot ulcers, and the lower limb amputation rates in diabetic subjects are 15 times higher than in the non-diabetic population. Early detection of DSP by screening is therefore of paramount importance[8]. This is particularly important as many patients with DSP are asymptomatic, or have only mild symptoms. In view of the causation pathways, the majority of amputations should be potentially preventable if appropriate screening and preventative measures were adopted.

Acute painful neuropathy

Acute painful neuropathy has been described as a separate clinical entity[16]. It is encountered infrequently in both type 1 and type 2 diabetic patients, presenting with continuous burning pain particularly in the soles of the feet ('like walking on burning sand'), with nocturnal exacerbation. A characteristic feature is a cutaneous contact discomfort to clothes and sheet, which can be objectified as hypersensitivity to tactile (allodynia) and painful stimuli (hyperalgesia). Motor function is preserved, and sensory loss may be only slight, being greater for thermal than for vibration sensation. Onset is associated with and preceded by precipitous and severe weight loss. Depression and impotence are constant features. The weight loss has been shown to respond to adequate glycemic control, and the severe manifestations subsided within 10 months in all cases. No recurrences were observed after follow-up periods of up to 6 years[16]. The syndrome of acute painful neuropathy seems to be equivalent to 'diabetic cachexia' as described by Ellenberg[17]. It has also been described in girls with anorexia nervosa and diabetes in association with weight loss[18].

The term 'insulin neuritis' was used by Caravati[19] to describe a case with precipitation of acute painful neuropathy several weeks following the institution of insulin treatment. Sural nerve biopsy showed signs of chronic neuropathy with prominent regenerative activity[20], as well as epineurial arterio–venous shunting and a fine network of vessels, resembling the new vessels of the retina, which may lead to a steal effect rendering the endoneurium ischemic[21]. This may happen in analogy to the transient deterioration of a preexisting retinopathy following rapid improvement in glycemic control.

Focal and multifocal neuropathies

Most of the focal and multifocal neuropathies tend to occur in long-term diabetic patients of middle age or older. The outlook for most of them is recovery, either partial or complete, and eventual resolution of the pain that frequently accompanies the conditions. With this in mind, physicians should always maintain an optimistic outlook in dealing with patients with these afflictions[22].

Cranial neuropathy

Palsies of the third cranial nerve (diabetic ophthalmoplegia) are painful in about 50% of the cases[23]. Onset is usually abrupt. The pain is felt behind and above the eye, and at times precedes ptosis and diplopia (with sparing of pupillary function) by several days. Oculomotor findings reach their nadir within a day, or at most a few days, persist for several weeks, and then begin gradually to improve. Full resolution generally takes place within 3–5 months[22]. The fourth, sixth, and seventh cranial nerves are in order of frequency of affliction.

Mononeuropathy of the limbs

Focal lesions affecting the limb nerves, most commonly the ulnar, median, radial, and peroneal, may be painful, particularly if of acute onset, as may entrapment neuropathies, such as carpal tunnel syndrome, which is associated with painful paresthesias[12].

Diabetic truncal neuropathy

Mononeuropathy of the trunk (thoracoabdominal neuropathy or radiculopathy) presents with an abrupt onset; pain or dysesthesias are the heralding feature, sometimes accompanied by cutaneous sensory impairment or hyperesthesia. Pain has been described as deep, aching, or boring, but also the descriptors jabbing, burning, sensitive skin, or tearing have been used. The neuropathy is almost always unilateral, or predominantly so. As a result, the pain felt in the chest or abdomen may be confused with pain of pulmonary, cardiac, or gastrointestinal origin. Sometimes it may have a radicular or girdling quality, half encircling the trunk in a root-like distribution. Pain may be felt in one or several dermatomal distributions and, almost universally, it is worst at night. Rarely, abdominal muscle herniation may occur, predominantly in middle-aged men, involving 3–5 adjacent nerve roots between T6 and T12 (Reference 24). The time from first symptom to the peak of the pain syndrome is often just a few days, although occasionally the spread of pain to adjacent dermatomes may continue for weeks or even months. Weight loss of 15–40 pounds occurs in > 50% of cases. The course of truncal neuropathy is favorable, and pain subsides within months to a maximum of 1.5–2 years[22].

Diabetic amyotrophy

Asymmetric or symmetric proximal muscle weakness and muscle wasting (iliopsoas, obturator, and adductor muscles) are easily recognized clinically in the syndrome of lower limb proximal motor neuropathy (synonyms: Bruns–Garland syndrome, diabetic amyotrophy, proximal diabetic neuropathy, diabetic lumbosacral plexopathy, ischemic mononeuropathy multiplex, femoral–sciatic neuropathy, femoral neuropathy). Pain is nearly universal in this syndrome. Characteristically, it is deep, aching, constant, and severe, invariably worse at night, and may have a burning, raw quality. It is usually not frankly dysesthetic and cutaneous. Frequently, pain is first experienced in the lower back or buttock on the affected side, or may be felt as extending from hip to knee. Although severe and tenacious, the pain of proximal motor neuropathy has a good prognosis. Concurrent distal sensory polyneuropathy is frequently present. Weight loss is also a frequently associated feature and may be as much as 35–40 pounds. The weight is generally regained during the recovery phase[22].

Patients with proximal or multifocal diabetic neuropathy show marked ischemic nerve lesions with vasculitis and inflammatory infiltration of mononuclear cells[25,26] and T-cells of the CD8+ cell type[27]. Activated endoneurial lymphocytes express immunoreactive cytokines and major histocompatibility Class II antigens[27]. To classify these changes, Krendel[28] coined the term 'diabetic inflammatory vasculopathy', which he describes as a 'multifocal axonal neuropathy' caused by inflammatory vasculopathy, predominantly encountered in type 2 diabetic patients, indistinguishable from diabetic proximal neuropathy or mononeuritis multiplex. Separated from this form is the 'demyelinating neuropathy' without vascular inflammation, predominantly encountered in type 1 diabetic patients, indistinguishable from chronic inflammatory demyelinating polyneuropathy (CIDP)[29]. These findings suggest that immunological mechanisms may be implicated in the pathogenesis of these neuropathies.

Central nervous system dysfunction

Relatively little attention has been directed toward impairment of the central nervous system (CNS) in diabetic patients with DSP. Autopsy studies in diabetic patients have demonstrated diffuse degenerative lesions in the CNS, including demyelination and loss of axon cylinders in the posterior columns[30,31], degeneration of cortical neurons[32], and abnormalities in the midbrain and cerebellum[32,33], which have been described as 'diabetic myelopathy'[31] and 'diabetic encephalopathy'[32,34].

Studies that evaluated CNS function in diabetic patients using evoked potentials in response to stimulation of peripheral nerves, event-related potentials, and neuropsychological tests have yielded variable results as to the existence of spinal or supraspinal (central) conduction deficits, or cognitive dysfunction. However, we have shown that the degree of dysfunction along the somatosensory afferent pathways in type 1 diabetic patients depends on the stage of peripheral neuropathy, is not related to the duration of diabetes or glycemic control, and can be characterized by an alteration of the cortical sensory complex and peripheral rather than spinal or supraspinal conduction deficits[35]. We also demonstrated evidence of cognitive dysfunction with increasing degree of DSP in diabetic patients, using event-related potentials (P300 latency) and neuropsychological tests. The P300 latency, as an electrophysiological index of cognitive dysfunction, was normal in diabetic patients without DSP, but was significantly prolonged in those with Stage 1 (asymptomatic) and Stage 2 (symptomatic) DSP[36]. Dejgaard *et al.*[37] using magnetic resonance imaging (MRI), have found an increased frequency of subcortical and brainstem lesions in type 1 diabetic patients with peripheral neuropathy. Using positron emission tomography (PET) and [^{18}F]-2-deoxy-2-fluoro-D-glucose (FDG), we have shown reduced cerebral glucose metabolism in type 1 diabetic patients with DSP, as compared with newly diagnosed diabetic patients and healthy subjects[38].

Recently, Eaton *et al.*[39] found a smaller cross-sectional chord area at C4/5 and T3/4, as assessed by MRI, in patients with DSP compared with those without DSP and controls. Thus, there is accumulating evidence suggesting that neuropathic involvement at central and spinal levels is a feature of DSP. However, it is not clear whether these are primary or secondary events.

PATHOGENETIC MECHANISMS

Recent experimental studies suggest a multifactorial pathogenesis of diabetic neuropathy. Most data have been generated in the diabetic rat model. On the basis of this, two approaches have been chosen to contribute to the clarification of the pathogenesis of diabetic neuropathy. Firstly, attempts have been made to characterize the pathophysiological, pathobiochemical, and structural abnormalities that result in experimental diabetic neuropathy. Secondly, specific therapeutic interventions have been employed to prevent the development of these alterations, to halt their progression, or to induce their regression, despite concomitant hyperglycemia. At present, the following six pathogenetic mechanisms are being discussed, which, however, are no longer regarded as separate hypotheses but as a complex interplay, with multiple interactions between metabolic and vascular factors[40]:

- Increased flux through the polyol pathway, which leads to accumulation of sorbitol and fructose, *myo*-inositol depletion, and reduction in Na^+-K^+-ATPase activity.
- Disturbances in n-6 essential fatty acid and prostaglandin metabolism, which result in alterations of nerve membrane structure and microvascular and hemorrheologic abnormalities.
- Endoneurial microvascular deficits with subsequent ischemia and hypoxia, generation of reactive oxygen species (oxidative stress), activation of the redox-sensitive transcription factor NF-κB, and increased activity of protein kinase C (PKC).

- Deficits in neurotrophism leading to reduced expression and depletion of neurotrophic factors, such as nerve growth factor (NGF), neurotrophin-3 (NT-3), and insulin-like growth factor (IGF), and alterations in axonal transport.
- Accumulation of non-enzymatic advanced glycation end-products (AGEs) on nerve and/or vessel proteins.
- Immunological processes with autoantibodies to vagal nerve, sympathetic ganglia, and adrenal medulla, as well as inflammatory changes.

From the clinical point of view it is important to note that, based on these pathogenetic mechanisms, therapeutic approaches could be derived, some of which have been evaluated in randomized clinical trials (see treatment section below).

DIAGNOSIS

Due to the increasing recognition of diabetic neuropathy as a major contributor to morbidity and the recent burst of clinical trials in this field, together with the lack of agreement on the definition and diagnostic assessment of neuropathy, several consensus conferences were convened to overcome the current problems.

Diagnostic assessment

The Consensus Development Conference on Standardized Measures in Diabetic Neuropathy[41] recommended the following five measures to be employed in the diagnosis of diabetic neuropathy:

- Clinical measures
- Morphological and biochemical analyses
- Electrodiagnostic assessment
- Quantitative sensory testing
- Autonomic nervous system testing.

Clinical measures
Clinical measures include:

- General medical history and neurological history

- Neurological examination consisting of
  Sensory (pain, light touch, vibration, position)
  Motor [graded as normal = 0, weak = 1–4 (25–100%)]
  Reflex (present or absent)
  Autonomic examination[41] (simple bedside tests, including heart-rate variation during deep-breathing and postural blood-pressure response).

Both the severity of symptoms and the degree of neuropathic deficits should be assessed using scores such as the Neuropathy Symptom Score (NSS) and Neuropathy Disability or Impairment Score (NDS, NIS), which appear to be sufficiently reproducible[42]. For routine clinical and epidemiological purposes the simplified versions of the NSS and NDS for assessment of DSP suggested by Young *et al.*[43] can be used (Tables 17.2 and 17.3). Minimum criteria for diagnosis of neuropathy according to the NSS and NDS are:

- Moderate signs with or without symptoms
- Mild signs with moderate symptoms.

Clinical measures are used to:

- Establish the presence or absence of neurological dysfunction in diabetes
- Exclude nonneuropathic causes of neurological dysfunction
- Eliminate nondiabetic causes of neuropathy
- Distinguish and classify the different forms of diabetic neuropathy
- Monitor progression and provide a clinical correlate of outcome in trials.

The limitations to clinical measures include:

- Lack of sensitivity to change once they become abnormal.
- Limited reliability and reproducibility.
- Positive symptoms may reflect different pathophysiology rather than deficits, i.e. pain or paresthesiae may be related to the degree of compensatory regeneration, rather than to the degree of nerve fiber damage.

Table 17.2 Neuropathy symptom score (NSS)	
Burning, numbness or tingling	2
Fatigue, cramping or aching	1
Distribution:	
Feet	2
Calves	1
Elsewhere	0
Nocturnal exacerbation	2
Day and night	1
Daytime alone	0
Woken from sleep	1
Reduction by:	
Walking	2
Standing	1
Sitting or lying down	0

NSS score: 3–4 = mild symptoms; 5–6 = moderate symptoms; 7–9 = severe symptoms.
After MJ Young et al.[43].

Table 17.3 Neuropathy disability score (NDS)	
Ankle reflexes	
Vibration perception threshold	
Pin-prick sensation	
Temperature sensation (cold tuning fork)	
Reflexes:	
Normal = 0	
Present with reinforcement = 1	
Absent = 2 at each side	
Sensory modalities:	
Present = 0	
Reduced or absent = 1 at each side	

NDS score: 3–5 = mild signs; 6–8 = moderate signs; 9–10 = severe signs of neuropathy.
After MJ Young et al.[43].

Hence, it has been suggested that symptom or pain scores should not be used to evaluate overall presence or progression of diabetic neuropathy, but only to assess pain severity[41].

Morphological and biochemical measures
Sural nerve biopsy does not represent a routine method in the diagnosis of diabetic neuropathy. It may be used to:

- Study the role of various pathogenetic mechanisms
- Enhance understanding of the natural history of diabetic neuropathy
- Examine drug levels in nerve tissue and to assess the structural effects of treatment (controversial issue)
- Establish the diagnosis when the etiology of the neuropathy is in doubt.

The limitations to this technique are derived from the fact that the information from the biopsy is of no direct benefit to the patient, and that the procedure is associated with a certain morbidity and may result in complications[41].

Electrodiagnostic measures
Electrophysiological techniques have the advantage of being the most objective, sensitive, specific, and reproducible methods available in many neurophysiological laboratories worldwide.
   Electrodiagnostic measures also have limitations, they:

- Measure function only in the largest, fastest conducting myelinated fibers
- Have relatively low specificity for detecting diabetic neuropathy
- Show relatively high intra-individual variability for certain parameters (amplitudes)
- Are vulnerable to external factors, such as electrode locations or limb temperature
- Provide only indirect information about symptoms and deficits[41].

Quantitative sensory testing
Quantitative sensory testing (QST) is the "determination of the absolute sensory threshold, defined as the minimal energy reliably detected for a particular modality"[41]. The Peripheral

Only a few smaller studies have evaluated the effects of intensive diabetes therapy on established polyneuropathy in type 1 diabetic patients. They indicate that improved glycemic control may improve some parameters of diabetic neuropathy, but imperfect study designs and methodology hamper the validity of most of these small-sample-size trials. At more advanced stages, improvement is still possible for some nerve function parameters, such as motor nerve conduction velocity (MNCV), but less likely for autonomic dysfunction. This may be due to the fact that true normoglycemia could not be achieved in many patients. A large-sample randomized controlled trial, to specifically show favorable effects of intensive diabetes therapy on diabetic polyneuropathy, is not available. In type 1 patients with most advanced stages of peripheral neuropathy, the progression of nerve conduction deficits is halted after 3–4 years of normoglycemia following pancreatic transplantation, but no effect is seen in autonomic neuropathy. However, successful pancreas transplantation results in long-term normoglycemia. Hence, the effect on nerve function that can be achieved with this method cannot be extrapolated to the widely used current methods of intensive diabetes therapy. Using these methods the majority of diabetic patients do not achieve sustained normoglycemia for various reasons. Although observational studies suggest a glycemic threshold for the development and progression of the long-term complications in type 1 diabetes, the DCCT data do not support such an assumption. Thus, attempts to achieve optimal glycemic control should not aim at a certain glycosylated hemoglobin (HbA1c) threshold within the diabetic range, but follow the goal of achieving normal glycemia as early as possible in as many type 1 patients as is safely possible. In general, intensive diabetes therapy is associated with a moderately increased risk of weight gain and hypoglycemia.

Treatment based on pathogenetic concepts

Aldose reductase inhibitors

An increased flux through the polyol pathway, resulting in multiple biochemical abnormalities in the diabetic nerve, is thought to play a major role in the pathogenesis of diabetic neuropathy. Aldose reductase inhibitors (ARI) block the increased activity of aldose reductase, the rate-limiting enzyme that converts glucose to sorbitol (Table 17.5). The first trials of ARI in diabetic neuropathy were published 20 years ago. The various compounds that have been evaluated are alrestatin, sorbinil, ponalrestat, tolrestat, epalrestat, zopolrestat, zenarestat, and fidarestat. Except for epalrestat, which is marketed in Japan, none of these agents could be permanently licensed due to serious adverse events (sorbinil, tolrestat, zenarestat) or lack of efficacy (ponalrestat, zopolrestat). A meta-analysis of 13 clinical trials with ARI revealed a marginal effect on peroneal motor NCV of 1.24 m s^{-1} and an even weaker effect on median motor NCV of 0.69 m s^{-1} after 1 year[47]. Data from 738 subjects for three trials of tolrestat showed a benefit equal to 1 m s^{-1} in a pooled analysis of NCV in all the nerves studied.

The following degrees of changes in motor and sensory NCV that are associated with a change in the NIS of two points have been considered to be clinically meaningful in controlled clinical trials:

- Median motor NCV 2.5 m s^{-1}
- Ulnar MNCV: 4.6 m s^{-1}
- Peroneal MNCV: 2.2 m s^{-1}
- Median SNCV: 1.9 m s^{-1}
- Sural SNCV: 5.6 m s^{-1} (Reference 48).

According to this standard, the changes in NCV obtained from the ARI trials so far do not appear to reflect a meaningful magnitude of treatment effect. In a recent 1-year Phase II trial of zenarestat in 208 patients with diabetic polyneuropathy, a dose-dependent improvement in small myelinated fiber loss and peroneal NCV was observed. However, subsequent large Phase III trials of zenarestat had to be prematurely terminated due to a significant deterioration in renal function in some patients. A recent 52-week controlled multicenter trial of fidarestat (1 mg day^{-1}), in 279 patients with diabetic polyneuropathy, showed an improvement in F-wave conduction velocity and reduction in neuropathic

Table 17.5 Treatment of diabetic neuropathy based on the putative pathogenetic mechanisms

Abnormality	Compound	Aim of treatment	Status of RCTs
Polyol pathway ↑	Aldose reductase inhibitors	Nerve sorbitol ↓	
	Sorbinil		Withdrawn (AE)
	Tolrestat		Withdrawn (AE)
	Ponalrestat		Ineffective
	Zopolrestat		Withdrawn (marginal effects)
	Zenarestat		Withdrawn (AE)
	Epalrestat		Marketed in Japan
	Fidarestat		Studies ongoing
myo-inositol ↑	*Myo*-inositol	Nerve *myo*-inositol ↑	Equivocal
GLA synthesis ↓	γ-linolenic acid (GLA)	EFA metabolism ↑	Withdrawn (effective: deficits)
Oxidative stress ↑	α-lipoic acid	Oxygen free radicals ↓	Effective in RCTs (studies ongoing)
	Vitamin E	Oxygen free radicals ↓	Effective in 1 RCT
Nerve hypoxia ↑	Vasodilators	NBF ↑	
	ACE inhibitors		Effective in 1 RCT
	Prostaglandin analogs		Effective in 1 RCT
	VEGF	Angiogenesis ↑	Studies ongoing
Protein kinase C ↑	PKC β inhibitor	NBF ↑	RCTs ongoing
C-peptide ↓	C-peptide	NBF ↑	Studies ongoing
Neurotrophism ↓	NGF	Nerve regeneration, growth ↑	Ineffective
LCFA metabolism ↓	Acetyl-L-carnitine	LCFA accumulation ↓	Ineffective
NEG ↑	Aminoguanidine	AGE accumulation ↓	Withdrawn

NEG = non-enzymatic glycation; AGE = advanced glycation end products; EFA = essential fatty acids; LCFA = long-chain fatty acids; AE = adverse events;
NBF = nerve blood flow; RCTs = randomized clinical trials.

Nerve growth factor

Nerve growth factor (NGF) selectively promotes the survival, differentiation, and maintenance of small fiber sensory and sympathetic neurons in the peripheral nervous system (Table 17.5). It is expressed in the skin and other target tissues of its responsive neuronal populations, binds to its high-affinity receptor (trk A) on nerve terminals, and exerts its trophic effects after being retrogradely transported back to the neuronal perikaryon. A 6-month Phase II trial, including 250 patients with symptomatic diabetic neuropathy, showed an improvement of the sensory component of the neurologic examination, and both cooling detection and heat as pain threshold, but no effect on neuropathic symptoms could be observed following treatment with recombinant human NGF. In contrast, a subsequent large 12-month Phase III trial failed to demonstrate a favorable effect of rhNGF on subjective and objective variables of diabetic neuropathy[53]. The reasons for the latter disappointing result could be:

- The DSP did not progress during the trial in the placebo group
- The dose chosen may have been below the threshold to produce an effect
- The most distal testing site (big toe) was selected for assessment, where the most advanced neuropathic changes are expected, which are less susceptible to intervention than more proximal sites
- The primary outcome measure (neuropathy impairment score at the lower limbs (NIS-LL) is not sensitive to small fiber sensory dysfunction
- The drug did not get to the target tissue
- The manufactoring process for NGF has been altered after the Phase II trial prior to the Phase III trial, giving rise to the possibility that the drug was not identical[53].

Protein kinase C beta inhibitors

Increased activity of protein kinase C (PKC), a family of serine-threonine kinases that regulate various vascular functions—including contractility, hemodynamics, and cellular proliferation—has been implicated in the pathogenesis of diabetic complications, including neuropathy (Table 17.5). Treatment with a PKC-beta-selective inhibitor ameliorated several neuropathic deficits in experimental diabetic neuropathy. Clinical trials using this agent are currently underway.

C-peptide

Recent studies suggest that C-peptide shows specific binding to cell-membrane binding sites and augments skin microcirculation in type 1 diabetic patients, possibly via an increase in both nitric oxide production and Na^+/K^+-ATPase activity. In experimental diabetic neuropathy, C-peptide administration prevented NCV deficit, axonal atrophy, and paranodal swelling and demyelination, it produced an increase in Na^+/K^+-ATPase activity and phosphorylation of the insulin receptor (Table 17.5). A pilot study showed an improvement in small fiber sensory and autonomic function in type 1 diabetic patients[54]. Phase II and Phase III trials with diabetic neuropathy patients are needed to confirm these preliminary data.

Vascular endothelial growth factor

Based on the experimental concept of endoneurial microvacular abnormalities and reduced nerve blood flow resulting in ischemia and hypoxia, it has recently been hypothesized that destruction of the vasa nervorum can be reversed by administration of vascular endothelial growth factor (VEGF), an endothelial cell mitogen that promotes angiogenesis in several animal models and in humans (Table 17.5). Intramuscular gene transfer of plasmid DNA encoding VEGF-1 or VEGF-2 reversed experimental neuropathy after 4 weeks in diabetic rats[55]. Preliminary data in patients with chronic ischemic neuropathy and critical limb ischemia indicate neurologic improvement in four out of six diabetic patients after 6 months following intramuscular *phVEGF165* gene transfer[56]. However, caution has been expressed regarding possible adverse effects of VEGF, such as retinal neovascularization and increased retinal vascular permeability, induction of peripheral edema, activation of the PKC pathway, and possible mitogenic effects in tumor development. Thus, if

VEGF is evaluated in larger scale clinical trials, a close monitoring of these and other possible consequences will be mandatory.

Symptomatic treatment of painful neuropathy

Painful symptoms in diabetic polyneuropathy may constitute a considerable management problem. The efficacy of a single therapeutic agent is not established, and simple analgesics are usually inadequate to control the pain. Various therapeutic schemes have therefore been proposed, but none has been validated. Nonetheless, there is agreement that patients should be offered the available therapies in a stepwise fashion. Effective pain treatment considers a favorable balance between pain relief and side effects, without implying a maximum effect.

A rational treatment algorithm, including various causal and symptomatic options is summarized in Table 17.7. Prior to any decision regarding appropriate treatment, the diagnosis of the underlying neuropathic manifestation should be established to allow the estimation of its natural history. In contrast to agents that have been derived from the pathogenetic mechanisms of diabetic neuropathy, those used for symptomatic therapy were designed to modulate pain, without favorably influencing the underlying neuropathy. A number of trials have been conducted to evaluate the efficacy and safety of these drugs, but few of them included large patient samples.

The relative benefit of an active treatment over a control in clinical trials is usually expressed as the relative risk, the relative risk reduction, or the odds ratio. However, to estimate the extent of a therapeutic effect (i.e. pain relief) that can be translated into clinical practice, it is useful to apply a simple measure, which allows the physician to select the appropriate treatment for the individual patient. Such a practical measure is the 'number needed to treat' (NNT), i.e. the number of patients that need to be treated with a particular therapy to observe a clinically relevant effect or adverse event in one patient. This measure is expressed as the reciprocal of the

absolute risk reduction, i.e. the difference between the proportion of events in the control group (Pc) and the proportion of events in the intervention group (Pi): $NNT = 1/(Pc–Pi)$. The 95% confidence interval (CI) of NNT can be obtained from the reciprocal value of the 95% CI for the absolute risk reduction. The NNT and NNH (number needed to harm) for the individual agents used in the treatment of painful diabetic neuropathy are given in Table 17.7.

Tricyclic antidepressants

Psychotropic agents, among which antidepressants have been evaluated most extensively, have constituted an important component in the treatment of chronic pain syndromes for more than 30 years. Several authors consider the tricyclic antidepressants (TCA) to be the drug treatment of choice for neuropathic pain. Putative mechanisms of pain relief by antidepressants include the inhibition of norepinephrine and/or serotonin reuptake at synapses of central descending pain control systems, and the antagonism of N-methyl-D-aspartate receptor, which mediates hyperalgesia and allodynia. Imipramine, amitriptyline, and clomipramine induce a balanced reuptake inhibition of both norepinephrine and serotonin, while desipramine is a relatively selective norepinephrine inhibitor. The NNT (CI) for a $\geq 50\%$ pain relief by TCA is 2.4 (2.0–3.0)[57]. The NNH is 2.8 for minor adverse events, and 19 for major adverse events (Table 17.7). Thus, among 100 diabetic patients with neuropathic pain who are treated with antidepressants, 30 will experience pain relief by $\geq 50\%$, 30 will have mild adverse events, and five will discontinue treatment due to severe adverse events. The mean NNT for drugs with balanced reuptake inhibition is 2.2, and 3.6 for the noradrenergic agents[57].

The most frequent adverse events of TCA include tiredness and dry mouth. The starting dose should be 25 mg (10 mg in frail patients) taken as a single night-time dose 1 h before sleep. It should be increased by 25 mg at weekly intervals, until pain relief is achieved or adverse events occur. The maximum dose is usually 150 mg per day. Amitriptyline is frequently the drug of first choice, but alternatively

Table 17.7 Treatment options for painful diabetic neuropathy

Approach	Compound/measure	Dose per day	Remarks	NNT	Author
Optimal diabetes control	Diet, OAD, insulin	Individual adaptation	Aim: HbA1c ≤ 6.5%	–	
Pathogenetically oriented treatment	α-lipoic acid (thioctic acid)[a]	600 mg i.v. infusion	Duration: 3 weeks	4.0[b]	Ziegler
Symptomatic treatment	*Tricyclic antidepressants (TCA)*	1200–1800 mg orally	AE rare		
	Amitriptyline	(10-)25–150 mg	NNMH: 15	3.0/2.0	Max
	Desipramine	(10-)25–150 mg	NNMH: 24	2.2/5.0	Max
	Imipramine	(10-)25–150 mg	CRR	1.4/1.7/3.0	Sindrup
	Clomipramine	(10-)25–150 mg	NNMH: 8.7	2.1	Sindrup
	Nortriptyline	(10-)25–150 mg	plus Fluphenazine	1.6[c]	Gomez-Perez
	SSRI				
	Citalopram	40 mg	Small sample	7.7	Sindrup
	Paroxetine	40 mg	CRR	2.9	Sindrup
	Other antidepressants				
	Venlafaxine	150–220 mg	Abstract	4.5	Kunz
	NMDA antagonists				
	Memantine	40 mg	Abstract	6.7	Pellegrino
	Ion channel blockers				
	Carbamazepine	200–800 mg	NNMH: 15	3.3	Rull
	Gabapentin	900–3600 mg	Less AE	3.7	Backonja
	Lamotrigine	200–400 mg	Less AE	4.0	
	Mexiletine	675 mg	Modest effect	10.3	Oskarsson
	Weak opioids				
	Tramadol	50–400 mg	NNMH: 7.8	3.1	Harati
	Local treatment				
	Capsaicin (0.075%) cream	q.i.d. topically	Max. duration: 8 weeks	4.2[d]	Meta-analysis
Ultima ratio in pain resistant to standard pharmacotherapy	*Strong opioids* Electrical spinal cord stimulation (ESCS)	Individual adaptation	Potential of dependence Invasive, complications		Tesfaye
Physical therapy	TENS, medical gymnastics, Balneotherapy, relaxation therapy		No AE No AE		Kumar
Acupuncture			Uncontrolled study		Abuaisha

[a] Available in only some countries.
[b] ≥ 30% symptom relief.
[c] Combined with fluphenazine.
[d] Analgesic effectiveness as ascertained by the physician; OAD = oral antidiabetic drugs; CRR = concentration–response relationship; AE = adverse events.

desipramine may be chosen, for its less pronounced sedative and anticholinergic effects. The effect is comparable in patients with and without depression, and is independent of a concomitant improvement in mood. The onset of efficacy is more rapid (within 2 weeks) than in the treatment of depression. The median dose for amitriptyline is 75 mg per day, and there is a clear dose–response relationship. In two studies of imipramine, the dose was adjusted to obtain the optimal plasma concentration of 400–500 nmol L^{-1}, to ensure maximum effect. The target concentration could be attained in 57% of patients[57].

Whether combined treatment with antidepressants and phenothiazines offers any advantage is not known. Nortriptyline has been evaluated in combination with fluphenazine, compared with placebo and carbamazepine. This combination resulted in significant pain relief, with a NNT of 1.6 against placebo, and both pain reduction and rates of adverse events similar to carbamazepine.

The notion that the character of the neuropathic pain is predictive of response, so that burning pain should be treated with antidepressants and shooting pain with anticonvulsants, is unfounded, since both pain qualities respond to TCA. Most evidence of efficacy of antidepressants comes from studies that have been conducted over only several weeks. However, many patients continue to achieve pain relief for months to years, although this is not true for all patients. Tricyclic antidepressants should be used with caution in patients with orthostatic hypotension, and are contraindicated in patients with unstable angina, recent (< 6 months) myocardial infarction, heart failure, history of ventricular arrhythmias, significant conduction system disease, and long QT syndrome.

Selective serotonin reuptake inhibitors

The relatively high rates of adverse effects and contraindications of TCA, has led to the question of whether patients who do not tolerate them due to adverse events could alternatively be treated with selective serotonin reuptake inhibitors (SSRI). SSRI specifically inhibit presynaptic reuptake of serotonin, but not norepinephrine and,

unlike the tricyclics, they lack postsynaptic receptor blocking effects and quinidine-like membrane stabilization. Three studies showed that treatment with paroxetine and citalopram, but not fluoxetine, resulted in significant pain reduction. Paroxetine appeared to influence both steady and lancinating pain qualities[57]. The therapeutic effect was observed within 1 week and was dependent on plasma levels, being maximal at concentrations of 300–400 nmol L^{-1}. As well as the relatively low rates of adverse events, the advantage of SSRI compared with the tricyclic compounds is the markedly lower risk of mortality due to overdose. However, a recent case-control study suggested that SSRI moderately increased the risk of upper gastrointestinal bleeding to a degree about equivalent to low-dose ibuprofen. The concurrent use of non-steroidal anti-inflammatory drugs or aspirin greatly increases this risk.

Venlafaxine

Venlafaxine is an antidepressant that inhibits the reuptake of serotonin, norepinephrine, and, weakly, dopamine, but unlike the TCA, it does not block the muscarinic, histaminergic, and adrenergic receptors. It has been suggested that drugs with a balanced inhibition of serotonin and norepinephrine, but without the postsynaptic and quinidine-like effects of TCA, could exert similar effects but be better tolerated[58]. In a 6-week trial including 244 patients, the analgesic response rates were 56%, 39%, and 34% in patients given 150–225 mg venlafaxin, 75 mg venlafaxin, and placebo, respectively. Patients with depression were excluded from the trial, the effect of venlafaxin (150–225 mg) was therefore attributed to an analgesic, rather than antidepressant, effect. The most common adverse effect was nausea[59].

Anticonvulsants

Carbamazepine   The successful treatment of trigeminal neuralgia with carbamazepine resulted in a more extensive use of this anticonvulsant in painful neuropathies. There have been three controlled clinical trials of carbamazepine (1–3 × 200 mg per day orally) in 30–40 patients that showed superiority over placebo treatment. In one study the NNT was 3.3 for pain reduction, and NNH was 1.9 for mild (somnolence, dizziness) and 15 for severe (allergic skin reactions) adverse events (Table 17.7). These relatively high rates of adverse events and the relative paucity of clinical trials somewhat limit the value of this remedy, so that it should find its place after the aforementioned drugs have been found to be unsuccessful (Table 17.7). Whether patients with certain pain qualities (shooting or stabbing pain) respond preferentially is not known. A recent, small, 4-week controlled study revealed no differences in pain relief between carbamazepine and a combination of nortriptyline–fluphenazine. The pain relief of carbamazepine is mediated presumably by stabilizing neuronal membranes through an effect on sodium conductance.

Gabapentin Gabapentin is an anticonvulsant structurally related to gamma-aminobutyric acid (GABA), a neurotransmitter that plays a role in pain transmission and modulation. The exact mechanisms of action of this drug in neuropathic pain have not been fully elucidated but, among others, involve interaction with L-amino acid transport and high-affinity binding to the alpha-2-delta subunit of voltage-activated calcium channels. The antihyperalgesic properties of gabapentin are, at least partially, modulated through spinal cord mechanisms. In an 8-week multicenter dose-escalation trial including 165 diabetic patients with painful neuropathy, 60% of the patients on gabapentin (3600 mg day^{-1} achieved in 67%) had at least moderate pain relief compared to 33% on placebo. Furthermore, gabapentin treatment was associated with improvement in quality-of-life. Dizziness and somnolence were the most frequent adverse events in about 23% of the patients each[60]. Gabapentin has been suggested to be the preferred drug for patients in whom TCA are contraindicated or who do not tolerate their adverse effects.

Lamotrigine A recent Phase II trial randomly assigned 59 patients to receive either lamotrigine (titrated from 25 to 400 mg day^{-1}) or placebo over a 6-week period. Primary outcome measure was self-recording of pain intensity twice daily, using a 0–10 numerical pain scale (NPS). Secondary efficacy measures included daily consumption of rescue analgesics, the McGill Pain Questionnaire (MPQ), the Beck Depression Inventory (BDI), the Pain Disability Index (PDI), and global assessment of efficacy and tolerability. Daily NPS in the lamotrigine-treated group was significantly reduced ($p < 0.001$ for lamotrigine doses of 200, 300, and 400 mg). The results of the MPQ, PDI, and BDI remained unchanged in both groups. The global assessment of efficacy favored lamotrigine treatment over placebo, and the adverse events profile was similar in both groups[61]. These findings should be confirmed in a large Phase III trial.

Antiarrhythmic agents

Mexiletine Mexiletine, a Class Ib antiarrhythmic agent, has been shown to be effective in a small 10-week study of 16 patients, using an increasing dose from 150 mg day^{-1} to 10 mg kg^{-1} body weight day^{-1} orally. However, another study over 3 weeks could not confirm this effect. In a 5-week multicenter trial, using 75–225 mg three times a day orally, no beneficial influence on the total pain-rating index could be demonstrated, but retrospective analysis indicated a favorable effect on burning and stabbing pain. An oral dose of 150 mg three times a day, which is well below that required for antiarrhythmic therapy (600–800 mg per day), was sufficient for this effect, and did not produce any adverse events or ECG abnormalities. In contrast, in a second multicenter trial for 3 weeks a dose of 675 mg day^{-1} was required to achieve a significant reduction in sleep disturbances and pain at night. This effect had a relatively rapid onset, within 1 week. A recent review of seven controlled trials of mexiletine in painful diabetic neuropathy concluded that the drug produces a modest analgesic effect[62]. Thus, short-term treatment with mexiletine should at best be reserved for a few patients with burning or stabbing pain during night-time, which is unresponsive to a multitude of drugs, such as antidepressants, anticonvulsants, or tramadol (see below); regular ECG monitoring is mandatory.

Lidocaine

In a controlled study of 15 diabetic patients with chronic painful neuropathy, a single intravenous infusion of lidocaine (5 mg kg^{-1} body weight over 30 min during continuous ECG monitoring) resulted in significant pain relief after 1 and 8 days. The individual effect was sustained for 3–21 days. The NNT for a pain reduction of > 30% after 3 days was 2.2. Since lidocaine resulted in an increase in the threshold for the nociceptive flexion reflex (M. biceps femoris) in diabetic patients with painful neuropathy, it is conceivable that this compound mediates its pain-relieving effect via spinal or supraspinal mechanisms. Thermal and pain thresholds are not influenced. The onset of the analgesic effect during the intravenous infusion (500 mg in 60 min) is abrupt over a narrow dosage and concentration range. It has recently been suggested that additional clinical trials are needed to obtain a rational, rather than empirical basis for this treatment option[63].

Phenytoin (diphenylhydantoin)
In the past, phenytoin (3 × 100 mg per day orally) has been frequently advocated on the basis of an open study. However, controlled trials have yielded controversial results. Due to the equivocal data for this compound, it should not be used for treatment of painful diabetic neuropathy.

Transdermal clonidine
A controlled 6-week study using a transdermal clonidine patch (dose titration from 0.1 to 0.3 mg per day) in 24 diabetic patients has shown a non-significant trend towards pain relief. The NNT for a moderate or marked pain reduction was 5.3, while the NNH for adverse events was relatively low, being 3.4 for dry mouth and drowsiness, respectively. In a 3-week trial in 41 patients no significant difference between clonidine and placebo regarding pain relief could be observed[64]. However, 12 responder were identified, who experienced a moderate to complete pain relief on clonidine compared with placebo patch. These patients were included in a second study using an 'enriched enrollment' design (in which only patients who had been screened as responders are entered). In this study a significant 20% pain reduction compared with placebo was noted. The NNH for adverse events (dry mouth, sedation, orthostatic symptoms) was 2.0

in the responders. On the basis of these data, transdermal clonidine cannot be generally recommended. The potential mechanisms for the analgesic effect of clonidine include actions at alpha$_2$-adrenergic or imidazoline receptors, to cause post-synaptic inhibition of spinal cord neurons, pre-synaptic inhibition of nociceptive afferents, facilitation of brain-stem pain-modulating systems, or peripheral or central suppression of sympathetic transmitter release.

Tramadol
Tramadol acts directly, via opioid receptors, and indirectly, via monoaminergic receptor systems. Development of tolerance and dependence during long-term tramadol treatment is uncommon and its abuse liability appears to be low, it is therefore an alternative to strong opioids in neuropathic pain. In painful diabetic neuropathy, tramadol (up to 400 mg per day orally, mean dose: 210 mg per day orally) has been studied in a 6-week multicenter trial including 131 patients[65]. Pain relief was 44% on tramadol versus 12% on placebo. The most frequent adverse events were nausea and constipation. The NNH of 7.8 for drop-outs due to adverse events was relatively low, indicating significant toxicity. In a 4-week study including patients with painful neuropathy of different origins, one-third of which were diabetes, tramadol significantly relieved pain [NNT: 4.3 (2.4–20)] and mechanical allodynia. One possible mechanism for the favorable effect of tramadol could be a hyperpolarization of postsynaptic neurons via postsynaptic opioid receptors. Alternatively, the reduction in central hyperexcitability by tramadol could be due to a monoaminergic or a combined opioid and monoaminergic effect. Trials to assess equivalence (e.g. versus antidepressants) should clarify the relative potency and toxicity of tramadol in painful neuropathy.

N-methyl-D-aspartate receptor antagonists
Dextromethorphan Inhibition of *N*-methyl-D-aspartate (NMDA) receptor-mediated CNS excitation alleviates neuropathic pain in animal models, but adverse effects of dissociative anesthetic channel blockers, such as ketamine, limit clinical application. It has been hypothesized

that relatively high doses of low-affinity, non-competitive channel-blocking NMDA receptor antagonists, such as dextromethorphan, may have a more favorable therapeutic ratio than dissociative anesthetic-like blockers[66]. In a 6-week study, seven out of 13 patients reported moderate or greater relief of pain during dextromethorphan treatment (mean dose: 381 mg day[-1]) compared with none with placebo, giving a NNT of 1.9 (CI: 1.1–3.7). However, five of 31 patients who took dextromethorphan dropped out due to sedation or ataxia during dose escalation[67].

Memantine In an 8-week multicenter study including 375 patients, the analgesic response rates defined as ≥ 50% pain relief were 44% in patients given 40 mg of the NMDA receptor blocker memantine, compared with 29% in those given placebo (NNT: 6.7). There was no difference between patients treated with 20 mg of memantine and placebo. Most frequent adverse effects were diarrhoea in 11% and dizziness in 26% of the patients treated with 40 mg memantine[68]. The NNT for this agent is comparable with that obtained for SSRI.

Topical capsaicin

Capsaicin (trans-8-methyl-N-vanillyl-6-nonenamide) is an alkaloid and the most pungent ingredient in red pepper. It depletes tissues of substance P, and reduces neurogenic plasma extravasation, the flare response, and chemically-induced pain. Substance P is present in afferent neurones innervating skin, mainly in polymodal nociceptors, and is considered the primary neurotransmitter of painful stimuli from the periphery to the CNS. Several studies have demonstrated significant pain reduction and improvement in quality-of-life in diabetic patients with painful neuropathy after 8 weeks of treatment with capsaicin cream (0.075%). On the basis of a meta-analysis of four controlled trials[69] the NNT for capsaicin was 4.2 for analgesic effectiveness, as ascertained by physicians[70]. However, a 12-week trial in painful neuropathy of different etiologies failed to demonstrate pain relief by capsaicin, and no effect on thermal perception was noted. It has been criticized that a double-blind design is not

feasible for topical capsaicin, due the transient local hyperalgesia (usually mild burning sensation > 50% of the cases) it may produce as a typical adverse event. Treatment should be restricted to a maximum of 8 weeks, as during this period no adverse effects on sensory function (resulting from the mechanism of action) were noted in diabetic patients. However, a recent skin blister study in healthy subjects showed that there is a 74% decrease in the number of nerve fibers as early as 3 days following topical capsaicin application, suggesting that degeneration of epidermal nerve fibers may contribute to the analgesia induced by the drug[71]. This finding, questioning the safety of capsaicin in the context of an insensitive diabetic foot, limits its use.

Symptomatic non-pharmacological treatment

There is no entirely satisfactory pharmacotherapy of painful diabetic neuropathy, non-pharmacological treatment options should therefore always be considered.

Psychological support The psychological component to pain should not be under-estimated. An explanation to the patient that even severe pain may remit will help, particularly in poorly controlled patients with acute painful neuropathy or in those painful symptoms precipitated by intensive insulin treatment. Thus, the emphatic approach addressing the concerns and anxieties of patients with neuropathic pain is essential for their successful management[72].

Physical measures The temperature of the painful neuropathic foot may be increased due to arterio–venous shunting. Cold water immersion may reduce shunt flow and relieve pain. Allodynia may be relieved by wearing silk pyjamas, or using a bed cradle. Patients who describe painful symptoms on walking, likened to walking on pebbles, may benefit from the use of more comfortable footwear[72].

Acupuncture In a 10-week uncontrolled study in diabetic patients on standard pain therapy 77% showed significant pain relief after up to 6 courses of traditional Chinese acupuncture, without any side effects. During a follow-up period of 18–52 weeks, 67% were able to stop or significantly reduce their medications and only 24% required further acupuncture treatment[73]. Controlled studies using placebo needles should be performed to confirm these findings.

Transcutaneous electrical nerve stimulation (TENS)
Transcutaneous electrical nerve stimulation (TENS) influences neuronal afferent transmission and conduction velocity, increases the nociceptive flexion reflex threshold, and changes the somatosensory evoked potentials. In a 4-week study of TENS applied to the lower limbs, each for 30 min daily, pain relief was noted in 83% of patients compared to 38% of a sham-treated group. In patients who only marginally responded to amitriptyline, pain reduction was significantly greater following TENS given for 12 weeks compared with sham treatment. Thus, TENS may be used as an adjunctive modality combined with pharmacotherapy to augment pain relief [74].

Electrical spinal cord stimulation It is generally agreed that electrical stimulation is effective in neurogenic forms of pain. Experiments indicate that electrical spinal chord stimulation (ESCS) is followed by a decrease in the excitatory amino-acids glutamate and aspartate in the dorsal horn. This effect is mediated by a GABAergic mechanism. In diabetic painful neuropathy that was unresponsive to drug treatment, ESCS with electrodes implanted between T9 and T11 resulted in a pain relief > 50% in eight out of 10 patients. In addition, exercise tolerance was significantly improved. Complications of ESCS included superficial wound infection in two patients, lead migration requiring reinsertion in two patients, and 'late failure' after 4 months in a patient who had initial pain relief[75]. This invasive treatment option should be reserved for patients who do not respond to drug treatment.

SEXUAL DYSFUNCTION IN DIABETES

Erectile dysfunction and female sexual dysfunction

Male erectile dysfunction (ED), defined as the "inability to achieve or maintain an erection sufficient for sexual intercourse"[76], is one of the most common sexual dysfunctions in men. ED becomes more common with advancing age and, as the aged population is increasing, its prevalence will continue to rise[77]. Diabetes mellitus is the most frequent organic cause of ED. In the Massachusetts male aging study, the age-adjusted prevalence of complete ED was 28% in diabetic men[78]. In a recent survey in Italy of 9868 men with diabetes 45.5% of those aged > 59 years reported ED[79], which may be the earliest clinical feature of autonomic neuropathy, with progression to complete loss of erection in > 2 years. Once ED develops, it persists in most patients. Risk factors and clinical correlates include duration of diabetes, glycemic control, each of the chronic diabetic complications, and smoking[79].

Cholinergic and noncholinergic nonadrenergic neurotransmitters mediate erectile function by relaxing the smooth muscle of the corpus cavernosum. A principal neural mediator of erection is nitric oxide, which activates guanyl cyclase to form intracellular guanosine monophosphate, a potent second messenger for smooth-muscle relaxation. The importance of this pathway is mirrored by the clinical effect of facilitated erection by a selective inhibitor of phosphodiesterase-5 (which breaks down cyclic guanosine monophosphate)[77]. *In vivo* studies of isolated corpus cavernosum tissue from diabetic men have shown functional impairment in autonomic and endothelium-dependent relaxation of corpus cavernosum smooth muscle.

A good clinical history and physical examination are the basis of assessment. It is important to establish the nature of the erectile problem, and to distinguish it from other forms of sexual difficulty, such as penile curvature or premature ejaculation. An interview with the partner is advisable, and will confirm the problem but may also reveal other causes of the difficulties, e.g. vaginal dryness. The relative importance of psychological and organic factors may be determined from the history. Drugs that may be associated with ED include tranquillizers (phenothiazines, benzodiazepines), antidepressants (tricyclics, selective serotonin reuptake inhibitors), and antihypertensives (beta-blockers, vasodilators, central sympathomimetics,

---

Table 17.8 Practical three-step algorithm for diagnosis of erectile dysfunction

Step 1	General sexual history
	Clinical examination; relevant laboratory parameters
	Information about treatment options
Step 2	Therapeutic trial with sildenafil
Step 3	Intracavernous pharmacotesting: color Doppler or duplex ultrasound of penile arteries

---

ganglion blockers, diuretics)[80]. Sophisticated investigation is unnecessary in most patients. A three-step diagnostic approach is shown in Table 17.8.

Diminished or absent testicular pain has been described as an early sign of autonomic neuropathy. Retrograde ejaculation from the prostatic urethra into the bladder may occur occasionally and follows loss of sympathetic innervation of the internal sphincter, which normally contracts during ejaculation. Complete loss of ejaculation probably indicates widespread pelvic sympathetic involvement and, like retrograde ejaculation, causes infertility, which may be overcome by insemination.

The scientific knowledge of sexual dysfunction in women with diabetes is rudimentary. Problems affecting sexuality in diabetic women are fatigue, changes in perimenstrual blood glucose control, vaginitis, decreased sexual desire, decreased vaginal lubrication, and an increased time to reach orgasm. Even minor episodes of depression, which is twice more frequent than in men, can result in a loss of libido. The degree to which these symptoms are related to autonomic neuropathy has been examined in a few studies, the results of these are, however, at variance. Examination of a diabetic woman with sexual dysfunction should include consideration of: the duration of symptoms; psychological state; concomitant medications; presence of vaginitis, cystitis, and other infections; frequency of intercourse; blood pressure; body mass index (BMI); retinal status; pelvic examination; presence of discharge; and glycemic control[81].

Management of erectile dysfunction

A stepwise therapeutic approach for ED is shown in Table 17.9. Initial management should advise the patient to reduce possible risk factors and to optimize glycemic control. However, no studies are available to show that improvement in glycemic control will exert a favorable effect on ED. In fact, a recent study could not demonstrate an effect of intensive diabetes therapy maintained for 2 years on ED in men with type 2 diabetes[82]. Even if the cause is organic, almost all men with ED will be affected psychologically. Sexual counselling is an important aspect of any treatment, and it is preferable to involve the partner as well.

Oral therapy

Most men consider this to be the treatment of choice. The oral treatment options and their mechanisms of action are summarized in Table 17.10.

Yohimbine Yohimbine has a weak $alpha_2$-adrenoreceptor blocking activity and acts presumably via the adrenergic receptors in the brain centers associated with libido and penile erection. In a meta-analysis this drug has been found to be more effective than placebo for all types of ED combined, but the effect was most prominent in non-organic ED[83]. Adverse events include palpitations, tremor, hypertension, and anxiety. As it has a marginal effect on organic ED, yohimbine cannot be generally recommended for treatment of ED in diabetic men.

Apomorphine Apomorphine is a potent emetic agent that acts via central dopaminergic (D1 or D2) receptors as well as central mu-, delta-, and kappa-receptors. A 4-week multicenter, crossover, placebo-controlled trial using the sublingual formulation of apomorphine (Uprima) evaluated 90 diabetic patients on the 4 mg dose, and 86 patients on the 5 mg dose. The percentages of attempts resulting in an erection firm

Table 17.9 Stepwise algorithm for treatment of erectile dysfunction

General management	Control of risk factors and diabetes, sexual counselling	
Pharmacological treatment	*First-line therapy*	*Dose range*
	Sildenafil (Viagra)	50–100 mg
	[Tadalafil (Cialis)][a]	10–20 mg
	[Vardenafil (Levitra)][a]	10–20 mg
	[Apomorphine (Uprima, Ixense)[b]]	2–4 mg s.l.
	Oral therapy inappropriate	
	Transurethral alprostadil (MUSE)	500–1000 µg
	Intracavernosal injection therapy	
	Alprostadil (Caverject)	5–20 µg
	Papaverine/phentolamine (Androskat)	
	Thymoxamine (Erecnos)	10–20 mg
	VIP/Phentolamine (Invicorp)	
	Papaverine/phentolamine/alprostadil (Trimix)	
	Pharmacological therapy inappropriate	
Mechanical treatments	Vacuum devices	
Surgery	Arterial/venous surgery	
	Penile prostheses	

[a]Market approval expected in 2003.
[b]Only marginally effective in unselected diabetic patients.

Table 17.10 Agents for oral treatment of erectile dysfunction

Central mechanism of action
Yohimbine (alpha$_2$ adrenergic antagonist)
Apomorphine (dopamine receptor agonist)

Peripheral mechanism of action
Phentolamine (non-selective adrenergic antagonist)
Phosphodiesterase isoenzyme type 5 inhibitors:
   Sildenafil
   Tadalafil
   Vardenafil

enough for intercourse (primary endpoint) were 14.5 and 24.6% for placebo and 4 mg, respectively ($p = 0.02$) and 27.2 and 34.1% for placebo and 5 mg, respectively ($p = 0.18$). In the *post hoc* combined analysis, the corresponding rates were 20.4 and 28.9%, respectively ($p = 0.009$). No dose–response correlation could thus be demonstrated in this trial. The Federal Drug Agency (FDA) concluded from these data that, even though the 4 mg dose and combined analysis showed statistical significance, the clinical significance is questionable due to the relatively modest benefits noted over placebo[24]. Indeed, the number needed to treat (NNT) for the 4 mg dose based on the aforementioned results is relatively high, i.e. 10 patients need to be treated in order to achieve an erection firm enough for intercourse in one of these patients. The rates of nausea, the most prominent adverse effect of apomorphine, were 21.2, 12.9 and 1.0% for 4 mg, 5 mg, and placebo, respectively. The corresponding rates of vomiting were 6.7, 1.0 and 0%, respectively. Moreover, three syncopal events and three episodes of significant hypotension were reported in patients taking apomorphine[84].

Phentolamine Oral phentolamine (Vasomax) (an alpha$_1$ and alpha$_2$-adrenergic receptor blocker) has been evaluated in a trial including 457 men with mild-to-moderate ED of various causes. Erections were improved in 45, 37, and 16% of the men treated with 80 mg phentolamine, 40 mg phentolamine, and placebo, respectively[85]. Adverse effects include headache, facial flushing, and nasal congestion.

Sildenafil Sildenafil (Viagra) is the first effective oral drug that has been approved for the treatment of ED, and is generally regarded as a first-line treatment of ED of various causes, including diabetes. It is a type-5 PDE inhibitor that prevents the intracorporeal breakdown of cyclic GMP. Sildenafil is taken 60 min before anticipated sexual activity and its effects last approximately 4 h. The drug is available in three doses (25, 50 or 100 mg). It does not stimulate sexual desire and provoke an erection as such, but enhances the continued relaxation of the cavernous smooth muscle initiated by the release of endogenous nitric oxide, with an improved quality of erection.

In a controlled, flexible-dose US multicenter trial including a mixed group of 268 type 1 and type 2 diabetic men, the rates of those with improved erections after 12 weeks of treatment with 25–100 mg sildenafil were 56%, compared with 10% in the placebo group[86]. In a 12-week European multicenter trial including 219 type 2 diabetic men the response rate was even higher, achieving 64.6% on sildenafil versus 10.5% on placebo[87]. The estimated percentages of intercourse attempts that were successful significantly improved from baseline to end of treatment in patients receiving sildenafil (14.4% to 58.8%) compared with those receiving placebo (13.2% to 14.4%). Three-quarters of the patients required the 100 mg sildenafil dose. The response rates were independent of the baseline HbA1c levels and number of chronic complications, suggesting

that sildenafil is effective in improving ED even in cases with poor glycemic control and in presence of angiopathy and neuropathy.

In a combined analysis of 11 controlled trials of sildenafil (25–100 mg) the percentages of maximum score for the six questions in the erectile function domain of the International Index of Erectile Function (IIEF) were 61.3% among 69 type 1 and 60.8% among 399 type 2 diabetic men on sildenafil, compared with 39.3% for 452 diabetic men on placebo[88].

Side effects consist mainly of headache (18%), facial flushing (15%), and dyspepsia (2%). A mild and transient disturbance of colour vision, and increased sensitivity to light, or blurred vision, has been found in 4.5% of diabetic men[87]. Concerns have been expressed regarding an increased number of deaths associated with sildenafil compared with other treatments for ED[89]. However, after an average follow-up of 4.9 months, the Prescription Event Monitoring (PEM) Study including 5391 sildenafil users from England showed a mortality rate of 3.2 per 1000 patient years for ischemic heart disease (IHD), and a rate of 7.2 per 1000 patient years for fatal and non-fatal myocardial infarctions (MI). The comparison figures in England for IHD are 2.6 per 1000 patient years and for MI are 2.7 and 7.0 per 1000 patient years, depending on the source used[90]. Moreover, acute administration of sildenafil (100 mg) to men with severe stenosis of at least one coronary artery did not result in adverse hemodynamic effects on coronary blood flow or vascular resistance, but coronary flow reserve was improved[91].

According to the recommendations of the American Heart Association, sildenafil is contraindicated in men taking nitrates, due to the risk of hypotension, and those with severe cardiovascular disease. Before sildenafil is prescribed, treadmill testing may be indicated in men with heart disease, to assess the risk of cardiac ischemia during sexual intercourse. Initial monitoring of blood pressure after the administration of sildenafil may be indicated in men with congestive heart disease who have borderline low blood pressure and low volume status, and men being treated with complicated, multidrug antihypertensive regimens[92].

As sildenafil treatment is costly and ED is not a life-threatening illness, the appropriateness of insurance coverage for sildenafil treatment has been questioned. However, recent cost–effectiveness studies using cost per quality-adjusted life-year (QALY) gained as outcome measures have shown that sildenafil treatment compared favorably with intracavernosal injection therapy[93], or with accepted therapies for other medical conditions[94].

Tadalafil and vardenafil Tadalafil (Cialis) and vardenafil (Nuviva) are novel PDE5 inhibitors due to be marketed in 2002 and 2003, respectively. In a 12-week multicenter trial including 216 diabetic men (type 2: 91%), but excluding sildenafil non-responders, the rates of men with improved erections were 64% with 20 mg tadalafil, 56% with 10 mg tadalafil, and 25% with placebo[95]. Both tadalafil 10 mg and 20 mg were superior to placebo in improving penetration ability (IIEF Question 3) and ability to maintain an erection during intercourse. Thus, although non-responders to sildenafil were excluded, the effect of tadalafil was not superior to that of sildenafil. Treatment-related adverse events (> 5%) on 20 mg, 10 mg and placebo were dyspepsia (8.3, 11.0 and 0%) and headache (6.9, 8.2 and 1.4%).

Vardenafil (Nuviva) was evaluated in a large 12-week multicenter trial including 439 diabetic men (type 2: 88%). The rates of men with improved erections were 72% with 20 mg vardenafil, 57% with 10 mg vardenafil, and 13% on placebo[96]. Both vardenafil 10 mg and 20 mg were superior to placebo in improving the IIEF erectile function domain score (Questions 1–5, and 15). Similar to tadalafil, despite the exclusion of non-responders to sildenafil, the effect of vardenafil was comparable to that reported previously for sildenafil. Treatment-related adverse events (> 5%) on 20 mg, 10 mg, and placebo were headache (10, 9 and 2%), flushing (10, 9 and < 1%), and headache (6, 3 and 0%). The relative efficacy and safety of these three PDE 5 inhibitors can only be answered by head-to-head comparison trials.

Vacuum devices

These have the merit of being non-invasive and may be used by many men. They create a vacuum around the penis and blood is drawn into the corporal spaces. A band is slipped off the plastic cylinder around the base of the penis to maintain penile tumescence without rigidity in the crura. The disadvantages are that they require some degree of dexterity in handling, and time spent in application of the device. They should only be used for 30 min at a time, and require the willing cooperation of the partner. There are few side effects, although there is some degree of discomfort and the penis feels cold. Ejaculation is usually blocked and some men find this makes orgasm less satisfactory. Bruising can occur in 10–15% of men. Vacuum devices are particularly useful in older men in stable relationships and when other treatment options are ineffective. They may also be used to augment the result of pharmacotherapy. Some men find that the constrictive ring is a useful aid in itself for maintaining erection without the use of a vacuum device. However, the long-term drop-out rates among users of vacuum constriction devices are relatively high. A recent study showed an overall drop-out rate over 3 years for the ErecAid system of 65%, i.e. 100% in men with mild ED, 56% in those with moderate ED, and 70% in those with complete ED. The main reasons for stopping use were that the device was ineffective (57%), too cumbersome (24%), and too painful (20%)[97].

Transurethral alprostadil

Alprostadil was first licensed for the treatment of erectile dysfunction by intracavernous injection. It is a synthetic preparation of the naturally occurring prostaglandin E1, and acts by initiating erection. In contrast to sildenafil, it initiates the relaxation of cavernous smooth muscle to bring about erection. This drug has been incorporated into a pellet that can be given by intraurethral application (MUSE: medical urethral system for erection). Patients need to be instructed in the use of MUSE, which is introduced into the urethra with a disposable applicator. The patient first passes urine, to act as a lubricant and facilitate the passage of the applicator and the absorption of the drug. Absorption of the drug is also facilitated by the patient rolling the penis between the palms of his hands. Some patients find that a constrictive ring around the base of the penis enhances the efficacy. The erection takes about ten min to develop, and the dose range varies between 125 and 1000 µg, although the majority of patients require 500 or 1000 µg. The use of MUSE without a condom is contraindicated when the partner is pregnant or likely to conceive.

In the US and European multicenter trials about 65% of men with different causes of ED who tried MUSE had erections sufficient for intercourse during in-clinic testing[98,99]. About one-half of the treatments at home were successful, but the drop-out rate after 15 months was 75%, the main reason being lack of efficacy[99]. The most common side effects are penile pain (30%), urethral burning (12%) or minor urethral bleeding (5%)[100]. Systemic side effects (such as hypotension or even syncope) were usually uncommon, but highlight the role of the physician in administering the first supervised dose. Disappointing results have recently been reported in a study conducted in a urology practice setting, in which an adequate rigidity score was achieved in only 13 and 30% of the patients using 500 and 1000 µg, respectively. Pain, discomfort, or burning in the penis were observed in 18%, but orthostatic hypotension (defined as a decrease in systolic/diastolic blood pressure by 20/10 mmHg or orthostatic symptoms) was present in 41% of the patients. The discontinuation rate was very high, reaching 81% after 2–3 months[101].

Intracavernosal injection therapy

Intracavernosal therapy requires some specialist knowledge and the ability to treat priapism, should it occur. Many specialists used to regard this as standard treatment and use it for both diagnostic and therapeutic reasons, although its role as first-line therapy has been replaced by less invasive treatment modalities. Patients need to be taught how to self-inject, and the dose needs to be chosen carefully to avoid prolonged erections or priapism. Some patients find it helpful to use one of the many autoinjector devices available. Erection occurs after ten min and may

be enhanced by sexual stimulation. The incidence of complications varies with the different pharmacological agents. Some pain is not uncommon, but long-term problems are limited to priapism or penile fibrosis.

Alprostadil is the most widely used agent[102,103]. It is effective in > 80% of patients with different etiologies of ED, and has a low incidence of side effects. In a recent comparative study of intracavernosal versus intraurethral administration of alprostadil the rates of erections sufficient for sexual intercourse were 82.5 versus 53.0%, respectively[103]. Patient and partner satisfaction was higher with intracavernosal injection, and more patients preferred this therapy. Penile pain occurs in 15–50% of patients, but is often not troublesome. The dose range is 5–20 µg, but some physicians will increase it further, or use a combination with papaverine and phentolamine. Priapism occurs in about 1% of patients. The cumulative incidence of penile fibrosis was 11.7% after a period of 4 years, and the risk of irreversible fibrotic alterations was 5%[104]. About half of the cases with fibrosis resolved spontaneously. Other less frequently used agents include thymoxamine [moxisylyte hydrochloride (Erecnos)], papaverine/phentolamine mixtures, (Androskat), papaverine/phentolamine/alprostadil mixtures (Trimix), and VIP/phentolamine (Invicorp).

Penile prostheses

This treatment is carried out only after careful patient selection and a trial of the less invasive options. There are a number of different devices available, ranging from the simple malleable prosthesis to more complex hydraulic prostheses. The choice of prosthesis is dependent upon the wishes of the patient and is often cost-related. A prosthesis does not restore a normal erection, but makes the penis rigid enough for sexual intercourse. The hydraulic prostheses have the advantage of flaccidity and are now mechanically reliable with revision rates of less than 5% per annum. Infection remains a major complication in approximately 3–5% of cases with different causes of ED and usually leads to removal of the device[80].

Surgery

Arterial reconstruction is associated with complication rates of > 30% and remains an experimental procedure that cannot be generally recommended for diabetic patients with ED.

CONCLUSION

Diabetic neuropathy

Despite the recently accelerating publication rate for controlled trials demonstrating significant pain relief in diabetic neuropathy with several agents, the symptomatic pharmacological treatment of chronic painful diabetic neuropathy remains a challenge for the physician. Major limiting factors are still the paucity of adequately large conclusive trials and the relatively high rates of adverse effects for several drug classes. Recent trials evaluating agents such as gabapentin or tramadol have included adequately large patient samples, but the effect on pain was not superior to the tricyclic compounds that have been used for many years. Thus, individual tolerability will be a major consideration in the physician's treatment decision. There is almost no information available from controlled trials on long-term analgesic efficacy and the use of drug combinations.

Combination drug use, or the addition of a new drug to a therapeutic regimen, may lead to increased drug toxicity or decreased efficacy. Drug interactions should be more predictable, based on the knowledge of which compounds induce inhibition or are metabolized by specific cytochrome *P450* enzymes. Drug combinations might also include those aimed at symptomatic pain relief and quality-of-life on one hand, and improvement or slowing the progression of the underlying neuropathic process on the other. Future trials should consider these aspects in order to optimize the current treatment strategies in painful diabetic neuropathy.

Erectile dysfunction

ED is present in one of every 2–3 men with diabetes mellitus. The annual incidence rate of ED in diabetes is twice as high as in the general population. The risk of ED is increased by a multitude of comorbidities and sequelas of diabetes. Thus, a practical multifactorial approach to managing ED in diabetes is required. Despite the enormous impact of ED on the quality-of-life, and the recent explosion of interest in ED, the number of diabetic patients seeking medical help is still low, as the topic remains a 'secret' in many cases.

REFERENCES

1 Consensus statement. Report and recommendations of the San Antonio conference on diabetic neuropathy. *Diabetes Care* 1988;11:592-597.

2 Thomas PK. Metabolic neuropathy. *J R Coll Phys London* 1973;7:154.

3 Sima AAF, Thomas PK, Ishii D, Vinik A. Diabetic neuropathies. *Diabetologia* 1997;40:B74–B77.

4 Shaw JE, Zimmet PZ. The epidemiology of diabetic neuropathy. *Diabetes Rev* 1999;7:245–52.

5 Resnick HE, Vinik AI, Schwartz AV *et al*. Independent effects of peripheral nerve dysfunction on lower-extremity physical function in old age. The Women's Health and Aging Study. *Diabetes Care* 2000;23:1642–7.

6 Forsblom CM, Sane T, Groop PH *et al*. Risk factors for mortality in Type II (non-insulin-dependent) diabetes: evidence of a role for neuropathy and a protective effect of HLA-DR4. *Diabetologia* 1998;4:1253–62.

7 Coppini DV, Bowtell PA, Weng C *et al*. Showing neuropathy is related to increased mortality in diabetic patients—a survival analysis using an accelerated failure time model. *J Clin Epidemiol* 2000;53:519–23.

8 Abbott CA, Vileikyte L, Williamson S *et al*. Multicenter study of the incidence of and predictive risk factors for diabetic neuropathic foot ulceration. *Diabetes Care* 1998;21:1071–5.

9 Chan AW, MacFarlane IA, Bowsher DR *et al*. Chronic pain in patients with diabetes mellitus: comparison with non-diabetic population. *Pain Clin* 1990;3:147–59.

10 Galer BS, Gianas A, Jensen MP. Painful diabetic neuropathy: epidemiology, pain description, and quality of life. *Diabetes Res Clin Pract* 2000;47:123–8.

11 Ward JD. Upright posture and the microvasculature in human diabetic neuropathy. A hypothesis. *Diabetes* 1997;46 (Suppl 2):S94–S97.

12 Thomas PK. Painful diabetic neuropathy: mechanisms and treatment. *Diab Nutr Metab* 1994;7:359–68.

13 Boulton AJM, Scarpello JHB, Armstrong WD, Ward JD. The natural history of painful diabetic neuropathy—a 4-year study. *Postgrad Med J* 1983;59:556–9.

14 Young RJ, Ewing DJ, Clarke BF. Chronic and remitting painful diabetic neuropathy. *Diabetes Care* 1988;11:34–40.

15 Benbow SJ, Chan AW, Bowsher D *et al.* A prospective study of painful symptoms, small-fibre function and peripheral vascular disease in chronic painful diabetic neuropathy. *Diabetic Med* 1993;11:17–21.

16 Archer AG, Watkins PJ, Thomas PK *et al.* The natural history of acute painful neuropathy in diabetes mellitus. *J Neurol Neurosurg Psychiat* 1983;46:491–9.

17 Ellenberg M. Diabetic neuropathic cachexia. *Diabetes* 1974;23:418–23.

18 Steele JM, Young RJ, Lloyd GG, Clarke BF. Clinically apparent eating disorders in young diabetic women: associations with painful neuropathy and other complications. *Br Med J* 1987;294:859–66.

19 Caravati CM. Insulin neuritis: a case report. *Va Med Mon* 1933;59:745–6.

20 Llewelyn JG, Thomas PK, Fonseca V *et al.* Acute painful diabetic neuropathy precipitated by strict glycaemic control. *Acta Neuropathol* 1986; 72:157–63.

21 Tesfaye S, Malik R, Harris N *et al.* Arterio–venous shunting and proliferating new vessels in acute painful neuropathy of rapid glycaemic control (insulin neuritis). *Diabetologia* 1996;39:329–35.

22 Asbury AK. Focal and multifocal neuropathies of diabetes. In: Dyck PJ, Thomas PK, Asbury AK *et al.* editors. *Diabetic neuropathy*. Philadelphia: Saunders, 1987: 45–55.

23 Zorilla E, Kozak GP. Ophthalmoplegia in diabetes mellitus. *Ann Intern Med* 1967;67:968–74.

24 Chaudhuri KR, Wren DR, Werring D, Watkins PJ. Unilateral abdominal muscle herniation with pain: a distinctive variant of diabetic radiculopathy. *Diabetic Med* 1997;14:803–7.

25 Said G, Goulon-Goeau C, Lacroix C, Moulonguet A. Nerve biopsy findings in different patterns of proximal diabetic neuropathy. *Ann Neurol* 1994;35:559–69.

26 Said G, Elgrably F, Lacroix C *et al.* Painful proximal diabetic neuropathy: inflammatory nerve lesions and spontaneous favorable outcome. *Ann Neurol* 1997;41:762–70.

27 Younger DS, Rosoklija G, Hays AP *et al.* Diabetic peripheral neuropathy: a clinicopathologic and immunohistochemical analysis of sural nerve biopsies. *Muscle Nerve* 1996;19:722–7.

28 Krendel DA. Diabetic inflammatory vasculopathy. *Muscle Nerve* 1997;20:520.

29 Krendel DA, Costigan DA, Hopkins LC. Successful treatment of neuropathies in patients with diabetes mellitus. *Arch Neurol* 1995; 52:1053–61.

30 Reske-Nielsen E, Lundbaek K. Pathological changes in the central and peripheral nervous system of young long-term diabetics. II The spinal cord and peripheral nerves. *Diabetologia* 1968;4:34–43.

31 Slager U. Diabetic myelopathy. *Arch Pathol Lab Med* 1978;102:467–9.

32 Olsson Y, Säve-Söderbergh J, Sourander P, Angervall L. A patho-anatomical study of the central and peripheral nervous system in diabetics of early onset and long duration. *Pathol Eur* 1968;3:62–79.

33 Reske-Nielsen E, Lundbaek K, Rafaelsen OJ. Pathological changes in the central and peripheral nervous system of young long-term diabetics. I Diabetic encephalopathy. *Diabetologia* 1965;1:233–41.

34 DeJong RN. The nervous system complications in diabetes mellitus with special reference to cerebrovascular changes. *J Nerv Ment Dis* 1950;111:181–206.

35 Ziegler D, Mühlen H, Dannehl K, Gries FA. Tibial nerve somatosensory evoked potentials at various stages of peripheral neuropathy in Type 1 diabetic patients. *J Neurol Neurosurg Psychiatry* 1993;56:58–64.

36 Ziegler D, Seemann-Monteiro M, Mühlen H, Gries FA. The degree of cognitive dysfunction is associated with the stage of peripheral neuropathy in Type 1 diabetic patients. *Diabetologia* 1993;36 (Suppl. 1):A185.

37 Dejgaard A, Gade A, Larsson H *et al.* Evidence for diabetic encephalopathy. *Diabetic Med* 1991;8:162–7.

38 Ziegler D, Langen K-J, Herzog H *et al.* Cerebral glucose metabolism in Type 1 diabetic patients. *Diabetic Med* 1994;11:205–9.

39 Eaton SE, Harris ND, Rajbhandari SM *et al.* Spinal-chord involvement in diabetic peripheral neuropathy. *Lancet* 2001;358:35–6.

40 Cameron NE, Cotter MA. Metabolic and vascular factors in the pathogenesis of diabetic neuropathy. *Diabetes* 1997;46 (Suppl 2):S31–S37.

41 Proceedings of a consensus development conference on standardized measures in diabetic neuropathy. *Diabetes Care* 1992;15;(Suppl 3):1080–107.

42 Dyck PJ. Detection, characterization, and staging of polyneuropathy: assessed in diabetics. *Muscle Nerve* 1988;11:21–32.

43 Young MJ, Boulton AJM, Macleod AF *et al.* A multicentre study of the prevalence of diabetic peripheral neuropathy in the United Kingdom hospital clinic population. *Diabetologia* 1993; 36:150–4.

44 Quantitative sensory testing: a consensus report from the Peripheral Neuropathy Association. *Neurology* 1993;43:1050–2.

45 The Diabetes Control and Complications Trial Research Group. The effect of intensive treatment of diabetes on the development and progression of long-term complications in insulin-dependent diabetes mellitus. *N Engl J Med* 1993;329:977–86.

46 UK Prospective Diabetes Study (UKPDS) Group. Intensive blood-glucose control with sulphonylureas or insulin compared with conventional treatment and risk of complications in patients with type 2 diabetes (UKPDS 33). *Lancet* 1998; 352:837–53.

47 Nicolucci A, Carinci F, Cavaliere D *et al.* on behalf of the Italian study group for the implementation of the St Vincent Declaration. A meta-analysis of trials on aldose reductase inhibitors in diabetic peripheral neuropathy. *Diabetic Med* 1996;13:1017–26.

48 Dyck PJ, O'Brien PC. Meaningful degrees of prevention or improvement of nerve conduction in controlled clinical trials of diabetic neuropathy. *Diabetes Care* 1989;12:649–52.

49 The γ-Linolenic Acid Multicenter Trial Group. Treatment of diabetic neuropathy with γ-linolenic acid. *Diabetes Care* 1993;16:8–15.

50 Ziegler D, Reljanovic M, Mehnert H, Gries FA. α-Lipoic acid in the treatment of diabetic polyneuropathy in Germany: current evidence from clinical trials. *Exp Clin Endocrinol Diabetes* 1999;107:421–30.

51 Malik RA, Williamson S, Abbott C *et al.* Effect of angiotensin-converting-enzyme (ACE) inhibitor trandolapril on human diabetic neuropathy: randomised double blind placebo controlled trial. *Lancet* 1998;352:1978–81.

52 Toyota T, Hirata Y, Ikeda Y *et al.* Lipo-PGE1, a new lipid-encapsulated preparation of prostaglandin E1: placebo- and prostaglandin E1-controlled multicenter trials in patients with diabetic neuropathy and leg ulcers. *Prostaglandins* 1993;46:453–68.

53 Apfel SC, Schwartz S, Adornato BT *et al.* Efficacy and safety of recombinant human nerve growth factor in patients with diabetic polyneuropathy. *J Am Med Assoc* 2000;284:2215–21.

54 Johansson B-L, Borg K, Fernqvist-Forbes E *et al.* Beneficial effects of C-peptide on incipient nephropathy and neuropathy in patients with Type 1 diabetes mellitus. *Diabetic Med* 2000; 17:181–9.

55 Schratzberger P, Walter DH, Rittig K *et al.* Reversal of experimental diabetic neuropathy by VEGF gene transfer. *J Clin Invest* 2001; 107:1083–92.

56 Simovic D, Isner JM, Ropper AH *et al.* Improvement in chronic ischemic neuropathy after intramuscular *phVEGF165* gene transfer in patients with critical limb ischemia. *Arch Neurol* 2001;58:761–8.

57 Sindrup SH, Jensen TS. Efficacy of pharmacological treatments of neuropathic pain: an update and effect related to mechanism of drug action. *Pain* 1999;83:389–400.

58 Sindrup SH, Jensen TS. Pharmacologic treatment of pain in polyneuropathy. *Neurology* 2000; 55:915–920.

59 Kunz NR, Goli V, Lei D, Rudolph R. Treating painful diabetic neuropathy with venlafaxine extended release. *Diabetes* 2000;49(Suppl 1):A165.

60 Backonja M, Beydoun A, Edwards KR *et al.* Gabapentin for the symptomatic treatment of painful neuropathy in patients with diabetes mellitus. *J Am Med Assoc* 1998;280:1831–6.

61 Eisenberg E, Lurie Y, Braker C *et al.* Lamotrigine reduces painful diabetic neuropathy: a randomized, controlled study. *Neurology* 2001;57:505–9.

62 Jarvis B, Coukell AJ. Mexiletine. A review of its therapeutic use in painful diabetic neuropathy. *Drugs* 1998;56:691–707.

63 Mo J, Chen LL. Systemic lidocaine for neuropathic pain relief. *Pain* 2000;87:7–17.

64 Byas-Smith MG, Max MB, Muir J, Kingman A. Transdermal clonidine compared to placebo in painful diabetic neuropathy using a two-stage "enriched enrollment" design. *Pain* 1995;60:267–74.

65 Harati Y, Gooch C, Swenson M *et al.* Double-blind randomized trial of tramadol for the treatment of the pain of diabetic neuropathy. *Neurology* 1998;50:1842–6.

66 Sindrup SH, Jensen TS. Efficacy of pharmacological treatments of neuropathic pain: an update and effect related to mechanism of drug action. *Pain* 1999;83:389–400.

67 Nelson KA, Park KM, Robinovitz E *et al.* High-dose oral dextromethorphan versus placebo in painful diabetic neuropathy and postherpetic neuralgia. *Neurology* 1997;48:1212–18.

68 Pellegrino RG. Memantine reduces neuropathic pain in diabetics. 52nd Annual Meeting of the American Academy of Neurology, San Diego, 2000.

69 Zhang WY, Li Wan Po A. The effectiveness of topically applied capsaicin. A meta-analysis. *Eur J Clin Pharmacol* 1994;46:517–22.

70 McQuay HJ, Moore RA. Using numerial results from systematic reviews in clinical practice. *Ann Intern Med* 1997;126:712–20.

71 Nolano M, Simone DA, Wendelschafer-Crabb G *et al.* Topical capsaicin in humans: parallel loss of epidermal nerve fibers and pain sensation. *Pain* 1999;81:135–45.

72 Tesfaye S. Painful diabetic neuropathy. Aetiology and nonpharmacological treatment. In: Veves A editor. *Clinical management of diabetic neuropathy.* Totowa, New Jersey: Humana Press, 1998: 133–46.

73 Abuaisha BB, Costanzi, Boulton AJM. Acupuncture for the treatment of chronic painful peripheral diabetic neuropathy: a long-term study. *Diabetes Res Clin Pract* 1998;39:115–21.

74 Kumar D, Alvaro MS, Julka IS, Marshall HJ. Diabetic peripheral neuropathy. Effectiveness of electrotherapy and amitriptyline for symptomatic relief. *Diabetes Care* 1998;21:1322–5.

75 Tesfaye S, Watt J, Benbow SJ *et al.* Electrical spinal-cord stimulation for painful diabetic peripheral neuropathy. *Lancet* 1996;348:1696–1701.

76 NIH consensus development panel on impotence. Impotence. *J Am Med Assoc* 1993;270:83–90.

77 Wagner G, Saenz de Tejada I. Update on male erectile dysfunction. *Br Med J* 1998;316:678–82.

78 Feldman HA, Goldstein I, Hatzichristou DG *et al.* Impotence and its medical and psychosocial correlates: results of the Massachusetts male ageing study. *J Urol* 1994;151:54–61.

79 Fedele D, Coscelli C, Santeusanio F *et al.* Erectile dysfunction in diabetic subjects in Italy. *Diabetes Care* 1998;21:1973–7.

80 European Society for Impotence Research. *Erectile dysfunction: a physicians' guide to the management of erectile dysfunction.* European Society for Impotence Research, 1998.

81 Jovanovic L. Sex and the woman with diabetes: desire versus dysfunction. *IDF Bull* 1998;43:23–8.

82 Azad N, Emanuele NV, Abraira C *et al.* and the VA CSDM Group. The effects of intensive glycemic control on neuropathy in the VA Cooperative Study on Type II diabetes mellitus. *J Diabetes Compl* 2000;13:307–13.

83 Vogt HJ, Brandl P, Kockott G *et al.* Double-blind, placebo-controlled safety and efficacy trial with yohimbine hydrochloride in the treatment of nonorganic erectile dysfunction. *Int J Impot Res* 1997;9:155–61.

84 Reproductive Health Drugs Advisory Committee. *Urology Subcommittee. FDA briefing package.* FDA, April 10, 2000: 42–110.

85 Goldstein I, Vasomax Study Group. Efficacy and safety of oral phentolamine (Vasomax) for the treatment of minimal erectile dysfunction [abstract]. *J Urol* 1998;159(Suppl):240.

86 Rendell MS, Rajfer J, Wicker PA, Smith MD. Sildenafil for treatment of erectile dysfunction in men with diabetes: a randomized controlled trial. Sildenafil Diabetes Study Group. *J Am Med Assoc* 1999;281:421–6.

87 Boulton AJM, Selam J-L, Sweeney M, Ziegler D. Sildenafil citrate for the treatment of erectile dysfunction in men with type II diabetes mellitus. *Diabetologia* 2001;44:1296–1301.

88 Sellam R, Ziegler D, Boulton AJM. Sildenafil citrate is effective and well tolerated for the treatment of erectile dysfunction in men with Type 1 or Type 2 diabetes mellitus [abstract]. *Diabetologia* 2000;43(Suppl 1):A253.

89 Mitka M. Some men who take Viagra die—Why? *J Am Med Assoc* 2000;283:590–3.

90 Shakir SAW, Wilton LV, Boshier A *et al.* Cardiovascular events in users of sildenafil: results from first phase of prescription event monitoring in England. *Br Med J* 2001;322:651–2.

91 Herrmann HC, Chang G, Klugherz BD, Mahoney PD. Hemodynamic effects of sildenafil in men with severe coronary artery disease. *N Engl J Med* 2000;342:1622–6.

92 Cheitlin MD, Hutter AM, Brindis RG *et al.* Use of sildenafil (Viagra) in patients with cardiovascular disease. *Circulation* 1999;99:168–77.

93 Stolk EA, Busschbach JJ, Caffa M *et al.* Cost utility analysis of sildenafil compared with papaverine-phentolamine injections. *Br Med J* 2000;320:1165–8.

94 Smith KJ, Roberts MS. The cost-effectiveness of sildenafil. *Ann Intern Med* 2000;132:933–7.

95 Saenz de Tejada I, Emmick J, Anglin G *et al.* The effect of as-needed tadalafil (IC351) treatment of erectile dysfunction in men with diabetes. *Int J Impot Res* 2001;13(Suppl 4):S46.

96 Goldstein I. Vardenafil demonstrates improved erectile function in diabetic men with erectile dysfunction. 4th Congress of the European Society

for Sexual and Impotence Research (ESSIR), Rome, 1 October 2001.

97 Dutta TC, Eid JF. Vacuum constriction devices for erectile dysfunction: a long-term, prospective study of patients with mild, moderate, and severe dysfunction. *Urology* 1999;54:891–3.

98 Padma-Nathan H, Hellstrom WJ, Kaiser FE *et al.* Treatment of men with erectile dysfunction with transurethral alprostadil. Medicated Urethral System for Erection (MUSE) Study Group. *N Engl J Med* 1997;336:1–7.

99 Porst H. Transurethrale Alprostadilapplikation mit MUSE ("medicated urethral system for erection"). *Urologe [A]* 1998;37:410–16.

100 Spivack AP, Peterson CA, Cowley C *et al.* VIVUS-MUSE Study Group. Long-term safety profile of transurethral alprostadil for the treatment of erectile dysfunction [abstract]. *J Urol* 1997;157(Suppl):203.

101 Fulgham PF, Cochran JS, Denman JL. Disappointing initial results with transurethral alprostadil for erectile dysfunction in a urology practice setting. *J Urol* 1998;160:2041–6.

102 Linet OI, Ogrinc FG. Efficacy and safety of intracavernosal alprostadil in men with erectile dysfunction. The Alprostadil Study Group. *N Engl J Med* 1996;334:873–7.

103 Shabsigh R, Padma-Nathan H, Gittleman M *et al.* Intracavernous alprostadil alfadex is more efficacious, better tolerated, and preferred over intraurethral alprostadil plus optional actis: a comparative, randomized, crossover, multicenter study. *Urology* 2000;55:109–13.

104 Porst H, Buvat J, Meuleman EJH *et al.* Final results of a prospective multi-center study with self-injection therapy with PGE$_1$ after 4 years of follow-up. *Int J Impot Res* 1996;6:151, D118.

18

Diabetic foot—assessment, management, and prevention

Arthur E Helfand

INTRODUCTION

Foot problems in the patient with diabetes mellitus represent one of the most distressing and disabling afflictions associated with the complications of this chronic disease[1]. Diabetic foot pathology is a major cause of morbidity and permanent disability[2]. Foot problems significantly change the quality-of-life in diabetic patients, and magnify those changes as the patient ages[3]. Foot problems are one of the most common complications leading to hospitalization and tissue loss[4]. In the USA, there are about 16 million people with diabetes, of whom 15% will probably develop a foot ulcer at some point in their lifetime[5]. For diabetic patients, a foot ulcer usually precedes about 85% of amputations[6]. Caring for the diabetic foot represents a serious and expensive complication[7]. In addition, minor changes in the foot of a diabetic serve as a predictor for other vascular and neuropathic changes, such as ocular pathology, cardiovascular disease, renal impairment and neuropathy.

In excess of 86 000 nontraumatic amputations occur in the USA, representing about 50% of the national total[8]. The cost-estimate exceeds more than one billion dollars per year. The usual clinical sequence includes minor and repetitive trauma, skin breakdown and ulceration, faulty wound healing, infection, peripheral neuro-pathy, foot deformities, and peripheral vascular disease, as well as skin and toenail changes[9].

As an example, in a report issued by the Pennsylvania Department of Health, in 1997, there were 5017 lower extremity amputations, an average of 13.77 amputations per day. The cost report issued by the Pennsylvania Cost Containment Council for the year 2000 estimated a length of stay of 11.0 days and hospital costs of $31 515. This cost includes only the hospital stay, and does not include professional fees, rehabilitation and long-term care costs, or the eventual cost in quality-of-life for older patients.

In many cases, because foot and related problems are the primary complaint, the patient may seek footcare initially[10]. Thus the concept of secondary prevention, i.e. finding the complications at their earliest manifestation and providing early intervention that includes, not only care[11], but also continuing assessment and surveillance, as well as education, become the cornerstone in the management of foot problems for patients with diabetes. Some of the keys to management include appropriate care of the disease itself, screening, assessment, evaluation, risk stratification, professional and practitioner education, patient education, primary podiatric care, therapeutic shoes and orthoses—and a recognition that preventing complications is a family affair[12].

IDENTIFYING COMPLICATING FOOT PROBLEMS

The management of foot problems in the diabetic patient requires the early recognition of their etiologic factors[13]. The complaints and symptoms of the patient, physical signs, and the clinical manifestations of disease and degenerative change, which may be local in origin or a complication of a related systemic or functional disease, should be considered. Degenerative joint diseases, as manifest in the diabetic foot, will be related to acute trauma, inflammation, metabolic change, repeated and chronic microtrauma, strain, obesity, osteoporosis and postmenopausal changes[14]. The primary manifestations of these alterations in the foot are noted in Table 18.1.

These changes increase pain, limit motion and reduce the ambulatory status of the patient. Chronic gouty changes result in painful joints, stiffness, soft tissue tophi, a loss of bone substance, gouty arthritis, joint deformity and excessive pain associated with acute episodes and exacerbation of the disease. Musculoskeletal change manifest as early morning stiffness, pain, fibrosis, ankylosis, contracture, deformity, impairment and the reduction of ambulation[15]. All are characteristic residuals in the foot.

The primary signs and symptoms of peripheral arterial impairment are those related to occlusion and/or vasospasm[16]. In general, many systemic diseases present in the elderly increase the prevalence and incidence of arterial insufficiency. The most common are diabetes mellitus, obesity, hypertension, congestive heart failure, cerebrovascular disease, renal disease and reduced activity tolerance, associated with chronic obstructive pulmonary disease. Given the fact that many diabetics present with other comorbid conditions, assessment and risk stratification are essential.

Common complaints from the patient usually consist of one or more of the following[17]; fatigue, rest pain, coldness, burning, color changes, tingling, numbness, ulcerations, a history of phlebitis, cramps, edema, claudication, and repeated foot infections. Primary physical findings in the foot include diminished or absent pedal pulses, with similar changes in the entire

Table 18.1 Alterations in the foot—primary manifestations

Plantar fasciitis
Spur formation
Calcaneal spurs
Periostitis
Decalcification
Stress fractures
Tendonitis
Tenosynovitis
Residual deformities
Pes planus
Pes valgo planus
Pes cavus
Hallux valgus
Hallux limitus
Hallux rigidus
Atrophy of the plantar fat pad
Metatarsal prolapse (prominent metatarsal heads)
Metatarsalgia
Hammertoes
Morton's syndrome (short first metatarsal segment)
Rotational digital deformities
Joint swelling
Anterior imbalance
Bursitis
Haugland's deformity (osseous enlargement of the posterior–superior surfaces of the calcaneus)
Neuritis
Entrapment syndrome
Neuroma

extremity, depending on the location and degree of occlusion. The hypertensive patient may demonstrate pulsations that are a false reflection of the vascular supply. The general appearance of the foot usually demonstrates color changes, which include rubor and/or cyanosis. The temperature of the foot is usually cool, and spastic changes are more pronounced in colder climates. The skin is usually dry, xerotic and atrophy of the skin and soft tissues is pronounced.

Table 18.2 Symptoms and signs
Paresthesias, e.g., abnormal spontaneous sensations in the feet
Burning
Claudication
Temperature changes, e.g. cold feet
Edema
Fatigue
Rest Pain
Signs
Absent posterior tibial pulse
Absent dorsalis pedis pulse
Advanced trophic changes
Hair growth – decrease or absent
Nail changes – thickening
Pigmentary changes – discoloration
Skin texture – thin and shiny
Skin color – rubor or cyanosis
Ulceration
Vasospasm
Gangrene
Useful scale for vascular risk stratification
0 = No change
1 = Mild claudication
2 = Moderate claudication
3 = Severe claudication
4 = Ischemic rest pain
5 = Minor tissue loss
6 = Major tissue loss

Table 18.3 Peripheral risk factors
Achilles reflex
Vibratory sensation
Sharp and dull response
Superficial plantar response
Paresthesia
Burning
Joint position
Monofilament (Semmes–Weinstein 5.07 gauge – 10 g)
A useful scale for neurosensory risk stratification
0 = No sensory loss
1 = Sensory loss
2 = Sensory loss and foot deformity
3 = Sensory loss and foot deformity with a history of ulceration

Superficial infections are more common and, with extension, pain becomes more significant[18]. A summary of 'at risk' signs and symptoms related to peripheral arterial function in the foot are given in Table 18.2[18A]. A summary of the peripheral risk factors in relation to neurologic function in the foot are noted in Table 18.3.

GENERAL PODIATRIC CONSIDERATIONS[19]

The toenails of diabetic patients demonstrate a variety of changes, including: onychodystrophy (nutritional changes, subungual hemorrhage, discoloration, and onycholysis), onychorrhexis (longitudinal striations), onycholysis (shedding from the distal portion), onychomadesis (shedding from the proximal portion), subungual hemorrhage (bleeding into the nail bed), onychophosis (keratosis), onychauxis (thickening with hypertrophy), onychogryphosis (thickening with gross deformity), onychia (inflammation), onychomycosis (fungal infection), subungual ulceration (ulceration in the nail bed), incurvation or involution (onychodysplesia), autoavulsion, subungual keratosis, and deformity.

Edema is usually a clinical sign of advanced occlusion, and must be related to edema from other conditions. Blebs are common in the later stages of local occlusion. Varicosities complicate management and ulcers related to arterial occlusion are usually painful, with a higher incidence of gangrenous changes. When necrosis and gangrene are evident, the type, onset, relationship to trauma and infection, must be considered in management. The clinical status and results of invasive and non-invasive studies, in particular, Doppler studies, can project the need for surgical consideration to attempt to re-vascularize the area. In addition, we must consider the degenerative changes of age and the pathomechanical and biomechanical changes that produce increased pressure on avascular areas. Early management and preventive measures are essential to minimize the potential for amputation. Tissue loss in the elderly and amputation can terminate the patient's independent life of usefulness to themselves and society.

The diabetic patient with neuropathy presents with sensitive feet, which will generally exhibit some degree of parasthesia, sensory impairment to pain and temperature, motor weakness, diminished or lost Achilles and patellar reflexes, decreased vibratory sense, a loss of proprioception, xerotic changes, anhidrosis, neurotrophic arthropathy, atrophy, neurotrophic ulcers, and the potential for a marked difference in size between two feet[20]. There is a greater incidence of infection, necrosis and gangrene. Vascular impairment adds pallor, a loss or decrease in the posterior tibial and dorsalis pedis pulse, dependent rubor, a decrease in the venous filling time, coolness of the skin and trophic changes. Numbness and tingling, as well as cramps and pain, are demonstrated. There is usually a loss of the plantar metatarsal fat pad, which predisposes the patient to ulceration in relation to the bony deformities of the foot.

Hyperkeratotic lesions form as space replacements, and provide a focus for ulceration due to increased pressure on the soft tissues, with an associated localized avascularity from direct pressure and counter-pressure[21]. Hemorrhage in the keratotic areas are pre-ulcerous lesions, and demonstrate a high-risk patient. Tendon contractures and claw toes (hammertoes) are common. A warm foot with pulsations in a diabetic with neuropathy is not uncommon.

When ulceration is present, the base is usually covered by keratosis, which retards and may prevent healing. Necrosis and gangrene are related to infection, with eventual occlusion and gangrene. Foot drop and a loss of position sense are usually present. Pretibial lesions are indicative of this change, as well as micro-vascular infarction. Arthropathy gives rise to deformity, altered gait patterns, and a higher risk of ulceration and limb loss.

Pruritis and cutaneous infections are more common in the diabetic. Dehydration, trophic changes, anhidrosis, xerosis, and fissures are predisposing factors to calcaneal ulceration.

Radiographic findings in the foot in diabetic patients usually demonstrate thin trabecular patterns, decalcification, joint position changes, osteophytic formation, osteolysis, deformities and osteoporosis. A summary of related diabetic foot-related findings and issues are identified in Table 18.4[22].

MANAGEMENT OF REPEATED TRAUMA TO THE FOOT

In addition to the relationship of vascular and neuropathic changes, ulceration must be related to trauma and, in particular, the effects of repeated micro-trauma. Hyperkeratosis related to keratin dysfunction, space replacement, bony abnormality, and/or pathomechanics, will react to pressure and trauma, which may be mechanical, thermal and/or chemical in nature[23]. Sub-hyperkeratotic hemorrhage is usually an early clinical sign of tissue breakdown[24]. Regardless of the cause, the general principles of management include a decrease of local trauma by the use of orthotics, shoe modifications, specialized footwear and efforts to maximize weight diffusion and weight dispersion. Physical modalities, vasomodifiers and exercise can be employed to improve the vascular supply, following adequate evaluation by Doppler and other techniques. Appropriate invasive techniques and by-pass surgical procedures should be considered. Local debridement of the ulcerative site and adequate home-care, with the use of Betadine compresses, topical antibiotics and enzymes, and tissue stimulants, should be considered. Radiographs and bone scans should be ordered early on in the management process, to deal with infection at its first signs. Culture and sensitivity, appropriate antibiotic therapy, and hospitalization should be considered to prevent, where possible, amputation.

Asymptomatic diabetic elderly patients should be evaluated at least twice a year to identify problems at their earliest development. Patients with foot conditions requiring primary

Table 18.4 Diabetic clinical findings related to podiatric care

Risk factors
Aging
Tobacco use – smoking
Diabetes present for more than
  10 years
Decreased peripheral arterial
  pulses
Decreased peripheral sensation
Deformities
Hallux valgus
Hammertoes
Prominent metatarsal heads
Atrophy of plantar fat pad
Metatarsal head prolapse
History of prior foot ulcer
Sensory loss
Peripheral neuropathy
Peripheral vascular disease
Diabetic neuropathy
Limited joint mobility
Visual impairment
History of alcohol abuse
Inability to bend easily
Patients who live alone

Diabetic foot assessment
Change since last evaluation
Current or prior foot ulcer
Change in foot shape or size
Weakness
Thickened nails with or without
  subungual hematoma
Callus with or without hematoma
Pre-ulcer
Sensory change and level
Skin changes: redness, swelling,
  warmth, dryness, or maceration
Appropriate footwear for risk
  category
Clinical foot-care needs

Dermatologic findings
Painful or painless wounds
Slow healing or non-healing
  wounds
Necrosis
Skin color changes
Cyanosis
Redness
Chronic itching, scaling or dryness
Recurrent infections
Paronychia
Tinea pedis
Keratotic lesions with or without
  hemorrhage, either plantar or
  digital
Trophic ulcers
Diminished or absent hair
Trophic nail changes
Onychomycosis
Onychodystrophy
Onychogryphosis

Musculoskeletal findings
Gradual change in foot shape or
  size
Sudden, painless change in foot
  shape with swelling, without a
  history of trauma
Cavus feet with claw toes
Drop foot
Rocker bottom foot – Charcot's
  Foot
Neuropathic arthropathy
Elevated plantar pressure

Vascular findings
Cold feet
Intermittent claudication involving
  the calf or foot
Pain at rest, especially nocturnal,
  relieved by dependency
Dry, atrophic skin

Rubor of toes
Dystrophic toenails
Prolonged capillary filling time
Absent pedal, popliteal or femoral
  pulses
Femoral bruits
Dependent rubor with plantar
  pallor on elevation
Decreased skin temperature

Neurologic findings
Sensory
Burning
Tingling
Clawing sensations
Pain
Hypersensitivity
Sensory deficits
Vibratory
Proprioceptive
Pain
Temperature perception
Hyperesthesia
Motor
Weakness and foot drop
Diminished to absent deep tendon
  reflexes
Achilles then patellar, and
  weakness
Autonomic
Diminished sweating
Hypohidrosis
Well perfused, warm, apparently
  healthy foot on initial inspection
Foot pulses palpable with
  prominent dorsal foot veins
Diabetic dermoathy or pre-tibial
  lesions
Dry, thickened skin
Xerosis
Calluses under high pressure area
Intrinsic or minus foot

management should be assessed every 30–60 days, depending on the degree of complications. A multidisciplinary care approach, which includes the patient and his/her family is an essential element in managing the elderly diabetics with foot problems.

PRIMARY FOOT PROBLEMS AND THEIR MANAGEMENT

The management of localized foot problems in the diabetic patient[25] requires a review of the etiologic considerations, the symptoms presented by the patient, physical signs and clinical manifestations, and appropriate diagnostic studies, including the use of weight-bearing and non-weight-bearing radiographs, vascular studies, etc[25A]. Complications, sequelae, relevant treatment, the prognosis and overall management of the geriatric patient should reflect a reasonable approach, which will reduce pain, improve the functional capacity of the patient, maintain that restored function and provide for the comfort of the patient in his or her activities of daily living[26,27].

Onychia and paronychia

The onychial changes that occur in the elderly patient[28] are the result of new disease, or are the residual of long-term disease, injury, and/or functional modification. Onychia is an inflammation involving the posterior nail wall and nail bed. It is usually precipitated by local trauma or pressure, or is a complication of systemic diseases, such as diabetes, and is an early sign of a developing infection[29]. Mild erythema, swelling and pain are the most prevalent findings. Treatment should remove all pressure from the area, and tepid saline or other appropriate antiseptic compresses should be used for 15 min, three times per day. With systemic complications, systemic antibiotics should be instituted early, along with radiographs and scans to detect bone change at its earliest sign. Lambswool, tube foam or shoe modification should also be considered, to reduce pressure on the toe and nail.

If the onychia is not treated early, paronychia may develop, with significant infection and abscess of the posterior nail wall. The infection progresses proximally, and deeper structures become involved. The potential for osteomyelitis is greater in the presence of diabetes and vascular insufficiency. Necrosis, gangrene and the potential for amputation become reality.

Management includes establishing drainage, culture and sensitivity, radiographs and scans as appropriate, together with the use of Betadine compresses and appropriate systemic antibiotics. Early follow-up is essential as these conditions can result in significant problems in management.

Toenail deformities

Deformities of the toenails are the result of repeated micro-trauma, degenerative changes, or disease[30]. For example, the continued rubbing of the toenails over the years against the inferior toe box of the shoe is sufficient trauma to produce change. The initial thickening is termed onychauxis. Onychorrhexis, with accentuation of normal ridging, trophic changes, and longitudinal striations are onychopathic when related to disease and/or nutritional etiology. When debridement is not completed on a periodic basis, the nail structure elongates, continues to thicken and becomes deformed with shoe pressure. Onychogryphosis or 'rams horn nail' is usually complicated by fungal infection. The resultant disability can prevent the elderly from wearing shoes. Pain is usually associated with shoe pressure and the deformity. In addition, a traumatic avulsion of the nail is more frequent with this condition. The exaggerated curvature may even penetrate the skin, with resultant infection and ulceration[31–33].

Management should be directed towards periodic debridement of the onychial structures, both in length and thickness, with as little trauma as possible. The degree of onycholysis (freeing of the nail from the anterior edge) and onychoschezia (splitting), help determine the level of debridement. With the excess pressure of deformity, the nail grooves tend to become onychophosed (keratotic). When this occurs, debridement and the use of mild keratolytics and emollients, such as Keralyt Gel and 10% to 20% urea preparations, provide some measure of home-care for the patient. With onycholysis, subungual debris and keratosis develop, which increase discomfort and may generate pain. However, the patient may not present complaints of pain and discomfort, and care should be provided with the deformity. In addition, with degenerative changes, the sense of pain may be lost, which tends to defer care by the patient until a complicating condition is presented.

Similar changes can be demonstrated with vascular insufficiency, hemophelia, heart disease, chronic renal failure and chronic obstructive pulmonary disease, which also place these patients at risk of infection, necrosis, gangrene and possible amputation.

Toenail infections

The most common non-bacterial infection of the toenails is onychomycosis[34]. It is a chronic and communicable disease, and clinically may appear as distal subungual, white superficial, proximal subungual, total dystrophic and candida onychomycosis[35]. In the superficial variety[36], the changes appear on the superior surface of the toenail and generally do not invade the deeper structures. In the distal, proximal and total dystrophic manifestations, the nail-bed, as well as the nail-plate, are infected. There is usually some degree of onycholysis (freeing of the nail from the distal edge) and subungual keratosis. In the elderly, due to the long-standing chronic nature of this condition, the posterior nail-wall and eponychium demonstrate xerotic changes and hypertrophy, as does the nail-plate. Candida is most common in patients with some form of chronic mucocutaneous manifestation.

The diabetic patient usually presents with a chronic infection involving one or more of the nail-plates. The entire thickness of the nail-plate is usually involved, with resultant hypertrophy and deformity. Pain is usually not a significant factor, due to the normal lessening of sensation in the elderly, but can be present when the deformity becomes excessive, and is related to external pressure. Mycoticonychia, auto-avulsion, subungual hemorrhage, a foul, musty odor, and

degeneration of the nail plate are common findings. The most practical form of treatment in the elderly is one of management. Due to the chronicity of the condition and the fact that once the matrix of the nail is involved and hypertrophy and deformity occur, the residuals cannot be reversed. In addition, multiple drug use for disease and vascular impairment may limit systemic management. Periodic debridement, the use of 20–40% urea to aid in debridement, and the use of a topical fungicide in a solution to permit penetration provides the best approach to management; to be augmented with oral medication if indicated and if laboratory studies are completed within normal limits. Onychomycosis must be viewed as a chronic infectious disease, deserving management as any other chronic condition, such as diabetes itself.

Ingrown nails

Ingrown toenails are usually the end result of deformity and improper self-care. When the nail penetrates the skin, an abscess and infection result. If not managed early, periungual granulation tissue may form, which complicates treatment[81]. Deformity and involution are also complicating factors. In the early stage, a segment of the nail can easily be removed utilizing an English Nail Splitter and an onychotome, drainage is established, Betadine or saline compresses employed for 15 min, three times a day, and antibiotics utilized as indicated[37]. Measures should be taken to prevent the problem in the future. When granulation tissue is present, excision, fulgeration, desiccation, or the use of caustics, such as silver nitrate (75%) and astringents are employed to reduce the granulation tissue. In all cases, removal of the penetrating nail is primary. Partial excision of the nail plate and matrix can be completed utilizing regional anesthesia, followed by chemical cautery of the matrix area with e.g. CP Phenol. With this procedure, post-operative management includes isopropyl alcohol compresses and topical steroid solutions, three times per day to healing[37A].

With aging, there are also changes in the nail-plate, which, when viewed distally, appear 'C' shaped. This abnormal curvature is incurvation

Table 18.5 Risk categories related to management

Risk category	0	1	2	3
	Has a disease that leads to insensitivity	Does not have protective sensation	Does not have protective sensation	Does not have protective sensation
	Has protective sensation	Has not had a plantar ulcer	Has not had a plantar ulcer	Has a history of plantar ulcer
	Has not had a plantar ulcer	Does not have foot deformity	Does have foot deformity	
Management	Examine feet at each visit or at least four times per year	Examine feet at each visit or at least four times per year	Examine feet at each visit or at least four times per year with comprehensive assessment	Examine feet at each visit or at least four times per year
	Clinical care annually as needed	Clinical care every 6 months as needed	Custom molded orthotics/insoles	Clinical care every 1–2 months as needed
	Patient education	Soft orthotics/insoles, Plastazote, PPT, etc.	Prescription footwear	Custom molded shoes as needed
		Patient education	Patient education	Prescription footwear with appropriate orthotics/insoles
				Patient education

Key issues of preventive strategies	**Goals in management**
Peripheral neuropathy	Relieve areas of excessive plantar pressure
Peripheral vascular disease	Reduce shock
Limited joint mobility	Reduce shear
Elevated plantar pressures	Accommodate deformities
Bony deformities	Stabilize and support deformities
Hyperkeratosis	Limit joint motion
Diabetic onychopathy/onychodystrophy	Weight diffusion
Prior ulceration as risk	Weight dispersion

or involution. When present, the pressure of the nail-plate on the nail-bed and folds produces onychophosis (hyperkeratosis in the nail-folds) and discomfort, with complaints similar to an ingrown toenail. The condition may precipitate pressure ulcerations and infection. When this condition is severe, early and total removal of the nail plate and matrix should be considered, to avoid complications as the patient ages.

In all cases of suspected bone pathology, radiographs properly positioned to isolate the area of pathology will provide an appropriate diagnostic approach. Bilateral weight and non-weight bearing studies are indicated when management needs to be considered from both a static and dynamic phase[38]. Onychopathies that occur in the diabetic which are associated with cutaneous and systemic disease, are outlined in Table 18.5[39].

Alterations in the moisture content of the skin

A common problem in the older diabetic patient is dryness of the skin and xerosis[40]. This is due to a lack of hydration and lubrication, and, to some degree, is a part of the normal aging and degenerative process. There is usually some evidence of keratin dysfunction, which can be associated with xerosis. Fissures develop as a result of dryness and, when present on the heel, with associated stress present a potential hazard for the development of ulceration. Initial management includes the use of an emollient, following hydration of the skin. Twenty percent urea is helpful to aid as a mild and safe keratolytic. A plastic or styrofoam heel cup can be of assistance in minimizing trauma to the heel, thus reducing the potential for complications.

Pruritus is also a common complaint, and is usually more severe in the colder weather. It is related to dryness, scaliness, decreased skin secretions, keratin dysfunction, environmental changes and defatting of the skin, which is usually precipitated by the constant use of hot foot soaks. The patient will scratch, with excoriations noted on examination. Chronic tinea, allergic, neurogenic and/or emotional dermatoses should be considered as part of the differential diagnosis and treated accordingly. Management consists of hydration, lubrication, protection, topical steroids if indicated and judicious use of antihistamines in minimal doses to control the itching, which is usually the primary complaint. If excoriations are infected, proper antibiotic therapy should be instituted.

The etiology of hyperhidrosis and bromidrosis, when present, should be identified[41]. If local, measures should be taken to control the excessive perspiration and odor. Hydrogen peroxide, isopropyl alcohol and astringents may be used topically. Neomycin powder will help control the odor, by reducing the bacterial decomposition of perspiration. Recommendations on footwear and stocking modifications should be considered. Particular care should be provided in colder climates, as dampness can predispose a patient to the vasospastic effects of cold.

Contact dermatitis may be the result of reactions to chemicals used in shoe construction, foot-wear fabrics and/or stockings. Limited, and usually bilateral distribution of the skin lesions are clinical findings. Skin-testing can be employed to identify the primary irritant. The general principles of management include removing the primary irritant, mild wet dressings and the use of topical steroids. Stasis dermatitis is the usual residual of venous insufficiency and chronic ulceration. It is more common in patients with dependent edema. Management locally consists of elevation, mild wet dressings, topical steroids, antibiotics as indicated, and supportive measures needed in the management of venous disease

Skin infections

Pyodermas and superficial bacterial infections should be managed locally in a similar manner and, when present with tinea, treatment directed towards both etiologies[42]. Tinea pedis is often an extension of onychomycosis, which serves as a focus of infection. It also may be the focus of a secondary bacterial infection. It is more common in warmer weather, with the chronic keratotic type more common clinically in the elderly. Poor foot hygiene in many older patients, and the inability to see their feet, may motivate the patient to seek care only when the condition becomes clinically significant[43]. The wide variety of topical medications available can usually control this condition[44]. Solutions and/or creams (water washable or miscible) should be utilized when the patient is unable to easily remove an ointment base.

Other common dermatological manifestations that can be demonstrated in the elderly are those associated with atopic dermatitis, nummular eczema, neurodermatitis, and psoriasis, and are managed according to their etiology.

Skin ulcerations

Simple and/or hemorrhagic bullae are related to shoe trauma and friction, or to systemic diseases such as diabetes[45]. Management is directed towards eliminating pressure, protection and drainage when appropriate. Supportive dressings and shoe modifications should be employed as appropriate. It should be noted that gait changes in the elderly can magnify many of the foot to shoe-last incompatibilities that can result in local foot lesions. Hemorrhagic and bullae related to diabetes are usually early ulcerative indicators.

The management of ulcerations in the diabetic patient depends on the etiology and related complications associated with the problem[46]. General principles include supportive measures to reduce trauma and pressure to the ulcerated area, such as dressings, orthoses and shoe modifications, and special shoes (Extra Depth, Thermold, and custom molded shoes). The prevention and control of infection, and maintaining a clean, healthy base to permit healing are essential. The debridement of keratosis, when indicated, is essential to prevent roofing of the ulcer. The use of physical modalities and measures, such as low voltage therapy (contractile currents) and exercises can assist in improving the local vascular supply to the ulcer, and in helping to establish a clean base. Pressure ulcers of local origin are usually associated with a bony prominence, biomechanical abnormality, external trauma or as the result of stress associated with gait change[47].

Atrophy of soft tissue, and the residuals of arthritis, provide a focus for the development of ulcerations. Those associated with diabetes disease usually are related to neuropathic change, vascular insufficiency, infection and mechanical factors creating pressure. Management focuses on identifying the underlying diagnosis, local supportive measures, adequate treatment of the related systemic diseases, and efforts to minimize the potential for osteomyelitis, maintaining the ambulatory status of the patient for as long as possible.

Removing pressure from weight-bearing areas can be attained by the use of orthoses and/or shoe-last changes, and/or the use of pads, bars, wedges, and other corrections. Increasing the sole thickness, and using shock absorbing material, such as a Vibram or Ripple sole can be of assistance. The Plastazote or Aliplast sandal, and the Thermold Shoe can permit local treatment when conventional foot wear will not compensate for the condition.

The mechanical factors leading to ulceration, include the following[48]: body mass; tissue trauma; weight diffusion; weight dispersion; pathomechanics, i.e. structural changes in relation to function; biomechanics, i.e. forces that change and affect the foot in relation to function; and imbalance, i.e. the inability to adapt to alterations of stress. Stress can be evaluated as:

- Force: an alteration in physical condition, shape or position
- Compression stress: one force moves towards another
- Tensile stress: pulling away of one part against another
- Shearing stress: gliding of one part on the other
- Friction: the force needed to overcome resistance and usually associated with a sheering stress
- Elasticity: weight diffusion and weight dispersion
- Fluid pressure: soft tissue adaptation and conformity to stress
- Mechanical stress (micro and macro trauma)
- Systemic stress: disease
- Adaptation: neurologic and vascular systems
- Other chronic diseases.

Other issues include vertical force; shear stress; time, i.e. the number of repetitions to which the foot is subjected; the relationship between focal high foot pressure and ulceration, and repetitive stress, i.e. micro trauma.

Diabetic patients, especially those with neuropathy, expose themselves to the potential for foreign bodies and foot injury. They should always wear proper foot protection and not go barefoot. Some foreign bodies will cause ulcerations and injuries, others may require debridement and/or excision to relieve pain.

Hyperkeratotic lesions

A common complaint of most diabetic patients are the many forms of hyperkeratotic lesions, such as tyloma (callous) and heloma (corn) and their varieties, such as hard, soft, vascular, neurofibrous, seed and subungual[49,50].

Intractable keratoma, ecrine poroma, porokeratosis, and verruca must be differentiated from these keratotic lesions, although each may present initially as a hyperkeratotic area. The biomechanical and pathomechanical factors that help create these problems are those associated with stress, i.e., compressive, tensile and/or shearing. The loss of soft tissue as part of the aging process, and atrophy of the plantar fat-pad increase pain and limit ambulation. Contractures, gait changes, deformities and the residuals of arthritis are all additional factors that need to be considered in management. The incompatibility of the foot-type (in-flare, straight or out-flare) to the shoe-last is another factor to be considered. It is important to recognize that there is usually not just one factor, but a multiplicity of conditions, including skin tone and elasticity, which result in the development of keratotic lesions in the elderly. Their management is not routine, and the term management signifies a period of continuing care, as with any other chronic condition in the elderly, to provide for ambulation and comfort. Mechanical keratosis can also be classified and stratified as follows[16,51].

The foot deformities are precipitating factors to foot to shoe-last incompatibilities, which produce excessive pressure on segments of the foot. Management and treatment should be directed towards the functional needs of the patients and on their activity needs for daily living. Considerations include debridement, padding, emollients, shoe modifications and last changes, orthoses and surgical revision, as indicated. Materials to provide soft tissue replacement, weight dispersion and weight diffusion are also indicated. It is also important to recognize that keratotic lesions of long-standing represent a hyperplastic and hypertrophic pathology, and that even when weight-bearing is removed, they tend to persist. In a sense, hyperkeratotic lesions are a form of body protection against pressure, and are symptoms of an abnormal state. If permitted to persist, enlarge and condense, they become primary irritants. With pressure, such as weight bearing and ambulation, they produce local avascularity, which can precipitate ulceration and their resultant sequelae.

Foot ulcers usually begin with subkeratotic hemorrhage. Once debrided and managed properly, they usually heal, but may be repetitive, unless adequate measures are instituted to reduce the pressure to the localized areas of ulceration. Even with all measures, the problem may persist due to residual deformity and systemic diseases, such as diabetes. Thus management and monitoring similar to any other chronic condition can have a significant impact on the social elements of society, for without ambulation, the diabetic and, in particular, the older diabetic patient is clearly institutionalized.

Biomechanical and pathomechanical abnormalities

The above deformities create functional problems in relation to gait and obtaining adequate footwear[52]. Treatment consists of both non-surgical and surgical considerations. Disease and age themselves should not be the final determining factor in considering surgery. What is important is to determine what can be done to maintain the quality-of-life for the patient[53]. Consideration must also be given to the patient's ability to adapt, to change in relation to ambulation, for to have an anatomically corrected joint, and a patient that cannot ambulate without pain, defeats the treatment needs of the elderly.

Conservative modalities include shoe-last changes, shoe modifications, orthoses, digital braces, physical medicine, exercises, and mild analgesics for pain. The residuals of these deformities can produce inflammatory changes[54], such as periarthritis, bursitis, myositis, synovitis, neuritis, tendonitis, sesamoiditis, and plantar myofasciitis, which need to be managed medically, physically and mechanically to keep the patient ambulatory and pain free.

Fractures of the foot and toes may be the result of direct trauma and/or stress, related to bone loss[55]. Most uncomplicated and closed fractures that are in good position can be managed with the use of a surgical shoe and supportive dressings, as long as the joints distally and proximally are immobilized[56]. Silicone molds can be utilized for digital fractures, and their use maintains position through healing, permitting the patient to maintain proper hygiene.

Shoe modifications that can be considered for the elderly[47] include mild calcaneal wedges, to limit motion and alter gait; metatarsal bars, to transfer weight; Thomas Heels to increase calcaneal support; long shoe counters to increase mid-foot support and control foot direction; heel flares to add stability; shank fillers or wedges to produce a total weight-bearing surface; steel plates to restrict motion; and rocker bars to prevent flexion and extension. Additional internal modifications include longitudinal arch pads, wedges, bars, lifts, and tongue or bite pads. Available orthoses include the rigid, semi-rigid and flexible varieties, using materials such as plastic, leather, laminates, polyurethane, sponge or foam rubber, Korex, felt, latex, wood flour, Plastazote, Aliplast, and silicone, to provide support, reduce pressure, and give weight diffusion and dispersion[57].

Diabetic ulcers—general principles

Diabetic patients are more likely to develop foot-related ulcers. About 15% of patients progress to ulceration and are 12 times more likely to undergo amputation than the non-diabetic patient[58]. Neuropathy significantly increases the risk of ulceration and, combined with ischemia, has a significantly greater potential for hospital admission than the non-diabetic patient[59]. Diabetic complications in the foot represent the leading cause of amputation. Diabetic patients are at greater risk for ulceration and amputation following minor trauma, are more likely to have a second amputation within 3 years of the first, and the real cost is difficult to estimate in terms of the quality-of-life. What is clear is that 50–75% of most foot ulcerations can be prevented with proper education, early assessment and risk stratification, primary preventive care and appropriate management of the ulcer and its complications[60].

The management of the diabetic ulcer includes a history of the duration, prior ulcer, pain, sensory deficit, vascular status and prior treatment[61]. The ulcer should be evaluated as to etiology, size, depth, and the involvement of deeper structures. The ulcer should be classified utilizing one or more of the current recognized categories. Infection should be ruled out, taking particular note of purulent exudate, necrosis, sinus tracts, odor, edema, cellulitis, abscess and fluctuation. Systemic signs of infection also include elevated temperature, fever and chills. Radiologic studies should be completed to exclude subcutaneous gas, the presence of a foreign body, osteomyelitis or a Charcot's foot[62]. Standard radiographs may also demonstrate periosteal resorption and osteolysis. A baseline radiograph, taken to determine biomechanical and pathomechanical changes, provides a good comparison to demonstrate change. Bone scans, magnetic resonance imaging (MRI), and computed tomography (CT) should be ordered as indicated. Cultures, antibiotics, wound care, metabolic control, evaluating the vascular status and off-loading pressure are all initial determining factors and part of a multidisciplinary approach to management[63].

For the non-infected ulcer, the general foot examination, sensory, vascular and ulcer evaluations are important initial approaches[64]. Wound-care includes debridement, drainage, dressings, total antibiotics and growth factors, and grafts. Off-loading procedures include total contact casts, cam walkers, braces, surgical shoes, crutches, and other procedures to limit weight-bearing at the ulcerative site. Once healed, measures must continue to prevent recurrence; these include surveillance, re-evaluation and pressure reduction measures, including patient education and compliance. For non-healing ulcers, surgical approaches should be considered for both vascular and deformity considerations.

Diabetic foot infections should be evaluated to include a history of trauma, puncture wound, foreign body, fever, chills, nausea, general malaise and ulceration[65]. Drainage, swelling, erythema, pain, sensory loss and elevated blood sugars need to be addressed. The initial determination for an infection, with or without ulceration, is to determine if the problem is limb threatening, or non-limb threatening.

For the non-limb threatening infection, the clinical presentation includes cellulitis, usually a superficial ulcer that does not probe to bone, no bone or joint involvement, a mild infection with no systemic toxicity or significant ischemia[66,67]. Diagnostic procedures include cultures and tissue specimens, diagnostic imaging such as radiography, MRI and nuclear scans as indicated, and appropriate blood laboratory studies.

Management includes debridement of necrotic and keratotic tissue, appropriate off-loading and pressure reduction, wound care and dressings, antibiotic coverage modified by culture results, outpatient management, wound care and dressings, hospitalization if the foot does not improve, with management to healing with appropriate shoes, orthotics, braces and education as needed.

For the limb-threatening infection, lymphangitis, edema, fever, odor, deep ulceration, drainage, systemic toxicity and ischemia may all be noted. Diagnostic procedures include deep cultures and tissue samples, diagnostic imaging including X-ray, MRI, nuclear, bone, and leukocyte scans, and arteriography, blood cultures and studies, renal and hepatic profiles as appropriate, and medical management of the patient's diabetes. Management includes hospital admission; surgical debridement; drainage; wound packing and care; appropriate antibiotic therapy, empiric and as determined by culture; long-term antibiotic management as appropriate; resection of osteomyelitis; reconstructive procedures; and general principles associated with ulcer management.

Charcot foot (neurotrophic osteoarthropathy)[68] is a progressive condition characterized by joint dislocation, pathologic fractures, debilitating deformity and changes that may be progressive or static[69]. Trauma, and in particular repetitive trauma, may precipitate the development of Charcot with sensory deficits that reduce pain and remove the natural protective mechanisms. The clinical diagnosis includes swelling, increased skin temperature, erythema, deformity, joint effusion, bone resorption, possible ulceration and advanced neuropathy and sensory loss. Radiographs and other imaging procedures are indicated on a serial basis given the complications that develop rapidly. Management includes weight-bearing restriction with crutches or wheelchairs; immobilization with splints, casts, or walkers until the acute phase becomes quiescent; appropriate footwear, orthotics, insoles and braces; and management of any related ulceration or infection (Table 18.6)[70].

Table 18.6 Therapeutic shoes and multidensity orthoses
1) A history of diabetes mellitus
2) Management under a comprehensive plan for diabetes and that shoe are needed and
3) Document that the patient has one or more of the following conditions
a) Peripheral neuropathy with evidence of callus formation
b) History of pre-ulcerative calluses
c) History of previous ulceration
d) Foot deformity
e) Previous amputation of the foot or part of the foot, or
f) Poor circulation

A sample comprehensive podogeriatric and chronic disease assessment protocol is given in the Appendix[71–73]. This protocol or index was developed under contract to the Pennsylvania Department of Health to Temple University School of Podiatric Medicine, in cooperation with the Pennsylvania Diabetes Academy (Project Director: Arthur E. Helfand).

CONCLUSION

Much of the ability to remain ambulatory for diabetic patients is directly related to foot health[74]. In order to accomplish this aim, practitioners must think comprehensively, and recognize that team-care must be an essential part of patient care[75,76]. Foot health education, such as the programs developed by the Pennsylvania Diabetes Academy ('Feet First' and 'If The Shoe Fits')[77], are available to both patients and professionals, and should be employed as a part of all diabetic patient education[78]. With the high prevalence and incidence of foot problems in the diabetic patient, much of their quality-of-life will depend on their ability to manage their diseases, remain mentally alert and ambulatory.

REFERENCES

1 National Institute of Health. *Prevent diabetes problems—keep your feet and skin healthy*. Bethesda, MD: National Institute of Health, 2000.

2 Bolton AJM, Connor H, Cavanagh PR. *The foot in diabetes*. 3rd edn. Chichester: John Wiley and Sons Ltd, 2000.

3 Bowker JH, Pfeifer MA. *Levin's and Oneal's the diabetic foot*. 6th edn. St Louis, MO: Mosby, 2001.

4 Cavanagh PR, Boone EY, Plummer DL. *The foot in diabetes: a bibliography*. Pennsylvania, PA: State University, State College, 2000.

5 Davidson JK. *Clinical diabetes mellitus*. 3rd edn. New York, NY: Thieme Inc., 1999.

6 Davidson MB. *Diabetes mellitus, diagnosis and treatment*. 4th edn. Philadelphia, PA: WB Saunders Co., 1998.

7 Mayfield JA, Reiber GE, Sanders LJ *et al. Diabetes Care* 1988;21:2161–77.

8 Bild DE *et al.* Lower extremity amputation in people with diabetes, epidemiology and prevention. *Diabetes Care* 1989;12:23–31.

9 American Diabetes Association. *Therapy for diabetes and related disorders*. Alexandria, VA: American Diabetes Association, 1991.

10 Brody SJ, Pawlson LG. *Aging and rehabilitation II, the state of the practice*. New York: Springer Publishing, 1990.

11 Calkins E, Davis PJ, Ford AB, Amasa B. editors. *The practice of geriatrics*. Philadelphia, PA: WB Saunders, 1986.

12 Sanders LJ. *The philatelic history of diabetes*. Alexandria, VA: American Diabetes Association, 2001.

13 McDermott JE. *The diabetic foot*. Rosemont, IL: American Academy of Orthopedic Surgeons, 1995.

14 American Diabetes Association. Preventive foot care in people with diabetes. *Diabetes Care* 2001;24(Suppl 1):556–7.

15 Benvenuti F, Ferrucci L, Gurlink JM *et al.* Foot pain and disability in older persons, an epidemiologic survey. *J Am Geriatr Soc* 1995;43:479.

16 Robbins JM. *Primary podiatric medicine*. Philadelphia, PA: WB Saunders Co., 1994.

17 Dyck PJ, Thomas PK. *Diabetic neuropathy*. 2nd edn. Philadelphia, PA: WB Saunders Co., 1991.

18 Tollafield DR, Merriman. *Clinical skills in treating the foot*. New York, NY: Churchill Livingstone, 1997.

18A Merriman LM, Tollafield DR. *Assessment of the lower limb*. New York, NY: Churchill Livingstone, 1995.

19 Lorimer D, French G, West S. *Neale's common foot disorders, diagnosis and management*. 5th edn. New York: Churchill Livingstone, 1997.

20 Eisdorfer C, editor. *Annual review of gerontology and geriatrics*. Vol. 4. New York: Springer Publishing Co., 1984.

21 Evans J, Grimley W, Franklin T *et al. Oxford textbook of geriatric medicine*. 2nd edn. Oxford, UK: Oxford University Press, 2000.

22 Scardinia RJ. Diabetic foot problems, assessment and prevention. *Clin Diabetes* 1983; 1:1–7.

23 Frykberg RG. Team approach toward lower extremity amputation prevention in diabetes. *J Am Podiatr Med Assoc* 1997;87:305–12.

24 Frykberg RG. *The high risk foot in diabetes mellitus*. New York: Churchill Livingstone, 1991.

25 Alexander IJ. *The foot, examination and diagnosis*. 2nd edn. New York, NY: Churchill Livingstone, 1997.

25A Collet BS. *Foot problems, the Merck manual of geriatrics*. Rahway, NJ: Merck and Co. Inc., 1990.

26 Sammarco GJ. *The foot in diabetes*. Philadelphia, PA: Lea and Febiger, 1991.

27 Sammarco GJ, Cooper PS. *Foot and ankle manual*. Baltimore, MD: Williams and Wilkins, 1998.

28 Helfand AE, editor. *Clinical podogeriatrics*. Baltimore, MD: Williams and Wilkins, 1981.

29 Samman PD, Fenton DA. *The nails in disease*. 4th edn. London UK: William Heinemann Medical Books, 1986.

30 Brenner MA. *Management of the diabetic foot*. Baltimore, MD: Williams and Wilkins, 1987.

31 Baran R, Dawber RPR, Tosti A, Haneke E. *A text atlas of nail disorders, diagnosis and treatment*. St Louis: Mosby, 1996.

32 Baran R, Hay R, Haneke E *et al. Onychomycosis, the current approach to diagnosis and therapy*. London: Martin Dunitz, 1999.

33 Beaven DW, Brooks SE. *Color atlas of the nail in clinical diagnosis*. Chicago, IL: Year Book Medical Publishers, Inc., 1984.

34 McCarthy DJ, editor. *Podiatric dermatology*. Baltimore, MD: Williams and Wilkins, 1986.

35 Meers MH, Berkow R. *The Merck manual of diagnosis and therapy*. 17th edn. Whitehouse Station, NJ: Merck and Co., 1999.

36 Neale D, Adams I, editors. *Common foot disorders, diagnosis and management*. 2nd edn. Edinburgh: Churchill Livingstone, 1985.

37 Pathy MSJ. *Principles and practice of geriatric medicine*. 3rd edn. Chichester, UK: John Wiley and Sons, 1998.

37A Yale JF. *Yale's podiatric medicine.* 3rd edn. Baltimore, MD: Williams and Wilkins, 1987.

38 Sims DS, Canvanagh P, Ulbrecht JS. Risk factors in the diabetic foot, recognition and management. *Phys Ther* 1988;68:1887–902.

39 Peterson KA, editor. Advances in managing the diabetic foot. *Journal of Family Practice* 2000; 49(11):S1–S48.

40 Dauber R, Bristow I, Turner W. *Text atlas of podiatric dermatology.* London: Martin Dunitz, 2001.

41 Harkless LB, Krych SM. *Handbook of common foot problems.* New York: Churchill Livingstone, 1990.

42 Witkowski JA, editor. *Diseases of the lower extremities.* Clinics in Dermatology, Vol. 1, No. 1. Philadelphia, PA: Lippincott, 1983.

43 Finucane P, Sinclair AJ. *Diabetes in old age.* Chichester: John Wiley and Sons, 1995.

44 Samitz MH. *Cutaneous disorders of the lower extremities.* 2nd edn. Philadelphia, PA: JB Lippincott Co., 1981.

45 Wieman TJ. Diabetic foot ulcers: epidemiology, current management, and new treatment strategies. Am J Surg 1998:176 (2A Suppl.):1S–82S.

46 Pinzur MS, Slovenkai M, Trepman E. Guidelines for diabetic foot care. *Foot Ankle Int* 1999;20:696–702.

47 Helfand AE, Bruno J, editor. *Rehabilitation of the foot.* Clinics in podiatry. Vol. 1, No. 2. Philadelphia, PA: WB Saunders Co., 1984.

48 Williams TF, editor. *Rehabilitation in the aging.* New York, NY: Raven Press, 1984.

49 Helfand AE, editor. *The geriatric patient and considerations of aging.* Clinics in podiatric medicine and surgery. Philadelphia, PA: WB Saunders Co., 1993.

50 Helfand AE. *The foot—geriatric overview.* Part I: 3: 58, 1993 and Part II: 5: 19, 1995.

51 Reichel W, editor. *Clinical aspects of aging.* 3rd edn. Baltimore, MD: Williams and Wilkins, 1989.

52 Birrer RB, Dellacorte MP, Grisafi PJ. *Common foot problems in primary care.* 2nd edn. Philadelphia: Henley and Belfus, Inc, 1998.

53 Jessett DF, Helfand AE. In: Pathy MSJ editor. *Foot problems in the elderly, principles and practice of geriatric medicine.* 2nd edn. Edinburgh: John Wiley and Sons, 1991.

54 Cailliet R. *Foot and ankle pain.* 3rd edn. Philadelphia, PA: FA Davis Co., 1997.

55 Hurwitz SR, Wiesel SW. *Foot and ankle pain.* New York, NY: Lexis Publishing, 1988.

56 Yale I, Yale JF. *The arthritic foot and related connective tissue disorders.* Baltimore, MD: Williams and Wilkins, 1984.57 Dahmen R, Haspels R,

Koomen N, Hoeksma AM. Therapeutic footwear for the neuropathic foot. *Diabetes Care* 2001;24:705–9.

58 American College of Foot and Ankle Surgeons. *Diabetic foot disorders—a clinical practice guideline.* Park Ridge, IL: American College of Foot and Ankle Surgeons, 2000.

59 Sanders LJ. *Diabetic foot ulcers and amputations.* Alexandria, VA: American Diabetes Association, 2001.

60 Armstrong DG, Lavery LA. Diabetic foot ulcers: prevention, diagnosis and classification. *Am Fam Phys* 1998;March 15:1325–37.

61 American Diabetes Association. Consensus Development Conference on Diabetic Foot Wound Care. *Diabetes Care* 1999;22:1354–60.

62 Jahss MH, editor. *Diseases of the foot.* Philadelphia, PA: WB Saunders Co., 1982.

63 Veves A, Falanga V. *Diabetic foot ulcers: prevention and treatment.* Wounds Vol. 12, No. 6, Suppl B. Wayne, PA: HMP Communications, 2000.

64 Shaw KM. *Diabetic complications.* Chichester: John Wiley and Sons, 1996.

65 Levin ME, O'Neal LW, Bowker JH, editor. *The diabetic foot.* 5th edn. St Louis, MO: The C V Mosby Co., 1993.

66 Kozak GP, Hoar CS Jr, Rowbotham JL *et al. Management of the diabetic foot.* Philadelphia, PA: WB Saunders Co., 1984.

67 Kozakm GP, Campbell DR, Frykbert RG *et al. Management of diabetic foot problems.* 2nd edn. Philadelphia, PA: WB Saunders Co., 1995.

69 Levin ME. *Foot complications due to diabetes.* Harrisburg, PA: Pennsylvania Diabetes Academy, 1996.

68 Klenerman L, editor. *The foot and its disorders.* 3rd edn. London: Blackwell Scientific Publications, 1991.

70 Helfand AE. What you need to know about therapeutic footwear. *Pract Diabetol* 1996;15:4–9.

71 Helfand AE, Jessett, DF. In: Pathy MSJ, editor. *Foot problems, principles and practice of geriatric medicine.* 3rd edn. Edinburgh: John Wiley and Sons, 1998.

72 Helfand AE. Public health strategies to develop a comprehensive chronic disease and podogeriatric protocol. *Natl Acad Pract Forum* 1999;1:49–57.

73 Helfand AE. *Health care strategies to assess the older 'at risk' patient with foot problems related to diabetes mellitus and comprehensive podogeriatric assessment.* Harrisburg, PA: Pennsylvania Diabetes Academy, 2001

74 Ahroni JH. 101 Foot care tips for people with

diabetes. Alexandria, VA: American Diabetes Association, 2000.

75 Helfand AE. *Feet first*. Harrisburg, PA: Pennsylvania Diabetes Academy, 1995.

76 Helfand AE. *If the shoe fits*. Harrisburg, PA: Pennsylvania Diabetes Academy, 1998.

77 US Department of Health and Human Services. *Feet first*. USPHS, NIH, No. 0–388–126, USGPO, 1970.

78 Helfand AE, editor. *Public health and podiatric medicine*. Baltimore: Williams and Wilkins, 1987.

APPENDIX

Podogeriatric Assessment and Chronic Disease Protocol

Date of Service .... MR # ....

Patient Name .... Date of Birth .... Social Security # ....

Address .... City .... State................. Zip Code ....

Sex M F   Race B W A L N/A   Weight .... lbs   Height ....in   Marital Status M S W D Sep

Name of Primary Physician/Health Care Facility .... Date of Last Visit ....

HISTORY OF PRESENT ILLNESS

__Swelling of Feet	__Infections	__Duration
__Painful Feet	__Cold Feet	__Context
__Hyperkeratosis	__Other	__Modifying Factors
__Onychial Changes	__Location	__Associated Signs & Symptoms
__Bunions	__Quality	
__Painful Toe Nails	__Severity	

PAST HISTORY

__Heart Disease	__Thyroid	__Hypercholesterol
__High Blood Pressure	__Allergy	__Gout
__Arthritis	__Diabetes Mellitus*	__History: Smoking: OH
__*Circulatory Disease	__IDDM __NIDDM	__Family – Social

SYSTEM REVIEW

__Constitutional	__Hematologic	__Neurologic
__ENT	__Card/Vasc	__Endocrine
__Eyes	__Musculo-Skeletal	__GI
__Skin/Hair	__GYN	__Immunologic
__Respiratory	__Lymphatic	
Psychiatric	GU	

MEDICATIONS

DERMATOLOGIC

__*Hyperkeratosis	__Onychodystrophy	__Hematoma
__Onychauxis B-2-b	__*Cyanosis	__Rubor
__Infection	__Xerosis	__*Preulcerative
__*Ulceration	__Tinea Pedis	__Discolored
__Onychomycosis	__Verruca	

FOOT ORTHOPEDIC

__*Hallux Valgus	__*Pes Valgoplanus	__*Prominent Met Head
__*Anterior Imbalance	__*Pes Cavus	__*Charcot Joints
__*Digiti Flexus	__*Hallux Rigidus Limitus	__ Other
__*Pes Planus	__*Morton's Syndrome Bursitis	

VASCULAR EVALUATION

__ *Coldness	C-2	__ *Night Cramps		__ *Amputation	
__ *Trophic Changes	B-2-a	__ *Edema	C-3	__ *AKA BKA FF T	A-1
__ *DP Absent	B-3	__ *Claudication	C-1	__ Atrophy	B-2-d
__ *PT Absent	B-1	__ Varicosities			

NEUROLOGIC EVALUATION

__ *Achilles	__ *Paresthesia	C-4	__ *Burning	C-5
__ *Vibratory	__ Superficial Plantar		__ Other	
__ *Sharp/Dull	__ *Joint Position			

RISK CATEGORY – NEUROLOGIC

__ - 0 = No Sensory Loss	__ * 2 = Sensory Loss & Foot Deformity
__ * I = Sensory Loss	__ * 3 = Sensory Loss, Hx Ulceration & Deformity

RISK CATEGORY – VASCULAR

__ 0 - 0 No Change	__ * I - 4 Ischemic Rest Pain
__ * I - 1 Mild Claudication	__ * II - 5 Minor Tissue Loss
__ * I - 2 Moderate Claudication	__ * III - 6 Major Tissue Loss
__ * I - 3 Severe Claudication	

CLASS FINDINGS

__ A1	Nontraumatic Amputation		__ B2e	Skin Color (rubor or redness)
__ B1	Absent Posterior Tibial		__ B3	Absent Dorsalis Pedis
__ B2	Advanced Trophic Changes		__ C1	Claudication
__ B2a	Hair Growth (decrease or absent)		__ C2	Temperature Changes (cold)
__ B2b	Nail Changes (thickening)		__ C3	Edema
__ B2c	Pigmentary Changes (discoloration)		__ C4	Paresthesia
__ B2d	Skin Texture (thin, shiny)		__ C5	Burning

Onychomycosis: Documentation of mycosis/dystrophy causing secondary infection and/or pain which result or would result in marked limitation of ambulation.

Discoloration	Onycholysis
Hypertrophy	Secondary Infection
Subungual Debris	Limitation of Ambulation and Pain

CLASSIFICATION OF MECHANICAL OR PRESSURE HYPERKERATOSIS

Grade	Description
0	No Lesion
1	No specific Tyloma Plaque, but diffuse or pinch Hyperkeratotic tissue present or in narrow bands.
2	Circumscribed, Punctate oval, or circular, well defined thickening of Kertinized Tissue
3	Heloma Milliare or Heloma Durum with no associated Tyloma
4	Well defined Tyloma Plaque with a definite Heloma within the Lesion
5	Extravasation, Maceration and early breakdown of structures under the Tyloma or Callus Layer
6	Complete breakdown of structure of Hyperkeratotic Tissue, Epidermis, extending to superficial Dermal involvement

PLANTAR KERATOMATA PATTERN

LT   1   2   3   4   5   RT   1   2   3   4   5

ULCER CLASSIFICATION
Grade - 0 - Absent Skin Lesions
Grade - 1 - Dense Callus but not Pre-Ulcer or Ulcer
Grade - 2 - Preulcerative Changes
Grade - 3 - Partial Thickness (Superficial Ulcer)
Grade - 4 - Full Thickness (deep) Ulcer but no involvement of Tendon, Bone, Ligament or Joint
Grade - 5 - Full Thickness (deep) Ulcer with involvement of Tendon, Bone, Ligament or Joint
Grade - 6 - Localized Infection (Abscess or Osteomyelitis)
Grade - 7 - Proximal spread of Infection (Ascending Cellulitis or Lymphadenopathy)
Grade - 8 - Gangrene of Forefoot only
Grade - 9 - Gangrene of Majority of Foot

ONYCHIAL GRADES AT RISK
Grade I   Normal   Grade IV Hypertrophic
Grade II   Mild Hypertrophy   Deformed
Grade III Hypertrophic   Onychogryphosis
           Dystrophic   Dystrophic
           Onychauxis   Mycotic
           Mycotic   Infected
           Infected
           Onychodysplasia

FOOTWEAR SATISFACTORY   ## HYGIENE SATISFACTORY
Yes   No   Yes   No

STOCKINGS: Nylon   Cotton   Wool   Other   None

ASSESSMENT

PLAN
__Podiatric Referral   __Medical Referral   __Vascular Studies   __Imaging
__Patient Education   __Special Footwear   __Clinical Lab   __Rx

19

Gastrointestinal and autonomic complications of diabetes mellitus

Adrian Vella and Michael Camilleri

INTRODUCTION

Gastrointestinal function is controlled in part by the vast extrinsic and intrinsic nervous systems. Extrinsic neural control is exerted by the parasympathetic and sympathetic nervous system, the autonomic nervous system. Intrinsic control is imposed by the enteric plexuses (the 'little brain' in the digestive tract) (Figure 19.1). Experimental models of gut motor function suggest a predominant modulatory role for the extrinsic nervous system, and primary control through the enteric nervous system[2]. Thus, derangements of the extrinsic nerves at any level may result in alterations of gastrointestinal motility and secretion[3].

Intrinsic control can occur quite independently of extrinsic control. The enteric nervous system consists of 100 million neurons that are organized in ganglionated plexi, including the submucous plexus (involved in absorption and secretion), myenteric plexus (involved in motility), and plexus of Cajal (which serves pacemaking functions). As with the somatic and autonomic nerves elsewhere, the gut's autonomic and enteric nervous system can be affected in diabetes mellitus.

Gastrointestinal (GI) tract symptoms are common in patients with diabetes seen at tertiary referral centers (Figure 19.2). In the absence of structural lesions in the gut, such patients are commonly assumed to have autonomic neuropathy. This is not unreasonable,

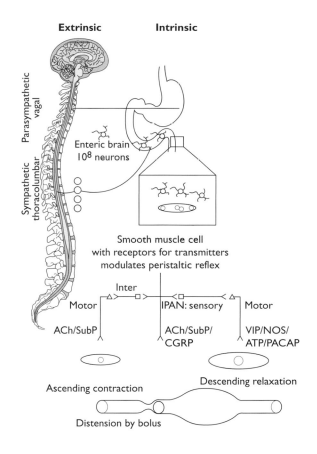

Figure 19.1 Control of gastrointestinal motility. Note the extrinsic or autonomic nervous system modulates the function of the enteric nervous system, which controls smooth muscle cells through transmitters. Adapted from Camilleri M, Phillips SF[1].

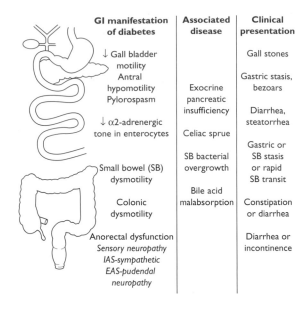

GI manifestation of diabetes	Associated disease	Clinical presentation
↓ Gall bladder motility		Gall stones
Antral hypomotility Pylorospasm	Exocrine pancreatic insufficiency	Gastric stasis, bezoars
↓ α2-adrenergic tone in enterocytes	Celiac sprue	Diarrhea, steatorrhea
Small bowel (SB) dysmotility	SB bacterial overgrowth	Gastric or SB stasis or rapid SB transit
Colonic dysmotility	Bile acid malabsorption	Constipation or diarrhea
Anorectal dysfunction Sensory neuropathy IAS-sympathetic EAS-pudendal neuropathy		Diarrhea or incontinence

Figure 19.2 Gastrointestinal manifestations of diabetes mellitus. Adapted from Camilleri[4].

since autonomic neuropathy is a common complication of diabetes. Although microvascular complications are less frequent in type 2 diabetes, compared with type 1 diabetes, the prevalence of autonomic neuropathy among type 2 diabetics is still significant. The degree of glycemic control affects the incidence and progression of neuropathic complications, including gastrointestinal neuropathy. Moreover, since the rate of gastric emptying and the nature of the ingested meal are important determinants of postprandial glucose concentrations, altered gastric emptying may impact on the ability to achieve good glycemic control in people with diabetes.

Gastrointestinal involvement is frequently associated with autonomic dysregulation of the eyes, blood pressure, heart and peripheral vessels and the urinary bladder and sexual organs. This chapter focuses on the gastrointestinal manifestations of diabetes mellitus; advances in understanding the mechanism and role of autonomic, enteric and hormonal dysfunctions; the autonomic symptoms and

tests that are indicative of autonomic denervation; and management of gastrointestinal manifestations of diabetes.

DEFINITIONS: DIABETIC ENTEROPATHY, GASTROPARESIS, DYSPEPSIA, DIARRHEA, INCONTINENCE

Gastrointestinal symptoms are frequently encountered in patients with diabetes. Diabetic enteropathy refers to all the gastrointestinal complications of diabetes, and may result in dysphagia, heartburn, nausea and vomiting, abdominal pain, constipation, diarrhea, and fecal incontinence[5]. Feldman and Schiller reported that 76% of referrals to a diabetic clinic had at least one gastrointestinal symptom[5]. Clouse also reported that GI symptoms were present in a high proportion (20%) of diabetic patients on the registry of a General Clinical Research Center[6]. A third study from a tertiary care center reported an increased incidence of GI symptoms in patients with diabetes, compared with control subjects[7]. However, in the Rochester Diabetic Neuropathy Study[8], only 1% of patients had symptoms of gastroparesis, and only 0.6% had nocturnal diarrhea. This discrepancy has been addressed in community-based epidemiological studies, which are discussed below.

Kassender recognized asymptomatic gastric retention in diabetics in 1958[9] and coined the term 'gastroparesis diabeticorum'. Since the original report, the term gastroparesis has been used to reflect symptomatic as well as asymptomatic gastric retention. More recently, the term 'diabetic dyspepsia' was used to reflect the spectrum of postprandial symptoms in diabetics that are attributable to upper gastrointestinal dysfunction, including those associated with delayed gastric emptying[10]. Thus, while nausea, vomiting and early satiation after meals were the classical symptoms of gastroparesis, the term diabetic dyspepsia also reflects bloating, fullness and pain in the upper abdomen[10].

Constipation among diabetic patients reflects the common etiologies: impaired rectal evacuation, slow transit or normal transit constipation[11].

The extrinsic parasympathetic supply to the colon forms the ascending intracolonic nerves, and is a major excitatory mechanism inducing transit of stool in the colon.

The pathogenesis of chronic diarrhea in patients with diabetes is incompletely understood. Several mechanisms may contribute to the development of the condition, including anorectal dysfunction, intestinal dysmotility, abnormal intestinal secretion, bacterial overgrowth, bile acid diarrhea and exocrine pancreatic insufficiency[12]. Celiac disease, which has been reported with increased frequency in type 1 diabetes, may also contribute to diarrhea.

The term 'diabetic diarrhea' was first coined in 1936 by Bargen[13] at the Mayo Clinic to describe unexplained diarrhea associated with severe diabetes. Typically, patients with diabetic diarrhea have poorly controlled diabetes and evidence of diabetic neuropathy, usually peripheral neuropathy and frequently autonomic neuropathy. Diarrhea is often nocturnal and may be associated with anal incontinence. Episodes of diarrhea may alternate with constipation or normal bowel movements. Symptoms of delayed gastric emptying, such as early satiety, nausea and vomiting, are often experienced by such patients with diarrhea.

Fecal incontinence is experienced by a substantial percentage of patients with chronic diabetes referred to tertiary referral centers. This does not necessarily correlate with the presence of diarrhea, although patients may sometimes describe fecal incontinence as 'diarrhea'. Fecal continence is maintained by the internal and external anal sphincters and the puborectalis sling, which maintains the rectoanal angulation. Anorectal sensation and reflex contractions of the sphincter mechanisms are essential for continence. Wald et al.[14] and Schiller et al.[15] have demonstrated that patients with diabetes and incontinence have a higher threshold (that is reduced sensation) for rectal perception of balloon distention when compared with continent diabetics and healthy controls. Patients with diabetes and incontinence also exhibit decreased resting anal sphincter pressure when compared with continent patients with diabetes. This reflects loss of

sympathetic nerve supply to the internal anal sphincter. Daytime fecal incontinence, aggravated by urgency or raised intra-abdominal pressure, is suggestive of external sphincter weakness and pudendal neuropathy.

In summary, diabetic constipation, diarrhea and incontinence refer to the occurrence of these symptoms in the absence of any disorder other than diabetes or neuropathy. For example, in patients with 'diabetic diarrhea', associated conditions, such as celiac sprue and bacterial overgrowth, are excluded. These disturbances of lower bowel function are closely linked with autonomic neuropathy. For example, colonic transit delay may result in constipation secondary to loss of extrinsic or intrinsic neural control of the colon, and diarrhea may result from loss of $alpha_2$ adrenergic 'tone' in enterocytes. Incontinence may result from loss of sensation, impaired sympathetic supply to the internal anal sphincter, or loss of pudendal innervation of the external sphincter.

EPIDEMIOLOGY OF GASTROINTESTINAL SYMPTOMS IN DIABETES

The first community-based epidemiological studies of symptoms in diabetics were performed in Germany and Finland by the groups of Enck et al.[7] and Janatuinen et al.[16]. These studies provided the surprising information that the only gastrointestinal problems with higher prevalence in diabetics than in controls were constipation, use of laxatives, and history of gallbladder surgery. The main findings were confirmed by a questionnaire-based study in Olmsted County, Minnesota[17]. This showed that only constipation and use of laxatives were more prevalent in type 1 (not type 2 diabetics) diabetics than in controls matched for age and gender[17] (Table 19.1).

The high prevalence of functional gastrointestinal disorders, such as irritable bowel syndrome, constipation, and functional dyspepsia, in Western civilizations confounds any estimates of the prevalence of diabetic enteropathy based on symptoms alone. Prevalence figures do

Table 19.1 Prevalence (%) of gastrointestinal and neurological symptoms among diabetic residents of Olmsted County, MN compared with their respective community controls

Symptoms/syndrome	IDDM Patients (*n* = 138)	IDDM Controls (*n* = 170)	NIDDM Patients (*n* = 217)	NIDDM Controls (*n* = 218)
Irritable bowel syndrome				
Rome criteria	10.9	7.6	5.1	8.3
Manning criteria	8.0	8.8	5.5	7.8
Constipation				
Symptoms only	16.7	13.5	10.1	11.5
Symptoms and/or laxatives	27.0	19.0	17.0	15.0
Dyschezia	2.9	3.5	2.3	2.3
Diarrhea	0	0	0	0
Fecal incontinence	0.7	1.2	4.6	1.8
Nausea/vomiting	11.6	10.6	6.0	5.5
Dyspepsia	18.8	20.6	13.4	17.4
Heartburn				
Symptoms only	11.6[a]	22.9	19.8	24.3
Symptoms and/or antacids	18.8[a]	36.5	24.0	36.2
PNeuro symptoms (overall)	50.0	47.1	65.9[a]	50.5
Numbness	34.8	28.2	41.5[a]	21.6
Muscular weakness	33.3	31.2	54.4[a]	43.6
ANeuro symptoms (overall)	9.4	5.9	7.8	7.3
Insufficient sweating	6.5[a]	1.8	5.5	5.5
Gustatory sweating	3.6	4.1	2.3	2.8

[a]$p < 0.05$ (univariate association, diabetes subgroup versus corresponding controls);

PNeuro = peripheral neuropathy; ANeuro = autonomic neuropathy; IDDM = insulin-dependent diabetes mellitus; NIDDM = noninsulin-dependent diabetes mellitus.

Note that people with IDDM have increased prevalence of constipation and/or use of laxatives and decreased prevalence of heartburn. Prevalence of dyspepsia is not greater in diabetics than in controls. Reproduced from Maleki D *et al.*[15].

not assess the impact or severity of the upper gastrointestinal symptoms suggestive of dyspepsia or gastroparesis. Thus, although Maleki *et al.* identified nausea, vomiting or dyspepsia in ~11% of type 1 diabetics and ~6% of controls, these prevalence figures were not significantly different from age- and gender-matched nondiabetic community controls[17]. A significant number of diabetics experienced impaired sweating, a marker of autonomic neuropathy relative to community controls[17].

Paradoxically, the Olmsted County study[17] demonstrated a lower prevalence of heartburn among the participants with type 1 diabetes. Factors that may contribute to this finding are the possibility of vagal neuropathy reducing the sensation of heartburn and the strong recommendation by diabetologists to patients to avoid nonsteroidal anti-inflammatory medications to protect their renal function.

A more recent questionnaire-based community study in South Eastern Australia reported more diarrhea, fecal incontinence, dysphagia and postprandial fullness among diabetics[18]. In contrast to the three prior studies[6-8], which included at least 10% type 1 diabetics, in the study from Australia, 95% of the cohort were type 2 diabetics. Constipation (other than the symptom of 'anal blockage') was not significantly more prevalent in diabetics, in contrast to the three other epidemiological studies. The odds ratio (OR) for nausea was close to significant (OR 0.98–2.35). The nature of these symptoms suggests that they may result from motor and sensory abnormalities of the gastrointestinal tract. Epidemiological studies attempted to identify risk factors for developing gastrointestinal symptoms among diabetics. In two Australian studies[18,19], a community evaluation found an association between self-reported poor glycemic control and gastrointestinal symptom complexes[18]. A clinic questionnaire-based study showed gastrointestinal symptoms were associated with diabetic complications, but not with current glycemic control (as reflected by blood glucose and glycosylated hemoglobin (HbA1c)[19]).

MECHANISM OF GASTROINTESTINAL COMPLICATIONS IN DIABETES

The presence of gastrointestinal symptoms in patients with diabetes does not correlate with glycemic control (assessed by measurement of HbA1c) at the time of presentation. Good glycemic control at the time of presentation may reflect poor caloric intake, secondary to gastroparesis or malabsorption, secondary to diarrhea. However, a history of poor glycemic control seems to be more closely associated with gastrointestinal symptoms than does the presence of diabetic complications, such as peripheral or autonomic neuropathy (assessed by tests of cardiovascular autonomic function). It is also important to consider the role of psychological factors in the perception of gastrointestinal symptoms. The Psychosomatic Symptom Checklist score is significantly associated with the reporting of gastrointestinal tract symptoms[17]. Several mechanisms interact to produce disordered gastrointestinal function in diabetes.

These are best documented in the function of the stomach; hence the following section addresses the mechanisms that are relevant in diabetic gastroparesis.

Hyperglycemia

Acute hyperglycemia reversibly influences upper-gut motor and sensory function. Since the rate of gastric emptying is a major determinant of postprandial blood glucose concentrations, altered gastric emptying can contribute to the progression of gastrointestinal symptoms, as well as diabetic complications[20]. Patients with type 2 diabetes mellitus and without neuropathic complications have been shown to exhibit accelerated gastric emptying of liquids when compared with healthy control subjects[21].

In patients with type 1 or type 2 diabetes, and in healthy subjects, acute hyperglycemia slows emptying of both solids and caloric liquids when compared with euglycemia[22,23]. This effect is also observed in patients with autonomic neuropathy. In patients with type 2 diabetes, emptying of liquids is related to the blood glucose concentration[24]. Conversely, hypoglycemia will lead to marked acceleration of gastric emptying when compared with euglycemia. Hyperglycemia has recently been shown to interfere with the prokinetic effect of intravenous erythromycin on gastric emptying in healthy subjects and patients with diabetes[25]. Extreme hyperglycemia (> 20 mmol L⁻¹) may contribute to the acute gastric dilatation sometimes observed at presentation of diabetic ketoacidosis.

Extrinsic neural control

Extrinsic neuropathy results in impaired gastrointestinal contractility or abnormal myoelectrical control[26]. The syndrome is typically seen in patients with type 1 or insulin-dependent diabetes mellitus (IDDM). Peripheral neuropathy is present in the majority of patients with enteropathy, and other forms of autonomic neuropathy (e.g., orthostatic hypotension) are common. Previous work has attributed these motility disorders mainly to vagal nerve dysfunction[27]. Motor abnormalities of the small intestine observed in symptomatic diabetic patients[28,29] are often indistinguishable from those seen in patients with other syndromes affecting postganglionic sympathetic function[30]. Vagal dysfunction is probably critical in gastric stasis of solid food. Electrolyte imbalances due to diabetic ketoacidosis (e.g., hypokalemia) and uremia may further aggravate impaired motor function in diabetic patients.

Vagal neuropathy was considered a likely cofactor preventing normal gastric accommodation or compliance in diabetics[31,32]. However, a recent study in patients with diabetes and vagal neuropathy showed normal postprandial change in gastric volume measured using SPECT imaging[33]. This is consistent with the normalization of gastric accommodation in rats within 30 days after vagotomy[34]. This normalization is suggestive of an adaptive response, which was inhibited in rats treated with tetrodotoxin, suggesting that enteric neurons are involved in the adaptation to chronic vagal denervation[34].

Intrinsic neural control

Nitrergic innervation
The importance of nitric oxide (NO) as an intestinal neurotransmitter regulating gastropyloric function is increasingly recognized. Mice with a targeted genomic deletion of neuronal nitric oxide synthase (nNOS) develop pyloric hypertrophy and gastric dilatation. Similarly, loss of pyloric nNOS is associated with infantile hypertrophic pyloric stenosis. This is supported by the observation that exogenous NO reduces the number and amplitude of isolated pyloric pressure waves in normal humans.

Abnormalities of nNOS have been observed in animal models of diabetes. Stomachs of spontaneously diabetic rats and rats with streptozotocin-induced diabetes exhibit decreased NO-mediated relaxation of gastric muscle strips and decreased expression of nNOS. Watkins *et al.*[35] have subsequently demonstrated that nNOS protein and mRNA are depleted in the pyloric myenteric neurons of diabetic mice. Insulin treatment restores pyloric nNOS protein and reverses the delay in gastric emptying observed

in such mice. Sildenafil, a cGMP phosphodiesterase inhibitor augments NO signaling and also reverses delayed gastric emptying in diabetic mice. These data suggest that reversible down regulation of NOS may play an important role in the pathogenesis of diabetic gastropathy.

Peptidergic and serotonergic innervation
Peptidergic and serotonergic[36–38] innervation is abnormal in animal models of diabetes.

Interstitial cells of Cajal
The interstitial cells of Cajal (ICC) play an important role in the regulation of gastrointestinal motility. ICC are distributed throughout the gastrointestinal tract, interspersed in the circular and longitudinal muscle layers and in the murine and human small intestine, and form a dense plexus at the level of the neuronal myenteric plexus. ICCs generate the electrical slow wave, required for normal gastrointestinal motility.

Defects of ICC have been associated with several human gut-motility diseases including slow transit constipation, hypertrophic pyloric stenosis, Hirschsprung's disease and pseudo-obstruction. Ordog *et al.*[39] demonstrated that spontaneously diabetic mice develop delayed gastric emptying, impaired electrical slow waves, and reduced motor neurotransmission. They also observed greatly reduced ICCs in the distal stomach. Moreover, the association of the ICC and enteric nerve cells was disrupted.

Recently, loss of ICC has been reported in a patient with type 1 diabetes[40] who underwent full-thickness jejunal biopsy. However, it remains to be ascertained whether defects of ICC are consistently present in patients with gastrointestinal dysmotility due to diabetes.

Hormonal control

Numerous peptide hormones play a role in the regulation of intestinal motility and gastric emptying and, directly or indirectly, in the control of satiety and caloric intake. Some of these peptides are also involved in glycemic control. These hormones may also influence the neural control of gut motility.

Glucagon-like peptide-1

Glucagon-like peptide-1 (GLP-1) arises from the differential post-transcriptional processing of the proglucagon gene that occurs in the intestinal L cells and in the hypothalamus. It is a putative incretin hormone, because of its potentiation of glucose-induced insulin secretion. When infused in pharmacological concentrations it markedly delays gastric emptying while increasing insulin and suppressing glucagon secretion in response to meal ingestion. Because of these actions, GLP-1 could be used to prevent and treat postprandial hyperglycemia. The effect of GLP-1 is at least partly dependent on inhibition of vagal cholinergic function[41].

Since the intestinal L cells are dispersed in the lower small intestine and colon and GLP-1 levels rise markedly in response to nutrient ingestion, it has been hypothesized that GLP-1 may contribute to the ileal brake effect, that is, the inhibition of upper gastrointestinal motility due to the presence of (unabsorbed) nutrients in the distal small intestine.

Amylin

Amylin is a 37 amino-acid polypeptide that is co-secreted with insulin by the pancreatic beta-cells in response to nutrient stimuli. Human studies have shown that the plasma concentrations of amylin and insulin rise and fall in parallel in both the fasted and fed states. Amylin secretion mirrors the abnormalities of insulin secretion observed in diabetes. People with type 1 diabetes typically do not have detectable amylin in the circulation during the fasting and fed states. Consequently, type 1 diabetes is a state of amylin, as well as insulin, deficiency. In contrast, amylin concentrations are more variable in people with type 2 diabetes. Amylin concentrations are elevated in early type 2 diabetes, but are decreased in the later stages as insulin secretion wanes.

Infusion of pharmacological concentrations of amylin, or the more stable analog pramlintide, in both animals and humans, has established that amylin can inhibit gastric emptying[42,43] and decrease glucagon secretion. The effects of amylin on gastric emptying are similar in type 1 and type 2 diabetes[43]. Studies in rats and, more recently, in humans suggest that the effects of pramlintide may be centrally mediated. Pramlintide inhibits meal-induced secretion of pancreatic polypeptide, a well-established marker of abdominal vagal activity[42,43]. The inhibition of gastric emptying produced by pramlintide is avoided during insulin-induced hypoglycemia, which is associated with vagal stimulation[44].

Psychological factors

Lustman, Clouse et al.[6,45] have provided evidence that symptoms in diabetics are significantly influenced by psychological factors.

CLINICAL EVALUATION OF PATIENTS WITH SUSPECTED DIABETIC ENTEROPATHY

The evaluation of upper gastrointestinal symptoms in patients with diabetes by means of esophagogastroduodenoscopy may document the presence of intercurrent conditions, such as peptic ulceration, peptic stricture or Mallory–Weiss tears (a result of repeated retching and vomiting). The presence of bezoars suggests delayed gastric emptying.

Confirmation of the diagnosis of gastroparesis requires documentation of delayed gastric emptying. Scintigraphic transit studies are typically used to measure gastric emptying. However, it is important to emphasize that measurements using labeled liquid meals are of limited value, because gastric emptying may be normal even in the presence of significant symptoms. Assessment of solid emptying by means of a radiolabel that tags the solid phase of the meal is a more sensitive test, with a well-defined normal range. The proportion of radioisotope retained in the stomach at 2 and 4 h distinguishes normal function from gastroparesis with a sensitivity of 90% and a specificity of 70%[46].

Another useful test for the measurement of solid-phase gastric emptying utilizes a standardized meal with biscuit enriched with ^{13}C, a substrate containing the stable isotope. When metabolized, the proteins, carbohydrates and lipids of the *S. platensis* or medium chain triglyceride octanoate give rise to respiratory CO_2 that is enriched with ^{13}C. Measurement of $^{13}CO_2$ breath content (a reflection of the amount of biscuit remaining in the stomach) by isotope ratio mass spectrometry allows estimation of gastric emptying $t_{1/2}$[47,48].

Gastropyloroduodenal manometry is a specialized technique that allows assessment of the pressure profiles in the stomach and small bowel. Hypomotility of the gastric antrum is an important cause of motor dysfunction and impaired emptying in diabetes. Patients with selective abnormalities of gastric function may be able to tolerate enteral feeding (delivered directly into the small bowel) whereas patients with a more generalized motility disorder may not be able to tolerate this.

Gastric accommodation in response to meal ingestion may be impaired in diabetes. This may contribute to the gastrointestinal symptoms of nausea, bloating and early satiety. Imaging of the stomach wall using ^{99m}Tc pertechnetate allows measurement of gastric volume after meal ingestion[49].

Diarrhea and fecal incontinence are often due to the effects of diabetes on the gastrointestinal tract. However, features suggestive of malabsorption, such as anemia, macrocytosis or steatorrhea, should lead to a consideration of underlying small bowel or pancreatic pathology. Celiac disease or bacterial overgrowth of the small intestine should be actively excluded[12].

Intestinal motor function can be evaluated by measurement of intestinal transit or, rarely, by small bowel manometry. Abnormal patterns of motility, however, are not reliable indicators of rapid or delayed intestinal transit. Scintigraphic methods that can simultaneously measure gastric, small bowel and colonic transit are accurate, noninvasive and relatively inexpensive.

Anorectal function can be evaluated by anorectal manometry, which allows measurement of sphincter strength at rest (sympathetic function) and during squeeze (pudendal nerve function), testing of sensation to balloon distention. Anorectal ultrasound may help identify defects in the anal sphincter, while a defecating proctogram allows evaluation of pelvic floor dysfunction or the functional significance of rectoceles or intussusception. However, most of these abnormalities can be successfully evaluated by careful rectal examination.

EVALUATING THE PATIENT FOR AUTONOMIC SYMPTOMS AND SIGNS

Evaluation of patients for autonomic dysfunction should start with a careful review of symptoms. Several symptoms are useful indicators of the possibility of autonomic nervous dysfunction. These include postural dizziness, lack of sweating, failure of erection or ejaculation, difficulty with emptying the urinary bladder or recurrent urinary tract infections, and dryness of the eyes, mouth or vagina. Table 19.2 shows the implications for sympathetic and parasympathetic dysfunction in such patients. An infrequently sought symptom in patients with diabetic autonomic neuropathy is gustatory sweating of the face, which reflects parasympathetic denervation. Postprandial hypotension is unlikely to occur except in severe autonomic neuropathies. It results from pooling of blood in the viscera and is aggravated by abrupt standing after meals.

Autonomic function tests in diabetics with enteropathy

While general autonomic reflex tests[50,51] are useful to assess the function of the autonomic control of the viscera (Table 19.3), tests that are specific for gut autonomic innervation are:

- Pancreatic polypeptide response to hypoglycemia or to modified sham feeding by the 'chew and spit' technique. Pancreatic polypeptide concentrations rise after meal ingestion and delivery of nutrients to the duodenum[52]. Atropine or vagotomy abolish this response. Normally, pancreatic polypeptide concentrations should increase by at least 25 pg mL^{-1} during sham feeding. The modified sham feeding test seems to be a more sensitive means of detecting vagal dysfunction than the postprandial response of plasma pancreatic polypeptide. The coexistence of antral hypomotility with abnormal pancreatic polypeptide responses to

Table 19.2 Symptoms and signs suggestive of autonomic dysfunction	
Sympathetic	**Parasympathetic**
Failure of pupils to dilate in the dark	Fixed dilated pupils
Fainting, orthostatic dizziness	Lack of pupillary accommodation
Constant heart rate with orthostatic hypotension	Sweating during mastication of certain foods
Absent piloerection	Decreased gut motility
Absent sweating	Dry eyes and mouth
Impaired ejaculation	Dry vagina
Paralysis of dartos muscle	Impaired erection
	Difficulty with emptying urinary bladder; recurrent urinary tract infections

Reproduced by permission from Camilleri[2].

sham feeding further supports the presence of vagal dysfunction or impaired gastric emptying of solids in these situations.

- R–R interval response to deep breathing. This is a test of cardiovagal reflexes[53,54]. However, Buyschaert et al.[55] showed that this is a good surrogate for the testing of abdominal vagal function, consistent with the concept that vagal denervation, as with most forms of diabetic neuropathy commences caudally and progresses in a cranial direction.

- Mesenteric flow in response to tilt-table tasting[56,57]. Splanchnic blood flow is under baroreflex control, and appropriate regulation is important in the maintenance of postural normotension. Evaluation of mesenteric flow in response to eating and head-up tilt provides important information on intra-abdominal sympathetic adrenergic function, and the ability of the patient to cope with orthostatic stress. Superior mesenteric artery flow in response to perturbations such as tilting and meal ingestion assesses sympathetic adrenergic function in the abdomen. While useful, this technique requires considerable expertise and is not widely available.

PRINCIPLES OF TREATMENT OF DIABETIC ENTEROPATHY

General principles in the management of diabetic enteropathy include optimal control of blood glucose, restoration of hydration, nutrition, and normal intestinal propulsion.

Gastroparesis and dyspepsia

Patients with severe exacerbation of symptoms should be hospitalized and may require nasogastric suction. Intravenous fluids should be provided, and metabolic derangements (ketoacidosis, uremia, hypo/hyperglycemia) corrected. Parenteral nutrition may become necessary in cases of malnutrition. Bezoars may be mechanically disrupted during endoscopy, followed by gastric decompression to drain residual nondigestible particles. Erythromycin at a dose of 3 mg kg^{-1} body weight intravenously every 8 h appears to be effective in accelerating gastric emptying[58]. A week's treatment with oral erythromycin, 250 mg, three times a day, is worthwhile once patients start to tolerate oral intake of food. Since both liquids and homogenized solids are more readily emptied from the stomach than solids, liquid or blended food will be better tolerated. Frequent monitoring of

Table 19.3 Commonly performed autonomic tests

Test	Physiologic functions tested	Rationale	Comments/pitfalls
Sympathetic function			
1. *Thermoregulatory sweat test (% surface area of anhidrosis)*	Preganglionic and postganglionic cholinergic	Stimulation of hypothalamic temp. control centers	Cumbersome, whole body test
2. *Quantitative sudomotor axon reflex test (sweat output, latency)*	Postganglionic cholinergic	Antidromic stimulation of peripheral fiber by axonal reflex	Needs specialized facilities
3. *Heart rate and blood pressure responses*			
Orthostatic tilt test	Adrenergic	Baroreceptor reflex	Impaired responses if intravascular volume is reduced
Postural adjustment ratio	Adrenergic	Baroreceptor reflex	Impaired responses if intravascular volume is reduced
Cold pressor test	Adrenergic	Baroreceptor reflex	Impaired responses if intravascular volume is reduced
Sustained hand grip	Adrenergic	Baroreceptor reflex	Impaired responses if intravascular volume is reduced
4. *Plasma norepinephrine response to:*			
Postural changes	Postganglionic adrenergic	Baroreceptor stimulation	Moderate sensitivity, impaired response if intravascular volume is reduced
Intravenous edrophonium	Postganglionic adrenergic	Anticholinesterase "stimulates" postganglionic fiber at prevertebral ganglia	False-negatives caused by contributions to plasma norepinephrine from many organs
Parasympathetic function			
1. *Heart rate (RR) variation with deep breathing*	Parasympathetic	Vagal afferents stimulated by lung stretch	Best cardiovagal test available, but not a test of abdominal vagus
2. *Supine/erect heart rate*	Parasympathetic	Vagal stimulation by change in central blood volume	Cardiovagal test
3. *Valsalva ratio (heart rate, max./min.)*	Parasympathetic	Vagal stimulation by change in central blood volume	Cardiovagal test
4. *Gastric acid secretory or plasma pancreatic polypeptide response to modified sham feeding or hypoglycemia*	Parasympathetic	Stimulation of vagal nuclei by sham feeding or hypoglycemia	Abdominal vagal test, critically dependent on avoidance of swallowing food during test
5. *Nocturnal penile tumescence*	Pelvic parasympathetic	Integrity of S_{2-4}	Plethysmographic technique requiring special facilities
6. *Cystometrographic response to bethanechol*	Pelvic parasympathetic	Increase in intra-vesical pressure suggests denervation supersensitivity	Tests parasympathetic supply to bladder, not bowel

Reproduced by permission from Camilleri M, Ford MJ[50].

blood glucose levels is essential during this phase. Rarely, it is necessary to bypass the stomach with a jejunal feeding tube if the motor dysfunction is limited to the stomach and there is no response to prokinetic therapy. This procedure should be preceded by a trial for a few days of nasojejunal feeding, with infusion rates of at least 60 mL iso-osmolar nutrient per hour. Jejunal tubes are best placed by laparoscopy or mini laparotomy, rather than via percutaneous endoscopic gastrostomy tubes. Such tubes allow restoration of normal nutritional status, but they are not without adverse effects.

If the patient remains symptomatic, other prokinetic agents may be considered as adjuncts. In the USA, the only available medication is metoclopramide, a peripheral cholinergic and antidopaminergic agent. During acute administration, it initially enhances gastric emptying of liquids in patients with diabetic gastroparesis, but its symptomatic efficacy is probably related with its central antiemetic effects. However, its long-term use is restricted by a decline in efficacy, and by a troubling incidence of central nervous system side effects.

Gastric pacing is still controversial, despite approval by the Food and Drug Administration. Diabetic gastroparesis has been attributed to impaired myoelectrical activity in the antrum. Two approaches have been proposed: McCallum et al. have used stimulation with an attempt to capture the pacesetter potentials[59]; in contrast, a multicenter study used electrical stimulation rather than pacing, and showed improved symptoms but no evidence of improved emptying[60]. In the absence of positive control treatments, it is still unclear whether the stimulation is effective in treatment of gastroparesis.

Diabetic diarrhea is treated symptomatically with loperamide, 2–8 mg per day. Second line approaches are clonidine, 0.1 mg orally[61], or by patch in patients who do not experience significant postural hypotension, and subcutaneous octreotide, 25–50 µg subcutaneously 5–10 min before meals[62].

Constipation is typically treated with osmotic and stimulant laxatives. One should avoid lactulose because of potential impact on glycemic control, and magnesium compounds in patients with impaired renal function because of risk of magnesium retention. Polyethylene glycol osmotic laxatives are useful (up to 17 g in 8 ounces of water per day), although care needs to be taken to avoid dehydration or sodium overload in patients requiring regular dosing. Pelvic floor disorders should be excluded before embarking on long-term polyethylene glycol therapy.

Incontinence may require physical medicine and biofeedback approaches to enhance rectal sensation, and to strengthen the external anal sphincter. A preliminary report has documented the use of phenylephrine suppositories for weak internal anal sphincter[63], but this needs to be confirmed. In the presence of a significant pudendal neuropathy or sensory loss, biofeedback may not work and the patient may have a better quality-of-life with a descending colostomy.

ACKNOWLEDGMENTS

This study was supported in part by grants RO1–DK54681 (MC) and K24–DK02638 (MC) from National Institutes of Health. We wish to thank Mrs Cindy Stanislav for excellent secretarial assistance.

REFERENCES

1 Camilleri M, Phillips SF. Disorders of small intestinal motility. In: Ouyang A, editor *Gastroenterol Clin NA*. Vol. 18. Philadelphia: WB Saunders, 1989: 405–24.

2 Wood JD. Enteric neurophysiology. *Am J Physiol* 1984;247:G585–98.

3 Camilleri M. Disorders of gastrointestinal motility in neurologic disease. *Mayo Clin Proc* 1990;65: 825–46.

4 Camilleri M. Gastrointestinal problems in diabetes. In: Brownlee MA, King GL, editors. *Endocrinology and metabolism clinics NA*. Vol. 25. Philadelphia. WB Saunders, 1996:361–78.

patients with gastroparesis. *Gastroenterology* 1998;114:456–61.

60 Anonymous. Long-term results of gastric stimulation four times higher than the slow wave frequency in patients with drug refractory gastroparesis. *Gastroenterology* 1999;116:A949 [Abstract].

61 Fedorak RN, Field M, Chang EB. Treatment of diabetic diarrhea with clonidine. *Ann Intern Med* 1985;102:197–9.

62 Mourad FH, Gorard D, Thillainayagam AV *et al.* Effective treatment of diabetic diarrhoea with somatostatin analogue, octreotide. *Gut* 1992;33:1578–80.

63 Carapeti EA, Kamm MA, Phillips RK. Randomized controlled trial of topical phenylephrine in the treatment of faecal incontinence. *Br J Surg* 2000;87:38–42.

20

Gestational diabetes

Maureen D Passaro and Robert E Ratner

INTRODUCTION

Gestational diabetes mellitus (GDM) is defined as any degree of glucose intolerance first recognized during pregnancy[1]. This definition applies regardless of treatment regimens and does not distinguish between those unrecognized cases of diabetes that may have preceded pregnancy. GDM occurs in 0.5–12.3% of pregnancies depending on the criteria used and the population being tested[2,3].

GDM conveys both short- and long-term risk to both mother and offspring. During the index pregnancy, women with GDM suffer from an increased prevalence of pregnancy-induced hypertension, toxemia and the need for primary Cesarian section delivery[4]. Although most women revert to normal glucose tolerance postpartum, approximately 20% have impaired glucose tolerance in the immediate postpartum phase[5,6], and the lifetime risk of development of type 2 diabetes exceeds 50%[7–11].

Maternal glucose values have been directly correlated with neonatal mortality[12–14]. Furthermore, fasting plasma glucose (FPG) showed an odds ratio (OR) of two for the development of macrosomia. For every 18 mg dL^{-1} increase in fasting value the likelihood of developing macrosomia doubles[15]. At delivery, GDM is associated with fetal macrosomia, with resultant shoulder dystocia and neonatal hypoglycemia. Long-term complications for infants of diabetic mothers include obesity and increased risk of abnormal glucose tolerance by adolescence.

PATHOPHYSIOLOGY

A thorough review of the pathophysiology of GDM can be found in other sources[16–18] and is beyond the scope of this chapter. A brief review of the normal adaptations in glucose homeostasis and maladaptations seen in GDM follows.

In normal pregnancy, glucose homeostasis changes in order to meet and maintain the demands of the growing fetus. Maternal adaptations ensure that there is an adequate nutrient supply of glucose and amino acids to the fetus, even at the expense of maternal glucose homeostasis. Increased levels of estrogen, human placental lactogen, growth hormone, corticotropin-releasing hormone and progesterone characterize the hormonal milieu during pregnancy[19]. These hormones play a major role in mobilizing maternal fuels and, either directly or indirectly increasing maternal insulin resistance. Subsequently, insulin requirements increase 1.5–2.5 fold in normal pregnancy over the non-pregnant state[20].

Overcoming the normal insulin resistance of pregnancy requires a compensatory increase in insulin secretion, to maintain maternal glucose concentrations within the normal range. When pancreatic beta cells are unable to compensate for the normal insulin resistance of pregnancy, GDM ensues. Individuals with GDM have both decreased insulin sensitivity and decreased insulin secretion. Although patients with GDM have insulin responses similar to those seen in normal pregnancy, their baseline glucose levels are higher indicating a diminished beta-cell response to glucose. In GDM, the insulin response to a glycemic stimulus is about half that of normal pregnancy[21]. It is unknown whether this defect in beta-cell function is a primary or secondary defect in GDM. Euglycemic clamp studies demonstrate diminished insulin secretion in women with GDM, despite the same or greater insulin resistance than that seen in pregnant women without GDM. Thus, failure of appropriate beta-cell compensation characterizes the onset of GDM[16].

The mechanism of insulin resistance is unclear. Studies by Garvey and colleagues suggest that the GLUT4 transporter may play a role in insulin resistance[22,23]. GLUT4 content is normal in skeletal muscle in women with GDM; however, in adipocytes, there is a decrease in number and sub-cellular distribution[22]. Fifty percent of women with GDM have significant decreases in GLUT4 concentration, with glucose transporter function depressed by 60%[23].

DIAGNOSTIC ISSUES

Since its first recognition, there has been considerable controversy and lack of consensus in the diagnosis of GDM. There remains no universal standard regarding screening and diagnosis of GDM. Although the 100 g oral glucose-tolerance test (oGTT) is preferred in the USA, much of the world uses the 75 g oGTT for diagnostic purposes.

Who to screen

Prior to the 4th International Workshop on Gestational Diabetes, universal screening for GDM was recommended. However, the Workshop and subsequent ADA recommendations advise screening only those women at high risk for GDM[24]. The risk factors associated with GDM include:

- Age > 25 years
- Elevated pre-pregnancy weight (greater than 110% IBW)
- Family history of diabetes, especially in a first degree relative
- History of macrosomia in prior pregnancy
- History of abnormal glucose tolerance
- History of poor obstetric outcome, or
- Member of minority population at increased risk for type 2 diabetes[25].

The ADA position statement suggests that it is not cost-effective to screen women at low risk, and recommends screening only be done in the presence of one or more risk factors[26,27]. This change in recommendation has been challenged, however, as universal screening appears to improve detection of as many as 10% of all cases of GDM[28].

Screening and diagnosis

Several different methods can be used to diagnose GDM. In the USA, the recommended approach to screening is taken in two steps. Pregnant women without a history of carbohydrate intolerance are screened with a randomly timed 50 g glucose challenge between 24 and 28 weeks of gestation. Those with elevated plasma glucose ≥ 140 mg dL^{-1} are subsequently referred for 100 g oGTT. Although the 50 g glucose challenge test can be done without regard to fasting, in the fed state the sensitivity is improved if the cut-off value is lowered to 130 mg dL^{-1} (Reference 29).

The 100 g oGTT is used for diagnostic purposes in most areas throughout the USA. This test is performed after 3 days of unlimited carbohydrate intake and 8–14 h of fasting. Evidence to support the use of the 100 g oGTT, includes the classic study by O'Sullivan and Mahan[11]. In this study, 752 pregnant women were evaluated with a 3 H oGTT. The mean blood glucose values were determined at each time-point. Using two standard deviations (SD) as normal, diagnostic criteria were set (see Table 20.1). These criteria not only predict future diabetes in the mother, but also reveal a four-fold increase in perinatal mortality in untreated

Table 20.1 Historical evolution of O'Sullivan–Mahan criteria for the diagnosis of gestational diabetes

	O'Sullivan–Mahan criteria	National Diabetes Data Group	Carpenter–Coustan modification
Fasting	5.0 (90)[a]	5.83 (105)	5.28 (95)
1 h	9.17 (165)	10.56 (190)	10.0 (180)
2 h	8.06 (145)	9.17 (165)	8.61 (155)
3 h	6.94 (125)	8.06 (145)	7.78 (140)

[a]Values in brackets give mM (mg dL^{-1}) whole blood.

GDM compared with control[30]. These original criteria for GDM were subsequently modified[3,31] due to changes in assay technique (see Table 20.1). However, these changes were merely mathematical, and are based on criteria that define subsequent diabetes in the mother.

The 75 g oGTT in pregnancy is used in much of the world, and the data supporting its use is even more controversial than that for the 100 g oGTT. The 4th International Workshop on Gestational Diabetes defined cut-off values for the 75 g oGTT in pregnancy as a FPG of 95 mg dL^{-1} and a 2 h plasma glucose of 155 mg dL^{-1}. These values were arbitrarily defined, based on the mean plus 1.5 SD of the oGTT values in a study of over 3500 patients[32]. However, the 2 h value was raised to 155 mg dL^{-1} to be more consistent with the 2 h value recommended for the 100 g oGTT[3] and the values of the European Association for the Study of Diabetes (162 mg dL^{-1})[33] (Table 20.2).

Contrary to the 4th International Workshop on Gestational Diabetes, the World Health Organization (WHO) defines GDM based on the 75 g oGTT in the same fashion as in the non-pregnant state, with a fasting level > 125 and 2 h > 200. However, they compensate by recommending treatment of those with IGT based on a 2 h glucose > 140 but < 200 (Reference 34). Moses et al.[35] suggest lowering the glucose cut-off values to a fasting value of 90 mg dL^{-1} and the 2 h value to 140 mg dL^{-1}, to significantly reduce the rate of large-for-gestational-age

Table 20.2 Glucose values recommended by 4th International Workshop on Gestational Diabetes

	100 g oGTT (mg dL^{-1})	75 g oGTT (mg dL^{-1})
Fasting	95	95
1 h	180	
2 h	155	155
3 h	140	

infants, and the need for obstetric interventions. In support of the 75 g oGTT, Pettitt found an increased perinatal mortality rate proportional to the height of the 2 h glucose response to 75 g in Pima Indians[36].

Aside from the debate concerning the appropriate oGTT criteria to be used for the diagnosis of GDM, there is increasing evidence to suggest that a single abnormal value on oGTT may better predict the occurrence of perinatal morbidity. Tallerigo et al.[37] examined the neonatal outcome in 249 women failing to meet O'Sullivan–Mahan criteria for GDM. They found that the 2 h plasma glucose concentration after a 100 g oGTT significantly correlated with the infant's birth weight; the higher the 2 h plasma glucose concentration, the greater the incidence of macrosomia, toxemia, and the need for cesarean section delivery. A significant increase was noted as 2 h plasma glucose concentrations exceeded 140 mg dL^{-1} compared with the 165 mg dL^{-1} cut-off level noted in traditional O'Sullivan–Mahan criteria. Lindsay et al.[38] found both maternal and fetal morbidity increased in women with only a single abnormal value on GTT. Toxemia was increased in the affected group, with an OR = 2.51, and macrosomia in the infants and subsequent shoulder dystocia were found to have OR of 2.18 and 2.97, respectively. Berkus and Langer[39] found the incidence of large-for-gestational-age infants among women with a single abnormal glucose value during the oGTT to be twice that of mothers in whom the oGTT was entirely normal.

The controversies over which oGTT to perform are further compounded by problems with poor reproducibility[40]. In studies performed during pregnancy in which high-risk pregnant women underwent two sequential oGTT 1 week apart, 24% were found to have discrepant test results on the two examinations[41]. Surprisingly, the majority (80%) of the discrepant tests reverted from abnormal to normal glucose tolerance at the second examination.

TREATMENT

Goals of therapy

The goals of therapy in GDM are to decrease both maternal and fetal morbidity and mortality attributed to the disease. In particular, to limit macrosomia, intrauterine demise and neonatal morbidity. Preventing macrosomia has been found to decrease birth trauma, and cesarean-section rate[42].

Maternal hyperglycemia conclusively poses a threat to the well-being of the fetus. Fasting hyperglycemia (FPG > 105 mg dL^{-1}) is associated with increased risk of fetal death[14,13]. Higher postprandial glucose values during weeks 29–32 are associated with fetal macrosomia[43]. One hour postprandial glucose is a strong predictor of infant birth weight and fetal macrosomia[44]. The risk of macrosomia is a continuum that increases further if 1 h postprandial glucose is > 120 mg dL^{-1} whole blood capillary glucose (plasma glucose of approximately 140 mg dL^{-1}). Controlling post-prandial glucose excursions can improve outcomes, by decreasing neonatal hypoglycemia, macrosomia and rates of cesarean-section delivery[45]. Despite aggressive treatment with diet, exercise and insulin therapy, which may normalize glycosylated hemoglobin (HbA1c), neonatal morbidities persist. The relative risk of neonatal hypoglycemia remains elevated at 5.7, while macrosomia is elevated 3.2 fold, polycythemia 2.7 fold, hypocalcemia, and hyperbilirubinemia 2.0 fold[4].

Attaining good glycemic control is the cornerstone of therapy (Table 20.3). Treatment is aimed at maintaining normoglycemia, and limiting maternal ketosis[46,47]. Controlling blood sugars using postprandial glucose monitoring goals (1 h postprandial whole blood glucose < 140 mg dL^{-1}) in combination with fasting blood glucose measurement (fasting blood glucose 60–90 mg dL^{-1}) can optimize glycemic control and significantly improve pregnancy outcomes, by decreasing neonatal hypoglycemia, macrosomia and

Table 20.3 Goals of therapy				
	Whole blood glucose (mg dL^{-1})	(mmol L^{-1})	**Plasma glucose** (mg dL^{-1})	(mmol L^{-1})
Fasting	95	5.3	105	5.8
1 h postprandial	140	7.8	155	8.6
2 h postprandial	120	6.7	130	7.2

cesarean-section rates[45]. However, 1990 dated provider surveys among obstetricians and maternal fetal specialists reveal that, despite recommendations, the goals of therapy were not met or agreed upon. Among those surveyed, 54% aimed for FPG < 105 mg dL[-1], 32% accepted FPG 110–150 mg dL[-1], while 13% aimed for FPG 90–104 mg dL[-1]. Only 30% of those surveyed aimed for postprandial glucose < 120 mg dL[-1] (Reference 48).

When to initiate self-monitoring of blood glucose

Self blood-glucose monitoring (SBGM) should be instituted as soon as possible after diagnosis. Studies using fetal ultrasound[49,50] have shown that accelerated growth begins early in the third trimester. So, to avoid fetal consequences, glycemic control should be obtained as soon as possible. Risk of fetal macrosomia increases with postprandial hyperglycemia[43–45]. In order to attain targeted goals, home SBGM is necessary. Initial therapy, medical nutrition therapy (MNT), requires blood-glucose monitoring four times daily, while women treated with insulin typically need to monitor at least six times per day. Care should be taken to give appropriate goals of therapy, since some reflectance meters are calibrated to plasma glucose values, while others reflect whole blood-glucose values.

The importance of SBGM is supported by a study of 153 women with GDM. These women were treated with intensive diet therapy and SBGM, with insulin therapy added only if therapeutic goals were not obtained. There was no difference in the birth weight or incidence of macrosomia between groups, showing that intensive dietary therapy with monitoring and insulin as needed can reduce macrosomia[51].

Medical nutrition therapy

MNT is the mainstay of treatment for women with GDM. The optimal diet should provide adequate nutrition without causing postprandial hyperglycemia or fasting ketosis. Approximately 70–80% of patients can achieve adequate glycemic control when MNT is aggressively applied. Meal plans vary with the practitioner, but often include three meals and one to two snacks per day. Caloric restriction is often necessary in obese women, to prevent hyperglycemia. Since insulin resistance is highest in the morning, carbohydrate intake at breakfast is usually limited.

Optimum weight at delivery is 120% ideal body weight. Recommended weight gain is 12.5 18 kg if the body mass index (BMI) is < 19.8 kg m[-2], 11.5–16 kg when BMI is 19.9–26 kg m[-2], 7–11.5 kg for BMI 26–29 kg m[-2] and only 6 kg if BMI is > 35 kg m[-2] (References 52–54).

Women with the least amount of weight gain typically have the best glycemic control and pregnancy outcome. However, caloric restriction must be done with caution. Protein malnutrition and ketosis should be avoided. A small study of 22 obese pregnant women demonstrated that moderate caloric restriction, not less than 25 kcal kg[-1] actual in obese women is acceptable, and does not result in ketonuria[55]. When obese women with GDM are subjected to caloric deprivation during late pregnancy there is a greater fall in plasma glucose compared with normal pregnant women, without a greater propensity to ketosis. This suggests that brief periods of fasting are well-tolerated and longer spacing can occur between meals[56].

Caloric restriction is limited by the occurrence of ketosis, when the carbohydrate intake is insufficient. Initial studies suggest that ketosis is associated with lower IQ scores in adolescents[57,58].

There are no large randomized trials of optimum dietary therapy in GDM. Studies suggest that intensive dietary therapy should be tailored to postprandial glucose. A small study of 14 overweight women with GDM between 32 and 36 weeks gestation looked at the effect of carbohydrate intake on postprandial glucose. All women were treated without insulin and received 24 kcal kg[-1]day[-1]. The calories were distributed such that they received 12.5% breakfast, 28% lunch, 28% dinner, and the remainder in snacks. In order to maintain 1 h postprandial capillary whole blood glucose levels < 140 mg dL[-1], carbohydrate intake needed to be < 45% at breakfast, < 55% at lunch and < 50% at dinner. Aggressive MNT, with < 33% carbohydrates at breakfast, < 45% at lunch and < 40% at dinner succeeded in achieving a blood glucose < 120 mg dL^{-1} (Reference 59). This suggests that postprandial glucose is directly dependent on the carbohydrate content consumed during a meal.

Original recommendations from the American Diabetes Association suggested a diet that consisted of 35 kcal kg^{-1} pregnant weight, with 50–60% of those calories coming from carbohydrates. This caused excessive weight gain and postprandial hyperglycemia. Fifty percent of women on this diet ultimately required insulin therapy[60]. A few small studies have looked at caloric restriction as a treatment for obese patients with GDM. Magee and colleagues[61] studied 12 patients. The women were all placed on 2400 kcal diets for 1 week. At the end of the first week, five were randomized to caloric restriction (1200 kcal day^{-1}), the remainder continued on the 2400 kcal day^{-1} diet. After 1 week, average glucose levels and fasting insulin levels were markedly declined in the restricted group. Fasting and postprandial glucose challenges were not different. However, ketonuria and ketonemia developed in those patients who received caloric restriction. When women were placed on a 1600 kcal diet, ketonuria did not occur, but there remained marked improvement in glycemic control[61]. In a nonrandomized trial of women treated for GDM, restriction of carbohydrates to 35–42% compared with carbohydrate intake > 45% resulted in improved maternal postprandial glucose with decreased need for insulin, fewer large-for-gestational-age infants and less need for cesarean sections[62]. Current dietary recommendations range from 24 kcal kg^{-1} for normal pregnant weight, to 12 kcal kg^{-1} for morbidly obese, with < 40% calories coming from carbohydrate[61,63,64].

Exercise

Exercise serves as an adjunct therapy to medical nutrition in patients with diabetes[65,66] and can be helpful in the primary prevention of GDM[67]. Exercise enhances insulin sensitivity and improves hepatic glucose production. However, little data is available on the use of exercise in treatment of GDM. Exercise should be monitored and should not increase fetal distress, lower infant birth weight, cause uterine contractions or maternal hypertension.

Obstetricians generally do not recommend initiation of exercise programs in pregnancy. Safe exercise programs for pregnancy have been developed, and include the recumbent bicycle, arm ergonomics and brisk walking. Contraindications to exercise include: pregnancy-induced hypertension, rupture of membranes, pre-term labor, bleeding, incompetent cervix, and intrauterine growth retardation. There are no data to indicate that pregnant women should limit exercise intensity and lower target heart-rates to avoid potential adverse events[68].

Initiation of pharmacologic therapy

Success of MNT is measured by weight gain and glycemic control. Blood glucose levels drop rapidly and dramatically in response to MNT. A 2 week trial to obtain and maintain fasting blood glucose < 95 mg dL^{-1} and postprandial blood glucose < 120 mg dL^{-1} is reasonable. Women with FPG level < 95 mg dL^{-1} have significantly higher levels of insulin production than those with glucose > 95 mg dL^{-1}. This suggests that women with fasting glucose > 95 mg dL^{-1} may not have adequate insulin secretion[69]. Fasting glucose > 95 mg dL^{-1}, together with increased body weight, predicts failure of diet therapy and, therefore, a shorter trial (1 week) of diet therapy may be indicated[70]. MNT is limited by the occurrence of starvation ketosis, and when MNT fails to attain normoglycemia in the absence of ketonuria in an adequate time-frame, pharmacologic therapy becomes necessary.

An argument can also be made for the use of third trimester fetal ultrasound in assessing the need for initiating insulin therapy. Seventy-three subjects with GDM treated with MNT, who obtained adequate glycemic control and had a fetal abdominal circumference by ultrasound > 75 percentile, were randomized to continue MNT or begin insulin therapy. Treatment with insulin reduced macrosomia, without an increased risk of hypoglycemia, suggesting that ultrasound can be useful in determining treatment strategies in pregnancies complicated by GDM[71]. Similarly, ultrasound can be used to identify those at low risk for macrosomia and perinatal complications. In a study using monthly ultrasound to measure fetal abdominal circumference, participants were randomized to standard therapy or monitoring with ultrasound and glycemic control. In the experimental group, insulin was only begun if the fetal abdominal circumference exceeded the 70th percentile for gestational age, or FPG was > 120 mg dL^{-1}. Of those randomized to the experimental group 38% did not meet study requirements for insulin therapy. Using the study guidelines, there was no difference in birth weight, incidence of macrosomia, duration of insulin therapy or pregnancy-induced hypertension. There was a slight increase in cesarean sections in the experimental group, which was not explained by birth weight. In the experimental group, birth weights were lower in those women who did not receive insulin therapy[72].

Oral hypoglycemic agents

Oral hypoglycemic agents are not approved or recommended in the USA for treatment of GDM. Older sulfonylureas, such as tolbutamide and chlorpropamide, cross the placenta and cause fetal hyperinsulinemia and macrosomia. They also have the potential to cause prolonged neonatal hypoglycemia. However, minimal amounts of glyburide cross the placenta[73]. Recently, 404 women with mild GDM participated in a trial and were randomly assigned to receive either glyburide or insulin. The results demonstrated that the groups achieved similar glycemic control, with no differences in the frequency of macrosomia, neonatal hypoglycemia, and neonatal morbidity, or cord insulin concentration levels, between groups[74]. The level of glycemic control achieved in the insulin-treated group, however, is considered to be inadequate by many clinicians, rendering the findings somewhat in doubt. These results should be confirmed before glyburide is widely used in women with GDM.

Although not approved, women with GDM have also been treated with metformin and two studies suggest that this is safe in pregnancy[75,76]. However, a recent retrospective analysis suggests that metformin increases the risk of pre-eclampsia and stillbirths[77]. This small study was not well controlled and included patients treated over a 25-year period of time, in which the treatment for GDM has undergone major advances. Other factors may, in fact, account for these small differences in pre-eclampsia and stillbirths.

Insulin therapy

Treatment with insulin has been shown to decrease fetal morbidity. Failure to maintain fasting blood glucose < 95 mg dL^{-1}, 1 h postprandial blood glucose < 140 mg dL^{-1}, and 2 h postprandial blood glucose < 120 mg dL^{-1} has been associated with increased fetal morbidity and mortality. The type and amount of insulin therapy should be individualized, based on blood glucose levels. Patients should be instructed on signs and symptoms of hypoglycemia and given appropriate adjustment algorithms for home use. Close contact with the physician and educator throughout pregnancy is needed. Adjustments in insulin therapy every 3–4 days can achieve targeted glycemic control in an optimum timeframe. There are a wide variety of management algorithms used by various practitioners, which require frequent home SBGM. No particular algorithm has proven better than others.

More frequent injections better mimic pancreatic function. Increasing the number of injections from 2 per day to 4 per day results in improved glycemic control and perinatal outcomes without increasing the risk of maternal hypoglycemia, pre-term labor or cesarean section rates[78]. Insulin requirements increase throughout pregnancy, as a result of increasing hormones of pregnancy and subsequent increasing insulin resistance[79].

Starting doses of insulin in massively obese women are typically 1.5–2 U kg^{-1}. Twin gestations frequently need twice these requirements. Aggressive use of insulin, with frequent monitoring (6 times per day) and appropriate titration of insulin, decreased macrosomia in one clinic from 18% to 7%[80].

No insulin is currently FDA approved for use in pregnancy, however only human insulin is recommended. Regular insulin and NPH insulin have long been used in treatment of diabetes in pregnancy, but Insulin lispro has been used with increasing frequency in pregnancy since its approval in 1996. Insulin lispro offers the benefit of closely controlling post-prandial glucose excursion, without causing late-postprandial or pre-prandial hypoglycemia.

To demonstrate that insulin lispro was more physiologic and provided better postprandial glucose control than human regular insulin, 42 women with GDM who failed control with diet alone were randomized to NPH and Regular human insulin or NPH and insulin lispro. The group that received insulin lispro had significantly lower glucose levels after meals without an increase in hypoglycemia[81].

One complication of insulin therapy during pregnancy has been the development of insulin antibodies. The presence of insulin antibodies has been associated with macrosomia in the infant, independent of maternal glucose concentration[82]. For this reason, animal source insulins such as Beef and Pork insulins are contraindicated in pregnancy. Antibodies have not been found in cord blood in patients receiving insulin lispro[81]. The newly approved insulin aspart is associated with the development of insulin antibodies initially after treatment. The long-term effects on the fetus are unknown, although studies are currently under way. This is a theoretical concern with insulin aspart, since it takes approximately 3 months for antibodies to form, at which point parturition has occurred and GDM has resolved. The use of the long-acting insulin analog, insulin glargine, is not recommended in pregnancy. Increased IGF-1 receptor binding by this analog carries theoretical risks and the preparation is considered Category C by the Food and Drug Administration.

TIMING AND NATURE OF DELIVERY

Contemporary efforts to maintain normoglycemia during pregnancy with diet, exercise, and aggressive insulin therapy may result in normalization of HbA1c and near-normal glucose profiles throughout the day by SBGM. Despite this degree of near-normalization of glycemia, neonatal morbidity persists[4].

The optimum timing of delivery is controversial. Most experts agree that women with GDM should be delivered at term. GDM is not an indication for elective cesarean delivery, nor for delivery prior to 38 weeks in the absence of fetal compromise[1]. Most deliveries in patients with GDM, however, occur at 38–39 weeks, with a resulting 30% cesarean section rate, without any outcome data to support this practice[83]. The Toronto Tri-Hospital study found that making the diagnosis of GDM alone increased cesarean delivery rates, without apparent explanation[84]. Similar results were seen by Buchanan, when women with GDM randomized to receive insulin had a higher Cesarean section rate, despite reduction in the percentage of large-for-gestational-age babies, compared with those who did not receive insulin therapy[71].

Nevertheless, indications for early delivery include macrosomia (estimated weight > 4000 g) or large-for-gestational-age infants, poor maternal compliance, history of previous stillbirth, and presence of vasculapathy or hypertension.

POST-NATAL CARE

With delivery, insulin resistance markedly declines as the hormones of pregnancy decline; insulin sensitivity returns within a few hours of delivery of the placenta. Most women with GDM no longer require insulin. The recurrence rate of GDM is reported as 30–70% depending on the study cited[85–88] and has been associated with infant birth weight in the index pregnancy[88], maternal fat intake[89], and maternal pre-pregnancy weight of the subsequent pregnancy[88]. The lifetime risk of developing type 2 diabetes remains high. The risk of progression to diabetes within 5 years approaches 50%[8,7] and is associated with gestational age at diagnosis, impairment of beta-cell function, severity of GDM, obesity and subsequent pregnancy.

The ADA recommends that an oGTT be repeated 6 weeks postpartum to ensure resolution of normal carbohydrate handling, and regular postpartum surveillance and annual assessment for diabetes[1]. All subsequent pregnancies carry a risk for GDM; therefore patients should be counseled about planning pregnancies with appropriate pre-pregnancy counseling and evaluation. Fasting plasma glucose should be measured annually.

SUMMARY

GDM affects approximately 1–13% of all pregnancies and results from a shift in counter-regulatory hormones in glucose homeostasis. Early screening and detection are important to optimize maternal and fetal outcomes. Screening can be done using a one- or two-step process. Although the 75 g oGTT is now recognized by the diabetes community for diagnosis, the majority of outcome data stems from results of the 100 g oGTT. Achieving the desired weight and glycemic goals requires aggressive management. MNT is the first line of treatment, and is successful for the majority of women. Failure to achieve the desired goals of therapy within a short period of time is an indication for insulin therapy. Small studies have been done in women using oral agents, but more data is needed before recommending the use of oral agents globally. Although most women revert to normal glucose-tolerance postpartum, the lifetime risk of developing type 2 diabetes remains high, and close surveillance of these women is indicated.

REFERENCES

1 Metzger BE, Coustan DR. The Organizing Committee. Summary and recommendations of the fourth international workshop–conference on gestational diabetes mellitus. *Diabetes Care* 1998;21(Suppl 2):B161–7.
2 Berkowitz GS, Lapinski RH, Wein R, Lee D. Racial/ethnicity and other risk factors for gestational diabetes. *Am J Epidemiol* 1992;135:965.
3 Carpenter MW, Coustan DR. Criteria for screening tests for gestational diabetes. *Am J Obstet Gynecol* 1982;144:768–72.
4 Hod M, Merlob P, Freidman S *et al.* Gestational diabetes mellitus a survey of perinatal complication in the 1980s. *Diabetes* 1991;40(Suppl 2):74–8.
5 Kjos SL, Buchanan TA, Greenspoon JS *et al.* Gestational diabetes mellitus: the prevalence of glucose intolerance and diabetes mellitus in the first two months post partum. *Am J Obstet Gynecol* 1990;163:93–8.
6 Catalano PM, Vargo KM, Bernstein IM *et al.* Incidence and risk factors associated with abnormal postpartum glucose tolerance in women with gestational diabetes. *Am J Obstet Gynecol* 1991;165:914.
7 Kjos SL, Peters RK, Xiang A *et al.* Predicting future diabetes in Latino women with gestational diabetes. *Diabetes* 1995;44:586.
8 Metzger BE, Cho NH, Roston SM *et al.* Prepregnancy weight and antepartum insulin secretion predict glucose tolerance 5 years after gestational diabetes mellitus. *Diabetes* 1993;16:1598.
9 O'Sullivan JB. Diabetes mellitus after GDM. *Diabetes* 1991;40:131.
10 O'Sullivan JB. Body weight and subsequent diabetes mellitus. *J Am Med Assoc* 1982;248:949.
11 O'Sullivan JB, Mahan CM. Criteria for the oral glucose tolerance test in pregnancy. *Diabetes* 1964;13:278–85.
12 Langer O, Levy J, Brustman L *et al.* Glycemic control in gestational diabetes mellitus: how tight is tight enough: small for gestational age versus large for gestational age? *Am J Obstet Gynecol* 1989;161:646–53.
13 Sermer M, Naylor CD, Gare DJ *et al.* Impact of increasing carbohydrate intolerance on maternal fetal outcomes in 3637 women without gestation diabetes: the Toronto Tri-Hospital Gestational Diabetes Project. *Am J Obstet Gynecol* 1995;173:146–56.
14 Jang HC, Cho NH, Min Y-K *et al.* Increased macrosomia and perinatal morbidity independent of maternal obesity and advanced age in Korean women with GDM. *Diabetes Care* 1997;20:1582–8.
15 Pettitt DJ, Bennett PH, Hanson RL *et al.* Comparison of World Health Organization and National Diabetes Data Group procedures to detect abormalities of glucose tolerance during pregnancy. *Diabetes Care* 1994;17:1264–8.
16 Catalano PM, Tyzbir ED, Wolfe RR *et al.* Carbohydrate metabolism during pregnancy in control subjects and women with gestational diabetes. *Am J Physiol* 1993;264:E60–E67.

17 Ciraldi TP, Kettel M, el-Roeil A *et al.* Mechanisms of cellular insulin resistance in human pregnancy. *Am J Obstet Gynecol* 1994;170:635–41.

18 Kuhl C. Aetiology of gestational diabetes. *Baillieres Clin Obstet Gynecol* 1991;5:279–92.

19 Freinkel N. Effects of the conceptus on maternal metabolism. In: Leibel BS, Wrenshall GA, editors. Amsterdam: Excerpta Medica, 1964: 675–91.

20 Freinkel N. The Banting Lecture 1980: Of pregnancy and progeny. *Diabetes* 1980;29:1023–35.

21 Hormes PJ, Kuhl C, Lauritsa KB. Gastro-enteral-pancreatic hormone in gestational diabetes: a response to protein rich meal. *Horm Metab Res* 1982;14:335–8.

22 Garvey WT, Maianu L, Hancock JA. Amsterdam Gene expression of GLUT 4 in skeletal muscle from insulin resistant patients with obesity, IGT, GDM and NIDDM. *Diabetes* 1992;41:465–75.

23 Garvey WT, Maianu L, Zhu JH *et al.* Multiple defects in the adipocyte glucose transport system cause cellular insulin resistance in gestational diabetes. *Diabetes* 1993;42:1773–85.

24 Report on the expert committee on the diagnosis and classification of diabetes mellitus. *Diabetes Care* 1997;20:1183–97.

25 Solomon CG, Willett WC, Carey VJ *et al.* A prospective study of pregravid determinants of gestational diabetes mellitus. *J Am Med Assoc* 1997;278:1078.

26 Metzgar BE, Coustan DR. The Organizing Committee. Summary and recommendations of the Fourth International Workshop Conference on Gestational Diabetes Mellitus. *Diabetes Care* 1998;21(Suppl. 2):B61.

27 American Diabetes Association. Gestational diabetes mellitus. *Diabetes Care* 2002;25(Suppl. 1):S94–S96.

28 Moses RG, Davis WS. Gestational diabetes: do lean young Caucasian women need to be tested? *Diabetes Care* 1998;21:1803–6.

29 Coustan DR, Widness JA, Marshall W *et al.* Should the fifty-gram, one-hour plasma glucose screening test for gestational diabetes be administered in the fasting for fed state? *Am J Obstet Gynecol* 1986;154:1031–5.

30 O'Sullivan JB, Charles D, Mahan CM *et al.* Gestational diabetes and perinatal mortality rate. *Am J Obstet Gynecol* 1973;116:901.

31 National Diabetes Data Group. Classification and diagnosis of diabetes mellitus and other categories of glucose intolerance. *Diabetes* 1979;28:1039.

32 Sacks DA, Greenspoon JS, Abu-Fadil S *et al.* Toward universal criteria for gestational diabetes: The 75–gram glucose tolerance test in pregnancy. *Am J Obstet Gynecol* 1995;172:607.

33 Lind T, Phillips PR. The DPSG of the EASD. Influence of pregnancy on the 75 g OGTT: a prospective multicenter study. *Diabetes* 1991; 40(Suppl 2):8.

34 World Health Organization. *Diabetes mellitus: report of a WHO study group. Technical Report Series.* Geneva: World Health Organization, 1985. Report No.: 727.

35 Moses RG, Moses M, Russell KG, Schier GM. The 75 g glucose tolerance test in pregnancy: a reference range determined on a low-risk population and related to selected pregnancy outcomes. *Diabetes Care* 1998;21:1807–11.

36 Pettitt DJ, Knowler WC, Baird HR, Bennett PH. Gestational diabetes: infant and maternal complications of pregnancy in relation to third-trimester glucose tolerance in Pima Indians. *Diabetes Care* 1980;3:458–64.

37 Tallarigo L, Giampietro O, Penno G *et al.* Relation of glucose tolerance test to complications of pregnancy in nondiabetic women. *N Engl J Med* 1986;315:989.

38 Lindsay MK, W. G, Klein L. The relationship of one abnormal glucose tolerance test value in pregnancy complications. *Obstet Gynecol* 1989;73:103–6.

39 Berkus MD, Langer O. Glucose tolerance test: Degree of glucose abnormality correlates with neonatal outcome. *Obstet Gynecol* 1993;81:344.

40 Freeman H, Looney JM, Hoskins RG. Spontaneous variability of oral glucose tolerance. *J Clin Endocrinol* 1942;2:431.

41 Catalano PM, Avallone D, Drago NM, Amini SV. Reproducibility of the oral glucose tolerance test in pregnant women. *Am J Obstet Gynecol* 1993;169:874.

42 Coustan DR, Imarah J. Prophylactic insulin treatment of gestational diabetes reduces the incidence of macrosomia, operative delivery and birth trauma. *Am J Obstet Gynecol* 1984;150: 836–42.

43 Combs CA, Gunderson E, Kitzmiller JL *et al.* Relationship of fetal macrosomia to maternal postprandial glucose control during pregnancy. *Diabetes Care* 1992;15:1251–7.

44 Jovanovic-Peterson L, Peterson CM, Reed GF *et al.* Maternal postprandial glucose levels predict infant birth weight: the diabetes in early pregnancy study. *Am J Obstet Gynecol* 1991;164: 103–11.

45 DeVeciana M, Major CA, Morgan M *et al.* Postprandial versus preprandial blood glucose monitoring in women with gestational diabetes mellitus requiring insulin therapy. *N Engl J Med* 1995;333:1237.

46 Pettitt DJ, Bennett PH, Saad MF *et al.* Abnormal glucose tolerance during pregnancy in Pima Indian women: long-term effects on offspring. *Diabetes* 1991;40(Suppl. l2):126–30.

47 Pettitt DJ, Nelson RG, Saad MF *et al.* Diabetes and obesity in the offspring of Pima Indian women with diabetes during pregnancy. *Diabetes Care* 1993;16:310–14.

48 Landon MB, Gabbe SG, Sachs L. Management of diabetes mellitus and pregnancy: a survey of obstetricians and maternal-fetal specialists. *Obstet Gynecol* 1990;75:635–40.

49 Ogata ES, Sabbagha R, Metzgar BE *et al.* Serial ultrasonography to assess evolving fetal macrosomia. *J Am Med Assoc* 1980;243:2405–8.

50 Langer O, Kozlowski S, Brustman L. Abnormal growth patterns in diabetes in pregnancy: a longitudinal study. *Israel J Med Sci* 1991;243: 2405–8.

51 Wechter D J, Kaufmann RC, Amankwah KS *et al.* Prevention of neonatal macrosomia in gestational diabetes by the use of intensive dietary therapy and home glucose monitoring. *Am J Perinatal* 1994;8:131–4.

52 King J, Allen H. Nutrition during pregnancy. In: *National Academy of Science 1990*. Washington DC: National Academy Press, 1990.

53 Ratner RE, Hamner LH, Isada NB. Effects of gestational weight gain in morbidly obese women: I. maternal morbidity. *Am J Perinatal* 1991;8:21–4.

54 Ratner RE, Hamner LH, Isada NB. Effects of gestational weight gain in morbidly obese women: fetal effects. *Am J Perinatal* 1990;7: 295–9.

55 Algert A, Shragg P, Hollingsworth DR. Moderate caloric restriction in obese women with gestational diabetes. *Obstet Gynecol* 1985;65:487–91.

56 Buchanan TA, Metzger BE, Freinkel N. Accelerated starvation in late pregnancy: A comparison between obese women with and without gestational diabetes mellitus. *Am J Obstet Gynecol* 1990;162:1015–20.

57 Churchill JA, Berrendes HW, Nemore J. Neuropsychological deficits in children of diabetic mothers: a report for the Collaborative Study of Cerebral Palsy. *Am J Obstet Gynecol* 1969;105:257–68.

58 Rizzo T, Metzger BE, Burns WJ, Burns K. Correlations between antepartum maternal metabolism and child intelligence. *N Engl J Med* 1991;325:911–6.

59 Peterson CM, Jovanovic-Peterson L. Percentage of carbohydrate and glycemic response to breakfast, lunch and dinner in women with gestational diabetes. *Diabetes* 1991;40(Suppl 2):172–4.

60 Jovanovic-Peterson L, Peterson CM. Dietary manipulation as the primary treatment strategy for pregnancies complicated by diabetes. *J Am Coll Nutr* 1990;9:320.

61 Magee MS, Knopp RH, Benedetti TJ. Metabolic effects of 1,200-kcal diet in obese pregnant women with gestational diabetes. *Diabetes* 1990;39:234–40.

62 Major CA, Henry MJ, DeVeciana M, Morgan MS. The effects of carbohydrate restriction in patients with diet-controlled gestational diabetes. *Obstet Gynecol* 1998;91:600–4.

63 Jovanovic-Peterson L, Peterson CM. Nutritional management of the obese gestational diabetic woman. *J Am Coll Nutr* 1996;11:246–50.

64 *Diabetes and pregnancy. Technical bulletin.* American College of Obstetricians and Gynecologists 1994: Report No.: 200.

65 Jovanovic-Peterson L, Peterson CM. Exercise and the nutritional management of diabetes during pregnancy. *Obstet Gynecol Clin N Am* 1996;23:75–86.

66 Bung P, Artal R. Gestational diabetes and exercise: a survey. *Semin Perinatal* 1996;20:328–33.

67 Dye TD, Knox KL, Artal R *et al.* Physical activity, obesity and diabetes in pregnancy. *Am J Epidemiol* 1997;146:961–5.

68 *Exercise during pregnancy and the postpartum period.* American College of Obstetrics and Gynecology committee opinion. No 267. *Obstet Gynecol* 2002;99:171–3.

69 Langer O, Hod M. Management of gestational diabetes mellitus. *Obstet Gynecol Clin N Am* 1996;23:137–59.

70 McFarland MR, Langer O, Conway DL, Berkus MD. Dietary therapy for gestational diabetes: how long is long enough? *Obstet Gynecol* 1999;93:978–82.

71 Buchanan TA, Kjos SL, Montoro MN *et al.* Use of fetal ultrasound to select metabolic therapy for pregnancies complicated by mild gestational diabetes. *Diabetes Care* 1994;17:275–83.

72 Kjos SL, Schaefer-Graf U, Sardesi S *et al.* A randomized controlled trial using glycemic plus fetal ultrasound parameters versus glycemic

parameters to determine insulin therapy in gestational diabetes with fasting hyperglycemia. *Diabetes Care* 2001;24:1904–10.

73 Elliot BD, Langer O, Shenker S, Johnson RF. Insignificant transfer of glyburide occurs in the human placenta. *Am J Obstet Gynecol* 1991;165: 807.

74 Langer O, Conway DL, Berkus MD *et al.* A comparison of glyburide and insulin in women with gestational diabetes mellitus. *N Engl J Med* 2000;343:1134–8.

75 Coetzee EJ, Jackson WPU. Metformin in management of pregnant insulin-dependent diabetics. *Diabetologia* 1979;16:241–5.

76 Coetzee EJ, Jackson WPU. Diabetes newly diagnosed during pregnancy. A 4-year study at Groote Schur Hospital. *S Afr Med J* 1979;56: 467–75.

77 Hellmuth E, Damm P, Molsted-Pedersen L. Oral hypoglycaemic agents in 188 diabetic pregnancies. *Diabet Med* 2000;7:507–11.

78 Nachum A, Ben-Shlomo I, Weiner E, Shalev E. Twice daily versus four times daily insulin dose regimens for diabetes in pregnancy: randomized controlled trial. *Br Med J* 1999;319:1223–7.

79 Jovanovic L, Druzen M, Peterson CM. Effects of euglycemia on the outcome of pregnancy in insulin-dependant diabetic women as compared with normal control subjects. *Am J Med* 1981;71:921–7.

80 Jovanovic-Peterson L, Bevier W, Petersen CM. The Santa Barbara County Health Services Program: birthweight change concomitant with screening for and treatment of glucose intolerance of pregnancy: a potential cost-effective intervention. *Am J Perinatal* 1997;14:221–8.

81 Jovanovic L, Ilic S, Pettitt D *et al.* The metabolic and immunologic effects of insulin lispro. *Diabetes Care* 1999;22:1422–7.

82 Menon RK, Cohen RM, Sperling MA *et al.* Transplacental passage of insulin in pregnant women with insulin-dependent diabetes mellitus. Its role in fetal macrosomia. *N Engl J Med* 1990;323:309–15.

83 Langer O, Rodrigues SA, Xenakis EM-J *et al.* Intensified versus conventional management of gestational diabetes. *Am J Obstet Gynecol* 1994;170:1036–47.

84 Naylor CD, Sermer M, Chen E, Sykora K. Cesarean delivery in relation to birth weight and gestational glucose tolerance. *J Am Med Assoc* 1996;275:1165–70.

85 Moses RG. The recurrence rate of gestational diabetes in subsequent pregnancies. *Diabetes Care* 1996;19:1348–50.

86 Major CA, DeVicianna M, Weeks J, Morgan MA. Recurrence of gestational diabetes: who is at risk? *Am J Obstet Gynecol* 1998;179:1038–42.

87 Phillipson EH, Super DM. Gestational diabetes mellitus: Does it reoccur in subsequent pregnancy? *Am J Obstet Gynecol* 1989;160:1324.

88 MacNeill S, Dodds L, Hamilton DC *et al.* Rates and risk factors for recurrence of gestational diabetes. *Diabetes Care* 2001;24:659–62.

89 Moses RG, Shand JL, Tapsell LC. The recurrence of gestational diabetes: could dietary differences in fat intake be an explanation? *Diabetes Care* 1997;20:1647–50.

21

Type 2 diabetes in children and adolescents

Arlan L Rosenbloom

EPIDEMIOLOGY OF TYPE 2 DIABETES IN CHILDREN AND ADOLESCENTS

In 1971, Harvey Knowles made the prescient observation that:

"A second type of diabetes in young persons closely resembles that of the stable middle-aged onset type. Herein the patients as a rule have no symptoms, are overweight, can secrete insulin, and respond to sulfonylurea therapy. Often the diagnosis is made serendipitously. In the Juvenile Diabetic Clinic at the Cincinnati General Hospital 11 of these patients have been followed along with 300 patients with the unstable insulin deficient type of diabetes. The age of these 11 patients at diagnosis ranged from 11 to 17 years. The prevalence of this type of diabetes very likely is higher than presently appreciated, because of lack of symptoms or signs leading to suspicion of diabetes."[1]

Twenty-five years later, one-third of all new cases of diabetes in patients age 10–19 years in the Cincinnati clinic were type 2 diabetes; the estimated age-specific incidence was 7.2/100 000, approximately one half the incidence rate for type 1 diabetes in the childhood population. This was a tenfold increase from 1982 to 1994. The proportion of new cases of diabetes in children diagnosed as type 2 went from 2–4% before 1992, unchanged from Knowles' 1971 prevalence figure of 3.7%, to 16% by 1994. For 10–19 year olds, one-third of new patients were type 2[2].

Between the 1970s and the 1990s, prevalence of type 2 diabetes increased more than fivefold in young Pima Indians, from 9/1000 15–24 year olds to 51/1000 15–19 year olds, and the disease emerged in the 10–14 year age group with a prevalence of 22/1000[3,4]. Type 2 diabetes is also frequent among indigenous people in Canada[5]. Affected females outnumber males 4–6 to 1 in the North American Indian populations[6].

African–Americans accounted for 70–75% of type 2 diabetes patients in the Cincinnati report[2], and in studies from Arkansas[7]. In a largely Mexican–American clinic population, 31% under the age of 17 with diabetes had type 2 diabetes[8]. The sex ratio in the African–American and Mexican–American groups with type 2 diabetes averages 1.5:1, far less distorted than in Native Americans[6].

In a study of 5–19 year old diabetic patients diagnosed between January 1 1994 and December 31 1998 at the three University diabetes centers in Florida, 86% of 682 subjects were type 1 and 14% type 2. Females accounted for 63% of type 2 diabetes, but only 47% of type 1 diabetes. Only 46% of type 2 diabetes were African–American, 22% Hispanic, and the rest

Table 21.1 Estimates of the frequency of type 2 diabetes in children and adolescents

Location	Race/ ethnicity	Year	Age (years)	Incidence per 10^5	Prevalence per 10^3	% of all DM	Ref
Arizona	Pima Indian	1979	< 15	0	0	—	
			15–24	—	9	—	3
		1996	10–14	—	22.3	—	
			15–19	—	50.9	—	4
Manitoba	First Nation		5–14	—	1	—	5
Ontario	First Nation		< 16	—	2.3	—	5
Cincinnati	White, African-	1971	0–19	—	—	3.5	1
	American	1994	0–19	—	—	16	
			10–19	7.2	—	33	2
California	Mexican-Amer.	1994	0–17	—	—	45	8
Libya	Arab	1990	10–14	1.8	—	22	
			15–19	5.9	—	39	10
Tokyo	Japanese	1980	6–11	0.2	—	—	
			12–15	7.2	—	—	
		1995	6–11	2.0	—	—	
			12–15	13.9	—	—	12
Bangladesh	Asian Indian	1997	15–19		0.6	—	13

non-Hispanic Caucasians. For African–Americans, the risk of developing type 2 diabetes was threefold that of Caucasians; for Hispanics the relative risk was 3.5. The percentage of newly-diagnosed diabetes that was type 2 increased over the 5-year period from 8.7 to 19 ($p = 0.004$)[9].

Reports over the past decade from Libya, Hong Kong, Japan, Bangladesh, Australia (Aborigines), New Zealand (Maoris), and England (South Asians and Arabs) have indicated that the emergence of type 2 diabetes in young persons is a worldwide phenomenon with ethnic specificities (Table 21.1)[10–16]. In the Tokyo prefecture in Japan, annual urine testing followed by oral glucose-tolerance testing when indicated, documented a tenfold increase in type 2 diabetes incidence, from 0.2 to 2/100 000 in primary school-children and a doubling among junior high-school children, from 7.3 to 13.9/100 000, between 1976–80 and 1991–95, paralleling increasing obesity rates[12].

CLASSIFICATION AND DIAGNOSIS OF NON-TYPE 1 DIABETES IN CHILDREN AND ADOLESCENTS

Classification

Type 2 diabetes accounts for most of the non-type 1 or non-autoimmune diabetes in children. Less commonly, other types occur, specifically MODY (maturity onset diabetes of the young)[17] and 'atypical diabetes mellitus' (ADM) in African–American youngsters[18]. Of these three forms of non-type 1 diabetes, there is evidence for increasing incidence in the pediatric population only for type 2 diabetes (Table 21.2).

Diagnostic criteria

Criteria for the diagnosis of diabetes, recently revised by the American Diabetes Association, are given in Table 21.3[19]. Earlier criteria differed between children and adults, but the rationale

Table 21.2 Classification of the types of diabetes seen in children (adapted from reference 6)

	Type 1	ADM*	MODY	Type 2
Age at onset	Throughout childhood	<40 yrs old	<25 yrs old	Pubertal
Predominant race/ethnic distribution	Caucasian	African American	Caucasian	Hispanic, African American, Native American
Onset	Acute, severe, insulin required	Acute, severe, insulin required	Subtle, insulin not required	Subtle (~25% severe), insulin usually not required
Islet auto-immunity	Present	Absent	Absent	Absent
Ketosis, DKA	Common	Common at onset	Rare	Up to 40% at onset
Obesity	Uncommon	40% (comparable to population)	Uncommon	>90%
Proportion of diabetes	~80%	>10% of youth-onset in African American	<5%	~20%
Probands with affected relative	5–10%	>75%	100%	45–80%
Mode of inheritance	Non-Mendelian, generally sporadic	Autosomal dominant	Autosomal dominant	Non-Mendelian, strongly familial

*ADM = Atypical diabetes mellitus of African–American youth

Table 21.3 Criteria for the diagnosis of diabetes mellitus (adapted from references 19 & 22)

- Symptoms of diabetes plus random plasma glucose concentration ≥200 mg/dL (ll.l mmol/L). Casual is defined as any time of day without regard to time since last meal. Typical symptoms of diabetes include polyuria, polydipsia, and unexplained weight loss.
  or
- FPG* ≥126 mg/dL (7.0 mmol/L). Fasting is defined as no caloric intake for at least 8 h.
  or
- 2-h PG ≥200 mg/dL (ll.l mmol/L) during an OGTT**. The test should be performed using a glucose load containing the equivalent of 75 g anhydrous glucose dissolved in water for those weighing >43 kg and 1.75 g/kg for those weighing <43 kg.

In the absence of unequivocal hyperglycemia with acute metabolic decompensation, these criteria should be confirmed by repeat testing on a different day. The third measure (OGTT) is not recommended for routine clinical use.

*Fasting plasma glucose
**Oral glucose tolerance test

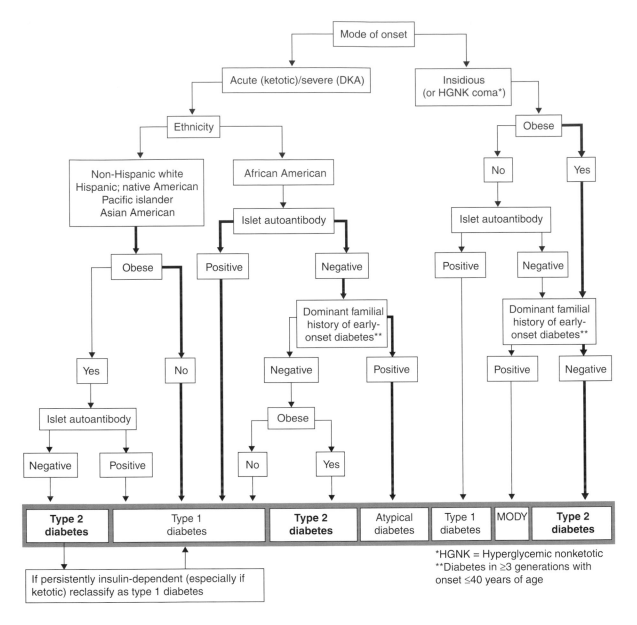

Figure 21.1 Decision tree for the clinical classification of diabetes in children.

for this difference was never clear[20]. The new criteria were based on epidemiologic evidence of risk thresholds for the long-term complications among several populations, including Pima Indians, other Americans participating in the National Health and Nutrition Survey (NHANES), and Egyptians. These risk relationships should also apply to a largely adolescent population developing type 2 diabetes.

Diagnostic strategy (Figure 21.1)

Islet cell auto-antibody testing is not yet widely available, is not always reliable, and the results are not immediately available. Thus, the physician must depend on clinical judgment in classifying new-onset diabetes patients. The pathways in bold in the decision trees provided in Figure 21.1 indicate the most likely outcomes. Classification may only be possible after months or longer of follow-up.

In African–American children with new, acute-onset diabetes, islet autoantibody testing can identify many of the children who have type 1 diabetes. If islet autoantibody studies are negative, a family history of early-onset diabetes in three or more generations suggests ADM. In the absence of such a family history, the absence of obesity suggests type 1 diabetes. Some children with new-onset type 1 diabetes, however, are overweight, because of the increasing prevalence of obesity in the society as a whole. Ketoacidosis or ketosis is not useful for distinguishing between type 1 diabetes, ADM, and type 2 diabetes, because as many as 25% of children with type 2 diabetes are initially seen with DKA and 40% with ketonuria[21, 22].

Obese children with insidious onset diabetes, commonly detected incidentally, most likely have type 2 diabetes. A family history of diabetes affecting at least one parent is found in 50–80%, and 75–100% have a first or second degree relative with type 2 diabetes[19].

The presence of islet cell autoantibodies strongly argues in favor of type 1 diabetes. Specific autoantibodies to insulin, glutamic acid dehydrogenase (GAD), or to the tyrosine phosphatase insulinoma antibody (IA)-2 and IA-2 beta, are seen at the time of diagnosis in 85–98% of patients with immune-mediated type 1 diabetes[23]. As MODY is rare, there is no routine value in testing for HNF-4 alpha, glucokinase, HNF-1 alpha, 1PF-1, or HNF-1 beta mutations[17]. Mitochondrial mutations account for < 2% of clinical type 2 (non-insulin dependent) diabetes in adults; therefore, studies of the mitochondrial genome and identification of genetic defects responsible for MODY remain research tools[6,17].

The Florida experience noted earlier provides a perspective on the difficulty of initial classification in a relatively small subset of patients and the importance of follow-up observation, with reconsideration of classification. Of the 723 patients newly diagnosed during the 5-year study period, 605 were classified as type 1 and 77 as type 2; 41 were considered either atypical or remained of uncertain classification. Of those initially diagnosed as type 1 diabetes, 17 (2.8%) were subsequently reclassified as type 2 diabetes, and six (8%) of those initially diagnosed as type 2 diabetes were reclassified as type 1 diabetes. Most of the 17 reclassified as type 2 had been diagnosed in DKA or with ketosis[9].

PATHOPHYSIOLOGY (Figure 21.2)

The epidemic of obesity, and the difficulty of losing accumulated weight suggest that there may have been an advantage to this metabolic phenotype during human evolution. The development of type 2 diabetes in susceptible individuals would not have been a disadvantage in the absence of opportunities to become obese. The thrifty genotype hypothesis was first advanced by JV Neel[24], nearly 40 years ago, and has recently been updated[25]. This hypothesis explains the insulin resistance and relative beta-cell insufficiency associated with the development of type 2 diabetes as an adaptation to conserve energy in times of famine. Changes in gene frequency, or in the genetic pool, cannot explain the rapid increases in type 2 diabetes prevalence within one or two generations in some populations, emphasizing the importance of environmental factors operating on this genetic background.

The role of fetal and childhood nutrition

When it was noted that impaired glucose tolerance (IGT), or type 2 diabetes, occurred in adults who had lower birthweight and smaller head circumference, and were thinner at birth, it was thought to indicate *in utero* programming that limited beta-cell capacity and induced insulin resistance in peripheral tissues. Maternal malnutrition was considered the cause of islet cell hypoplasia[26]. Later study demonstrated that the glycemic response to insulin was also reduced in individuals who had been thin at birth[27]. Large studies in Sweden and the USA have confirmed

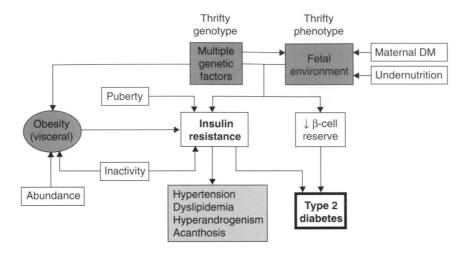

Figure 21.2 Factors in the development of type 2 diabetes in children.

the association of fetal under-nutrition with later type 2 diabetes risk[28,29]. The adult offspring of women who had starved in the last trimester of pregnancy during the Dutch famine at the end of World War II have also been noted to have an increased risk of IGT[30].

Underweight for gestational age has also been associated with increased cortisol axis activity in urbanized South African 20-year-olds who were not obese. They also had IGT compared with normal birthweight controls[31].

Two studies in young subjects from high-risk populations support findings in older subjects on the effect of fetal nutrition on the risk for development of the insulin resistance syndrome (type 2 diabetes, hypertension, hyperlipidemia) in adulthood. The relationships between birthweight, present weight, fasting and post-load glucose and insulin concentrations were examined by multiple regression analysis in 3061 Pima Indians aged 5–29 years. Their current weight correlated with their birthweight. A U-shaped relationship was noted between 2 h glucose concentrations and birthweight in those over 10 years of age, unrelated to present weight. When adjustment was made for height and weight, negative correlations were found between birthweight and insulin concentrations at baseline and 2 h, and insulin resistance in the 2272 subjects without diabetes. These observa-

tions supported the hypothesis that insulin resistance has a survival advantage for low birthweight babies[32]. In a study of 477 8-year old Indian children, the cardiovascular risk factors of insulin resistance and plasma total and LDL cholesterol concentrations were strongly related to current weight. With adjustment for current weight, age, and sex, lower birthweight was associated with elevated systolic BP, fasting plasma insulin and 32–33 split proinsulin concentrations, glucose and insulin concentrations 30 min after glucose, and plasma lipids. Lower birthweight was also associated with increased calculated insulin resistance. Children who had low birthweight but high-fat mass at 8 years had the highest risk for insulin resistance syndrome variables and hyperlipidemia[33].

The thrifty phenotype hypothesis has been developed to explain how low birthweight, reflecting fetal undernutrition, is a risk factor for the later development of the insulin resistance syndrome. Poor nutrition in fetal and early infant life would restrict the development and function of the beta-cells and insulin sensitive tissues, primarily muscle, leading to insulin resistance. Obesity in later life, with the attendant insulin resistance, would overcome the limited beta-cell capacity, leading to type 2 diabetes. These findings could, however, be interpreted as a reflection of the thrifty genotype, in which genetically determined defective insulin action *in utero* results in decreased fetal growth and obesity-induced impaired glucose-tolerance in later childhood or adulthood[6].

RACIAL AND FAMILIAL INFLUENCES

A number of studies comparing African–American and European–American children suggest a genetic basis for the apparently greater susceptibility to type 2 diabetes in certain racial/ethnic groups. African–Americans had greater insulin responses to oral glucose than European–Americans after adjustment for weight, age, ponderal (obesity) index, and pubertal stage, in a study of 377 children aged 5–17 years[34]. In another study of nearly 1200 11–18 year olds, African–Americans had higher insulin levels and lower glucose-to-insulin ratios than did European–Americans, after correction for ponderal index, further indicating reduced insulin sensitivity in African–American youngsters[35]. African–American prepubertal and pubertal youngsters have higher fasting and stimulated insulin concentrations during glucose clamp studies than do European–American youngsters[36]. Rates of lipolysis have also been found to be significantly lower in African–American children than in Caucasian children, further suggesting an energy conservation phenotype that would be detrimental with a surfeit of nutrition[37].

Prepubertal healthy children had 3 h hyperinsulinemic clamp studies to assess insulin sensitivity. Nine children with a family history of type 2 diabetes were matched for age; pubertal status; total body adiposity, determined by dual energy X-ray absorptiometry; abdominal obesity, determined by computed tomography (CT) scan; and physical fitness measured by $VO_{2\,max}$ with those without such history ($n = 13$). Those with a family history of type 2 diabetes had lower insulin-stimulated glucose disposal and non-oxidative glucose disposal. There were no differences in glucose oxidation, fat oxidation, or free fatty acid (FFA) suppression[38]. These data indicate that family history of type 2 diabetes is a risk factor for insulin resistance.

The familial clustering of type 2 diabetes can indicate environmental rather than genetic causation. In a study of physical, behavioral, and environmental characteristics of 42 parents and siblings in 11 families of adolescents with type 2 diabetes, five mothers and four fathers had diabetes before the study and it was diagnosed in three of the remaining fathers during the study. All 42 relatives had BMI > 85th percentile, and skin-fold measurements > 90th percentile. Fat intake was high, fiber intake low, and physical activity nil to low. Eating disorders were common and diabetes control poor[39].

MATERNAL DIABETES

Fetal beta-cell function was assessed by amniotic fluid insulin (AFI) concentration at 32–38 weeks gestation in 88 pregnancies with pre-gestational or gestational diabetes. Offspring had oral glucose tolerance testing annually from 18 months of age. At < 5 years of age IGT was present in 1.2%, in 5.4% at 5–9 years, and in 19.3% at 10–16 years of age. There was no association between IGT and the type of maternal diabetes or macrosomia at birth. One-third of those with elevated AFI had IGT during adolescence, in contrast with only one of 27 with normal AFI[40].

Studies in the Pima Indian population have also indicated that the diabetic intrauterine environment is an important contributor to the risk of type 2 diabetes. The prevalence of diabetes in the offspring of Pima women with diabetes during pregnancy is significantly greater than in non-diabetic mothers, or those who develop diabetes after delivery[41]. These studies of the effect of diabetic pregnancy on altered beta-cell function and glucoregulation later in life are of great concern, because of the possible cumulative effect from generation to generation.

INSULIN RESISTANCE IN CHILDREN

Puberty

The mean age at diagnosis in all studies of type 2 diabetes in children, including the Florida series, is approximately 13.5 years, corresponding to the time of peak adolescent growth and development[6,42]. Puberty is a time of relative insulin resistance, with normally a 2–3 fold increase in peak insulin response to oral glucose and, for those with type 1 diabetes, substantial increases in insulin dose[43]. Insulin-mediated glucose disposal averages 30% less in adolescents compared with prepubertal children or young adults[44]. This physiologic insulin-resistance of puberty is readily countered by increased insulin secretion in the absence of predisposition to type 2 diabetes and the additional stress of obesity. Increased activity of the GH–IGF axis is the likely cause of this physiologic insulin resistance of puberty, because it is transitory and coincident[22].

Obesity

Approximately 55% of the variance in insulin sensitivity can be explained by total adiposity. Obese children have hyperinsulinism and 40% decrease in insulin-stimulated glucose metabolism compared with the nonobese[44]. There is a direct correlation between the amount of visceral fat in obese adolescents and basal and glucose-stimulated insulinemia, and an inverse correlation with insulin sensitivity. Body mass index (BMI) increase results in decrease of insulin-stimulated glucose metabolism and increase of fasting insulinemia. This inverse relationship between insulin sensitivity and abdominal fat is greater for visceral than abdominal subcutaneous fat[44].

Ovarian hyperandrogenism and premature adrenarche

Polycystic ovarian syndrome (PCOS) is being increasingly recognized in adolescents, often as part of the 'syndrome X', also known as the metabolic syndrome or 'diabesity'. The syndrome includes, in addition to obesity and hyperinsulinism, hypertension, hyperuricemia, PCOS, acanthosis nigricans, dyslipidemia, and elevated plasminogen activator inhibitor-1[45]. Adolescents with PCOS have an approximate 40% reduction in insulin-stimulated glucose disposal, in comparison to body composition matched non-hyperandrogenic control subjects[46,47]. Girls with premature adrenarche are at increased risk of ovarian hyperandrogenism and PCOS[48].

It is of considerable interest that children born small-for-gestational-age are at increased risk of premature adrenarche, similar to the increased risk for insulin resistance from intrauterine undernutrition[49,50]. This link between premature adrenarche and insulin resistance has been further explored by examining 60 first-degree adult relatives of girls with precocious adrenarche. Seven of the relatives (11.6%) had type 2 diabetes and another 14 (23.3%) had glucose intolerance, compared with the reported figures for the population of the same age of 2.5% and 7.5%, respectively. At least two abnormal lipid levels were found in 40% of subjects. Gestational diabetes was common, and female relatives had lower steroid-hormone binding globulin levels than did population controls[51].

CASE FINDING

Epidemiologic criteria

Screening is testing applied to a group of individuals to separate those who are well from those who have an undiagnosed disease or defect, or who are at high-risk. Considerations of testing for type 2 diabetes in children begins with the assumption that this will be done in obese youngsters. Thus, determination of obesity is the screening test. Case finding, the more appropriate designation for testing obese children for type 2 diabetes, is defined as diagnostic testing in a population at risk[52].

Case finding is justified if the condition tested for is sufficiently common to justify the investment; type 2 diabetes is sufficiently common in obese children and youth to justify testing such youngsters, especially those with high-risk ethnicity or family history. Another criterion for case finding is that the condition tested for be serious, in terms of morbidity and mortality, which is unquestionably true of type 2 diabetes in children because of the association with increased cardiovascular risk factors of hypertension and dyslipidemia, hyperandrogenism/infertility, and early onset of microvascular disease. The condition being tested for should have a prolonged latency period without symptoms, during which abnormality can be detected.

Type 2 diabetes in children is often detected in the asymptomatic state, and albuminuria may already be present at the time of diagnosis, indicative of a prolonged latency period[53].

Further requirements for case finding include the availability of a test that is sensitive (few false negatives) and accurate, with acceptable specificity for the test (minimal number of false positives). The fasting plasma glucose (FPG) and two-hour plasma glucose (2HPG) have been applied to risk populations and are acceptably sensitive and specific, depending on criteria selected. There must also be an intervention able to prevent or delay disease onset, or to more effectively treat the condition detected in the latency phase[53]. Intervention to reverse hyperglycemia and associated dyslipidemia, or to prevent the development of overt disease in those with IGT involves the daunting challenge of changing lifestyle in asymptomatic individuals, who are at an age when long-term health goals are not on their agenda.

Testing recommendations

A consensus panel of the American Diabetes Association recommended that individuals who are overweight, as defined in Table 21.4, and with any two of the other risk factors indicated in the table should be tested every 2 years, starting at age 10 or at the onset of puberty if that begins earlier[22]. In the absence of data making definitive recommendations possible, the consensus panel considered it appropriate for the individual physician to test a specific child with any of the risk factors noted. Most instances of type 2 diabetes in children have occurred in the 10–19 year age group, although patients have been reported as young as 5 years. The FPG and oral glucose tolerance test (FPG + 2HPG) were both considered suitable means of testing, and the FPG was thought preferable by the ADA consensus panel because of lower-cost and greater convenience[22]. If one is testing for glucose intolerance in those at risk, however, the 2HPG will be elevated before the FPG. If necessary, for convenience, PG can be measured in individuals who have taken food or drink shortly before testing. A random PG concentration ≥ 140 mg dL^{-1} (7.8 mmol L^{-1}) is considered an indication for further testing, requiring FPG or 2HPG for confirmation on a different day[19].

Population-based studies have been done only in the Native North American population. School-based screening programs for investigational

---

Table 21.4 Testing for type 2 diabetes in children

- Criteria*: overweight (BMI>85th percentile for age and sex, weight for height >85th percentile, or weight >120% of ideal for height)
  plus

  Any two of the following risk factors:
  - Family history of type 2 diabetes in first- or second-degree relative
  - Race/ethnicity (American Indian, African American, Hispanic, Asian/Pacific Islander)
  - Signs of insulin resistance or conditions associated with insulin resistance (acanthosis nigricans, hypertension, dyslipidemia, PCOS)

- Age of initiation: age 10 or at onset of puberty, if puberty occurs at a younger age
- Frequency: every two years
- Test: fasting plasma glucose preferred

*Clinical judgment should be used to test for diabetes in high-risk patients who do not meet these criteria

purposes are needed. Such studies could establish the strength and risk level of various factors that might influence the development of type 2 diabetes [blood pressure, obesity (BMI), fat distribution, acanthosis nigricans, family history, race/ethnicity, socioeconomic status]. They would also provide useful information about the testing tools, including FPG, 2HPG, random glucose, and glycosylated hemoglobin (HbA1c). These school-based studies should be in populations with sufficient numbers of high-risk youth, and must be ongoing for several years, in order to track subjects with IGT, as well as those with risk factors who test normal, and to establish the predictability of various concentrations of PG and HbA1c[22].

PREVENTION

The US National Health and Nutrition Examination Survey of 1988–91 found 20% of children aged 12–17 years to be overweight (> 85th percentile of BMI for age and sex) and 8–17% were obese (> 95th percentile BMI), in various ethnic groups. This was an ~40% increase in the prevalence of obesity since the previous survey (1966–70)[54]. A 1996 survey in the UK found an even higher frequency of overweight, 31% at age 15 years, and obesity, 17% at age 15 years[55]. As noted earlier, similar trends have been documented in Japan[12]. The public-health implications of these trends, increasing the risk of problems associated with insulin resistance and the long-term complications of diabetes, are ominous. That there does not appear to be any reduction in the incidence of diabetes in the Pima population, despite extensive involvement of investigators and health workers for nearly 40 years, is of grave concern.

Prevention of the emergence of type 2 diabetes and other complications of hyperinsulinism that comprise the metabolic syndrome requires lifestyle changes that are as basic as they are difficult—decreased caloric intake and increased physical activity. This active eucaloric lifestyle is a challenge in a culture that promotes a hypercaloric diet, excessive TV watching, video game playing, and Internet surfing, combined with lack of attractive opportunities for vigorous activity in many places.

Summer camps and school-based education and prevention programs for Native American youth, who have been recognized with type 2 diabetes for > 15 years, have been carried out in Canada and the USA. School-based programs attempt to modify food supply in school meals, provide classroom education, and create a health- and physical-activity-promoting school environment. Programs for children in Headstart and kindergarten through sixth grade encourage family involvement, whereas high school-based programs use social networks and peer pressure to promote behavior change and reduce risk factors. Thus far, these programs have been successful in promoting short-term behavioral change, but long-term studies are needed to determine whether persistent behavior change and reduction in the risk for type 2 diabetes occur[5,56–58].

Culturally relevant programs for diabetes prevention require careful analysis of the health beliefs and behaviors, and the level of knowledge about the disease in the community[6]. For example, a study of American–Indian youth with family members having diabetes found that they did not relate the complications of retinopathy or amputation to diabetes, despite their presence in the community. Over half of the youth thought that diabetes was contagious or caused by bad blood, and more than one-third attributed it to 'weakness'[59].

The use of pharmacologic agents to reduce weight is not indicated in children until more safety and efficacy data become available[60]. Neither are fad diets, such as very low calorie or high protein, appropriate for growing children. Such programs, in any case, do not promote long-term healthy eating behavior.

The prevention of type 2 diabetes can be considered as a public-health approach directed to the general population, promoting improved dietary and physical activity behavior for all children and their families. At the next level, those children who are already at risk because of obesity, regardless of race/ethnicity, need to be identified, tested for diabetes and, if they are normal or have IGT, a lifestyle modification program undertaken for prevention of diabetes[22].

TREATMENT

Treatment goals

The goals of therapy are weight loss, normalization of glycemia and HbA1c, and control of hypertension and hyperlipidemia[22,61]. Pharmacologic therapy is directed at decreasing insulin resistance, increasing insulin secretion, or slowing postprandial glucose absorption.

Available hypoglycemic agents (Table 21.5)

Biguanides

The biguanides decrease blood glucose levels by acting on insulin target cells in the liver, muscle and fat. Hepatic glucose production is reduced, by decreasing gluconeogenesis, and insulin-stimulated glucose uptake in peripheral tissues, particularly muscle, contributes to decreasing blood glucose levels[62]. The biguanides also have an anorectic effect, which may promote weight loss. Long-term use of biguanides has resulted in 1–2% reduction in plasma HbA1c, with side effects being transient abdominal pain, diarrhea, and nausea. The major risk is the potential for lactic acidosis if the drug is given to patients with renal impairment, hepatic disease, cardiac or respiratory insufficiency, or not stopped with the administration of radiographic contrast materials.

The only treatment study of type 2 diabetes in pediatric patients has been with metformin. Newly diagnosed 8–16 year olds were randomized to placebo or metformin. By the time of the interim analysis at 8 weeks, few placebo cases remained, having been rescued according to protocol. At Week 16 or the last double-blind visit before rescue, placebo subjects had increased their mean FPG 20 mg dL^{-1} while metformin subjects had decreased theirs by 44 mg dL^{-1} with mean corresponding HbA1c 8.6% versus 7.5%. Lipid profiles improved, and there were no serious adverse effects[63].

Sulfonylureas and meglitinide

Sulfonylureas increase insulin secretion and are most useful when there is partial beta-cell failure. When plasma glucose levels rise, there is rapid phosphorylation of glucose to glucose-6-phosphate, which is rapidly metabolized to convert ADP to ATP. When the ATP:ADP ratio increases, K$^+$ channels close, resulting in depolarization of the adjacent cell membrane, with opening of the calcium channels. The secretion of insulin is controlled by the intracellular concentration of calcium. The higher the plasma glucose level, the greater the number of K$^+$ channels that close, resulting in more Ca^{2+} channels opening, with increased insulin release. Sulfonylureas bind to receptors on the K$^+$/ATP

Table 21.5 Drug treatment of type 2 diabetes					
Drug type	**Action**	**Effect on BG**	**Risk of low BG**	**Weight ↑**	**Lipid ↓**
Biguanides (metformin)	↓ hepatic glucose output; ↑ hepatic insulin sensitivity	+ +	0	0	+
Sulfonylureas	↑ insulin secretion & sensitivity	+ + +	+	+	0
Meglitinide (repaglinide)	short-term ↑ insulin secretion	+ + +	+	+	0
Glucosidase inhibitors (acarbose, miglitol)	slow hydrolysis & absorption of complex CHO	+	0	0	+
Thiazolidinediones (rosi-, pio-glitazone)	↑ insulin sensitivity in muscle and fat tissue	+ +	0	+	+
Insulin	↓ hepatic glucose output; overcome insulin resistance	+ + +	+	+ +	+

channel complex. A separate site on the K+/ATP channel complex binds meglitinide. Activation of ATP, sulfonylurea, or meglitinide binding sites causes K+ channels to close. The ATP binding sites equilibrate very rapidly, sulfonylurea sites equilibrate slowly and binding persists for prolonged periods, and meglitinide has an intermediate time of equilibration. Thus, the traditional sulfonylureas have prolonged effects, whereas the newer agent, metiglinide results in brief increases in insulin secretion[64]. The major adverse effects of the traditional sulfonylureas are hypoglycemia and weight gain.

Thiazolidinediones
Thiazolidinediones (TZDs) bind to nuclear proteins, activating peroxisome proliferator activator receptors (PPAR), orphan steroid receptors found primarily in adipocytes. Once activated by a TZD, PPAR forms a heterodimer with a retinoid X receptor, enabling it to bind to the promoter region of target genes, resulting in increased formation of proteins involved in nuclear-based actions of insulin, including cell growth and adipose cell differentiation, regulation of insulin receptor activity and glucose transport into the cell. This action increases insulin sensitivity in the liver, muscle, and adipose tissue and decreases hepatic glucose output[65]. During long-term therapy with TZD in adults, a reduction in HbA1c levels of 0.5–1.3% has been shown. The major side effects are edema, weight gain, anemia, and liver enzyme elevations, occurring in approximately 1% of subjects. The latter problem led to fatalities in adults who were taking the first available drug of this group, troglitazone, and it has been withdrawn from the US market. Newer thiazolidinediones, rosi- and pio-glitazone promise to be safer; pediatric trials are underway.

Alpha-glucosidase inhibitors
Alpha-glucosidase inhibitors (acarbose, miglitol) reduce the absorption of carbohydrates in the upper small intestine by inhibiting the breakdown of oligosaccharides, resulting in their delayed absorption in the lower small intestine. This delay reduces the postprandial rise of plasma glucose. A reduction in HbA1c levels of approximately 0.5–1% is expected during long-term therapy with acarbose[66]. The most frequent side effect is flatulence, making these agents unacceptable to most children and adolescents.

Insulin
There is a greater readiness to use insulin in the treatment of type 2 diabetes in children and adolescents, which may be related to the greater experience of pediatric practitioners with insulin than with oral agents. In the UK Prospective Diabetes Study (UKPDS), adults with type 2 diabetes had already lost 50% of their beta-cell function at the time of diagnosis, and by 6 or 7 years afterwards had little or no reserve, consistent with the failure of all oral hypoglycemic regimens to maintain early gains in control of HbA1c[67].

TREATMENT APPROACHES

The UKPDS demonstrated that intensive treatment of adults with type 2 diabetes resulted in improved metabolic control and this, in turn, resulted in decreased risk of microvascular disease[67]. The HbA1c goal inferred from the UKPDS data is < 7%. This study further demonstrated that aggressive treatment of blood pressure resulted in even greater reduction in the risk of both microvascular and macrovascular disease over 8.5 years, with a 37% reduction in microvascular disease, 44% reduction in stroke, and 56% reduction in heart failure[68].

There is evidence that the microvascular complications of diabetes are extraordinarily aggressive in type 2 diabetes in youth and it is, therefore, essential to strive for normal blood glucose levels[69,70]. Among 100 Pima Indian children and adolescents at the time of diagnosis of type 2 diabetes mellitus, 7% had hypercholesterolemia, 18% hypertension, and 22% microalbuminuria. Ten years after diagnosis, the mean HbA1c level was 12%; 60% had microalbuminuria and 17% had macroalbuminuria[70].

Initial therapy is determined by symptoms at diagnosis (Figure 21.3). Children who are asymptomatic, diagnosed following a routine physical exam in a doctor's office or by community or family testing, can be treated by non-pharmacologic

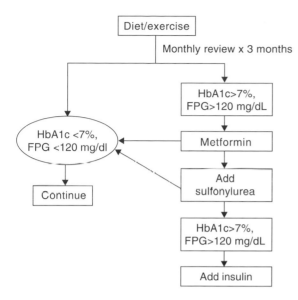

Figure 21.3 Treatment of type 2 diabetes mellitus in children.

means. These children need basic education about diabetes and its risks, and must be taught to monitor blood glucose levels, be given dietary counseling, and be encouraged to exercise daily.

The essentials of therapy are improved eating habits and increased physical activity, requiring behavior modification. A psychologist is therefore an important part of the treatment team, along with a dietician, and, if possible, an exercise specialist. The involvement of the parents and extended family is critical. The entire family should adopt the same healthy eating patterns, and exercise either together or individually. Physical activity does not need to be organized sports, but may involve walking to school, not using the elevator, bicycling, etc. Patients should exercise at least 30 min daily.

Patients who have not achieved glycemic goals, or whose blood glucose and HbA1c values are not improving after 3 months of an exercise/diet modification program, should be started on oral hypoglycemic agents. In the UKPDS, only 3% of patients were able to achieve treatment goals with diet and exercise alone; diet plus metformin resulted in reductions in HbA1c levels comparable to those resulting

from sulfonylureas or insulin, but without the weight gain and with fewer episodes of hypoglycemia than observed with the other therapies[67].

There can be an anorectic effect of metformin, with weight loss in some people, resulting in increased insulin sensitivity with consequent improved metabolic control. Intensive glycemic control with metformin as a single mode of therapy in the UKPDS trial was associated with a significant reduction in risk of long-term diabetes complications. The magnitude of this reduction was 32%, greater than that seen with sulfonylureas or insulin alone, which reduced the diabetes-related endpoints by only 12%[67]. In addition, metformin has very few side effects other than transient abdominal discomfort and diarrhea. As metformin increases insulin sensitivity, it is not associated with the risk of hypoglycemia that is attendant on the use of sulfonylureas, insulin, and benzoic acid derivatives (meglitinide). If monotherapy with metformin is not successful over a period of 3–6 months, sulfonylurea or meglitinide may be added to the regimen. Until more is known about the newer thiazolidinediones, it may be prudent to avoid their use in children. Insulin is added if oral agents are not able to achieve treatment goals.

Survey respondents from 130 pediatric endocrine practices in the USA and Canada reported that a mean 12% of their diabetes patients had type 2 diabetes and that approximately 48% of them were being treated with insulin, 44% with oral hypoglycemic agents. Those children with type 2 diabetes taking insulin were generally treated with two injections per day. Most children being treated with oral hypoglycemic agents received metformin (71%), with 46% using sulfonylureas, 9% thiazolidinediones and 4% meglitinide[61]. In the Florida diabetes centers study, 50% of the children with type 2 diabetes were being treated with oral hypoglycemic agents, 23% received insulin alone, 9% were treated with combination oral hypoglycemic/insulin and 11% with diet and exercise alone[9].

Patients who are mildly symptomatic at onset, but who have blood glucose levels < 17 mM are often started on oral hypoglycemic agents. Patients who have substantial ketosis, ketoacidosis, or markedly elevated blood-glucose levels are begun on insulin, usually twice a day, until blood-glucose control is established and symptoms subside. Metformin is added while the insulin dose is gradually reduced and stopped.

Patients receiving insulin should have blood-glucose checked before meals and at bedtime. Patients treated with exercise/diet or oral hypoglycemics are asked to monitor fasting BG levels and 2 h postprandial levels after dinner daily. Once target blood-glucose levels are achieved, fasting blood-glucose and 2 h postprandial (dinner) blood-glucose should be monitored three times a week.

TREATMENT OF COMORBIDITIES

The major goal of therapy is to reduce the risk of microvascular and macrovascular complications. The coexistence of type 2 diabetes with obesity, hypertension and hyperlipidemia place these patients at great risk for development of early cardiovascular disease. Lipid-lowering agents have been shown to reduce the risk of number of coronary events in patients with coronary heart disease and diabetes[71]. Hypertension is also an independent risk factor for the development of albuminuria and retinopathy[68]. Both blood pressure control (UKPDS) and blood glucose control are therefore important for decreasing the frequency and severity of the late complications of diabetes. Patients should have lipid levels and urine albumin checked annually. Dilated eye examination should also be performed annually in adolescents with type 2 diabetes. Unlike in children with type 1 diabetes, these examinations should begin at the time of diagnosis, rather than with puberty and after 3–5 years of disease[22].

Blood pressure should be monitored and treated aggressively with angiotensin-converting enzyme (ACE) inhibitors if either the systolic or diastolic pressures is above the child's usual percentile or above the 85th percentile for age and sex. Children with type 2 diabetes may have hyperlipidemia as an indication of insulin resistance, which will improve with exercise, weight loss, and glycemic control. Nutritional changes are made with initiation of a reduced fat diet, consistent with Step 1 American Heart Association guidelines. Should such attempts to normalize lipids fail after 2–3 months of intensive efforts, however, lipid-lowering medications are appropriate. The most commonly used lipid-lowering agents are the HMG CoA reductase inhibitors. They are contraindicated in pregnancy or if there is a risk of pregnancy.

TZD binding to PPAR-gamma receptors is ubiquitous, and includes arterial wall smooth muscle, inhibiting growth and migration in response to growth factors. This effect may be important in reducing the enhanced risk of macrovascular disease associated with type 2 diabetes[72].

REFERENCES

1 Knowles HC. Diabetes mellitus in childhood and adolescence. *Med Clin N Am* 1971;55:975–87.

2 Pinhas-Hamiel O, Dolan LM, Daniels SR *et al.* Increased incidence of non-insulin-dependent diabetes mellitus among adolescents. *J Pediatr* 1996;128:608–15.

3 Savage PJ, Bennett PH, Senter RG, Miller M. High prevalence of diabetes in young Pima Indians. *Diabetes* 1979;28:937–42.

4 Dabelea D, Hanson RL, Bennett PH *et al.* Increasing prevalence of type 2 diabetes in American Indian children. *Diabetologia* 1998;41:904–10.

5 Dean HJ. NIDDM-Y in First Nation children in Canada. *Clin Pediatr* 1998;39:89–96.

6 Rosenbloom AL, Joe JR, Young RS, Winter WE. The emerging epidemic of type 2 diabetes mellitus in youth. *Diabetes Care* 1999;22:345–54.

7 Scott CR, Smith JM, Cradock MM, Pihoker C. Characteristics of youth-onset noninsulin-dependent diabetes mellitus and insulin-dependent diabetes mellitus at diagnosis. *Pediatrics* 1997;100:84–91.

8 Neufeld ND, Raffal LF, Landon C *et al.* Early presentation of type 2 diabetes in Mexican–American youth. *Diabetes Care* 1998;21:80–6.

9   Macaluso CJ, Bauer UE, Deeb LC *et al.* Type 2 diabetes mellitus among Florida children and adolescents, 1994 through 1998. *Public Health Reports* 2002;117:373–9.

10 Kadiki OA, Reddy MR, Marzouk AA. Incidence of insulin-dependent diabetes (IDDM) and non-insulin-dependent diabetes (NIDDM) (0–34 years at onset) in Benghazi, Libya. *Diabetes Res Clin Pract* 1996;32:165–73.

11 Chan JCN, Cheung CK, Swaminathan R *et al.* Obesity, albuminuria, and hypertension among Hong Kong Chinese with non-insulin-dependent diabetes mellitus (NIDDM). *Postgrad Med J* 1993;69:204–10.

12 Kitagawa T, Owada M, Urakami T, Yamauchi K. Increased incidence of non-insulin dependent diabetes mellitus among Japanese schoolchildren correlates with an increased intake of animal protein and fat. *Clin Pediatr* 1998;37:111–15.

13 Sayeed MA, Hussain MZ, Banu A *et al.* Prevalence of diabetes in a suburban population of Bangladesh. *Diabetes Res Clin Pract* 1997;34: 149–55.

14 Braun B, Zimmerman MB, Kretchmer N *et al.* Risk factors for diabetes and cardiovascular disease in young Australian aborigines. A 5-year follow-up study. *Diabetes Care* 1996;19:472–9.

15 McGrath NM, Parker GN, Dawson P. Early presentation of type 2 diabetes mellitus in young New Zealand Maori. *Diabetes Res Clin Pract* 1999;43:205–9.

16 Ehtisham S, Barrett TG, Shawl NJ. Type 2 diabetes mellitus in UK children—an emerging problem. *Diabetic Med* 2000;17:867–71.

17 Winter WE, Nakamura M, House DV. Monogenic diabetes mellitus in youth: the MODY syndromes. *Endoc Metab Clin N Am* 1999;28: 765–85.

18 Winter WE, Maclaren NK, Riley WJ *et al.* Maturity onset diabetes of youth in black Americans. *N Engl J Med* 1987;316:285–91.

19 The Expert Committee on the Diagnosis and Classification of Diabetes Mellitus. Report of the Expert Committee on the Diagnosis and Classification of Diabetes Mellitus. *Diabetes Care* 2001;24:S5–S20.

20 Rosenbloom AL, Kohrman A, Sperling M. Classification and diagnosis of diabetes mellitus in children and adolescents. *J Pediatr* 1981;98: 320–3.

21 Pinhas-Hamiel O, Dolan LM, Zeitler PS. Diabetic ketoacidosis among obese African American adolescents with NIDDM. *Diabetes Care* 1997;28: 484–6.

22 American Diabetes Association. Type 2 diabetes in children and adolescents: consensus conference report. *Diabetes Care* 2000;23:381–9.

23 Feeney SJ, Myers MA, Mackay IR *et al.* Evaluation of ICA512As in combination with other islet cell autoantibodies at the onset of IDDM. *Diabetes Care* 1997;20:1403–7.

24 Neel JV. Diabetes mellitus: a 'thrifty' genotype rendered detrimental by 'progress'? *Am J Hum Genet* 1962;14:353–62.

25 Lev-Ran A. Thrifty genotype: how applicable is it to obesity and type 2 diabetes? *Diabetes Rev* 1999;7:1–22.

26 Phipps K, Barker DJP. Fetal growth and impaired glucose tolerance in men and women. *Diabetologia* 1993;36:225–8.

27 Philips DIW, Barker DJP, Hales CN *et al.* Thinness at birth and insulin resistance in adult life. *Diabetologia* 1994;37:150–4.

28 Lithell HO, McKeigue PM, Gerglund L *et al.* Relation at birth to non-insulin-dependent diabetes and insulin concentrations in men aged 50 60 years. *Br Med J* 1996;312:406–10.

29 Curhan GC, Willett WC, Rimm EB *et al.* Birth weight and adult hypertension, diabetes mellitus, and obesity in US men. *Circulation* 1996;94:3246–50.

30 Ravelli AC, van der Meulen JH, Michels RP *et al.* Glucose tolerance in adults after prenatal exposure to famine. *Lancet* 1998;351:173–7.

31 Levitt NS, Lambert EV, Woods D *et al.* Impaired glucose tolerance and elevated blood pressure in low birth weight, nonobese, young South African adults: early programming of cortisol axis. *J Clin Endocrinol Metab* 2000;85:4611–18.

32 Dabelea D, Pettitt DJ, Hanson RL *et al.* Birthweight, type 2 diabetes, and insulin resistance in Pima Indian children and young adults. *Diabetes Care* 1999;22:944–50.

33 Bavdekar A, Yajnik CS, Fall CHD *et al.* Insulin resistance syndrome in 8-year old Indian children. Small at birth, big at 8 years, or both? *Diabetes* 1999;48:2422–9.

34 Svec F, Nastasi K, Hilton C *et al.* Black–white contrasts and insulin levels during pubertal development: the Bogalusa Heart Study. *Diabetes* 1992;41:313–17.

35 Jiang X, Srinivasan SR, Radhakrishnamurthy B *et al.* Racial (black–white) differences in insulin secretion and clearance in adolescents: the Bogalusa heart study. *Pediatrics* 1996;97:357–60.

36 Arslanian S. Insulin secretion and sensitivity in healthy African–American vs. American–white children. *Clin Pediatr* 1998;37:81–8.

37 Danadian K, Lewy V, Janosky JJ, Arslanian S. Lipolysis in African–American children: is it a metabolic risk factor predisposing to obesity? *J Clin Endocrinol Metab* 2001;86:3022–6.

38 Danadian K, Balasekaran G, Lewy V *et al.* Insulin sensitivity in African–American children with and without a family history of type 2 diabetes. *Diabetes Care* 1999;22:1325–9.

39 Pinhas-Hamiel O, Standiford D, Hamiel D *et al.* The type 2 family. A setting for development and treatment of adolescent type 2 diabetes mellitus. *Arch Pediatr Adolesc Med* 1999;153:1063–7.

40 BL Silverman, BE Metzger, NH Cho, CA Loeb. Impaired glucose tolerance in adolescent offspring of diabetic mothers. Relationship to fetal hyperinsulinism *Diabetes Care* 1995;18:611–17.

41 Pettitt DJ, Aleck KA, Baird HR *et al.* Congenital susceptibility to NIDDM: role of intrauterine environment. *Diabetes* 1988;37:622–8.

42 Fagot-Campagna A, Pettitt DJ, Engelgau MM *et al.* Type 2 diabetes among North American children and adolescents: An epidemiological review and a public health perspective. *J Pediatr* 2000;136:664–72.

43 Rosenbloom AL, Wheeler L, Bianchi R *et al.* Age adjusted analysis of insulin responses during normal and abnormal oral glucose tolerance tests in children and adolescents. *Diabetes* 1975;24:820–8.

44 Caprio S, Tamborlane WV. Metabolic impact of obesity in childhood. *Endocrinol Metab Clin North Am* 1999;28:731–47.

45 Legro RS, Kunselman AR, Dodson WC, Dunaif A. Prevalence and predictors of risk for type 2 diabetes mellitus and impaired glucose tolerance in polycystic ovary syndrome: a prospective, controlled study in 254 affected women. *J Clin Endocrinol Metab* 1999;84:165–9.

46 Lewy V, Danadian K, Arslanian SA. Early metabolic abnormalities in adolescents with polycystic ovarian syndrome (PCOS). *Pediatr Res* 1999;45:93A.

47 Lewy V, Danadian K, Arslanian SA. Roles of insulin resistance and B-cell dysfunction in the pathogenesis of glucose intolerance in adolescents with polycystic ovary syndrome. *Diabetes* 1999;48:A292.

48 Banerjee S, Raghavan S, Wasserman EJ *et al.* Hormonal findings in African–American and Caribbean Hispanic girls with premature adrenarche: implications for polycystic ovarian syndrome. *Pediatrics* 1998;102:E36.

49 Vuguin P, Linder B, Rosenfeld RG *et al.* The roles of insulin sensitivity, insulin-like growth factor I (IGF-I), and IGF-binding protein-1 and -3 in the hyperandrogenism of African American and Caribbean Hispanic girls with premature adrenarche. *J Clin Endocrinol Metab* 1999;84: 2037–42.

50 Ibañez L, Potau N, Marcos MV, deZegher F. Exaggerated adrenarche and hyperinsulinism in adolescent girls born small for gestational age. *J Clin Endocrinol Metab* 1999;84:4739–41.

51 Ibañez L, Castell C, Tresserras R, Potau N. Increased prevalence of type 2 diabetes mellitus and impaired glucose tolerance in first-degree relatives of girls with a history of precocious pubarche. *Clin Endocrinol* 1999;51:395–401.

52 Fletcher RH, Fletcher SW, Wagner EH. *Clinical epidemiology, the essentials.* 2nd edn. Baltimore: Williams and Wilkins, 1988.

53 Sackett DL, Holland WW. Controversy in detection of disease. *Lancet* 1965;2:357–9.

54 Troiano RP, Flegal KM. Overweight children and adolescents: description, epidemiology, and demographics. *Pediatrics* 1998;101 (Suppl): 497–504.

55 Reilly JJ, Dorosty AR. Epidemic of obesity in UK children. *Lancet* 1999;354:1874–5.

56 Cook VV, Hurley JS. Prevention of type 2 diabetes in childhood. *Clin Pediat* 1998;37:123–9.

57 Teufel NI, Ritenbaugh CK. Development of a primary prevention program: insight gained in the Zuni Diabetes Prevention Program. *Clin Pediat* 1998;37:131–41.

58 Macaulay AC, Paradis G, Potvin L *et al.* The Kahnawake Schools Diabetes Prevention Project: intervention, evaluation and baseline results of a diabetes primary prevention program with a native community in Canada. *Prevent Med* 1997;26:779–90.

59 Joe JR. Perceptions of diabetes by Indian adolescents. In: Joe JR, Young RS, editors. *Diabetes as a disease of civilization: the impact of culture change on indigenous peoples.* Berlin: Mouton de Gruyter, 1994: 329–56.

60 Daniels S. Pharmacological treatment of obesity in paediatric patients. *Paediatr Drugs* 2001;3: 405–10.

61 Silverstein JH, Rosenbloom AL. Treatment of type 2 diabetes in children and adolescents. *J Ped Endocrinol Metab* 2000;13:1403–9.

62 DeFronzo RA, Goodman AM. Efficacy of metformin in patients with non-insulin dependent diabetes mellitus. The multicenter metformin study group. *N Engl J Med* 1995;333: 541–9.

63 Jones K, Arslanian S, Peterokova VA *et al.* Effect of metformin in pediatric patients with type 2

diabetes: a randomized controlled trial. *Diabetes Care* 2002;25:89–94.

64 Lebovitz HE. Insulin secretagogues, old and new. *Diabetes Rev* 1999;7:139–52.

65 Schwartz S, Raskin P, Fonseca V, Graveline JF. Effect of troglitazone in insulin treated patients with type 2 diabetes. *N Engl J Med* 1998;338:861–6.

66 Chiasson J, Josse R, Hunt J *et al.* The efficacy of acarbose in the treatment of patients with non-insulin-dependent diabetes mellitus. A multi-center controlled clinical trial. *Ann Int Med* 1994;121:928–35.

67 UKPDS Group. Intensive blood glucose control with sulphonylureas or insulin compared with conventional treatment and risk of complications in patients with type 2 diabetes (UKPDS 33). *Lancet* 1998;352:837–53.

68 UKPDS Group. Tight blood pressure control and risk of macrovascular and microvascular complications in type 2 diabetes: UKPDS 38. *Br Med J* 1998;317:703–13.

69 Yokoyama H, Okudaira M, Otani T *et al.* High incidence of diabetic nephropathy in early-onset Japanese NIDDM patients. Risk analysis. *Diabetes Care* 1998;21:1080–5.

70 Fagot-Compagna A, Knowler WC, Pettitt DJ. Type 2 diabetes in Pima Indian Children: cardio-vascular risk factors at diagnosis and 10 years later. *Diabetes* 1998;47 (Suppl 1):A155.

71 Haffner SM, Alexander CM, Cook TJ *et al.* for the Scandinavian Simvastatin Survival Study Group. Reduced coronary events in Simvastatin treated patients with coronary heart disease and diabetes or impaired fasting glucose levels. *Arch Int Med* 1999;59:2661–7.

72 Law RE, Goetze S, Xi X-P *et al.* Expression and function of PPARγ in rat and human vascular smooth muscle cells. *Circulation* 2000;101: 1311–18.

22

The insulin resistance syndrome and its vascular complications

Cyrus Desouza, Merri Pendergrass and Vivian Fonseca

INTRODUCTION

The insulin resistance syndrome (IRS), also known as the metabolic syndrome, is a 'cluster' of cardiovascular (CV) risk factors frequently, but not always, associated with obesity. Reaven *et al.* first drew attention to the association of insulin resistance and obesity, type 2 diabetes, high plasma triglycerides and low plasma high-density lipoprotein (HDL) cholesterol[1]. Since its original description, there has been much experimental, clinical and epidemiological data to support the association of this syndrome with cardiovascular disease (CVD)[2]. Additionally, other cardiovascular risk factors have been frequently included in the description of the syndrome. These include inflammation, abnormal fibrinolysis, and endothelial dysfunction[3]. Figure 22.1 summarizes the relationship of these risk factors and their link with CVD. It is unclear whether the components of this syndrome develop independently of each other, or spring from 'common soil' genetic abnormalities[4]. The frequency of co-existence of these abnormalities has resulted in this syndrome becoming a major clinical and public-health problem.

Historically, research studies have used complex experimental techniques to quantify insulin sensitivity/resistance (Table 22.1). Epidemiological studies utilize hyperinsulinemia to

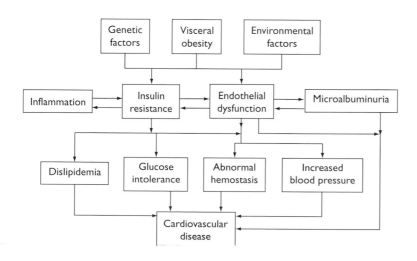

Figure 22.1 Potential links between insulin resistance and cardiovascular disease.

Table 22.1 Laboratory methods of measuring insulin sensitivity/resistance

Hyperinsulinemic-euglycemic clamp

Fasting insulin and insulin/glucose ratio[a]

Oral glucose tolerance test with plasma glucose and insulin measured[a]

Intravenous glucose tolerance test with minimal model analysis

Homeostatic model assessment (HOMA-IR)

Constant infusion of glucose with model assessment

[a]Several formulae based on these measurements have been proposed and validated against the euglycemic hyperinsulinemic clamp.

define insulin resistance. Since plasma insulin-concentrations are a reflection of both ambient glucose and pancreatic beta-cell function (which decreases even before the onset of type 2 diabetes), it is a poor marker of insulin resistance.

Furthermore, lack of standardization of the insulin assay makes interpretation of plasma insulin concentration difficult. More recently, the World Health Organization (WHO) and the National Cholesterol Education Program Adult Treatment Panel III (NCEP-ATP III) have attempted to define the syndrome for clinicians (see Table 22.2 and NCEP ATP III internet site http://www.nhlbi.nih.gov/guidelines/ cholesterol/atp_iii.htm). Subjects identified using these clinical definitions have been shown to be at increased risk of CVD. Waist circumference correlated with insulin levels and insulin resistance in several studies. Recently, a standardized method for measurement of waist circumference has been described (Internet site http://www.nhlb.nih.gov/guidelines/obesity/e_txtbk/index.htm).

Insulin resistance in the context of type 2 diabetes is discussed elsewhere in this book. This chapter discusses:

- The interaction of the various components of the syndrome and the associated CVD
- The pathophysiology of the syndrome
- Its clinical evaluation and treatment.

Table 22.2 Criteria for the diagnosis of IRS

WHO criteria

- Hypertension: on antihypertensive medication and/or BP > 160/90
- Dyslipidemia: plasma triglycerides > 1.7 mmol L^{-1} and/or HDL cholesterol < 0.9 mmol L^{-1} in men and < 1.0 mmol L^{-1} in women
- Obesity: BMI > 30 and/or WHR (> 0.90 in males, 0.85 in females)
- Microalbuminuria (overnight urinary albumin excretion rate > 20 μg min^{-1})

WHO requires a person to have type 2 diabetes or impaired glucose tolerance and any two of the above criteria. A person with normal glucose tolerance must demonstrate insulin resistance (see Table 22.1)

NCEP ATP III criteria

- Hypertension: BP > 130/85
- Dyslipidemia: plasma triglycerides > 150 mg dL^{-1}
- HDL cholesterol < 40 mg dL^{-1} in men and < 50 mg dL^{-1} in women
- Obesity: waist circumference > 40 cm in males and > 50 cm in females
- Fasting blood sugar > 110 mg dL^{-1}

NCEP requires any three of the above criteria to be met

IRS AS A RISK FACTOR FOR CVD

Prospective studies suggest that hyperinsuline-mia may be an important risk factor for ischemic heart disease. The Quebec Heart Study studied 45–76 year-old men who did not have ischemic heart disease[5]. A first ischemic event occurred in 114 men who were then matched for age, body-mass index (BMI), smoking habits, and alcohol consumption with a control selected from among the 1989 men who remained free of ischemic heart disease during follow-up. Fasting insulin concentrations at baseline were 18% higher in the case patients than in the controls. High fasting-insulin concentrations were an independent predictor of ischemic heart disease in these men, after adjustment for systolic blood pressure, family history of ischemic heart disease, plasma triglyceride, apolipoprotein B, LDL cholesterol, and high-density lipoprotein (HDL) cholesterol concentrations.

Similarly, hyperinsulinemia was associated with increased all-cause and cardiovascular mortality in Helsinki policemen, independent of other risk factors[6]. Correlation of insulin with other risk factors makes interpretation difficult. Factor analysis was carried out to study the clustering of risk factors in the baseline data of the Helsinki Policemen Study. When including only risk factor variables proposed to be central components of IRS, factor analysis predicted the risk of coronary heart disease (CHD) and stroke independently of other risk factors[7].

Other population studies, as well as a recent met-analysis, have supported these studies[8–10], confirming that components of the syndrome are present for several years before the onset of type 2 diabetes and that the "clock for coronary heart disease starts ticking before the onset of clinical diabetes"[10].

ASSOCIATION OF IRS WITH OTHER CARDIOVASCULAR RISK FACTORS

In addition to being a precursor of type 2 diabetes and an independent risk factor for CVD, insulin resistance is also closely associated with several other cardiovascular risk factors, some of which are discussed below.

Obesity

Obesity is frequently associated with several of the components of IRS, and may be critical for the development of the syndrome. Several mechanisms have been proposed for the link between obesity and IRS[11]. Cardiovascular morbidity and mortality are increased in obese individuals, independently of other risk factors. Insulin resistance is very common in obese individuals. However, some non-obese individuals demonstrate hyperinsulinemia and the other features of the IRS[12]. Thus, obesity may not be essential for the expression of the syndrome, but the presence of obesity or weight gain may accentuate the pathophysiological changes associated with the syndrome.

Body fat distribution, rather than body mass, may actually be a better predictor of insulin resistance and cardiovascular risk[13]. Insulin resistance, type 2 diabetes and hypertension are more closely associated with a central distribution of adiposity than with general increases in fat mass. Waist circumference serves as a clinical predictor of intra-abdominal fat.

DYSLIPIDEMIA

One of the earliest relationships between insulin resistance and a cardiovascular risk factor is with 'diabetic dyslipidemia'. The hallmark of the syndrome is hypertriglyceridemia and low plasma HDL cholesterol concentration. Plasma LDL cholesterol concentrations in insulin-resistant subjects are no different from those in insulin-sensitive subjects. However, there are qualitative changes in LDL cholesterol, resulting in 'pattern B' distribution of LDL particles— which consist of smaller LDL particles, are more susceptible to oxidation and thus, are potentially more atherogenic[14].

Several hypotheses have been proposed for the mechanism of association between IRS and dyslipidemia. Insulin resistance at the level of adipose tissue may result in increased activity of hormone sensitive lipase and, therefore, increased breakdown of stored triglycerides. Free fatty acids (FFA) released from adipocytes, particularly intra-abdominal adipocytes, can be transported to the liver, where they stimulate synthesis of triglycerides and assembly and secretion of very-low-density lipoprotein (VLDL). Increased plasma VLDL triglycerides exchange with cholesterol esters from HDL, resulting in a lower plasma HDL cholesterol. On the other hand, an increase in circulating FFA has been proposed as having an etiological role in the development of IRS[15]. The effect of treatment of insulin resistance on dyslipidemia is discussed below.

Hypertension

Although it is well-established that essential hypertension is frequently associated with insulin resistance, the impact of this abnormality on blood pressure homeostasis is still a matter of debate. Fasting plasma insulin is frequently higher in hypertensive subjects and glucose disposal during a euglycemic clamp is decreased. The association between hypertension and insulin resistance is more convincing in obese subjects. Significant decreases in blood pressure have been observed in obese subjects who lose modest amounts of weight, correlating closely with the decline in fasting plasma insulin concentrations. Plasma insulin concentrations are higher, and insulin-mediated total-body glucose disposal is reduced in young, normal weight individuals with essential hypertension[2]. The impairment in insulin-mediated glucose disposal was closely related to the increase in blood pressure. Multiple potential mechanisms by which IR may cause hypertension have been proposed[16]. These include resistance to insulin-mediated vasodilatation, impaired endothelial function, sympathetic nervous system over-activity, sodium retention, increased vascular sensitivity to the vasoconstrictor effect of pressor amines, and enhanced growth-factor activity, leading to proliferation of smooth muscle walls. However, some studies do not support the association of metabolic insulin resistance with essential hypertension. Clearly, hypertension is itself a complex disorder with many etiologies, and not all subjects with essential hypertension are insulin resistant.

Prothrombotic state

Factors contributing to a prothrombotic state in diabetes are summarized in Table 22.3. The endogenous fibrinolytic system represents equilibrium between activators of plasminogen [primarily tissue-type plasminogen activator (tPA)] and inhibitors of these activators [such as plasminogen activator inhibitor type 1 (PAI 1)][17]. Coagulation is a continuous process, and the fibrinolytic system maintains fluidity of blood. Excessive inhibition of fibrinolysis will lead to coagulation and thrombosis, a critical process in cardiovascular events. Impaired fibrinolytic function in diabetes correlates with severity of vascular disease in diabetes, and is a risk factor for myocardial infarction in both diabetic and non-diabetic subjects.

Impaired fibrinolysis is now recognized as being an important component of the IRS, and probably contributes considerably to the increased risk of cardiovascular events[17]. Plasma PAI 1 antigen and activity are elevated in a wide variety of insulin-resistant subjects, including obese subjects with and without diabetes, and women with the polycystic ovarian syndrome

---

Table 22.3 Potential impact of insulin resistance and diabetes on thrombosis and fibrinolysis

Factors predisposing to thrombosis
↑ platelet hyperaggregability
↑ platelet cAMP and cGMP
↑ thromboxane synthesis
Elevated concentrations of procoagulants
↑ fibrinogen
↑ von Willebrand factor and procoagulant activity
↑ thrombin activity
Decreased concentration and activity of antithrombotic factors
↓ antithrombin III activity
Factors attenuating fibrinolysis
Decreased t-PA activity
Increased PAI-1 synthesis and activity
Increased blood viscosity

(PCOS). Immuno-histochemical analysis of coronary lesions from patients with coronary artery disease have demonstrated an imbalance of the local fibrinolytic system, with increased coronary artery tissue PAI–1 in patients with type 2 diabetes. Many studies have attempted to elucidate the mechanistic link between insulin resistance and abnormal fibrinolysis. Insulin, proinsulin, abnormal cholesterol and various cytokines regulate PAI-1 synthesis and release. The greatest elevations in PAI-1 occur when there is a combination of hyperinsulinemia, hyperglycemia and increased FFA, in obese insulin-resistant subjects[18].

Other factors predisposing to thrombosis associated with insulin resistance, include increased platelet hyper-aggregation, elevated concentrations of pro-coagulants, particularly fibrinogen and von Willebrand factor, and a decrease in anti-thrombotic factors, such as antithrombin III[17]. Many of these abnormalities are non-specific and the association of insulin resistance with coagulation abnormalities is less robust than that with abnormal fibrinolysis.

ENDOTHELIAL FUNCTION AND VASCULAR ABNORMALITIES

The importance of the endothelium in maintaining vascular health has been widely recognized. The endothelium is a critical determinant of vascular tone, reactivity, inflammation, vascular remodeling, maintenance of vascular patency and blood fluidity[19]. Many of these functions of the endothelium are maintained through regulatory substances secreted from endothelial cells, which may often have opposing actions. For example, nitric oxide (NO) is the most potent known vasodilator and is secreted by endothelial cells, having been synthesized from arginine by nitric oxide synthase (NOS). Endothelial cells also secrete other important vasodilators, such as prostacyclin. The vasodilatory actions are opposed by secretion of potent vasoconstrictors such as endothelin 1. Similarly, these and other endothelial products are involved in maintaining the balance between smooth muscle cell growth, promotion and inhibition, thrombosis and fibrinolysis, inflammation and cell adhesion.

Endothelial dysfunction is now recognized as being an early abnormality in the natural history of CVD and may be a good predictor of cardiovascular events. Abnormalities in production of NO, increased inactivation of NO, along with increased activation of angiotensin-converting enzyme (ACE) and local mediators of inflammation, may be key precursors of clinical events in IRS.

The ability of blood vessels to dilate in response to stimuli, including ischemia, is termed vascular reactivity, or flow-mediated dilatation. Brachial artery vascular reactivity is a non-invasive method of assessing arterial endothelial function *in vivo*. Since endothelial injury is an early event in atherogenesis, it has been suggested that abnormal flow-mediated dilatation may precede the development of structural changes in the vessel wall. Abnormal flow-mediated dilatation has been shown in several insulin-resistant states and is present in relatives of patient with type 2 diabetes who have normal glucose tolerance. It has even been proposed that endothelial dysfunction may be a precursor of IRS[20]. Figure 22.2 summarizes this hypothesis and illustrates the various determinants and consequences of insulin resistance. Table 22.4 lists various endothelial abnormalities associated with insulin resistance.

Insulin itself has vasodilatory actions via an NO-dependent mechanism[21]. In healthy subjects, insulin dilates arterioles supplying skeletal muscle, probably through enhancement of NO production. Some *in vitro* studies have documented that insulin regulates NOS, and that this action maybe impaired in insulin resistant subjects—an abnormality that might be attributable to either impairment in the ability of the endothelium to produce NO, or enhanced inactivation of NO[21]. Since NO plays a critical role in the maintenance of vascular health[19], this abnormality may explain much of the increased CVD in IRS. Impairment of insulin action on glucose metabolism, assessed by glucose clamp, parallels impairment of insulin action on the vasculature (Figure 22.3). Thus, obesity and type 2 diabetes are associated with resistance to insulin's vascular effects.

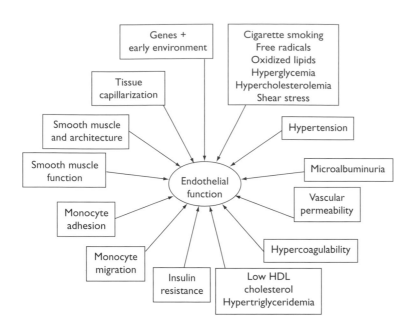

Figure 22.2 Determinants and consequences of endothelial function (adapted from Reference 20).

Table 22.4 Alterations in the vascular endothelium associated with diabetes mellitus and insulin resistance

Abnormality	Significance
↓ Release of and responsiveness to NO	Impaired endothelial function and reactivity
↑ Expression, synthesis, and plasma levels of endothelin-1	Vasoconstriction and hypertension
↓ Prostacyclin release	Impaired vasodilatation
↑ Adhesion-molecule expression	Increased monocyte adhesion to vessel wall
↑ Adhesion of platelets and monocytes	Foam cell formation, thrombosis and inflammation
↑ Pro-coagulant activity	Thrombosis
↑ Advanced glycosylated end products	Increased stiffness of arterial wall
Impaired fibrinolytic activity	Decreased clot breakdown

Finally, insulin resistance is associated with increased carotid intima–media thickness (IMT)[23]. This finding is compatible with the possible effect of hyperinsulinemia on growth of vascular smooth-muscle cells and extracellular matrix[24]. Carotid IMT is increased in newly diagnosed patients with type 2 diabetes, without cardiovascular disease[25]. This finding is important since IMT represents a structural abnormality in the arterial wall and is a good predictor of subsequent cardiovascular risk[26].

Microalbuminuria

Microalbuminuria is recognized as a complication of diabetes due to changes in the kidney secondary to hyperglycemia. Recent data suggests that it may occur even in non-diabetics, be a precursor of cardiovascular disease and may be related to insulin resistance[27]. It is possible that in individuals who are insulin resistant, microalbuminuria may be a manifestation of endothelial dysfunction, indicating endothelial

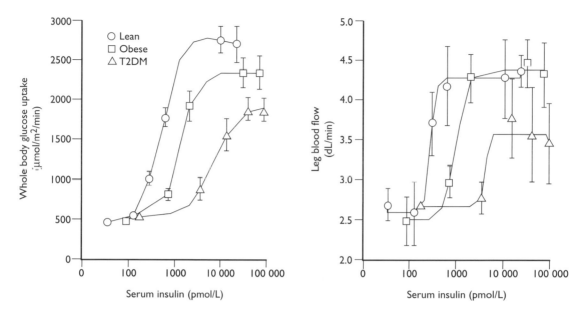

Figure 22.3 Insulin effects on glucose uptake parallels (adapted from Reference 22).

permeability, and is also related to increased carotid IMT[28]. Microalbuminuria is included in the criteria used by the WHO to define IRS.

PATHOGENESIS OF IRS

Physical activity

Habitual physical activity is an important determinant of insulin resistance. Epidemiological studies have shown a strong correlation between a sedentary lifestyle and type 2 diabetes, hypertension and CVD[29-31]. Exercise has been shown to have significant therapeutic value in treating most of the components of IRS (see below).

Genetic abnormalities associated with IRS

Although IRS appears to have a strong genetic basis, the precise genetic abnormalities in the common form of the syndrome have not been well-characterized. It is likely that the syndrome, as well as its components, is a polygenic disorder. A few single-point mutations associated with the IRS have been identified, but

these are rare. Examples include mutations of the leptin receptor, insulin receptor substrate-1 (*IRS-1*) gene and peroxisome proliferator activator receptor gamma (*PPAR-gamma*)[32]. Individuals with these mutations appear to have several components of IRS, including diabetes, dyslipidemia and hypertension.

Cytokines and inflammation

Several studies have suggested a role for inflammation in the etiology of IRS and its complications. Observations suggest that cytokines arising from adipose tissue may be partly responsible for the metabolic, hemodynamic and hemostatic abnormalities associated with insulin resistance. Studies show a close relationship between obesity and circulating C-reactive protein (CRP), tumor necrosis factor alpha (TNF-alpha) and interleukin-6 (IL-6). Plasma CRP is elevated in obese subjects who have other features of IRS[33]. It has been recently recognized that some of these cytokines are predictors of CVD. Thus, inflammation originating from excess adipose tissue cytokine production may contribute not only to the development of IRS but also to the associated CVD. Increased expression of TNF-alpha in adipose tissue has been reported in obese subjects. TNF-alpha inhibits the action of lipoprotein lipase and stimulates lipolysis. It also impairs the function of the insulin-signaling pathway, by effects on phosphorylation of both the insulin receptor and IRS-1. IL-6 may also induce endothelial expression of cytokines, thereby contributing to endothelial dysfunction.

ABNORMAL INSULIN SIGNALING, HYPERINSULINEMIA AND THE VASCULATURE

As outlined above, insulin resistance with resultant hyperinsulinemia is an independent risk-factor for CVD. However, the specific role of insulin in the pathogenesis of atherosclerosis remains unclear. Several mechanistic hypotheses have been proposed to explain this association[2,34]. Firstly, insulin is a growth factor that stimulates vascular cell growth and synthesis of matrix proteins. Secondly, the insulin-signaling pathway, thought to be responsible for abnormalities in glucose metabolism, is also involved in NO production. Thus, the abnormal intracellular signaling that causes hyperglycemia may also be responsible for vascular disease, due to loss of insulin's anti-atherogenic properties, while hyperinsulinemia continues to stimulate growth-promoting enzymes such as MAP kinase[34]. Although some controversy remains, this hypothesis (see Figure 22.4) has been supported by many studies. In addition, imbalances in insulin homeostasis are associated with abnormalities in expression and action of various peptides, growth factors and cytokines. These include angiotensin II, endothelin-1 and insulin-like growth factor-1[34].

While the exact role of peroxisome proliferator-activated receptors in the pathogenesis of this syndrome is unclear, several studies support the concept that they may have a role in the development of not only insulin resistance, but also atherosclerosis[35]. For example, these receptors are present in vascular tissue, heterozygous mutations in the ligand-binding domain of PPAR-gamma are occasionally associated with

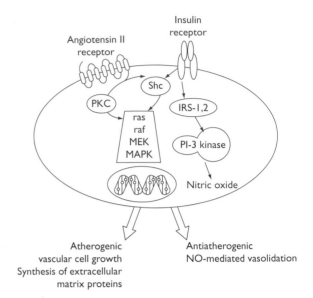

Figure 22.4 Mechanisms of insulin signalling and potential atherogenic and antiatherogenic actions of insulin in vascular cells (adapted from Reference 34). Activation of the tyrosine kinase of the insulin receptor results in tyrosine phosphorylation of intracellular substrates such as insulin receptor substrate-1 (IRS-1), IRS-2, and Shc. These docking proteins couple the receptor to several signalling pathways, including the ras pathway that activates mitogen-activated protein kinase (MAPK) and phosphatidylinositol-3-kinase (PI-3-kinase). Insulin resistance in vascular cells can impair insulin's ability to activate the latter pathway. Certain cytokines and vasoactive peptides, such as angiotensin II, can both activate the MAPK pathway and inhibit insulin's ability to activate PI-3-kinase. IRS = insulin receptor substrate; PKC = protein kinase C; IRS-1,2 = insulin receptor substrate; MAPK = mitogen activated protein kinase; MEK = MAP kinase–kinase; PI-3-kinase = phosphatidylinositol-3-kinase.

insulin resistance, and agonists of these receptors have a significant impact on the syndrome. Thus, it is possible that PPARs play a role in the pathogenesis of the complete syndrome: this is the subject of much current research.

Drug induced

Several classes of drugs have been associated with insulin resistance. These include corticosteroids, which frequently cause insulin resistance and type 2 diabetes. Recent data have shown that protease inhibitors, used for the treatment of human immunodeficiency virus (HIV) infection, frequently cause several manifestations of IRS[36].

Hypertriglyceridemia appears to be an early manifestation of protease inhibitor-induced lipodystrophy, and is associated with changes in body-fat distribution and marked insulin resistance. The long-term effects of these drugs on CVD are unknown.

Intrauterine/postpartum growth and development

Some data have suggested that a low birthweight and/or rapid gain of weight in early life are associated with the later development of multiple features of IRS, including type 2 diabetes and other risk factors for CVD[37,38]. It has become increasingly evident that impaired intrauterine growth plays a decisive role in the future physiology and function of many organs and body systems.

MANAGEMENT OF IRS

The use of insulin sensitizers and lifestyle modifications to improve insulin resistance in the treatment of type 2 diabetes is discussed elsewhere in this book. Any therapeutic maneuver that improves insulin sensitivity should also have beneficial effects on all the metabolic and cardiovascular abnormalities associated with IRS. This section concentrates on management of the syndrome as a whole, particularly its link with CVD.

Lifestyle changes

Since obesity and physical activity are important precursors of the syndrome, lifestyle change may be critical in its prevention and treatment. The NCEP has strongly endorsed the concept of 'total lifestyle change' in the prevention of CVD due to the syndrome. Recent clinical trials have demonstrated that modest reductions in calorie and fat intake, and a small increase in physical activity, can prevent the development of type 2 diabetes[39].

While a reduction in cardiovascular events has not yet been documented, a significant improvement in cardiovascular risk factors is possible.

Since many individuals with the metabolic syndrome are overweight, dietary treatment should be primarily focused on weight reduction. While the effect of weight reduction on the components of IRS are widely accepted, there remains some controversy about specific diets to achieve weight loss.

Insulin sensitivity can also be influenced by diet composition[40,41]. There is evidence that a higher saturated-fat intake is associated with impaired insulin action, some of which may be mediated by changes in body weight. In contrast, a high monounsaturated-fat diet significantly improves insulin sensitivity, compared with a high saturated-fat diet. Independent of its effects on insulin sensitivity, diet composition can influence the factors clustering in the metabolic syndrome. Dietary carbohydrate increases blood glucose levels, particularly in the postprandial period. Insulin levels and plasma triglycerides consequently rise. The detrimental effects of a high-carbohydrate diet on plasma glucose/insulin, triglyceride/HDL or fibrinolysis occur only when carbohydrate foods with a high glycemic index are consumed; they are abolished if the diet is based largely on fiber-rich, low-glycemic-index foods. Mono-unsaturated fats and omega-3 fatty acids can reduce plasma triglycerides. Such diets may also improve endothelial function.

Moderate physical activity (brisk walking for up to 30 min day^{-1}) should be feasible for most patients. One of the major anticipated benefits of an active lifestyle is a reduction in cardiovascular mortality. Exercise improves insulin sensitivity and glucose tolerance rapidly, and independent of weight loss. Exercise training results in preferential loss of fat stores from central regions of the body[42]. Aerobic exercise training has been shown to lower systolic and diastolic blood pressure, together with plasma triglycerides, and to increase HDL cholesterol.

PHARMACOLOGICAL THERAPY

Unfortunately, no clinical trial data is available to show a reduction in cardiovascular events

Table 22.5 Effect of pharmacological therapy on cardiovascular risk factors and markers in IRS

Drug type	Drug class	Body weight	Blood pressure	HDL	LDL	Tg	PAI-1	Endothelial function	Plasma insulin
Diabetes treatments	SFU/meglitidnide	↑	—	—	—	↓	—	—	↑
	TZD	↑	↓	↑	↑*	↓	↓	I	↓
	Metformin	—	↓	↑	↓	↓	↓	I	↓
	Acarbose	—	—	—	—	↓	—	I	↓
	Insulin	↑	—	—	—	↓	↓	—	—
Lipid lowering	HMGCoA	—	↓	↓	↓	↓	—	I	↓
Anti-hyper- tensive	ACE I	—	↓	—	↓	—	—	I	↓
Weight reduction	Orlistat	↓	—	—	↓	↓	—	—	—
	Sibutramine	↓	↑	↑	—	↓	—	—	↓

(—) indicates no change or insufficient data; Tg = plasma triglycerides. (*) decreases LDL particle size and decreases LDL oxidation. (I) improved endothelial function.

with pharmacological treatment of IRS *per se*. However, current pharmacological strategies for established risk factors, such as hyperglycemia, hypertension, dyslipidemia and platelet aggregation, have been shown to mitigate much of the consequences of the syndrome. Nevertheless, this leads to the prescription of complex multi-drug regimens, and there is a need for therapy that will directly treat the syndrome. Insulin sensitizers are approved for treatment of hyperglycemia in type 2 diabetes (discussed elsewhere). This chapter considers their role in IRS and its vascular complications. The effects of pharmacological therapy on some components of IRS are summarized in Table 22.5.

Metformin

Metformin is a biguanide that has been approved for the treatment of type 2 diabetes and has also been shown to prevent diabetes in obese subjects with impaired glucose tolerance. The primary glucose-lowering effect of metformin results from a decrease in hepatic gluconeogenesis, with some effect on peripheral glucose disposal[43]. The mechanism of action is different from, and complementary to, that of the thiazolidinediones.

Obese patients in the UK Prospective Diabetes Study (UKPDS) treated with metformin had a 36% lower risk of all cause mortality, and a 39% lower risk of myocardial infarction[44]. Since there was no difference in glycemic control in subjects treated with metformin compared with that achieved using other treatment modalities, it is possible that other effects of the drug, including its effects on IRS, may have decreased cardiovascular events. Most importantly, patients in the UKPDS gained less weight compared with those treated with other agents[44]. Potential mechanisms by which metformin may decrease cardiovascular events, include reduced plasma triglycerides and LDL concentration, reduced postprandial lipemia and plasma free fatty acid (FFA) concentration[45,46]. In addition, metformin has a favorable effect on several non-traditional cardiovascular risk factors, including PAI-1, fibrinogen and endothelial function[45,46] (Table 22.5).

Thiazolidinediones

Thiazolidinediones (TZDs) are oral antidiabetic agents developed to improve insulin sensitivity. Thiazolidinediones primarily exert their insulin-sensitizing effect by increasing peripheral uptake of glucose, especially at skeletal muscles[47]. Drugs of this class act as ligands for PPAR-gamma, which functions as a transcription factor involved in the regulation of genes involved in glucose homeostasis and lipid metabolism. These receptors have several potential effects in different tissues, including the vasculature. Since PPAR-gamma plays a role endothelial and vascular smooth muscle cells, ligands of these receptors, such as TZDs may play a role in atherosclerosis. For example, the TZDs inhibit vascular smooth-muscle cell proliferation and migration[35].

TZDs have been shown to have many other effects, other than reduction of hyperglycemia, some of which are summarized in Table 22.5[48]. They decrease the release of cytokines and peptides, such as TNF-alpha, from adipose tissue that are associated with insulin resistance and vascular inflammation. TZDs have been shown to improve endothelial function and inflammation, and to have an inhibitory effect on carotid artery IMT in patients with type 2 diabetes[49] (Figure 22.5). However, TZDs cause weight gain, although a decrease in visceral fat may help explain the concomitant decrease in insulin resistance[48]. They also increase plasma LDL concentration, although studies suggest that they change LDL particle size to the less atherogenic, large buoyant LDL cholesterol[48]. Thus,

thiazolidinediones may have beneficial effects against cardiovascular disease, although reductions in cardiovascular events have not yet been demonstrated. Clinical trials are in progress to determine whether they will prevent cardiovascular events.

Other hypoglycemics

Insulin secretagogues, such as sulfonylureas and meglitinides, do not directly improve insulin sensitivity. However, by reducing glucose concentrations they reduce the effect of 'glucose toxicity' on insulin sensitivity. They have very little impact on the components of the metabolic syndrome[46]. They also cause weight gain, which may explain some of the differences between this class of agents and metformin on cardiovascular events in the UKPDS. Exogenous insulin has similar effects, but in addition may have some more potent effect on lowering plasma triglycerides and PAI-1.

Alpha glucosidase inhibitors have significant lipid-lowering effects, especially on triglycerides. Some small studies have also suggested that they may improve insulin sensitivity (Table 22.5). The clinical benefits of these effects on CVD are unclear.

Anti-obesity agents

For individuals who do not respond to lifestyle modification, anti-obesity drugs probably improve insulin resistance through weight loss, or decreased food intake, rather than by a direct effect on insulin sensitivity. As a result of the weight loss, these drugs have a significant effect on various components of the syndrome[50]. Sibutramine, a serotonin-receptor inhibitor, improves glycemic control and the lipid profile[51]. Orlistat is a lipase inhibitor that decreases the absorption of dietary fat. Even modest weight loss with Orlistat results in a significant improvement in glucose tolerance, plasma insulin, LDL and HDL cholesterol concentrations[50].

Other drugs affecting insulin resistance

Several studies have shown that many pharmacological agents impact different components of

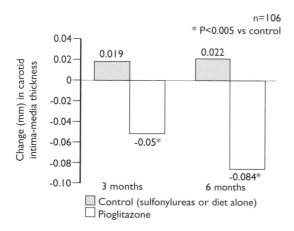

Figure 22.5 Inhibitory effect of piogliazone on carotid arterial ITM (adapted from Reference 49).

the syndrome, but very few have been shown to have an effect on the syndrome as a whole. Most intriguing among these are ACE inhibitors and HMG-Co-A reductase inhibitors (statins). ACE inhibitors are antihypertensive agents that inhibit the conversion of angiotensin I to angiotensin II. Several studies have demonstrated a small but statistically significant reduction in insulin resistance by ACE inhibitors. They have also been shown to decrease the incidence of new onset type 2 diabetes, in addition to preventing cardiovascular events[52]. The mechanism of action is unclear, but may be related to vasodilatory effects on vessels supplying skeletal muscle, as well as improving insulin sensitivity.

HMG-Co-A reductase inhibitors are useful drugs in the control of dyslipidemia. Studies have recently shown that simvastatin and atorvastatin improved insulin resistance in type 2 diabetics. Analysis of data from the West of Scotland coronary primary prevention trial has demonstrated that treatment with pravastatin reduced the incidence of new onset type 2 diabetes, in addition to decreasing coronary events[53]. Since these drugs improve endothelial function and decrease inflammation, it is possible that they may have an effect on IRS; this requires further investigation.

SUMMARY AND CONCLUSIONS

IRS is a major public health problem contributing to considerable morbidity related to diabetes and CVD. Consensus-based definition of the syndrome should lead to greater recognition in clinical practice. Several components of the syndrome are routinely evaluated in practice, and frequently cluster in patients.

Our understanding of the pathophysiological processes involved has improved considerably. This has resulted in the development of new treatments directly targeting insulin resistance, which have significant benefits on several aspects of the syndrome. Current research is focused on improving our understanding of the etiology of the syndrome, and finding new therapeutic interventions.

REFERENCES

1 Reaven GM. Banting lecture 1988. Role of insulin resistance in human disease [Review]. *Diabetes* 1988;37:1595–607.

2 McFarlane SI, Banerji M, Sowers JR. Insulin resistance and cardiovascular disease. *J Clin Endocrinol Metab* 2001;86:713–18.

3 Fonseca VA. Risk factors for coronary heart disease in diabetes. *Ann Intern Med* 2000;133:154–6.

4 Stern MP. Diabetes and cardiovascular disease. The 'common soil' hypothesis. *Diabetes* 1995;44: 369–74.

5 Despres JP, Lamarche B, Mauriege P *et al.* Hyperinsulinemia as an independent risk factor for ischemic heart disease. *N Engl J Med* 1996;334:952–7.

6 Pyorala M, Miettinen H, Laakso M, Pyorala K. Plasma insulin and all-cause, cardiovascular, and noncardiovascular mortality: the 22-year follow-up results of the Helsinki Policemen Study. *Diabetes Care* 2000;23:1097–102.

7 Pyorala M, Miettinen H, Halonen P *et al.* Insulin resistance syndrome predicts the risk of coronary heart disease and stroke in healthy middle-aged men: the 22-year follow-up results of the Helsinki Policemen Study. *Arterioscler Thromb Vasc Biol* 2000;20:538–44.

8 Ruige JB, Assendelft WJ, Dekker JM *et al.* Insulin and risk of cardiovascular disease: a meta-analysis. *Circulation* 1998;97:996–1001.

9 Folsom AR, Szklo M, Stevens J *et al.* A prospective study of coronary heart disease in relation to fasting insulin, glucose, and diabetes. The Atherosclerosis Risk in Communities (ARIC) Study. *Diabetes Care* 1997;20:935–42.

10 Haffner SM, Stern MP, Hazuda HP *et al.* Cardiovascular risk factors in confirmed prediabetic individuals. Does the clock for coronary heart disease start ticking before the onset of clinical diabetes? *J Am Med Assoc* 1990;263:2893–8.

11 Kahn BB, Flier JS. Obesity and insulin resistance. *J Clin Invest* 2000;106:473–81.

12 Ruderman N, Chisholm D, Pi-Sunyer X, Schneider S. The metabolically obese, normal-weight individual revisited. *Diabetes* 1998;47: 699–713.

13 Abate N, Garg A, Peshock RM *et al.* Relationship of generalized and regional adiposity to insulin

sensitivity in men with NIDDM. *Diabetes* 1996;45:1684–93.

14 Reaven GM, Chen YD, Jeppesen J *et al.* Insulin resistance and hyperinsulinemia in individuals with small, dense low density lipoprotein particles. *J Clin Invest* 1993;92:141–6.

15 Boden G, Lebed B, Schatz M *et al.* Effects of acute changes of plasma free fatty acids on intramyocellular fat content and insulin resistance in healthy subjects. *Diabetes* 2001;50:1612–17.

16 DeFronzo RA, Ferrannini E. Insulin resistance. A multifaceted syndrome responsible for NIDDM, obesity, hypertension, dyslipidemia, and atherosclerotic cardiovascular disease. *Diabetes Care* 1991;14:173–94.

17 Sobel BE. Insulin resistance and thrombosis: a cardiologist's view. *Am J Cardiol* 1999;84:37J–41J.

18 Calles-Escandon J, Mirza SA, Sobel BE, Schneider DJ. Induction of hyperinsulinemia combined with hyperglycemia and hypertriglyceridemia increases plasminogen activator inhibitor 1 in blood in normal human subjects. *Diabetes* 1998;47:290–3.

19 Calles-Escandon J, Cipolla M. Diabetes and endothelial dysfunction: a clinical perspective. *Endocrinol Rev* 2001;22:36–52.

20 Pinkney JH, Stehouwer CD, Coppack SW, Yudkin JS. Endothelial dysfunction: cause of the insulin resistance syndrome. *Diabetes* 1997;46 Suppl 2:S9–13.

21 Baron AD. Hemodynamic actions of insulin. *Am J Physiol* 1994;267:E187–E202.

22 Laakso M, Edelman SV, Brechtel G, Baron AD. Impaired insulin-mediated skeletal muscle blood flow in patients with NIDDM. *Diabetes* 1992;41:1076–83.

23 Howard G, O'Leary DH, Zaccaro D *et al.* Insulin sensitivity and atherosclerosis. The Insulin Resistance Atherosclerosis Study (IRAS) Investigators. *Circulation* 1996;93:1809–17.

24 Hsueh WA, Law RE. Insulin signaling in the arterial wall. *Am J Cardiol* 1999;84:21J–24J.

25 Wagenknecht LE, D'Agostino RJ, Savage PJ *et al.* Duration of diabetes and carotid wall thickness. The Insulin Resistance Atherosclerosis Study (IRAS). *Stroke* 1997;28:999–1005.

26 O'Leary DH, Polak JF, Kronmal RA *et al.* Carotid-artery intima and media thickness as a risk factor for myocardial infarction and stroke in older adults. Cardiovascular Health Study Collaborative Research Group [see comments]. *N Engl J Med* 1999;340:14–22.

27 Pinkney JH, Denver AE, Mohamed-Ali V *et al.* Insulin resistance in non-insulin-dependent diabetes mellitus is associated with microalbuminuria independently of ambulatory blood pressure. *J Diabetes Compl* 1995;9:230–3.

28 Agewall S, Wikstrand J, Ljungman S, Fagerberg B. Urinary albumin excretion is associated with the intima-media thickness of the carotid artery in hypertensive males with non-insulin-dependent diabetes mellitus. *J Hypertens* 1995;13:463–9.

29 Kronenberg F, Pereira MA, Schmitz MK *et al.* Influence of leisure time physical activity and television watching on atherosclerosis risk factors in the NHLBI Family Heart Study. *Atherosclerosis* 2000;153:433–43.

30 Folsom AR, Kushi LH, Hong CP. Physical activity and incident diabetes mellitus in postmenopausal women. *Am J Publ Health* 2000;90:134–8.

31 Hu FB, Stampfer MJ, Solomon C *et al.* Physical activity and risk for cardiovascular events in diabetic women. *Ann Intern Med* 2001;134:96–105.

32 Barsh GS, Farooqi IS, O'Rahilly S. Genetics of body-weight regulation. *Nature* 2000;404:644–51.

33 Festa A, D'Agostino RJ, Howard G *et al.* Chronic subclinical inflammation as part of the insulin resistance syndrome: The Insulin Resistance Atherosclerosis Study (IRAS). *Circulation* 2000;102:42–7.

34 Feener EP, King GL. Vascular dysfunction in diabetes mellitus. *Lancet* 1997;350(Suppl 1): SI9–13.

35 Hsueh WA, Jackson S, Law RE. Control of vascular cell proliferation and migration by PPAR-gamma: a new approach to the macrovascular complications of diabetes. *Diabetes Care* 2001;24:392–7.

36 Gan SK, Samaras K, Carr A, Chisholm D. Anti-retroviral therapy, insulin resistance and lipodystrophy. *Diabetes Obes Metab* 2001;3:67–71.

37 Osmond C, Barker DJ. Fetal, infant, and childhood growth are predictors of coronary heart disease, diabetes, and hypertension in adult men and women. *Environ Health Perspect* 2000;108 (Suppl 3):545–53.

38 Godfrey KM, Barker DJ. Fetal nutrition and adult disease. *Am J Clin Nutr* 2000;71:1344S–1352S.

39 Tuomilehto J, Lindstrom J, Eriksson JG *et al.* Prevention of type 2 diabetes mellitus by changes in lifestyle among subjects with impaired glucose tolerance. *N Engl J Med* 2001;344:1343–50.

40 Riccardi G, Rivellese AA. Dietary treatment of the metabolic syndrome—the optimal diet. *Br J Nutr* 2000;83 (Suppl 1):S143–S148

41 Reaven GM. Diet and Syndrome X. *Curr Atheroscler Rep* 2000;2:503–7.

42 Ross R, Dagnone D, Jones PJ *et al.* Reduction in obesity and related comorbid conditions after diet-induced weight loss or exercise-induced weight loss in men. A randomized, controlled trial. *Ann Intern Med* 2000;133:92–103.

43 Stumvoll M, Nurjhan N, Perriello G *et al.* Metabolic effects of metformin in non-insulin-dependent diabetes mellitus. *N Engl J Med* 1995;333:550–4.

44 Turner RC. The UK Prospective Diabetes Study. A review. *Diabetes Care* 1998;21(Suppl 3):C35–C38.

45 Bailey CJ, Turner RC. Metformin. *N Engl J Med* 1996;334:574–9.

46 Lebovitz HE. Effects of oral antihyperglycemic agents in modifying macrovascular risk factors in type 2 diabetes. *Diabetes Care* 1999;22(Suppl 3):C41–C44.

47 Saltiel AR, Olefsky JM. Thiazolidinediones in the treatment of insulin resistance and type II diabetes. *Diabetes* 1996;45:1661–9.

48 Parulkar AA, Pendergrass ML, Granda-Ayala R *et al.* Nonhypoglycemic effects of thiazolidine-diones. *Ann Intern Med* 2001;134:61–71.

49 Koshiyama H, Shimono D, Kuwamura N *et al.* Rapid communication: inhibitory effect of pioglitazone on carotid arterial wall thickness in type 2 diabetes. *J Clin Endocrinol Metab* 2001;86:3452–6.

50 Jones PH. Diet and pharmacologic therapy of obesity to modify atherosclerosis. *Curr Atheroscler Rep* 2000;2:314–20.

51 Fujioka K, Seaton TB, Rowe E *et al.* Weight loss with sibutramine improves glycaemic control and other metabolic parameters in obese patients with type 2 diabetes mellitus. *Diabetes Obes Metab* 2000;2:175–87.

52 Yusuf S, Sleight P, Pogue J *et al.* Effects of an angiotensin-converting-enzyme inhibitor, ramipril, on cardiovascular events in high-risk patients. The Heart Outcomes Prevention Evaluation Study Investigators. *N Engl J Med* 2000 20;342:145–53.

53 Freeman DJ, Norrie J, Sattar N *et al.* Pravastatin and the development of diabetes mellitus: evidence for a protective treatment effect in the West of Scotland Coronary Prevention Study. *Circulation* 2001;103:357–62.

23

Obesity—influence on diabetes and management

Hans Hauner

INTRODUCTION

Obesity is now recognized as a common chronic disorder of excessive body fat. This condition increases the risk of developing a variety of adverse consequences to human health, ranging from metabolic disturbances, including type 2 diabetes, and cardiovascular complications, to disorders of the locomotor system among others. In addition, obesity impairs the subjective quality-of-life in affected people and can reduce life expectancy[1].

The diagnosis of obesity is based on the body mass index (BMI). This simple anthropometric index can be calculated from body weight and height, is rather independent of body height, and correlates reasonably well with body fat mass ($r = 0.4$–0.7). The current classification of body weight according to WHO is presented in Table 23.1.

EPIDEMIOLOGY OF OBESITY

Obesity has become a global epidemic that is present not only in the industrialized world but also in many developing countries. At present, the prevalence of obesity (BMI ≥ 30 kg m^{-2}) is 15–25% in the adult population in Europe and North America, with an unequivocal trend for further increase. The most dramatic rise in these regions is currently observed in children and adolescents. In addition, there is also an alarming increase in the number of affected people in many developing countries[1].

Table 23.1 Classification of human obesity based on BMI (according to WHO[1])

Classification	BMI (kg m^{-2})
Underweight	< 18.5
Normal weight	18.5 24.9
Overweight	≥ 25.0
Obesity Grade I	30–34.9
Grade II	35–39.9
Grade III	≥ 40

OBESITY AS A RISK FACTOR FOR TYPE 2 DIABETES

There is a large body of clinical data demonstrating a close relationship between body fat mass and the risk of diabetes. In contrast with other obesity-associated metabolic disturbances, the diabetes risk is already increased in the upper normal range of BMI. In the Nurses' Health Study[2], women in the upper normal range, with a BMI 23.0–24.9 kg m^{-2} had a 4–5-fold increased risk of developing diabetes over a 14-year observation period, compared with women with a BMI < 22 kg m^{-2}. In those with a BMI of 29.0–30.9 kg m^{-2}, the risk of diabetes was 27.6-fold higher than in the lean reference group. Almost two-thirds of newly diagnosed women with type 2 diabetes were obese at the time of diagnosis[2]. Similar observations were reported for males in the Health Professionals' Study[3]. Interestingly, a change in body weight strongly predicts risk of diabetes. Weight gain since the age of 18 between 11.0 and 19.9 kg, which is the average range of weight change between adolescence and menopause for women in industrialized countries, was found to be correlated with a 5.5-fold higher risk of diabetes compared with weight-stable women, whereas weight reduction of the same extent reduced the risk of diabetes by almost 80%[2]. Similar data have been reported for men[3]. Duration of obesity also has a strong impact on the development of type 2 diabetes.

The health risks of obesity, particularly the risk of developing diabetes, depends not only on the extent and duration of obesity, but is also potently influenced by the fat distribution pattern. Enlarged visceral fat depots, which can be easily assessed by measuring the waist circumference, are closely associated with metabolic disturbances. In an early study in men, an abdominal pattern of fat distribution was found to be an independent risk factor for type 2 diabetes[4]. Subsequent studies confirmed this observation. Particularly at low degrees of overweight, the fat distribution pattern strongly predicts the risk for diabetes and the metabolic syndrome.

It is now accepted for Caucasians that a waist circumference > 80 and > 88 cm, respectively, in women and > 94 and > 102 cm, respectively, in men is associated with a moderately and highly elevated risk of metabolic complications[1]. Therefore, waist circumference should be routinely assessed when estimating the risk of diabetes. Other more precise measures of the visceral fat mass are computed tomography (CT), nuclear magnetic resonance (NMR) imaging and, with some limitations, dual energy X-ray absorptiometry (DEXA)[5].

GENETIC PREDISPOSITION FOR TYPE 2 DIABETES

Despite the major role of body fat as a risk factor for diabetes there is clear evidence that type 2 diabetes has a strong genetic basis. According to

family studies, every third offspring of one parent with diabetes is expected to develop this disease later in life. If both parents suffer from diabetes, this risk is over 50% and the concordance for type 2 diabetes in monozygotic twins is close to 100%. For this reason, it is currently assumed that only those obese subjects will develop the disease who have a genetic failure of the pancreas to compensate for insulin resistance[6]. Among severely obese subjects (BMI $\geq$ 40 kg m^{-2}) only 30–50% will develop diabetes throughout life.

PATHOPHYSIOLOGY

Type 2 diabetes is characterized by an impaired insulin action, or a defective secretion of insulin, or both. Both defects are thought to be required for the manifestation of the disease, they augment each other and are present many years prior to the clinical onset of the disease[6]. The mechanisms by which obesity affects these two central processes are far from being understood, but there is agreement that obesity mainly promotes and aggravates insulin resistance. One of the earliest hypotheses to explain the relationship between obesity and diabetes is the 'glucose–fatty acid cycle', which is based on the observation of a competition between glucose and fatty acid oxidation in the heart muscle[7]. The higher the supply of fatty acids from enlarged fat cells and adipose tissue depots, the more fatty acids are used as fuel in muscle, the main organ of glucose utilization. As a consequence, the rate of glucose oxidation is reduced. In addition, mechanisms have been described whereby elevated free fatty acids (FFA) can impair insulin action. Elevated FFA were found to reduce insulin-stimulated glucose uptake, and to decrease muscle glycogen synthesis. Finally, it is well-known that fatty acids promote hepatic glucose production, another key disturbance leading to glucose intolerance[8]. Recent studies suggest that obese and type 2 diabetic subjects have a high intramyocellular lipid accumulation, which interferes with muscle glucose metabolism and could play an important role in the pathogenesis of type 2 diabetes[9]. There are also studies of beta-cells indicating that long-

Table 23.2 Secretory factors from adipocytes possibly involved in the pathophysiology of obesity-associated insulin resistance
FFA
TNF-alpha
Leptin
Resistin
Interleukin-6
Angiotensin II
Adiponectin
Others (?)

chain fatty acids may exert an adverse effect on insulin secretion, via overproduction of ceramide[10]. A new observation is that over-expression of uncoupling protein 2 (UCP2) in the beta cell, possibly due to elevated fatty acids, may contribute to the development of obesity-linked diabetes, by decreasing mitochondrial coupling and impairing insulin secretion[11].

A recent hypothesis is that secretory products from enlarged adipose tissue depots and fat cells may directly contribute to insulin resistance. Table 23.2 summarizes currently discussed factors produced from fat cells that have been related to the pathophysiology of insulin resistance. Among these candidates, most data have been collected for a mediator role of tumor necrosis factor-alpha (TNF-alpha). TNF-alpha is a multifunctional cytokine that has been shown to exert a variety of catabolic effects in adipose tissue. It has been demonstrated by several groups that TNF-alpha and its two receptor subtypes are over-expressed in adipose tissue of obese subjects[12–14]. The up-regulated TNF-alpha induces multiple effects at the local level, such as inhibition of glucose uptake due to an impairment of insulin signalling, and suppression of GLUT4 expression, a reduction of lipoprotein lipase expression and activity, and an increase in lipolysis. Taken together, all these catabolic effects of TNF-alpha promote a state of insulin resistance[15,16]. However, it is questionable whether adipose over-expression of TNF-alpha

also contributes to muscle insulin resistance. There is no clear evidence from clinical studies for elevated circulating levels of the cytokine[17]. On the other hand, infusion of a soluble TNF-alpha antibody and neutralization of the cytokine had no effect on insulin sensitivity in subjects with type 2 diabetes[18,19].

Using an *in vitro* co-culture system of human adipocytes and muscle cells we were recently unable to demonstrate a role for TNF-alpha secreted from adipocytes in the development of muscle insulin resistance, although the presence of adipocytes induced a state of insulin resistance, indicating a role for fat-cell secretory products (Dietze *et al.*, submitted). However, there is currently little information on the nature of these factors. So far, there is also no clear evidence that the recently discovered resistin is involved in the pathophysiology of muscle insulin resistance in humans[20].

Taken together, and irrespective of many interesting new data on the relationship between fat-cell function and muscular insulin resistance, the dominating underlying mechanism(s) are still enigmatic and remain to be elucidated.

ANTIDIABETIC DRUGS AND BODY WEIGHT

It has long been recognized that antidiabetic drugs can promote weight gain in subjects with type 2 diabetes. The strongest weight-promoting effect is exerted by insulin. In the Diabetes Complications and Control Trial (DCCT), intensified insulin treatment was associated with substantial weight gain that resulted in unfavourable changes of lipid levels and blood pressure, similar to those seen in the insulin resistance syndrome (IRS)[21]. In the UK Prospective Diabetes Study (PDS), insulin treatment caused a mean weight gain of approximately 7 kg over 12 years of treatment in newly diagnosed subjects with type 2 diabetes[22]. In addition, sulfonylureas are known to promote weight gain due to their insulin-secretory action. In the UKPDS, the average weight gain under glibenclamide treatment amounted to about 5 kg[22]. It was recently reported that peroxisome proliferative activator receptor-gamma (PPARgamma)-agonists lead to weight gain. However, there is growing evidence that weight gain occurs only in the subcutaneous depots, but not in the visceral depot—which should have less deleterious metabolic consequences[23]. Furthermore, weight gain under administration of thiazolidinediones (TZDs) is not only due to an increase in fat mass, but also to enhanced fluid retention. In contrast, metformin and alpha-glucosidase inhibitors have a modest weight-lowering potential[24].

OBESITY AND GLYCEMIC CONTROL

It is noteworthy that BMI is the most important predictor of deterioration in glycemic control, regardless of the treatment regimen[25]. In the latter study from Finland, glycosylated hemoglobin (HbA1c) levels decreased almost three-fold more in patients whose baseline weight was below the mean BMI of 28.1 kg m^{-2} than in those whose weight was above this cut-off value (1.7 versus 0.5%, $p < 0.01$). For this reason, there is now agreement that prevention of weight gain is an important target when drug treatment is initiated in obese subjects with type 2 diabetes. This aspect is particularly significant in insulin-treated patients, independent of the type of diabetes.

MANAGEMENT OF OBESITY IN SUBJECTS WITH TYPE 2 DIABETES

The management of obesity represents a central component in the treatment strategy for type 2 diabetes, as obesity is not only a major predisposing factor of the disease and its accompanying disorders, but also aggravates the achievement of a good metabolic control. Moreover, it was repeatedly shown that reducing excessive body weight in individuals with type 2 diabetes improves metabolic control and prolongs life[26-28]. However, currently available weight reduction programs for patients suffering from diabetes turned out to have only limited success, particularly in the long run. An essential prerequisite for successful treatment are realistic goals. This is particularly important for this group, as treatment of obese subjects

with type 2 diabetes is usually more difficult than treating obese subjects without diabetes for several reasons. Type 2 diabetic subjects are usually older than non-diabetic obese subjects, which means a smaller weight loss as energy expenditure decreases with age. Another reason is that subjects with diabetes are focussing more on blood glucose control, which could result in the neglecting of other health problems. Finally, the weight increasing and weight-loss preventing potential of antidiabetic agents has to be considered. Irrespective of these specific considerations, the indications, goals and principles of treatment are the same in obese subjects with and without type 2 diabetes (Tables 23.3 and 23.4). Table 23.5 summarizes current evidence-based

---

Table 23.3 Treatment targets in the management of obese individuals with type 2 diabetes

Weight loss of 3–10 kg (depending on weight, age and gender)

Improvement of cardiovascular risk factors

Healthy lifestyle (healthy eating, regular physical activity)

High quality-of-life

Table 23.4 Treatment principles for weight management in obese individuals with type 2 diabetes

Dietary therapy
  Low-calorie diet (energy deficit: 500–1000 kcal day^{-1})
  VLCD
  Low-fat, carbohydrate-*ad libitum* diet
Increase in physical activity
Behaviour modification
Adjuvant drug treatment
Surgical treatment

therapeutic approaches for the prevention and treatment of obesity, depending on the degree of overweight and the presence of comorbidities that are also valid for overweight/obese subjects with type 2 diabetes[26].

Non-pharmacological therapy

The cornerstones of every weight reduction program are a moderately hypocaloric diet, an increase in physical activity and behaviour modification. There are numerous studies that applied and examined such concepts, but most of them were short-term and had disappointing long-term results[27,29].

Dietary approaches

The 'gold standard' in the dietary treatment of obese patients with type 2 diabetes is a balanced moderately energy-restricted diet. The energy deficit is between 500 and 1000 kcal per day. The most important single measure is the reduction in fat intake, particularly in saturated fatty acids. A low-fat high-carbohydrate diet is generally recommended. As shown recently, a diet rich in fiber and complex carbohydrates has some beneficial effects on parameters of glucose and lipid metabolism, but these effects may be small and possibly of limited clinical importance[30]. The concept of a high-carbohydrate, low-fat diet was, however, challenged by clinical studies showing that replacement of saturated fat by monounsaturated fat compared with high-carbohydrate intake is equally favourable, or has even some minor advantages with regard to glycemic response and lipids[31]. For these reasons, there is convincing evidence that energy content, rather than nutrient composition, is the major determinant of weight reduction in obese subjects with type 2 diabetes.

From a practical point of view it is extremely important to assess the habitual diet of a patient with type 2 diabetes and to focus counselling on punctual changes of his/her eating habits in order to approach current dietary recommendations[32,33]. It should be stressed that all efforts for dietary changes should be made as simple

as possible for the patients, as they are burdened by many requirements to manage their diabetes[34]. For obese subjects with type 2 diabetes, the frequent recommendation to distribute their allowed calories over 5–6 meals is difficult to meet, and may even hinder weight loss without being of any advantage for metabolic control[35]. Therefore, in many cases 3–4 meals a day may be more appropriate to reach the individual dietary goals.

Another possible dietary approach is the use of a very-low-calorie diet (VLCD) for initial weight loss. This option may be particularly valuable for patients with poor metabolic control and/or 'dietary failure'. Usually, there is a rapid improvement of insulin resistance and glycemic control, after even short periods of VLCD. However, this approach can only be applied for a limited number of weeks and requires intense medical care. One has also to keep in mind that the long-term results of VLCD are not better than those of conventional diets[29]. There is need, therefore, for new sophisticated solutions, such as intermittent VLCD in combination with conventional hypocaloric diets, to obtain better long-term results[36]. Another potentially promising strategy is to establish a long-term meal-replacement concept, which substitutes one or two meals daily by balanced formula diets of reduced calorie content, as recently demonstrated in a 4-year clinical study in non-diabetic obese subjects[37]. There is no doubt that more research is urgently required to develop strategies that may help to provide better individual solutions and to manage the weight problem of many patients more efficiently.

Increase of physical activity

Current approaches to increasing physical activity in patients with obesity and type 2 diabetes have also shown only partial efficacy. As most patients are completely sedentary, or immobilized due to other health problems, such as osteoarthritis, regular physical activity is difficult to establish on a regular basis. There is no doubt that most obese type 2 diabetic subjects would benefit from at least some level of

Table 23.5 Obesity prevention and treatment flowchart (modified according to Reference 26)

Health status	Treatment goals	Treatment steps
Normal weight (BMI 18.5–24.9)	Weight maintenance	Consider periodic weight monitoring
Normal weight (BMI 18.5–24.9) plus risk factors(s) and/or comorbidity(ies)	Weight maintenance. Prevention of a > 3 kg weight gain. Risk factor management, e.g. smoking cessation, healthy lifestyle	Weight monitoring, risk-factor management, treatment of co-morbidities, advice for a healthy lifestyle
Pre-obesity (BMI 25–29.9)	Prevention of further weight gain or, preferably, induction of modest weight loss	Best practice program*
Pre-obesity (BMI 25–29.9) plus risk factors(s) and/or comorbidity(ies)	5–10% weight reduction in 3–6 months (especially if success in controlling risk factors is only moderate after 3 months) and weight maintenance thereafter	Best practice program*, risk-factor management, treatment of comorbidities
Obesity Class I (BMI 30–34.9)	5–10% sustained weight reduction	Best practice program*
Obesity Class I (BMI 30–34.9) plus risk factors(s) and/or comorbidity(ies)	5–10% sustained weight reduction	1. Best practice program*, risk-factor management, treatment of comorbidities 2. If not successful, consider additional drug therapy no earlier than after 12 weeks
Obesity Class II (BMI 35–39.9)	≥ 10% sustained weight reduction	Best practice program*
Obesity Class II (BMI 35–39.9) plus risk factors(s) and/or comorbidity(ies)	10–20% sustained weight reduction	1. Best practice program*, risk-factor management, treatment of comorbidities 2. If not successful, consider additional drug therapy no earlier than 12 weeks 3. If conservative treatment is not successful, consider surgical treatment
Obesity Class III (BMI > 40)	10–30% sustained weight reduction	1. Best practice program*, risk factor management, treatment of comorbidities 2. If conservative treatment is not successful, consider surgical treatment

[a]The best practice program consists of a combination of dietary therapy, increased physical activity and behavioral modification.

physical activity. As almost all of these patients have low physical fitness, as assessed by $VO_{2\,max}$, only low intensity training is possible and appropriate. Among the low-intensity activities that should be recommended are walking at a self-selected speed, swimming or gymnastics/aerobics. There are sufficient data available to demonstrate an improvement of insulin resistance by low-to-moderate physical activity in men and women with and without type 2 diabetes[38]. Although there is still some debate about how much low-intensity activities are needed, to have a detectable impact on metabolic parameters and body weight, there is compelling evidence that even modest physical activity is very beneficial for subjective well-being, as well as long-term cardiovascular morbidity and mortality[29].

Weight-lowering drugs

Another component in the treatment of obesity is the adjunct administration of weight-lowering drugs. As limited experience is available, drug treatment is only recommended if the non-pharmacological treatment program is not sufficiently successful and if the benefit–risk ratio justifies drug administration[39]. At present, only two compounds are available that have demonstrated efficacy and safety in obese subjects with and without type 2 diabetes.

Orlistat is a gastric and pancreatic lipase inhibitor that impairs the intestinal absorption of ingested fat. In a 1-year study in obese type 2 diabetic subjects, orlistat treatment produced a greater weight loss compared to placebo treatment (6.2 versus 4.3%, $p < 0.001$). In addition, orlistat-treated patients had a small improvement in HbA1c compared with controls (–0.28 versus +0.18%, $p < 0.001$). Furthermore, the average dose of sulfonylureas needed decreased more in the orlistat than in the placebo group (–23 versus –9%, $p = 0.002$)[40]. This study, as well as others, indicate that adjunct treatment of obese type 2 diabetic patients by orlistat is followed by clinically significant improvements in glycemic control and other risk factors, due to additional weight loss[41].

Sibutramine is a selective serotonin- and noradrenaline-reuptake inhibitor that enhances satiety and slightly increases thermogenesis. There are data from two published studies with a duration of 3–6 months. On average, there was a net decrease in body weight between 3 and 9 kg, which was accompanied by an improvement in glycemic and lipid parameters[42,43]. As sibutramine is known to increase sympathetic nerve activity, this drug should not be used in diabetic patients with uncontrolled hypertension and/or clinically significant coronary artery disease.

Bariatric surgery

Bariatric surgery is now an established method of reducing body weight in subjects with extreme obesity (≥ 40 kg m^{-2}), but there is growing consensus[29] that this method can also be applied in subjects with type 2 diabetes at a BMI ≥ 35 kg m^{-2}. In this group of patients, surgery is by far the most effective treatment mode, with excellent long-term results compared to all other methods. In the Swedish Obese Subjects (SOS) study, a large prospective trial comparing bariatric surgery with conventional dietary treatment, sustained weight loss ≥ 20 kg was exclusively achieved in the operated subjects, with practically no significant weight change in the control group. Preliminary analysis of the data revealed that the 8-year cumulative incidence of diabetes, but not the 8-year incidence of hypertension was reduced by $> 80\%$ in the operated group compared with the control group[44]. Other studies have shown that bariatric surgery of extremely obese subjects with clinical diabetes is associated with a dramatic improvement in glycemic control. In up to 80% of the operated patients, insulin treatment was no longer required after substantial weight loss, and all other medications for diabetes and other cardiovascular risk factors could be considerably reduced or discontinued[45]. In another analysis from the same group, sustained weight reduction in obese type 2 diabetic subjects was associated with a remarkable lower mortality and healthcare utilization compared with patients on the waiting list[46].

IMPACT OF WEIGHT LOSS ON TYPE 2 DIABETES

Numerous studies investigated the consequences of short-term and long-term weight reduction on health. Meta-analyses of the available literature clearly suggest that intentional weight loss using appropriate methods is beneficial. A 5–10% weight loss appears to be sufficient to obtain significant health effects[47.] Nevertheless, the favorable effects depend on the methods applied and, most importantly, on the degree of weight loss[27,48]. In the recently published Finnish Diabetes Prevention Study, a comprehensive lifestyle modification program proved to be highly effective in preventing the development of type 2 diabetes in subjects with impaired glucose tolerance (IGT). The beneficial effect was positively influenced by the concomitant weight loss of 4 kg on average[49]. Concerning the prognosis of obese individuals with type 2 diabetes, weight loss has been shown to reduce the risk of death from comorbid diabetes. Each loss of 1 kg was estimated to add 3–4 months to life expectancy in newly diagnosed subjects with type 2 diabetes[50]. In a recent prospective analysis of a subgroup of overweight individuals with diabetes, from the American Cancer Society's Cancer Prevention Study I, intentional weight loss was associated with a 25% reduction in total mortality and a 28% reduction in coronary heart disease and diabetes mortality[28]. These positive changes in the risk factor profile and mortality, along with weight loss, should encourage efforts to look for more effective strategies for weight reduction in obese diabetic subjects.

LONG-TERM WEIGHT STABILIZATION

The long-term result of any weight-management program is critically dependent on the long-term strategy. Since a hypocaloric diet causes a decrease in energy expenditure, a return to previous eating habits will rapidly result in weight regain. Therefore, the patient has to recognize that long-term weight loss is only possible if a new energy balance is achieved at a lower level. To maintain a weight loss of about 10 kg, a long-term reduction in energy intake of about 500 kcal/day is required to compensate for the reduction in total energy expenditure[51]. To support weight stabilization and to prevent weight relapse the following strategies have proven useful: a low-fat diet rich in complex carbohydrates, an increase in physical activity, social support from family and friends, group support and continued contact with trusted medical-care professionals[26,29].

SUMMARY

Most patients with type 2 diabetes are overweight or obese. Weight management must be a central component of any treatment strategy, as weight loss has been convincingly shown to provide a marked improvement in metabolic control. However, as conventional concepts combining an energy-reduced diet and an increase in physical activity frequently have poor long-term results, more effective weight-loss strategies should be developed and applied. Such components with additional benefit are VLCD, weight-lowering drugs and bariatric surgery, the latter particularly for severely obese subjects. Long-term studies are urgently needed to obtain more precise information on the relative success of the various strategies in the management of obese diabetic patients.

REFERENCES

1 World Health Organization. *Obesity: preventing and managing the global epidemic. Report of a WHO consultation.* WHO Technical Report Series 894. Geneva: World Health Organization, 2000.

2 Colditz GA, Willett WC, Rotnitzky A, Manson JE. Weight gain as a risk factor for clinical diabetes in women. *Ann Intern Med* 1995;122:481–6.

3 Chan JM, Rimm EB, Colditz GA *et al.* Obesity, fat distribution, and weight gain as risk factors for clinical diabetes in men. *Diabetes Care* 1994;17:961–9.

4 Ohlson LO, Larsson B, Svärdsudd K *et al.* The

influence of body fat distribution on the incidence of diabetes mellitus. 13.5 years of follow-up of the participants in the study of men born in 1913. *Diabetes* 1985;34:1055–8.

5 Jebb SA, Elia M. Techniques for the measurement of body composition: a practical guide. *Int J Obes Rel Metab Dis* 1993;17:611–21.

6 Polonsky KS, Sturis SJ, Bell GI. Non-insulin-dependent diabetes mellitus—a genetically programmed failure of the beta cell to compensate for insulin resistance. *N Engl J Med* 1996; 334:777–83.

7 Randle P, Garland P, Hales C, Newsholme E. The glucose-fatty acid cycle. Its role in insulin sensitivity and the metabolic disturbances of diabetes mellitus. *Lancet* 1963;I:785–9.

8 Boden G. Role of fatty acids in the pathogenesis of insulin resistance and NIDDM. *Diabetes* 1997;45:3–10.

9 Storlien LH, Kriketos AD, Jenkins AB *et al.* Does dietary fat influence insulin action. *Ann NY Acad Sci* 1997;827:287–301.

10 Shimabukuro M, Higa M, Zhou YT *et al.* Lipoapoptosis in beta-cells of obese prediabetic fa/fa rats. Role of serine palmitoyltransferase overexpression. *J Biol Chem* 1998;273:32487–90.

11 Langin D. Diabetes, insulin secretion, and the pancreatic beta-cell mitochondrion. *N Engl J Med* 2001;345:1772–4.

12 Hotamisligil GS, Arner P, Caro JF *et al.* Increased adipose tissue expression of tumor necrosis factor-α in human obesity and insulin resistance. *J Clin Invest* 1995;95:2409–15.

13 Kern PA, Saghizadeh M, Ong JM *et al.* The expression of tumor necrosis factor in human adipose tissue. Regulation by obesity, weight loss and relationship to lipoprotein lipase. *J Clin Invest* 1995;95:2111–99.

14 Hube F, Birgel M, Lee Y-M, Hauner H. Expression pattern of tumour necrosis factor receptors in subcutaneous and omental human adipose tissue: role of obesity and non-insulin-dependent diabetes mellitus. *Eur J Clin Invest* 1999;29:672–8.

15 Hauner H, Petruschke T, Russ M *et al.* Effects of tumor necrosis factor-alpha (TNF) on glucose transport and lipid metabolism of newly differentiated human fat cells in culture. *Diabetologia* 1995;38:764–71.

16 Hube F, Hauner H. The role of TNF-α in human adipose tissue. Prevention of weight gain at the expense of insulin resistance? *Horm Metab Res* 1999;31:626–31.

17 Hauner H, Bender M, Haastert B, Hube F. Plasma concentrations of soluble TNF-alpha receptors in obese humans. *Int J Obes* 1998;22:1239–43.

18 Ofei F, Hurel S, Newkirk J *et al.* Effects of an engineered human anti-TNF-α antibody (CDP571) on insulin sensitivity and glycemic control in patients with NIDDM. *Diabetes* 1996;45:881–5.

19 Paquot N, Castillo MJ, Lefebvre PJ, Scheen AJ. No increased insulin sensitivity after a single intravenous administration of a recombinant human tumor necrosis factor receptor: Fc fusion protein in obese insulin-resistant patients. *J Clin Endocrinol Metab* 2000;85:1316–9.

20 Savage DB, Sewter CP, Klenk ES *et al.* Resistin/Fizz3 expression in relation to obesity and peroxisome proliferator-activated receptor-gamma action in humans. *Diabetes* 2001; 50:2199–202.

21 Purnell JQ, Hokanson JE, Marcovina SM *et al.* Effect of excessive weight gain with intensive therapy of type 1 diabetes on lipid levels and blood pressure. Results from the DCCT. *J Am Med Assoc* 1998;280:140–6.

22 UKPDS. Intensive blood-glucose control with sulphonylureas or insulin compared with conventional treatment and risk of complications in patients with type 2 diabetes (UKPDS 33). *Lancet* 1998;12:837–52.

23 Akazawa S, Fuyans S, Ito M *et al.* Efficacy of troglitazone on body fat distribution in type 2 diabetes. *Diabetes Care* 2000;32:1067–71.

24 Hauner H. Current pharmacological approaches to the treatment of obesity. *Int J Obes Rel Metab Dis* 2001;25 (Suppl. 1):S102–S106.

25 Yki-Järvinen H, Ryysy L, Kauppila M *et al.* Effect of obesity on the response to insulin therapy in non-insulin-dependent diabetes mellitus. *J Clin Endocrinol Metab* 1997;82.4037–43.

26 Hauner H, Westenhöfer J, Wirth A, Lauterbach K. Obesity guideline for the attending physician. User version of the evidence-based guideline on the treatment of obesity in Germany.

27 Brown SA, Upchurch S, Anding R *et al.* Promoting weight loss in type II diabetes. *Diabetes Care* 1996;19:613–24.

28 Williamson DF, Thompson TJ, Thun M *et al.* Intentional weight loss and mortality among overweight individuals with diabetes. *Diabetes Care* 2000;23:1499–51.

29 Expert Panel on the Identification, Evaluation, and Treatment of Overweight and Obesity in Adults. *Clinical guidelines on the identification, evaluation, and treatment of overweight and obesity in*

adults. The evidence report. Bethesda: National Institute of Health National Heart, Lung and Blood Institute, 1998.

30 Chandalia M, Grag A, Lutjohann D *et al.* Beneficial effects of high fiber intake in patients with type 2 diabetes mellitus. *N Engl J Med* 2000;342:1392–8.

31 Garg A, Bonanome A, Grundy SM *et al.* Comparison of a high-carbohydrate diet with high-monounsaturated-fat diet in patients with non-insulin-dependent diabetes mellitus. *N Engl J Med* 1988;319:829–34.

32 Mann J, Lean M, Toeller M *et al.* Recommendations for the nutritional management of patients with diabetes mellitus. *Eur J Clin Nutr* 2000;54:353–5.

33 American Diabetes Association. Nutrition recommendations and principles for people with diabetes mellitus. *Diabetes Care* 2001;24 (Suppl 1):544–7.

34 Campbell L, Rössner S. Management of obesity in patients with type 2 diabetes. *Diabet Med* 2001;18:345–54.

35 Arnold L, Mann JI, Ball MJ. Metabolic effects of alterations in meal frequency in type 2 diabetes. *Diabetes Care* 1997;20:1651–4.

36 Williams KV, Mullen ML, Kelley DE, Wing RR. The effect of short periods of caloric restriction on weight loss and glycemic control in type 2 diabetes. *Diabetes Care* 1998;21:2–8.

37 Ditschuneit HH, Flechtner-Mors M, Johnson TD, Adler G. Metabolic and weight-loss effects of long-term dietary intervention in obese patients. *Am J Clin Nutr* 1999;69:198–204.

38 Mayer-Davis EJ, D'Agostino R, Karter AJ *et al.* Intensity and amount of physical activity in relation to insulin sensitivity. The insulin resistance atherosclerosis study. *J Am Med Assoc* 1998;279:669–74.

39 National Task Force on the Prevention and Treatment of Obesity. Long-term pharmacotherapy in the management of obesity. *J Am Med Assoc* 1996;276:1907–15.

40 Hollander PA, Elbein SC, Hirsch IB *et al.* Role of orlistat in the treatment of obese patients with type 2 diabetes. *Diabetes Care* 1998;21:1288–98.

41 Keating GM, Jarvis B. Orlistat in the prevention and treatment of type 2 diabetes mellitus. *Drugs* 2001;61:2107–19.

42 Finer N, Bloom SR, Frost GS *et al.* Sibutramine is effective for weight loss and diabetic control in obesity with type 2 diabetes: a randomised, double-blind, placebo-controlled study. *Diab Obes Metab* 2000;2:105–12.

43 Gokcel A, Karakose H, Ertorer EM *et al.* Effects of sibutramine in obese female subjects with type 2 diabetes and poor blood glucose control. *Diabetes Care* 2001;24:1957–60.

44 Sjöström CD, Peltonen M, Wedel H, Sjöström L. Differentiated long-term effects of intentional weight loss on diabetes and hypertension. *Hypertension* 2000;36:20–5.

45 Pories WJ, MacDonald KG, Morgan EJ *et al.* Surgical treatment of obesity and its effect on diabetes: 10-y follow-up. *Am J Clin Nutr* 1992;55:582S–585S.

46 MacDonald KG, Long SD, Swanson MS *et al.* The gastric bypass operation reduces the progression and mortality of non-insulin-dependent diabetes mellitus. *J Gastrointest Surg* 1997;1:213–20.

47 Goldstein DJ. Beneficial health effects of modest weight loss. *Int J Obes Relat Metab Disord* 1991;16:397–415.

48 Wing RR, Koeske R, Epstein LH *et al.* Long-term effects of modest weight loss in type II diabetic patients. *Arch Intern Med* 1987;147:1749–53.

49 Tuomilehto J, Lindström J, Eriksson JG *et al.* Prevention of type 2 diabetes mellitus by changes in lifestyle among subjects with impaired glucose tolerance. *N Engl J Med* 2001;344:1343–9.

50 Lean ME, Powrie JK, Anderson AS, Garthwaite PH. Obesity, weight loss, and prognosis in type 2 diabetes. *Diab Med* 1990;7:228–33.

51 Leibel RL, Rosenbaum M, Hirsch J. Changes in energy expenditure resulting from altered body weight. *N Engl J Med* 1995;332:621–8.

24

Dyslipidemia and diabetes

D John Betteridge, Wilhem Krone and Dirk Müller-Wieland

INTRODUCTION

Disorders of lipid and lipoprotein metabolism in individuals with insulin resistance or type 2 diabetes mellitus increase cardiovascular risk, a feature associated with the metabolic syndrome or syndrome X. The most common characteristics of lipid disorders in insulin-resistant individuals are elevations of triglycerides and low levels of high-density lipoprotein (HDL)-cholesterol. This dyslipidemia appears to be causally related to the reduced insulin sensitivity, and appears to be an early marker of the metabolic syndrome. Accordingly, the American Diabetes Association recommends searching for underlying glucose intolerance in individuals with dyslipidemia [HDL cholesterol ≤ 35 mg dL^{-1} (0.90 mmol L^{-1}) and/or a triglyceride level ≥ 250 mg dL^{-1} (2.82 mmol L^{-1})] with an oral glucose tolerance test[1].

The epidemiology linking dyslipidemia to coronary heart disease (CHD) risk has long been recognized to fulfill the criteria for a causal relationship. However, until relatively recently there has been dispute concerning the overall benefits of lipid-lowering and possible non-cardiovascular adverse events of low plasma cholesterol and cholesterol-lowering[2]. The advent of the statin (HMG-CoA reductase inhibitors) drugs, which are highly effective and well tolerated, enabled definitive endpoint trials to be performed in populations with and without established CHD. These trials[3-7] have provided a huge evidence base for clinical practice, and national and international bodies have proposed various guidelines and treatment algorithms to enable the results of research to be translated into clinical practice for those patients at high risk of vascular events.

Diabetes mellitus, particularly type 2 diabetes, is associated with a markedly increased risk of cardiovascular events secondary mainly to premature and extensive atherosclerosis. This is not fully explained by the known major CHD risk factors. CHD is increased two- to three-fold and accounts for three-quarters of all cardiovascular deaths[8] among patients with type 2 diabetes. This increased risk appears to be present at the time of diagnosis, and diabetes has a relatively greater impact on CHD risk[9]. Diabetic patients who develop CHD have a much worse prognosis than non-diabetics and are more likely to die acutely with the first myocardial infarction (MI)[10]. In the GUSTO-I trial (Global Utilization of Streptokinase and Tissue Plasminogen Activator for Occluded Coronary Arteries) diabetes remained an independent determinant of 30-day mortality after adjustment for both clinical and angiographic variables[11]. In the longer term, the outlook is also poor – the 5-year mortality in a Swedish study was 55% in diabetic patients compared with 30% in non-diabetic patients[12].

The outcome for diabetic patients undergoing revascularization procedures is less good than for non-diabetics. In a subgroup analysis of the BARI study (Bypass Angioplasty Revascularization Investigation) the survival rate after percutaneous transluminal coronary angioplasty (PTCA) was only 65%, and after coronary artery bypass graft surgery (CABG) the survival rate was 6% in diabetics over 5 years[13]. In a recent follow-up report from the BARI investigators, diabetic patients who had previously undergone CABG, as compared to PTCA, showed a significantly improved prognosis after MI[14].

This massive burden of morbidity and mortality from the development of CHD, together with the poor outcome associated with large increases in the risk of cerebrovascular and peripheral vascular disease, provides a huge challenge to the physician caring for diabetic patients. This short review discusses dyslipidemia in relation to CHD risk.

EPIDEMIOLOGY OF DYSLIPIDEMIA IN TYPE 2 DIABETES

Given the predicted increase in the prevalence of diabetes worldwide and the progressive 'Westernization' of lifestyles in developing countries, cardiovascular disease, which is increased 2–5 times in people with diabetes, has and will continue to have major implications for health and healthcare provision[15,16]. Although the development of atherosclerosis and clinical vascular disease is multifactorial, it is likely that dyslipidemia is a major contributing risk factor[9].

Dyslipidemia is common in patients with type 2 diabetes; it is present at the time of diagnosis, and indeed in the pre-diabetic phase. It persists despite usual hypoglycemic therapy and its expression will be affected by genetic and lifestyle characteristics, such as gender, obesity, exercise levels, diet, alcohol intake, poor glycemic control, smoking, hypothyroidism, renal and hepatic function. It is also affected by concomitant drugs and the presence of primary dyslipidemia, such as familial combined hyperlipidemia and homozygosity for apoprotein E_2/E_2 predisposing to Type III dyslipidemia[17–21].

The hallmarks of diabetic dyslipidemia are moderate hypertriglyceridemia (usually 1.5 to 3-fold increased) and reduced HDL cholesterol (approximately 10–20%); total and low-density lipoprotein (LDL) cholesterol is generally not different quantitatively from non-diabetics drawn from the same population. For example, in the Prospective Cardiovascular Munster (PROCAM) study in the north of Germany 39% of diabetics had triglyceride concentrations > 2.3 mmol L^{-1} (versus 21% in non-diabetics) and 27% had low HDL cholesterol (< 0.9 mmol L^{-1}), compared with 16% in non-diabetics[22]. Similarly, in 2045 diabetic patients with established vascular disease screened to take part in a CHD secondary prevention trial, low HDL cholesterol (< 0.9 mmol L^{-1}) was found in 45% of diabetics compared with 46% of non-diabetics, and hypertriglyceridemia (> 2.3 mmol L^{-1}) in 30.5% versus 21.9%[23].

Although quantitatively there is little difference between total and LDL cholesterol concentrations in type 2 diabetic patients and controls, cholesterol (as LDL cholesterol) remains a very important risk factor for CHD. Furthermore, qualitative changes in LDL suggest increased atherogenicity. Of the 347 978 men screened for participation in the Multiple Risk Factor Intervention Trial (MRFIT), 5163 were identified as having diabetes through reporting of medication. Clearly, this under-estimates the number of diabetics, nevertheless this large cohort has provided very useful information. In the 12-year follow-up of these screened men, the absolute risk of cardiovascular death was increased three-fold in the diabetics after adjustment for age, race, income, serum cholesterol, systolic blood pressure and cigarette smoking. In both non-diabetic and diabetic men, cardiovascular deaths increased with increasing serum cholesterol; however, for a given cholesterol level, diabetic men had a two- to three-fold excess risk of cardiovascular disease. This was also true for two other major risk factors, cigarette smoking and hypertension, and for the three factors combined[24]. On the basis of these observations, Stamler and colleagues argued for rigorous intervention to control risk factors, including cholesterol levels, in diabetes[24].

It is mainly LDL cholesterol that accounts for the association between cholesterol and CHD, and this is an important predictor of risk in diabetes. In the UK Prospective Diabetes Study (UKPDS), LDL cholesterol was the major determinant for CHD[25]. LDL cholesterol is also an important risk factor in populations with low LDL concentrations[26].

Of considerable interest in relation to the pathogenicity of LDL in diabetes are the qualitative changes. LDL apoprotein B is susceptible to glycation[27], this decreases its affinity for the LDL receptor and increases its susceptibility to oxidative modification. In addition, the LDL subfraction distribution is altered. The important observations of Krauss[28] pointed to the lack of homogeneity in LDL and described it as, rather, a spectrum of particles varying in size, density and lipid content. In type 2 diabetes LDL is smaller and denser[17,29] (designated pattern B on electrophoretic separation and LDL_3 on ultracentrifugation), which is associated with increased vascular risk[30]. Like glycated LDL, small dense LDL is more susceptible to oxidation[31] and oxidized LDL is central to many of the processes of atherogenesis[32].

Triglycerides and CHD have been the subjects of much debate over the last two decades[33,34], particularly in relation to the independence of their relationship. However, given the complex metabolic interactions between triglycerides and other lipid parameters, especially HDL metabolism and small dense LDL, some investigators have examined CHD risk in relation to triglyceride, LDL and HDL. In both the PROCAM population[35] and the Helsinki Heart Study[36], hypertriglyceridemia was associated with CHD risk in individuals with an LDL:HDL cholesterol ratio > 5. This clustering of lipid abnormalities is often referred to as the atherogenic lipoprotein profile. Factor analysis and principal component analysis have recently been used to show that the 'hyperinsulinemia cluster' (a factor having high positive loadings for BMI, triglycerides and insulin, and a high negative loading for HDL cholesterol) was predictive of CHD death in type 2 diabetes[37].

Hypertriglyceridemia is associated with several important atherogenic mechanisms in type 2 diabetes. Some triglyceride-rich particles are directly atherogenic, namely remnant particles. These particles, which are also cholesterol-rich and contain apoproteins B and C-III, accumulate in diabetes[20]. These are the particles that accumulate in the rare Type III dyslipidemia (remnant particle disease or broad beta disease), which is associated with premature and extensive atherosclerosis[38]. Hypertriglyceridemia is also associated with important abnormalities in thrombosis and coagulation, particularly increased levels of plasminogen activator inhibitor-1[39], and prolonged, as well as elevated postprandial lipemia. Postprandial lipemia is central to important changes in the metabolism of other lipoproteins, with reductions in HDL cholesterol and the formation of small dense LDL[17]. Dyslipoproteinemia, including postprandial elevated plasma lipid levels, therefore appears to be an early and sensitive indicator of an underlying reduced insulin sensitivity.

Haffner et al.[41] investigated 1734 individuals prospectively over 7 years in the San Antonio Heart Study. They have shown recently that the 195 individuals who developed type 2 diabetes had a higher BMI, as well as waist-to-hip ratio, higher levels of blood pressure, elevated plasma triglyceride levels and lower HDL-cholesterol levels in plasma.

Kuja et al.[42] have shown that high triglyceride levels and low HDL-cholesterol concentrations in plasma are associated with postprandial hyperlipidemia. Sixty-three men with low fasting HDL-cholesterol levels and low or higher triglyceride levels were investigated. A significant relation between postprandial triglyceride increase and HDL-cholesterol levels in the fasting state was shown. Normal lipemic control individuals and men with low HDL-cholesterol levels showed a comparable postprandial lipid increase and no signs of insulin resistance. Individuals with low HDL-cholesterol levels, but also higher triglyceride levels, had a greater increase in postprandial lipemia associated with visceral obesity and insulin resistance.

LIPID AND LIPOPROTEIN METABOLISM IN INSULIN-RESISTANT STATES

Insulin resistance is central to the dyslipidemia of type 2 diabetes[20]. A simplified overview of

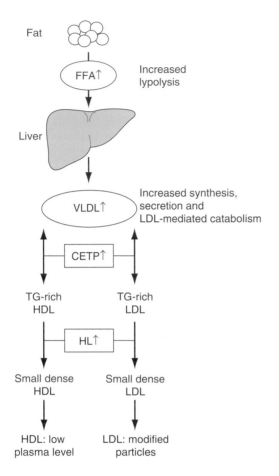

Figure 24.1 Essential steps in the development of diabetic dyslipidemia. Cholesteryl ester transfer protein (CETP) transfers triglycerides from VLDL to HDL and LDL for the exchange of cholesterol, thereby generating triglyceride-rich HDL and LDL particles. These particles are substrate for hepatic lipase (HL), which cleaves triglycerides and leaves small dense HDL and LDL. For further details see text.

current thinking that accounts for the various abnormalities and their relationship to insulin resistance is shown in Figure 24.1. In the presence of insulin resistance there is an increased flux of free fatty acids from adipose tissue to the liver, as a result of decreased inhibition of hormone-sensitive lipase. Fatty acids stimulate increased hepatic production and secretion of very low-density lipoprotein (VLDL), which is also increased by insulin resistance and hyperinsulinemia. Increased hepatic output of VLDL continues in the postprandial state and competes with exogenously-derived triglyceride carried in chylomicrons for the enzyme lipoprotein lipase. As a result, there is accumulation of triglyceride-rich lipoproteins and prolonged postprandial lipemia. The lipemia stimulates increased lipid transfer, via cholesterol ester transfer protein, with the exchange of triglyceride for cholesterol ester between triglyceride-rich lipoproteins and lipoproteins of higher density. As a result, LDL and HDL are enriched in triglycerides and become substrates for hepatic lipase, which hydrolyzes triglyceride, producing small dense LDL and small dense HDL. The importance of small dense LDL has been discussed above in relation to atherogenesis. Small dense HDL is more rapidly catabolized than other HDL species, leading to lower plasma HDL concentrations.

HDL represents a heterozygous group of lipoproteins that can be separated into different subfractions by various isolation techniques. Low HDL cholesterol concentrations are a strong predictor of vascular risk in diabetes, as in the general population[9]. It is therefore an ongoing research issue to determine how HDL-particles might play a role in atherogenesis. The role of HDL-particles in reverse cholesterol transport probably explains the epidemiological link between HDL and cardiovascular risk[43]. Reverse cholesterol transport involves HDL-mediated uptake of cholesterol from peripheral cells, such as macrophages or other vascular cells, followed by HDL-mediated transport of the cholesterolesters to the liver, from where it is excreted as bile acids. Research on the molecular basis of patients with low HDL-cholesterol levels in plasma resulting from Tangier disease has recently led to the identification of a novel protein family, the ATP cassette binding proteins. These proteins can interact with HDL-particles and might play an essential role in the extrusion of cellular cholesterol and the initial steps of reverse cholesterol transport[44].

The other side of the coin in reverse cholesterol transport and possibly regression of atherosclerosis, is selective uptake of cholesterolesters from HDL-particles by the liver. It has been shown that one major molecular mechanism of selective cholesterolester uptake from HDL-particles in liver utilizes the scavenger receptor class B type I (SR-B-I)[45]. SR-B-I is a protein with carveolin-resembling structures that is expressed at the cell surface. In mice, SR-B-I plays a pivotal role in maintaining the plasma level of HDL-cholesterol and the efficiency of reverse cholesterol transport. Mice with an inactivating mutation in the promotor region of the *SR-B-I* gene, which leads to only half of the expression of the receptor in the liver, have a highly elevated HDL-cholesterol level in plasma[46]. Knock-out mice, lacking the SR-B-I or HDL-receptor, also have an elevated plasma cholesterol level and a dramatically accelerated or enhanced manifestation of atherosclerosis on an ApoE knock-out mice background[47].

Elevation of the hepatic SR-B-I activity therefore appears to be a key element in reverse cholesterol transport. Accordingly, over-expression of SR-B-I in liver is associated with a reduction of atherosclerotic lesions in mice[48]. These two key steps of reverse cholesterol transport are therefore not only interesting potential novel drug targets, but might also be regulated by insulin and metabolites that are altered in states of insulin resistance.

IMPACT OF LIPID-LOWERING ON CARDIOVASCULAR ENDPOINTS

As yet, there are no major cardiovascular endpoint trials reported that have specifically targeted diabetic populations. However, many of the statin trials, particularly those in secondary prevention, have included sufficient diabetic patients to allow reasonable conclusions to be drawn. The recent results of the Health Protection Study, including 5963 diabetic patients, have significantly enhanced the clinical endpoint database in the high-risk population.

Secondary prevention

There are sufficient numbers of diabetic patients in the major secondary prevention trials with statins to allow meaningful subgroup analyses. In the Scandinavian Simvastatin Survival Study (4S)[49] an initial analysis described the impact of simvastatin (20–40 mg/day) on 202 diabetic patients out of a total of 4444 patients with established CHD and raised cholesterol concentrations (5.5–8.0 mmol L^{-1}). In the diabetic subgroup, simvastatin produced similar effects on serum lipid and lipoprotein concentrations over the course of the trial as in non-diabetics, with reductions in total and LDL-cholesterol of 24% and 34%, respectively: an 8% increase in HDL and a 9% reduction in triglyceride. It should be pointed out that the entry criteria for 4S stipulated total serum triglycerides ≤ 2.5 mmol L^{-1}. These changes were associated with a significant reduction in major coronary events – relative risk (RR) reduction 0.45 [95% confidence interval (CI) 0.27–0.74, P = 0.002]. The reduction in the primary endpoint of 4S – all-cause mortality – was not significant given the small numbers, but did approach significance. RR reduction was 0.57 (95% CI 0.30–1.08, P = 0.087). A further analysis of 4S data using the new diagnostic criterion for diabetes from the American Diabetes Association, i.e. a fasting plasma venous glucose of ≥ 7 mmol L^{-1}, revealed 483 diabetic patients[50]. In this larger group, the RR reduction for major coronary events was 0.58 (P = 0.001), with a highly significant reduction in revascularizations. Total and coronary mortality were also reduced, but these reductions did not reach statistical significance due to the small sample sizes. In 678 patients with impaired fasting glucose (6.0–6.9 mmol L^{-1}) there was a significant reduction in coronary events (RR = 0.62; P = 0.003) and total mortality (RR = 0.57; P = 0.02). These results have been analysed with regard to cost-effectiveness and resource utilization, and have been found to be highly cost-effective, with estimated cost savings[51,52].

Subgroup analysis of 586 diabetic patients included in the Cholesterol and Recurrent Events (CARE) trial provides additional evidence of the benefit of statin therapy[53]. Pravastatin 40 mg/day was associated with a RR reduction in major coronary events of 25% (P = 0.05). Further evidence of the benefit of pravastatin therapy in diabetic patients comes from the subgroup analysis of 782 diabetic patients in the Long-Term Intervention with Pravastatin in Ischemic Disease (LIPID) trial[54].

Taken together, these results point to the benefits of statin therapy in diabetic patients with established CHD.

Recent trials using fibrates have suggested benefits for diabetic patients with CHD. In the Veterans Affairs HDL Intervention Trial (VA-HIT), 2531 men with CHD and relatively normal LDL-cholesterol concentrations, but low HDL-cholesterol (≤ 1 mmol L^{-1}) were randomized to gemfibrozil or placebo[55]. Baseline lipid concentrations were LDL-cholesterol 2.9 mmol L^{-1}, HDL cholesterol 0.8 mmol L^{-1} and triglycerides 1.8 mmol L^{-1}. As expected, HDL cholesterol was 6% higher and serum triglycerides 31% lower in the placebo-treated group. There was no significant change in LDL-cholesterol. Overall, there was a reduction in the primary endpoint (non-fatal MI or death from coronary causes) of 22%. The risk reduction was 24% for the combined outcome of death from CHD, non-fatal MI and stroke. VA-HIT included 627 diabetic patients identified by clinical history and in this group the RR reduction was 24%. However, in the recent report of the Bezafibrate Infarction Prevention (BIP) study, no overall benefit was seen with the fibrate in 3090 patients with previous MI[56].

Primary prevention

Much less information is available on the benefits of lipid-lowering in diabetics without established CHD. Very few diabetic patients were included in the two major primary prevention trials using statins: the West of Scotland Coronary Prevention Study (WOSCOPS)[4] and the Air Force/Texas Coronary Atherosclerosis Prevention Study (AFCAPS/TexCAPS)[6]. In WOSCOPS there were 76 people with diabetes and in AFCAPS/TexCAPS 155 were included, making it difficult to draw meaningful conclusions. Similarly, few diabetics (*n = 135)* were included in the Helsinki Heart Study (HHS) of gemfibrozil. Although there was a reduction in events (60%) this did not achieve statistical significance given the small numbers involved[57].

Two trials have provided information on the progression of atherosclerosis in specific diabetic populations. In the St Mary's, Ealing, Northwick Park Diabetes Cardiovascular Disease Prevention (SENDCAP) Study, the progression of carotid atherosclerosis in carotid arteries was assessed by ultrasonic measurement[58]. Over 3 years, bezafibrate therapy versus placebo in 164 patients did not significantly affect intima-medial thickness. However, there was a significant reduction in events – albeit based on small numbers.

In the Diabetes Atherosclerosis Intervention Study (DAIS), 418 men and women with type 2 diabetes received fenofibrate or placebo for at least 3 years[59]. Eligible patients were in good glycemic control (mean HbA1c 7.5%) and showed 'mild' lipid and lipoprotein abnormalities; total cholesterol: HDL-cholesterol ratio ≥ 4 plus either LDL-cholesterol 3.5–4.5 mmol L^{-1} or a triglyceride concentration of 1.7–5.2 mmol L^{-1} and LDL-cholesterol ≤ 4.5 mmol L^{-1}. This was a coronary angiographic study and patients had at least one visible coronary lesion; roughly half of the patients had a history of coronary disease. Fenofibrate therapy was associated with significantly less increase in percentage diameter stenosis, and less decrease in minimum lumen diameter. Mean segment diameter, the primary endpoint on which power calculations were based, showed a smaller decrease, but this did not reach statistical significance. This trial was not based on clinical endpoints, but there were fewer events (not statistically significant) in the fenofibrate group (38 versus 50).

Heart protection study

A major study was conducted by the Heart Protection Study (HPS) collaborative group in the UK[60-62]. The study objective was to assess the effectiveness of 40 mg simvastatin per day, with and without antioxidant vitamin supplementation (vitamin E 650 mg, vitamin C 250 mg, beta-carotene 20 mg) on total and course-specific mortality in a wide range of patients at high risk of complications of CHD. A total of 20 536 patients aged 40–80 years, at high risk of vascular events due to existing cardiovascular disease, diabetes, or hypertension, were followed in the study for 5 years. A history of MI existed for 8510 individuals and 4876 had some other history of coronary disease. A total of 5963 patients with diabetes mellitus were included, of whom 3982 had no known coronary heart disease. There were no effects of vitamins on total mortality or cancer. The RR reduction for all-cause mortality in the simvastatin-treated group was 12.9% (1.328 versus 1.507 events). There was a highly significant 24% reduction in the event rate (absolute risk 18.8% or event number 2.033 versus 2.585) for the first occurrence of non-fatal MI or coronary death, non-fatal or fatal stroke, and for coronary or non-coronary revascularization. Interestingly, 3421 individuals were included who had a plasma LDL-cholesterol levels < 100 mg dL^{-1} (2.6 mmol L^{-1}) at study entry. The reason for this is that individuals were included unless their total cholesterol level was < 3.6 mmol L^{-1}. Therefore, 7882 individuals had a total cholesterol level < 212 mg L^{-1} or 5.5 mmol L^{-1}.

Interestingly, the RR reduction for cardiovascular events was irrespective of initial plasma LDL-cholesterol levels, i.e. RR reduction in the subgroup of individuals with an LDL-cholesterol level below 116 mg dL^{-1} (3.0 mmol L^{-1}) was comparable to the subgroup with LDL-cholesterol levels of 116 mg dL^{-1} or higher. Absolute RR among the 3421 individuals with LDL-cholesterol < 100 mg dL^{-1} by treatment (mean LDL-cholesterol of 97 mg dL^{-1} versus 65 mg dL^{-1}) was 4.6%. The RR reduction of cardiovascular events in patients with diabetes was significant and similar to the whole group. Initial analyses revealed 279 events in the treatment group, versus 369 in the placebo group.

On-going trials

Several on-going studies will provide further insights into the potential benefit of lipid-lowering in diabetic populations by using statins and fibrates[63,64]. The Collaborative Atorvastatin Diabetes Study (CARDS) in the UK (funded through a collaboration between Diabetes UK, the NHS Research and Development Directorate and Pfizer UK) compares atorvastatin 10 mg/day with placebo in approximately 2800 patients with type 2 diabetes, normal or moderately elevated LDL-cholesterol and no previous CHD. At entry, patients are aged 40–75 years and have one additional risk factor, hypertension, retinopathy, microalbuminuria or cigarette smoking (all patients are counselled to quit). Serum LDL-cholesterol concentration is ≤ 4.14 mmol L^{-1} (160 mg dL^{-1}) and serum triglycerides ≤ 6.78 mmol L^{-1} (600 mg dL^{-1}). The primary efficacy parameter is the time to first occurrence of: CHD death, resuscitated cardiac arrest and non-fatal MI, including silent infarction; coronary revascularization; stroke; and unstable angina. The trial is fully recruited and patients will be followed until at least 304 primary endpoints have accrued.

The Atorvastatin as Prevention of Coronary Heart Disease in Patients with Type 2 Diabetes (ASPEN) study involves approximately 2250 patients, mainly in the USA but also in Europe and Australia. It is a combined primary and secondary prevention trial comparing 10 mg atorvastatin with placebo. The primary end-points are similar to those of CARDS, which means that combined subgroup analyses will be feasible.

The Fenofibrate Intervention and Event Lowering in Diabetes (FIELD) trial is currently recruiting in Australia, New Zealand and Finland. It will compare micronized fenofibrate (200 mg/day) with placebo in 8000 men and women with type 2 diabetes. It is a combined primary and secondary prevention study of 8000 patients (2000 patients with established disease). The primary endpoints are coronary mortality and coronary events. Lipid entry criteria are total: HDL-cholesterol ratio of ≥ 4, total cholesterol 3.0–6.5 mmol L^{-1} and triglycerides ≤ 5 mmol L^{-1}. Follow-up is expected to be 5–7 years.

These on-going trials should provide an evidence base for clinical guidelines, particularly in primary prevention, together with cost-benefit assessments. On the basis of current clinical trial evidence, statin therapy is the treatment of choice for the majority of patients. The results of VAHIT suggest a place for fibrate therapy in high-risk individuals with low HDL-cholesterol, raised triglycerides and an LDL-cholesterol below target. However, in HPS benefit was seen with simvastatin in individuals with low LDL, low HDL and raised triglycerides.

Table 24.1 Recommendations of target values for LDL-cholesterol in plasma, and optimal or desirable values for other plasma lipids and lipoprotein in patients with diabetes

	Europe	International	ADA
Triglyceride	<150	<150	<150
Total cholesterol	<185	No recommendation	No recommendation
LDL-cholesterol	<115	<130/<100*	<100
HDL-cholesterol	>46	>35	>40

Treatment goals recommended by the European Diabetes Policy Group[65], the International Task Force for Prevention of Coronary Heart Disease[66] and the ADA[67]. Plasma values are shown in mg dL^{-1}. The International Task Force suggests target LDL-cholesterol levels in diabetic patients < 100 mg dL^{-1} with evidence and < 130 mg dL^{-1} without evidence of macrovascular disease[66]. *The National Cholesterol Education Program (NCEP) expert panel on detection, evaluation and treatment of high blood cholesterol in adults [Adult Treatment Panel (ATP) III] recommends LDL-cholesterol < 100 mg dL^{-1} in individuals with CHD or equivalent (10-year risk > 20%) and regards diabetes as such a CHD risk equivalent[70].

MANAGEMENT CONSIDERATIONS

Given the importance of diabetic dyslipidemia in diabetic macroangiopathy, lipid and lipoprotein indices have been incorporated into metabolic targets for diabetic control in Europe[65], internationally[66] and in the USA[67], see Table 24.1. In the European Diabetes Policy Group guide to management of type 2 diabetes, blood lipid control target levels are shown not only for total and LDL-cholesterol levels, but also for triglycerides and HDL-cholesterol levels, acknowledging their contribution to vascular risk. Categories of risk for adults with diabetes, based on lipoprotein levels, have been proposed by the American Diabetes Association (ADA). Although similar to the European guidelines, the LDL-cholesterol target is lower and the triglyceride target is higher in the ADA document. These authors strongly support the lower triglyceride target and the lower-LDL cholesterol target – the 'best' of all guidelines!

A fasting lipid profile should be incorporated into the annual assessment of all type 2 diabetic patients. In most laboratories, total cholesterol and triglycerides are measured directly: HDL-cholesterol is measured in the supernatant after precipitation of apoprotein B-containing lipoproteins. LDL-cholesterol is calculated using the Friedewald formula[68]:

$$\text{LDL cholesterol} = \text{total cholesterol} - \text{HDL cholesterol} - \left(\frac{\text{total triglyceride}}{2.19}\right)$$

(all concentrations in mmol L^{-1}).

The formula is reasonably accurate if total triglycerides are 4 mmol L^{-1}. Some authorities, acknowledging the importance of cholesterol-rich remnants in diabetes, have advocated using non-HDL cholesterol as a potentially better indicator of atherogenic cholesterol[69]. Indeed, in the recent report from the Adult Treatment Panel III of the National Cholesterol Education Program in the USA, non-HDL cholesterol is proposed as a secondary target [set at 130 mg dL^{-1} (3.4 mmol L^{-1})] of therapy in patients with hypertriglyceridemia[70]. In addition, normal triglycerides are now defined as ≤ 150 mg dL^{-1} (1.7 mmol L^{-1}).

In the majority of diabetic patients with established symptomatic CHD, or other vascular disease, statin therapy will be indicated; under the European guidelines if the LDL-cholesterol is ≥ 3 mmol L^{-1}, or under the American guidelines ≥ 2.6 mmol L^{-1}. In the European guidelines fibrate therapy is advised if total triglycerides are ≥ 2.2 mmol L^{-1} with LDL-cholesterol ≤ 3.0 mmol L^{-1}, although it is likely that these guidelines will be revised following HPS. In some high-risk patients, combination therapy with a statin and fibrate is required to achieve optimal LDL-cholesterol, non-HDL-cholesterol and triglyceride concentrations. Combination therapy requires more careful safety monitoring to avoid rare side-effects of myositis and hepatic dysfunction.

Among diabetic patients without established disease, many will fulfill the absolute CHD risk criteria of 20% over 10 years, which is sufficient to justify statin therapy[71]. The ADA recommends the same goals of therapy in both primary and secondary prevention, and an initiation level of 130 mg dL^{-1} (3.4 mmol L^{-1}) for drug therapy. However, in the presence of another risk factor [low HDL-cholesterol (< 3.5 mg dL^{-1}; 0.9 mmol L^{-1}), hypertension, smoking, family history of CHD or microalbuminuria or proteinuria] they suggest the same drug initiation level (100 mg dL^{-1}; 2.6 mmol L^{-1}) as for secondary prevention[67]. This approach has been taken a step further in the new ATP III report[70]. In these guidelines, diabetes is considered a CHD risk equivalent, because of the high risk it confers and, in part, because of its frequent association with multiple risk factors. Whether these recommendations will be adopted in Europe remains to be seen.

Interestingly, in the recently published Heart Protection Study[62], RR reduction of cardiovascular complications was similar in all patients, independent of initial LDL-cholesterol in plasma levels. Indications for statin treatment should therefore be set by clinical risk, and not lipid values alone. Recommended treatment targets for high-risk individuals still remain to be determined, but HPS implies that statin-induced reduction of LDL cholesterol should be at least 1 mmol L^{-1}, whatever the baseline level. For the moment it is likely that physicians will continue to use risk charts to determine statin usage, until

further evaluation of the HPS diabetic cohort and on-going trial reports enable full cost-benefit analysis of lipid-lowering therapy, especially in patients without symptomatic cardiovascular disease. However, the first published data from HPS show that there was an absolute RR of 4.6% in the rate of major vascular events in 3421 individuals with initial LDL-cholesterol levels < 100 mg dL^{-1}. This resulted in a number needed-to-treat (NNT) of about 20–25.

The management of diabetic dyslipidemia should be part of an overall risk management approach to the prevention and treatment of macrovascular disease in type 2 diabetes. In addition to lipid-lowering drug therapy, attention to lifestyle measures is essential[67,70,71]. Dyslipidemia is most likely to be due to the metabolic syndrome, however, where appropriate, other causes of dyslipidemia should be excluded, including both primary (familial hypercholesterolemia, familial combined hyperlipidemia, dysbetalipoproteinemia, familial hypertriglyceridemia) and secondary causes (hypothyroidism, obstructive liver disease, chronic renal disease and concomitant drug therapy).

Surveys from Europe and America[72,73] have emphasized the wide treatment gap with respect to appropriate lipid-lowering therapy, despite overwhelming evidence of benefit – particularly in secondary prevention and for high-risk individuals without established disease. Physicians caring for diabetic patients should ensure that their patients receive high-quality evidence-based care, which is likely to reduce substantially their risk of macrovascular disease. In the future it is likely that the attention of physicians will turn to the prevention of diabetes in high-risk individuals as an optimal means of reducing the burden of macrovascular disease. The exciting results from the Finnish Diabetes Prevention Study Group[74] show that type 2 diabetes can be prevented by lifestyle measures. In addition, treatment of glucose-intolerant individuals with metformin[75], or acarbose[76] can reduce or delay the development of clinically overt type 2 diabetes. However, there are data available that suggest there is also a related reduction in concomitant cardiovascular risk factors or events, a question discussed in Chapter 2.

Furthermore, the intriguing findings from the HOPE trial with ramipril[77], the LIFE trial with losartan[78], and the West of Scotland study with pravastatin[79] suggest a reduced incidence of diabetes. Understanding of the mechanisms of these effects may lead to further therapeutic developments to prevent both diabetes development and related disorders.

New advances in the prevention of diabetes may arise from the identification of novel transcription factors regulating the expression of many different genes. Altered nutrition, the use of hormones as well as drugs (e.g. the peroxisome proliferator activated receptors, PPARs)[80], sterol regulatory element binding proteins (SREBPs)[6,81] and other orphan receptors[82] and their relationships to insulin resistance, glucose, fatty acid and adipose tissue metabolism[83,84] may also open the way to other possible targets of treatment and prevention.

REFERENCES

1 American Diabetes Association. Screening for Diabetes. *Diabetes Care* 2002;25(Suppl.);521–4.

2 Law M, Wald WJ, Thompson SG. By how much and how quickly does reduction in serum cholesterol concentration lower risk of ischaemic heart disease? *Br Med J* 1994;308:367–72.

3 Scandinavian Simvastatin Survival Study Group. Randomized trial of cholesterol lowering in 4444 patients with coronary heart disease: the Scandinavian Simvastatin Survival Study (4S). *Lancet* 1994;344:1383–9.

4 Shepherd J, Cobb SM, Ford I *et al.* for the West of Scotland Coronary Prevention Study Group. Prevention of coronary heart disease with pravastatin in men with hypercholesterolaemia. *N Engl J Med* 1995;20:1301–7.

5 Sacks FM, Pfeffer MA, Moge LA *et al.* The effect of pravastatin on coronary events after myocardial infarction in patients with average cholesterol levels. *N Engl J Med* 1996;335:1001–9.

6 Downs JR, Clearfield M, Weis S *et al.* for the AFCAPs/TexCAPs Research Group. Primary prevention of acute coronary events with lovastatin in men and women with average cholesterol levels. Results of AFCAPs/TexCAPs. *J Am Med Assoc* 1998;279:1615–61.

7 The Long-Term Intervention with Pravastatin in Ischaemic Disease (LIPID) Study Group. Prevention of cardiovascular events and death with pravastatin in patients with coronary heart disease and a broad range of initial cholesterol levels. *N Engl J Med* 1998;339:1349–57.

8 Grundy SM, Benjamin IJ, Burke GL *et al.* AHA Scientific Statement. Diabetes and Cardiovascular Disease. A statement for healthcare professionals from the American Heart Association. *Circulation* 1999;100:1134–46.

9 Laakso M, Lehto S. Epidemiology of macrovascular disease in diabetes. *Diabetes Rev* 1997;5: 295–315.

10 Aronson D, Rayfield EJ, Chesebro JH. Mechanisms determining course and outcome of diabetic patients who have had acute myocardial infarction. *Ann Intern Med* 1997;126:296–306.

11 Woodfield SL, Lundergan CF, Reiner JS *et al.* for the GUSTO-1 angiographic investigators. Angiographic findings and outcome in diabetic patients treated with thrombolytic therapy for acute myocardial infarction: the GUSTO-1 experience. *J Am Coll Cardiol* 1996;28:1661–9.

12 Herlitz J, Malmberg K, Karlsson B *et al.* Mortality and morbidity during a five-year follow-up of diabetics with myocardial infarction. *Acta Med Scand* 1998;24:31–8.

13 Bypass Angioplasty Revascularization Investigation (BARI) Investigators. Comparison of coronary bypass surgery with angioplasty in patients with multivessel disease. *N Engl J Med* 1996;355:217–25.

14 Detre KM, Lombardero MS, Brooks MM *et al.* for the Bypass Angioplasty Revascularization Investigation Investigators. The effect of previous coronary-artery bypass surgery on the prognosis of patients with diabetes who have acute myocardial infarction. *N Engl J Med* 2000;342:989–97.

15 King H, Aubert RE, Herman WH. Global burden of diabetes, 1995–2025. Prevalence, numerical estimates and projections. *Diabetes Care* 1998;21:1414–31.

16 Zimmet PZ, Alberti KG. The changing face of macrovascular disease in non-insulin dependent diabetes mellitus: an epidemic in progress. *Lancet* 1997;350(Suppl 1):1–4.

17 Syvanne M, Taskinen M-R. Lipids and lipopro-

teins as coronary risk factors in non-insulin-dependent diabetes mellitus. *Lancet* 1997;350 (Suppl 1):S120–S123.

18　Duell PB. Diabetes mellitus. In: Betteridge DJ, Illingworth DR, Shepherd J, editors. *Lipoproteins in health and disease*. London: Arnold, 1999: 897–930.

19　Betteridge DJ. Risk factors for arterial disease in diabetes: dyslipidaemia. In: Tooke JE, editor. *Diabetic angiopathy*. London: Arnold, 1999:65–92.

20　Ginsberg HN. Insulin resistance and cardiovascular disease. *J Clin Invest* 2000;106:453–8.

21　Haffner SM. American Diabetes Association technical review: management of dyslipidaemia in adults with diabetes. *Diabetes Care* 1998;21: 160–78.

22　Assmann E, Schulte H. The prospective cardiovascular Munster (PROCAM) study: prevalence of hyperlipidaemia in persons with hypertension and/or diabetes mellitus and the relationship to coronary heart disease. *Am Heart J* 1988;116: 1713–24.

23　Behard S, Benderly M, Reicher-Reus H *et al.* for the Bezafibrate Infarction Prevention (BIP) Study. Lipid profile and outcome of diabetic patients with coronary artery disease in the BIP Study Registry. Proceedings of the American College of Cardiology; 1997 March; Anaheim, California.

24　Stamler J *et al.* for the Multiple Risk Factor Intervention Trial Research Group. Diabetes, other risk factors and 12 year cardiovascular mortality for men screened in the Multiple Risk Factor Intervention Trial. *Diabetes Care* 1993;16: 434–44.

25　Turner RC, Millns H, Neil HAW *et al.* for the United Kingdom Prospective Diabetes Study Group. Risk factors for coronary artery disease in non-insulin-dependent diabetes mellitus: United Kingdom prospective diabetes study (UKPDS: 23). *Br Med J* 1998;316:823–8.

26　Howard BV, Robbins DC, Sievers ml *et al.* LDL cholesterol as a strong predictor of coronary heart disease in diabetic individuals with insulin resistance and low LDL. The Strong Heart Study. *Arterioscler Thromb Vasc Biol* 2000;20:830–5.

27　Steinbrecher UP, Witztum JL. Glycosylation of low-density lipoproteins to an extent comparable to that seen in diabetes slows their catabolism. *Diabetes* 1984;33:130–4.

28　Krauss RM, Burke DJ. Identification of multiple subclasses of plasma low-density lipoproteins in normal humans. *J Lipid Res* 1982;23:97–104.

29　Betteridge DJ. LDL heterogeneity: implications for atherogenicity in insulin resistance and NIDDM. *Diabetologia* 1997;40:S149–S151.

30　Austin A, Breslow JL, Hennekens CH *et al.* Low density lipoprotein subclass patterns and risk of myocardial infarction. *JAMA* 1988;260:1917–21.

31　Chait A, Brazg RL, Tribble D, Krauss RM. Susceptibility of small dense low-density lipoproteins to oxidative modification in subjects with the atherogenic lipoprotein phenotype. *Am J Med* 1993;94:350–6.

32　Steinberg D. Oxidative modification of LL and atherogenesis. *Circulation* 1997;95:1062 71.

33　Hulley SB, Rosenman RH, Bawal RD *et al.* Epidemiology as a guide to clinical decisions: the association between triglyceride and coronary heart disease. *N Engl J Med* 1980;302:1383–9.

34　Hokanson E, Austin MA. Plasma triglyceride is a risk factor for cardiovascular disease independent of high-density lipoprotein cholesterol level: a meta-analysis of population-based prospective studies. *J Cardiovasc Risk* 1996;3:213–19.

35　Assmann G, Schulte H. Relation of high-density lipoprotein cholesterol and triglycerides to incidence of atherosclerotic coronary artery disease (the PROCAM experience). *Am J Cardiol* 1992; 70:733–7.

36　Manninen V, Tenkanen H, Koskinen P *et al.* Joint effects of triglycerides and LDL cholesterol and HDL cholesterol concentrations on coronary heart disease risk in the Helsinki Heart Study. Implications for treatment. *Circulation* 1992;85: 37–45.

37　Lehto S, Ronnemaa T, Pyorala K, Laakso M. Cardiovascular risk factors clustering with endogenous hyperinsulinaemia predict death from coronary heart disease in patients with type 2 diabetes. *Diabetologia* 2000;43:148–55.

38　Mahley RW, Rall Jr SC. Type III hyperlipoproteinaemias (dysbetalipoproteinaemia; remnant particle disease). In: Betteridge DJ, Illingworth DR, Shepherd J, editors. *Lipoproteins in health and disease*. London: Arnold, 1999:719–36.

39　Hamsten A, Karpe F. Triglycerides and coronary heart disease – has epidemiology given us the right answer? In: Betteridge DJ, editor. *Lipids: current perspectives*. London: Martin Dunitz, 1996:43–68.

40　Foger B, Patsch JR. Postprandial lipaemia. In: Betteridge DJ, editor. *Lipids and vascular disease: current issues*. London: Martin Dunitz, 2000:1–14.

41　Haffner SM, Mykkanen L, Festa A *et al.* Insulin-resistant prediabetic subjects have more atherogenic risk factors than insulin-sensitive prediabetic subjects: implications for preventing coronary heart disease during the prediabetic state. *Circulation* 2000;191:975–80.

42 Couillard C, Bergeron N, Bergeron J *et al.* Metabolic heterogeneity underlying postprandial lipemia among men with low fasting high density lipoprotein cholesterol concentrations. *J Clin Endocrinol Metab* 2000;85:4575–82.

43 Wang N, Tall AR. Therapeutic modulation of cellular cholesterol efflux. *Curr Atheroscler Rep* 2001;3:345–7.

44 Schmitz G, Kaminski WE. ATP-binding cassette (ABC) transporter in atherosclerosis. *Curr Atheroscler Rep* 2002;4:243–51.

45 Krieger M. Scavenger receptor class B type I is a multiligand HDL receptor that influences diverse physiologic systems. *J Clin Invest* 2001;108:793–7.

46 Rigotti A, Trigatti BL, Penman M *et al.* A target mutation in the murine gene encoding the high density lipoprotein (HDL) receptor scavenger receptor class B type I reveals its key role in HDL metabolism. *Proc Natl Acad Sci USA* 1997;94:12610–15.

47 Braun A, Trigatti BL, Post MJ *et al.* Loss of SR-BI expression leads to the early onset of occlusive atherosclerotic coronary artery disease, spontaneous myocardial infarctions, severe cardiac dysfunction, and premature death in apolipoprotein E-deficient mice. *Circ Res* 2002;90:270–6.

48 Ueda Y, Gong E, Royer L *et al.* Relationship between expression levels and atherogenesis in scavenger receptor class B, type I transgenics. *J Biol Chem* 2000; 275:20368–73.

49 Pyorala K, Pedersen TR, Kjeksus J *et al.* Cholesterol lowering with simvastatin improves prognosis of diabetic patients with coronary heart disease: a subgroup analysis of the Scandinavian Simvastatin Survival Study (4S). *Diabetes Care* 1997;20:614–20.

50 Haffner SM, Alexander CM, Cook TJ *et al.* for the Scandinavian Simvastatin Survival Study Group. Reduced coronary events in simvastatin-treated patients with coronary heart disease and diabetes or impaired fasting glucose levels. Subgroup Analysis in the Scandinavian Simvastatin Survival Study. *Archiv Intern Med* 1999;159:2661–7.

51 Jonsson B, Cook JR, Pedersen TR. The cost-effectiveness of lipid lowering in patients with diabetes: results from the 4S trial. *Diabetologia* 1999;42:1293–301.

52 Herman WH, Alexander CM, Cook JR *et al.* for the 4S Study Group. Effect of simvastatin treatment on cardiovascular resource utilization in impaired fasting glucose and diabetes. Findings from the Scandinavian Simvastatin Survival Study. *Diabetes Care* 1999;22:1771–8.

53 Goldberg R, Mellies MJ, Scaks FM *et al.* for the CARE Investigators. Cardiovascular events and their reduction with pravastatin in diabetic and glucose-intolerant myocardial infarction survivors with average cholesterol levels. Subgroup analysis in the Cholesterol and Recurrent Events (CARE) Trial. *Circulation* 1998;98:2513–19.

54 The Long-Term Intervention with Pravastatin in Ischaemic Disease (LIPID) Study Group. Prevention of cardiovascular events and death with pravastatin in patients with coronary heart disease and a broad range of initial cholesterol levels. *N Engl J Med* 1998;339:1349–57.

55 Rubins HB, Robins SJ, Collins D *et al.* for the Veterans Affairs High-Density Lipoprotein Cholesterol Intervention Trial Study Group. Gemfibrozil for the secondary prevention of coronary heart disease in men with low levels of high-density lipoprotein cholesterol. *N Engl J Med* 1999;341:410–18.

56 The BIP Study Group. Secondary prevention by raising HDL cholesterol and reducing triglycerides in patients with coronary artery disease. The Bezafibrate Infarction Prevention (BIP) Study. *Circulation* 2000;102:21–7.

57 Koskinen P, Lanthari M, Manninen V *et al.* Coronary heart disease in NIDDM patients in the Helsinki Heart Study. *Diabetes Care* 1992;15:820–5.

58 Elkeles RS, Diamond JR, Poulter C *et al.* The SENDCAP Study Group. Cardiovascular outcomes in Type 2 diabetes. A double-blind placebo-controlled study of bezafibrate: the St Mary's, Ealing, Northwick Park Diabetes Cardiovascular Disease Prevention (SENDCAP) Study. *Diabetes Care* 1998;21:641–8.

59 Diabetes Atherosclerosis Intervention Study Investigators. Effect of fenofibrate on progression of coronary-artery disease in type 2 diabetes: The Diabetes Atherosclerosis Intervention Study, a randomised study. *Lancet* 2001;357:905–10.

60 MRC/BHF Heart Protection Study Collaborative Group. MRC/BHF Heart Protection Study of cholesterol-lowering therapy and of antioxidant vitamin supplementation in a wide range of patients at increased risk of coronary heart disease death: early safety and efficacy experience. *Eur Heart J* 1999;20:725–41.

61 Collins R. The MRC/BHF Heart Protection

Study: preliminary results. *Int J Clin Pract* 2002;56:53–6.

62 MRC/BHF Heart Protection Study Collaborative Group. MRC/BHF Heart Protection Study of cholesterol lowering with simvastatin in 20 536 high-risk individuals: a randomised placebo-controlled trial. *Lancet* 2002;360:7–22.

63 Betteridge DJ, Colhoun H, Armitage J. Status report of lipid-lowering trials in diabetes. *Curr Opin Lipidol* 2000;11:621–6.

64 Steiner G. Diabetes, lipids and coronary heart disease: what have we learnt from lipid lowering trials. In: Betteridge DJ, editor. *Lipids and vascular disease: current issues*. London: Martin Dunitz, 2000:159–72.

65 European Diabetes Policy Group 1998–99. *Guidelines for diabetes care. A desktop guide to type 2 diabetes mellitus*. Brussels: International Diabetes Federation (Europe), 1999.

66 The International Task Force for Prevention of Coronary Heart Disease. Coronary heart disease: reducing the risk. The scientific background for primary and secondary prevention of coronary heart disease. *Nutr Metab Cardiovasc Dis* 1998;8:205–71.

67 American Diabetes Association. Management of dyslipidemia in adults with diabetes. *Diabetes Care* 2003;26(Suppl 4):S83–7.

68 Friedewald WT, Levy R, Frederickson DS. Estimation of the concentration of low-density lipoprotein in plasma without use of the preparative ultracentrifuge. *Clin Chem* 1972;18:499–502.

69 Garg A, Grundy SM. Diabetic dyslipidaemia and its therapy. *Diabetes Rev* 1997;5:425–33.

70 Expert Panel on Detection, Evaluation and Treatment of High Blood Cholesterol in Adults. Executive summary of the third report of the National Cholesterol Education Program (NCEP) expert panel on detection, evaluation and treatment of high blood cholesterol in adults (Adult Treatment Panel III). *J Am Med Assoc* 2001;285:2486–97.

71 Wood DA, De Backer G, Faergeman O *et al*. Prevention of coronary heart disease in clinical practice. Recommendations of the second joint task force of the European Society of Cardiology, European Atherosclerosis Society and European Society of Hypertension. *Eur Heart J* 1998;19:1434–8.

72 Euroaspire II Study Group. Lifestyle and risk factor management and use of drug therapies in coronary patients from 15 countries. Principal results from Euroaspire II Euro Heart Survey Programme. *Eur Heart J* 2001;22:554–72.

73 Pearson TA, Peters TD. The treatment gap in coronary artery disease and heart failure: community standards and the post discharge patient. *Am J Cardiol* 1997;80(8B):45H-52H.

74 Tuomilehto J, Lindstrom J, Eriksson JG *et al*. for the Finnish Diabetes Prevention Study Group. *N Engl J Med* 2001;344:1343–50.

75 Knowler WC, E Barrett-Connor, SE Fowler *et al*. for The Diabetes Prevention Program Research Group. Reduction in the incidence of type 2 diabetes with lifestyle intervention or metformin. *N Engl J Med* 2002;346:393–403

76 Chiasson JJ, RG Josse, R Gomis *et al*. for the STOP-NIDDM Trial Research Group. Acarbose for prevention of type 2 diabetes mellitus: the STOP-NIDDM randomized trial. *Lancet* 2002;359:2072–77.

77 The Heart Outcomes Prevention Evaluation Study Investigators. Effects of an angiotensin converting enzyme inhibitor, ramipril on cardiovascular events in high-risk patients. *N Engl J Med* 2000;342:145–53.

78 Dalöv B, Devereux RB, Kjeldsen SE *et al*. Cardiovascular morbidity and mortality in the Losartan Intervention for Endpoint Reduction in Hypertension Study (LIFE): a randomised trial against Atenolol. *Lancet* 2002;359:995–1003.

79 Freeman DJ, Norrie J, Sattar N *et al*. Pravastatin and the development of diabetes mellitus. Evidence for a protective treatment effect in the West of Scotland Coronary Prevention Study. *Circulation* 2001;103:357–62.

80 Desvergne B, Wahli W. Peroxisome proliferator-activity receptors: nuclear control of metabolism. *Endocr Rev* 1999;20:649–88.

81 Mueller-Wieland D, J Kotzka. *SREBP-1*: gene regulatory key to syndrome X? *Ann NY Acad Sci* 2002;967:19–27

82 Willson TM, JT Moore. Minireview: genomics versus orphan nuclear receptors – a half-time report. *Mol Endocrinol* 2002;16:1135–44.

83 McGarry JD. Dysregulation of fatty acid metabolism in the etiology of type 2 diabetes. *Diabetes* 2002;51:7–18.

84 Unger RH. Lipotoxic disesases. *Ann Rev Med* 2002;53:319–336.

25

Anti-hypertensive therapy in diabetes mellitus

Guntram Schernthaner

INTRODUCTION

Diabetes and hypertension are interrelated diseases that, if untreated, strongly predispose the patient to atherosclerotic cardiovascular disease (CVD) and renal disease. The combination of hypertension and diabetes is an important public health problem[1] since about 35–75% of diabetic complications can be attributed to hypertension. Patients who have both diabetes and hypertension have more renal disease and atherogenic risk factors, including dislipidemia, hyperuricaemia, elevated fibrinogen and left ventricular hypertrophy. Hypertension contributes to the leading causes of morbidity and mortality in people with diabetes, including coronary heart disease (CHD), stroke, peripheral vascular disease, lower extremity amputations and end-stage renal disease (ESRD). Hypertension also contributes to diabetic retinopathy, which is the leading cause of newly diagnosed blindness in the western world. For all these reasons, hypertension and diabetes should be recognized and treated early and aggressively.

PATHOGENESIS AND PATHOPHYSIOLOGY OF HYPERTENSION IN TYPE 1 AND TYPE 2 DIABETES

There are substantial differences in the causes of hypertension in type 1 and type 2 diabetes. In patients with type 1 diabetes, diabetic nephropathy appears to be the most common cause of hypertension[2]. A strong family history of essential hypertension and diabetes appears to identify those people with type 1 diabetes who are most likely to develop renal disease and hypertension[3]. Probably an equal number of people with type 2 diabetes mellitus develop renal disease[4], but hypertension often occurs associated with obesity or older age, even with normal renal function. Various hypotheses have been suggested to account for the increased prevalence of hypertension, particularly in type 2 diabetic patients[5]. Hypertension may be related, in part to central obesity and increased sympathetic nervous system stimulation and catecholamine production seen in diabetics[5]. It is now generally believed that essential hypertension is a part of the insulin resistance syndrome (IRS)[6]. In a considerable number of patients hypertension precedes the development of type 2 diabetes[7]. A recent epidemiologic study[8] has confirmed that patients with hypertension have a significantly increased risk [relative risk (RR) = 2.43] for the development of type 2 diabetes within a follow-up period of 6 years.

The risk for hypertensive patients of the later development of type 2 diabetes seems to be influenced by the type of antihypertensive treatment. According to a recent report by Gress *et al*[8], hypertensive patients who were taking beta-blockers had a 28% higher risk of diabetes than those taking no medication. In contrast, patients with hypertension who received thiazide diuretics, angiotensin-converting enzyme (ACE)-inhibitors or Ca^{2+} antagonists were found not to be at greater risk for subsequent diabetes than were patients who were not receiving any antihypertensive medications. It is important to mention that the study of Gress[8] was not prospective or randomized, and that other randomized prospected trials have not shown an increase in the development of diabetes with beta-blockers or low-dose diuretic treatment of hypertension. Recent studies have reported that ACE-inhibitor therapy reduced the propensity of hypertensive patients to develop type 2 diabetes by 21%[9] and 34%[10] in trials extending for 4–6 years, suggesting that the type of antihypertensive treatment may have a significant impact on the propensity for the development of diabetes.

ABNORMAL CIRCADIAN VARIATION OF BLOOD PRESSSURE (NONDIPPING)

Recent studies clearly indicate that in diabetic patients, measurement of ambulatory 24 h blood pressure (BP) is a much better predictor of microvascular and macrovascular complications than conventional BP measurement[11–13]. This is presumably due to better reproducibility, complete assessment of the circadian profile and exclusion of the 'white coat phenomenon'. An abnormal circadian variation of BP ('nondipping') can be demonstrated in a considerable number of diabetic patients, and was found to be related to microalbuminuria and diabetic nephropathy[11,12]. Nondipping was also found in nondiabetic patients, associated with glucose intolerance, insulin resistance and enhanced nocturnal sympathetic activity[13]. A disturbed diurnal variation of BP is a predicting marker for progression of both diabetic retinopathy[14] and diabetic nephropathy[12] in type 1 diabetic patients. A 20-fold risk of dying within the next 5 years was found in those type 2 diabetic patients who had a 'reversed' circadian BP profile, compared with patients who had a

normal decrease in BP during nighttime[15]. Interestingly, most sudden deaths or strokes in that study occurred during nighttime or early morning[15]. More research is needed to clarify whether the increased risk for end-organ damage can be lowered in diabetic patients with abnormal circadian variation of BP, by specific intervention strategies[16].

NONPHARMACOLOGICAL TREATMENT OF HYPERTENSION IN DIABETIC PATIENTS

The goal of treating hypertension in patients with diabetes is to prevent associated morbidity and mortality[17]. Lifestyle modification—including weight management, diet, salt reduction, moderation of alcohol intake, increased physical activity and smoking cessation are the cornerstones of therapy.

Weight loss in overweight individuals can improve control of both hypertension and diabetes. Studies have shown that even modest reductions of body weight can improve BP and glycemic control[18]. Reduction in weight may be associated with BP reductions because of reduction of insulin levels, sympathetic nervous system activity, and vascular resistance.

PHARMACOLOGICAL TREATMENT OF HYPERTENSION

Pharmacological therapy should be initiated when lifestyle modifications are unsuccessful in controlling hypertension. In stages 1 and 2 hypertension, lifestyle modifications may be continued for 3 months before initiating drug therapy. In more severe hypertension, drug therapy should be instituted at the time of diagnosis. All six classes of antihypertensive drugs (thiazide diuretics, beta-adrenergic blockers, calcium antagonists, ACE inhibitors, angiotensin II receptor blockers and alpha$_1$ specific blockers) are effective in controlling BP of diabetic patients, and can be principally used for single-agent therapy, or in combination with other classes of antihypertensive drugs. However, each drug class has potential advantages and disadvantages (Table 25.1).

Table 25.1 Metabolic and organoprotective effects of antihypertensive drugs in patients with diabetes

Metabolic effects	Thiazides	Beta-blockers	Alpha-blockers	Calcium antagonists	ACE inhibitors	Angiotensin II antagonists
Glucose	↑	↑	N	N	N	N
Lipids	↑	↑	N	N	N	N
Insulin resistance	↑	↑	↓	N	↓	↓
Complications of diabetes						
Cardioprotection	+	+	N/–	+	+	+
Stroke protection	+	+	—	+	+/–	+
Nephroprotection	ND	+	ND	ND	+	+
Impotence	—	—	N	N	N	N

AT1 = angiotensin II antagonists; ↑ = deterioration; ↓ = improvement; + = protection; — = worsening; N = neutral; ND = no data available

Diuretics

Thiazide diuretics are effective in lowering BP in hypertensive type 1 and type 2 diabetic patients, with and without diabetic nephropathy[19]. Thiazides normalize total body sodium and water in these patients. Loop diuretics are frequently required to control sodium and fluid retention in patients with diabetic nephropathy. It has been suggested that thiazides may lead to deterioration of glycemic control of type 2 diabetic patients[20,21], but the degree of deterioration is dose-related. Several mechanisms contribute to thiazide-induced hyperglycemia: reduced insulin secretion (hypokalemia), insulin resistance and the accelerating effect on hepatic glucose production[22]. With the use of lower doses of thiazide diuretics, glycemic deterioration may be less of a problem[7]. Thiazides may aggravate dyslipidaemia in diabetic patients, although low dosages probably carry a small risk. A number of different diuretics can be used in diabetic hypertension, including hydrochlorothiazide, bendrofluazide, indapamide, furosemide, and spironolactone. If diuretics are not effective enough alone, they should be combined with another first-line drug, for example an ACE inhibitor or/an angiotensin II receptor antagonist, rather than increasing the dosage of diuretics. The combination of spironolactone and ACE inhibitor should be avoided, as this increases the risk of hyperkalemia.

Beta-adrenergic blockers

Beta-adrenergic blockers are among the most commonly used first-line drugs in diabetics with essential hypertension. They also have a beneficial effect on kidney function in incipient and overt diabetic nephropathy[23]. Beta-adrenergic blockers may impair recognition of hypoglycaemia in insulin-treated type 1 and type 2 diabetic patients, and may delay blood glucose recovery and pressure response to hypoglycaemia[24]. Consequently, patients lacking hypoglycemic warning symptoms should not be treated with beta-blockers. These adverse effects are less pronounced with the use of cardioselective beta-adrenergic blockers. The interaction between beta-adrenergic blockers and glycemic control in diabetes has been used as an argument against the use of beta-blockers in the antihypertensive treatment of diabetic patients[25]. Their hyperglycaemic effect is attributed to inhibition of $beta_2$-adrenergic-mediated insulin release, as well as decreased insulin action in peripheral tissues[26]. Observational studies reported a six-fold increased risk of developing diabetes associated with the use of beta-adrenergic blocking agents in nondiabetic persons, and a 15-fold increased risk if given together with thiazides[20]. However, the overall deterioration of glycemic control in overt diabetic patients is small, and most pronounced with non-selective beta-blockers[25].

ACE inhibitors

ACE inhibitors may be used in hypertensive diabetic patients, even when the general renin angiotensin–aldosterone system (RAS) is not activated. A potential explanation may be interference with local tissue-specific RAS. ACE inhibitors have no adverse metabolic effects, and may even improve insulin sensitivity[21,27]. Many studies have demonstrated that ACE inhibition diminishes albuminuria and reduces the rate of decline in glomerular filtration rate (GFR) in type 1 diabetic patients suffering from diabetic nephropathy[28,29]. Reduction in microalbuminuria during ACE inhibition has also been reported in normotensive type 1[30] and type 2 diabetic patients[31]. Their antiproteinuric effect may be specifically due to relaxation of the afferent arterioles in the glomerulus, resulting in a reduction of intraglomerular hypertension[32]. ACE inhibitors are also indicated in cardiac failure, in combination with relatively low dosages of diuretics. A dry cough is reported by about 10% of patients treated with ACE inhibitors, probably caused by interference with bradykinin-mediated mechanisms in the bronchial epithelium. ACE inhibitors can precipitate acute renal failure, particularly in elderly patients taking non-steroidal-anti-inflammatory agents, as well as in patients with bilateral renal artery stenosis.

Calcium antagonists

The effect of calcium-channel blockers (calcium antagonists; CCBs) on BP, glycemic control and plasma lipids has been evaluated in many studies[33]. CCBs decrease the elevated peripheral vascular resistance that is characteristic of diabetic patients with hypertension. They also induce a transient natriuresis, which may be apparent to the patient during initial therapy. They generally have no adverse affect on serum lipids or insulin sensitivity. There are two groups of CCBs: the dihydropyridines and the non-dihydropyridines. The non-dihydropyridines have been developed more recently, and have a longer elimination half-life. These drugs provide 24 h activity with a single daily dose and have fewer side effects. They not only lower BP, but have, in addition, antianginal, cardioprotective and anti-arrhythmic properties. There has been controversy recently over whether the use of short-acting CCBs might be associated with an increase in the risk of cardiovascular events[34]. In two recently published studies it has been claimed that CCBs are inferior to ACE inhibitors in reducing cardiovascular events in diabetic hypertensive patients[35,36]. However, both studies have some weaknesses that make the conclusions doubtful.

In the ABCD (Appropriate Blood Pressure Control in Diabetes) study, significantly more patients assigned to enalapril required additional therapy with diuretics and beta-blockers than those assigned to the CCBs[35]. Moreover, significantly more patients in the enalapril group discontinued the study because of uncontrolled BP. The FACET (Fosinopril versus Amlodipine Cardiovascular Events Randomised Trial) study[36] was small, uncontrolled, open labelled, and had been extensively criticized. More recently published studies [Hypertension Optimal Treatment (HOT), Systolic Hypertension in Europe (Syst-EUR)] indicate that long-acting CCBs are very effective in the prevention of cardiovascular morbidity/mortality in type 2 diabetic patients[37,38].

Angiotensin II receptor antagonists

The angiotensin II receptor antagonists (e.g. losartan, valsartan, candesartan, irbesartan) interfere with binding of angiotensin II to angiotensin type-1 receptors. Their efficacy in BP lowering is comparable with ACE inhibitors and other antihypertensive agents, and they have an excellent metabolic profile[39]. They are often useful in patients with ACE inhibitor-induced cough. Information about the use of these relatively new drugs in diabetic patients has recently been reviewed[39]. Three large intervention studies in type 2 diabetic patients with early or advanced diabetic nephropathy[40–42] have recently demonstrated important renal protective effects of the angiotensin II receptor antagonists. Recent data also suggest that angiotensin II-receptor blockers promote regression of left ventricular hypertrophy.

Alpha-1 specific blockers

Postsynaptic or peripheral alpha-sympathetic blockers have been used for the treatment of hypertension for more than two decades. Postsynaptic alpha-blockers have been well documented to exert a beneficial effect on the hypertensive metabolic syndrome, particularly with regard to reduction in insulin resistance. Among all hypertensive drugs, doxazosin has been reported to have the strongest effect on insulin resistance[43]. Positive effects on dyslipidaemia and improvement of decreased fibrinolytic activity were further arguments for

analysing the potential advantageous long-term effects of this drug in the Antihypertensive and Lipid-Lowering Treatment to Prevent Heart-Attack Trial (ALLHAT)-study[44].

ANTIHYPERTENSIVE INTERVENTION STUDIES IN DIABETIC PATIENTS

During recent years, 10 antihypertensive intervention studies[9,10,37,38,44–55] have been published that included representative numbers of diabetic patients. All these interventions studies illustrate that BP lowering is very important for improving the poor prognosis of diabetic patients. Disagreements in the outcome of different clinical trials can be explained by the heterogeneity of these studies, summarized in Table 25.2. The included patients showed a wide variation in initial BP values and lowering of BP. Most of the patients had long-standing diabetic disease, however, the exact duration of diabetes and/or hypertension was not reported in most of the studies. The follow-up of the hypertensive patients ranged from 2 to 8 years, and newly diagnosed patients were only enrolled in the UK Prospective Diabetes Study (UKPDS) trial. The

Table 25.2 Antihypertensive intervention studies obtained in patients with type 2 diabetes

Study	Number of patients	Follow-up (years)	Initial BP Systolic (mmHg)	Initial BP Diastolic (mmHg)	Lowering of systolic BP (mmHg)	Lowering of diastolic BP (mmHg)
UKPDS	1148	8.4	160	94	−6/ −16 (Δ10)	−7/ −12 (Δ5)
HOT	1501	3.8	169.8	105.4	−26/ −28/ −30 (Δ4)	−20/ −22.3/ −24.3 (Δ4)
CAPP	572	6.1	163.6	97.3	−13	−10
SYST-EUR	492	2.0	175.3	84.5	−13.5/ −22.1	−2.9/ −6.9
STOP-2	719	4.5	194	98	−34.5	−16/ −17
HOPE	3577	4.5	142	80	−3	−1
ALLHAT	42433	4.9	146	87	−12/ −11/−11	−8/ −9/−9
NORDIL	727	5.0	173.5	105.8	−20.3/ −23.3 (Δ3)	−18.7/ −18.7 (Δ0)
INSIGHT	1302	4.0	173.0	99.0	−12/ −14 (Δ2)	−7/ −8 (Δ1)
LIFE	1195	4.7	177	96	−29/ −31 (Δ2)	−17/ −17 (Δ0)

Table 25.3 Antihypertensive intervention studies in type 2 diabetic patients: comparison of different BP target values or different antihypertensive drugs		
	Comparison of diabetic patients with different BP target values	**Comparison of different antihypertensive drugs**
UKPDS	Yes	Yes
HOT	Yes	No
CAPP	No	Yes
SYST-EUR	Yes	No
STOP-2	No	Yes
NORDIL	No	Yes
INSIGHT	No	Yes
LIFE	No	Yes
ALLHAT	No	Yes

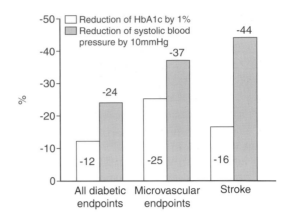

Figure 25.1 Reduction of endpoints in diabetic patients by lowering of HbA1c or blood pressure (UKPDS).

importance of different BP target levels on the outcome of type 2 diabetic patients has been evaluated in three trials; different drug treatment strategies were compared in six BP intervention studies (Table 25.3).

UKPDS hypertension study

In a sub-study of the UKPDS[46], 1148 newly detected type 2 diabetic patients with a mean BP of 160/94 mmHg were randomized to either 'tight BP control' ($n = 758$) or 'usual care' in BP control ($n = 390$). The mean difference in the achieved BP level of 10/5 mmHg between the two groups (144/82 versus 154/87 mmHg) resulted in a significant reduction in diabetes-related end points (–24%), diabetes-related death (–32%), stroke (–44%) and microvascular endpoints (–37%). Myocardial infarction and all-cause mortality, however, were not significantly reduced by BP-lowering in the UKPDS. The patients in the 'tight BP' arm were randomized to either treatment based on the ACE inhibitor captopril ($n = 400$) or the beta$_1$-selective blocker atenolol ($n = 358$).

The beneficial effects of tight BP control was shown irrespective of whether captopril or atenolol was the basis of antihypertensive treatment[47]. Interestingly, significantly more patients remained on captopril (80%) than atenolol (74%) at the end of the study. More patients needed additional antidiabetic drug treatment in the atenolol group (81%) compared with the captopril group (71%). The latter finding may be explained by the more pronounced weight gain over 9 years in the atenolol group compared with the captopril group (3.4 versus 1.6 kg), an effect well-known to decrease insulin sensitivity. Lowering of systolic BP by 10 mmHg induced a much higher effect on reduction of all diabetes-related endpoints, microvascular endpoints and strokes in comparison with lowering of glycosylated hemoglobin (HbA1c) by 1% (Figure 25.1). Remarkably, the risk reductions associated with the reduction of 10 mm reduction in BP was significantly higher in the clinical trial[46,47] compared with the observational analysis[50], indicating that the risk reductions via both ACE-inhibitor and beta-adrenergic blocker was mediated, at least in part, by additional effects of the two drugs, independent of BP lowering.

Systolic Hypertension in Elderly Program

The effect of low-dose diuretic-based antihypertensive treatment[45] on major CVD event rates was evaluated in older non-insulin-treated diabetic patients ($n = 583$) with isolated systolic hypertension (ISH) in comparison with nondiabetic patients in the Systolic Hypertension in Elderly Program (SHEP). Four thousand seven hundred and thirty-six patients with ISH (systolic BP ≥ 160 mmHg; diastolic BP ≤ 90 mmHg at baseline) received either a low dose of chlorthalidone (2.5–25.0 mm day^{-1}), with a step-up to atenolol (25.0–50.0 mg day^{-1}) or reserpine (0.05–0.10 mg day^{-1}) if needed. The 5-year major CVD rate was 34% lower for active treatment compared with placebo, both for diabetic patients and nondiabetic patients. Remarkably, the absolute risk reduction with active treatment compared with placebo was twice as great for diabetic versus nondiabetic patients (101/1000 versus 51/1000) patients at the 5-year follow-up, reflecting the higher risk of diabetic patients. The authors concluded that a low-dose diuretic-based (chlorthalidone) treatment is effective in preventing major CVD events, cerebral and cardiac, in both non-insulin treated diabetic and nondiabetic patients with ISH.

Hypertension Optimal Treatment

The HOT Study[37] included 1501 diabetic patients (total number: 18 790 patients) with hypertension who were randomly allocated to three different diastolic BP targets (< 90, < 85 and < 80 mmHg). The calcium antagonist felodipine was used as basic treatment. The group of diabetic patients ($n = 1501$) with hypertension, a mean systolic BP of 139.7 mmHg and a mean diastolic BP of 81.1 mmHg had a 51% reduction in major cardiovascular events and a 67% reduction in cardiovascular mortality (Figure 25.2) compared with the group with less tight control (143.7 mmHg, 85.2 mmHg), although the absolute difference in diastolic BP was only 4 mmHg. Remarkably, the enormous risk reduction was only seen in the diabetic, but not in the nondiabetic patients.

Systolic Hypertension in Europe

The Syst-Eur trial was initiated to study the effect of the CCB dihydropyridine nitrendipine on the outcome of cardiovascular mortality and morbidity in 4695 patients with systolic BP of 160–219 mmHg and diastolic BP < 95 mmHg. Very positive results were reported for the subgroup of older type 2 diabetic patients ($n = 492$) with systolic hypertension, randomized to treatment with either the CCB nitrendipine or placebo[38]. In the diabetic patients, active treatment

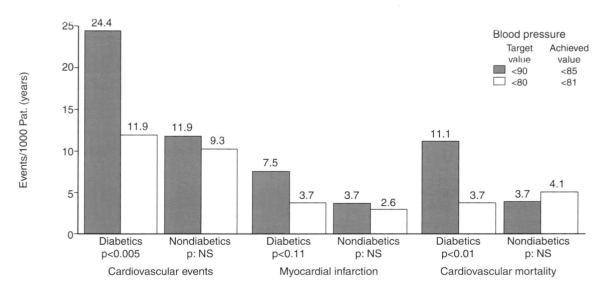

Figure 25.2 Significant risk reduction in diabetic patients (n=1501) with target value for diastolic blood pressure ≤ 80 mmHg.

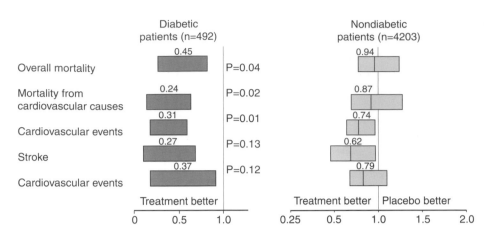

Figure 25.3 Adjusted relative hazards associated with active treatment as compared with placebo in diabetic and nondiabetic patients (SYST-EUR). Tuomiletho *et al.* *N Engl J Med* 1999;340:677–84.

reduced overall mortality by 55%, cardiovascular events by 76%, and strokes by 73%, compared with placebo, although the median follow-up was only 2 years. Active treatment with nitrendipine reduced the rate of all cardiovascular events by 69% in the diabetic patients, but by only 26% in the patients without diabetes (Figure 25.3).

CAPtopril Prevention Project

In the CAPtopril Prevention Project (CAPPP) Study[9], 10 985 patients (age 25–66 years) with diastolic BP > 100 mg Hg were allocated to receive either captopril or conventional treatment (thiazide diuretic and beta-receptor blocker). Over a follow-up period of about 6 years, there was a small increase in stroke in the captopril group, and a reduction of myocardial infarction (MI) and other cardiovascular death for the nondiabetic patients. In the diabetic subgroup ($n = 572$) there was a significant reduction in the cardiovascular disease (CVD) endpoints ($p = 0.002$) in the group receiving captopril. In the diabetic patients all fatal (–46%) and all cardiac events (–33%) were significantly lower in the patients treated with captopril compared with those on conventional treatment. However, the results for the group assigned to conventional therapy were not analysed separately for beta-blockers and diuretics, and it is

known that, at least in elderly hypertensive patients, diuretics are superior to beta-blockers. Moreover, patients assigned to captopril received diuretics if their BP did not reach the goal. Therefore, one cannot firmly conclude from the CAPPP study that ACE inhibitors are superior to either beta-blockers or diuretics in diabetic hypertensive patients. In contrast to the CAPPP trial, equivalence was found for ACE inhibitors, CCBs and conventional therapy in reducing morbidity and mortality in diabetic patients in the STOP-2 Study[54].

Heart Outcomes Prevention Evaluation

In the HOPE Study (Heart Outcomes Prevention Evaluation), which lasted 4.5 years, the role of ACE inhibition in patients at high risk of cardiovascular events was assessed[10]. A total of 9297 high-risk patients were randomly allocated to receive placebo or ACE inhibition therapy (Ramipril 10 mg per day). The diabetic patients ($n = 3577$)—with a mean age of 65 years and a mean duration of diabetes of 11.6 years at onset of the study—had at least one other cardiovascular risk factor, or a history of previous cardiovascular event (Micro-HOPE). Ramipril treatment was associated with risk reduction of MI (22%), stroke (33%), cardiovascular death (37%) and total mortality (24%) compared with placebo[51]. Combined microvascular endpoints (overt nephropathy, dialysis or laser therapy for retinopathy) were also significantly reduced (16%). For the interpretation of the Micro-Hope Study[51] two facts are important:

- Forty-four per cent of the included diabetic patients did not have hypertension
- Blood pressure levels of the hypertensive diabetic patients were relatively well-controlled by antihypertensive pretreatment.

The initial mean BP values of 141.9 mmHg systolic and 79.6 mmHg diastolic were only reduced by respectively 2.4 and 1.0 mmHg in the ramipril group. The benefit was seen irrespective of presence or lack of microalbuminuria, left ventricular dysfunction or presence or absence of hypertension.

Losartan Intervention For End Point Reduction in Hypertension Study

In the Losartan Intervention For End Point Reduction in Hypertension Study (LIFE) 9153 patients with essential hypertension and left ventricular hypertrophy (LVH) were randomly assigned to either once daily losartan-based or atenolol-based antihypertensive treatment for 4 years[52]. During the 4-year follow-up, the rate of new-onset diabetes was significantly lower (RR: 25%; $p < 0.001$) in the losartan-treated hypertensive nondiabetic patients (6%), compared with patients under atenolol (8%) therapy, confirming earlier studies with ACE-inhibitors (CAPPP, HOPE).

As a part of the LIFE-study, 1195 patients with diabetes, hypertension and LVH, with a mean age of 67 years and a mean BP of 177/96 mmHg, were randomly assigned to losartan-based or atenolol-based treatment[53]. Mean BP fell to 146/79 mmHg (17/11) in losartan patients and 148/69 mmHg (19/11) in atenolol patients. Diabetic patients treated with losartan showed a significant reduction of cardiovascular mortality (RR: 36.5%; $p = 0.028$) as well as total mortality (RR: 38.7%; $p = 0.002$) in comparison with patients treated with atenolol. In addition, myocardial infarction (RR: 17.1%) as well as stroke (RR: 21.2%) occurred also less often in the losartan-treated patients, however the difference with atenolol treatment did not reach levels of significance. Interestingly, losartan was significantly more effective than atenolol in reversing LVH ($p < 0.0001$), which is likely to result from more complete protection against angiotensin II with losartan, whether generated via the circulating renin–angiotensin system or other mechanisms, especially since angiotensin II is a myocardial growth factor and an independent risk factor for cardiovascular disease.

International Nifedipine GITS Study: Intervention as a Goal in Hypertension Treatment

In the INSIGHT (International Nifedipine GITS Study: Intervention as a Goal in Hypertension Treatment) study, the effects of the CCB nifedipine (30 mg in a long-acting gastro-intestinal transport system formulation) once daily on cardiovascular mortality and morbidity[48] was compared with the diuretic co-amilozide (hydrochlorothiazid 25 µg + amiloride 2.5 mg) in 6321 high risk patients (age: 45–80 years) with hypertension (BP $\geq 150/95$ mmHg or > 160 mmHg systolic). A comparable and significant fall of the mean BP from 173/99 mmHg to 138/82 mmHg was observed in both treatment groups. Nifedipine once daily and co-amilozide were equally effective in preventing overall cardiovascular or cerebrovascular complications. In the diabetes subgroup ($n = 1302$), primary endpoint rates were 8.3% in the nifedipine and 8.4% in the co-amilozide group. In the diabetic subgroup more patients needed an 'add on' treatment compared with the nondiabetics. In addition, more patients receiving enalapril than those receiving atenolol had diabetes (32% versus 19%). New diabetes occurred in 136 (4.3%) patients receiving nifedipine, and in 176 (5.6%) receiving co-amilozide ($p = 0.02$). The overall frequency was 14.1 cases per 1000 patients/years.

Nordil-Diltiazem study

In the Nordil-Diltiazem (Nordil) study, the effectiveness of diltiazem, a non-dihydropyridine calcium antagonist in reducing cardiovascular morbidity and mortality was compared with diuretics, beta-blockers or both in hypertensive patients[49]. Out of the 10181 enrolled patients, 727 had diabetes. All patients with diastolic BP ≥ 100 mmHg were randomly assigned to diltiazem, diuretics, beta-blockers or both. Fatal and non-fatal stroke occurred significantly less in the diltiazem compared with the diuretic and beta-blocker group (6.4 versus 7.9 events per 100 patients/years; RR:0.80; p = 0.04), whereas fatal and nonfatal myocardial infarctions did not significantly differ between the two groups. In the diabetic patients, no endpoint differed between the two treatment groups. The results of the Nordil Study are in agreement with those of the STOP Hypertension II Study[54], in which cardiovascular morbidity did not differ between the calcium antagonist regimen and the diuretic and beta-blocker regimen in patients with type 2 diabetes at baseline.

Swedish Trial in Old Patients with Hypertension-II

In the STOP Hypertension-II (Swedish Trial in Old Patients with Hypertension-II) Study[54], 6614 elderly patients aged 70–84 years were randomly assigned to one of three treatment strategies: conventional antihypertensive drugs (diuretics or beta-blockers), calcium antagonists, or ACE inhibitors. Of the patients, 719 had diabetes at the start of the study (mean age 75.8 years). Reduction in BP was similar in the three treatment groups of diabetic patients. The prevention of cardiovascular mortality was similar, and the frequency of this primary endpoint did not differ significantly between the three groups. There were, however, significantly fewer (p = 0.025) myocardial infarctions during ACE inhibitor treatment (n = 17) than during calcium antagonist treatment [n = 32; relative risk (RR) 0.51], but a (non-significant) trend to more stroke during ACE inhibitor treatment (n = 34 compared with n = 29; RR = 1.16). The researchers concluded that treatment of elderly hypertensive diabetic patients with conventional antihypertensive drugs (diuretics, beta-blockers, or both) seemed to be as effective as treatment with newer drugs, such as calcium antagonists or ACE inhibitors.

Antihypertensive and Lipid-Lowering Treatment to Prevent Heart Attack Trial (ALLHAT)

The ALLHAT study[44,55,56] compared 3 distinct antihypertensive drugs – amlodipine (representing calcium channel blockers), lisinopril (representing ACE inhibitors) and doxazosin (representing α-blockers) – with chlorthalidone (representing conventional thiazide diuretics). A total of 42 433 patients aged 55 years or older with hypertension and at least one other risk factor for coronary heart disease (CHD) were randomized to receive chlorthalidone 12.5–25 mg/day (n = 15 255), amlodipine 2.5–10 mg/day (n = 9048), or lisinopril 10–40 mg/day (n = 9054) or 2–8 mg/day doxazosin (n = 9076). Mean follow-up was 4.9 years. Mean age of patients was 67 years; 47% were women, 35% were black and 36% were diabetic; 90% of the patients were on antihypertensive treatment at entry.

Blood pressure (BP) control rates (< 140/90 mmHg) at study end were 68.2%, 66.3% and 61.2% for the chlorthalidone, amlodipine and lisinopril groups, respectively. Remarkably, systolic BP < 140 mmHg and diastolic BP < 90 mmHg were found in 67% and 92% of all patients, respectively[56]. Drugs added as needed to achieve target blood pressure included atenolol, reserpine and hydralazine. About 70% of patients required more than one drug for control of BP. Compared to chlorthalidone, systolic BP was higher in the amlodipine group (0.8 mmHg, p = 0.03) and in the lisinopril group (2 mmHg, p < 0.001), whereas diastolic BP was lower in the amlodipine group (0.8 mmHg, p < 0.001).

For the primary outcome (combined fatal CHD or non-fatal myocardial infarction) as well as for all-cause mortality there was no difference among the treatment groups[55]. For amlodipine, secondary outcomes were similar to chlorthalidone except for a higher rate of heart failure (10.2% vs 7.7%; RR 1.38). Lisinopril had a higher rate of combined cardiovascular disease (33.3% vs 30.9%; RR 1.10), stroke (6.3% vs 5.6%; RR 1.15;

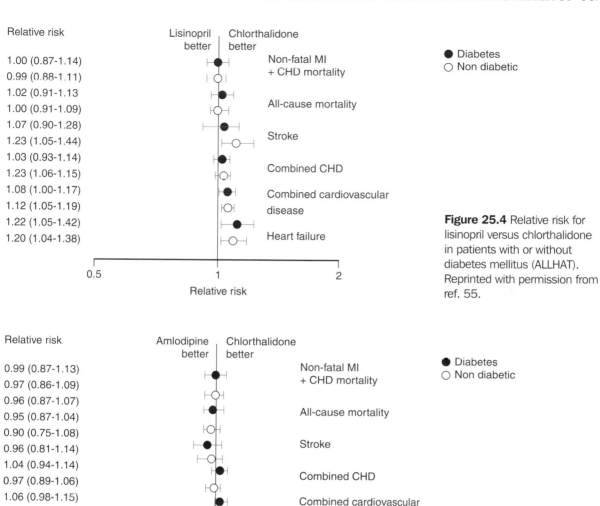

Figure 25.4 Relative risk for lisinopril versus chlorthalidone in patients with or without diabetes mellitus (ALLHAT). Reprinted with permission from ref. 55.

Figure 25.5 Relative risk for amlodipine versus chlorthalidone in patients with or without diabetes mellitus (ALLHAT). Reprinted with permission from ref. 55.

95%) and heart failure (8.7% vs 7.7%; RR 1.19). The primary and secondary outcome results for the amlodipine vs chlorthalidone group comparisons were consistent for all subgroups, including the large subgroup of diabetic patients (Figure 25.4). For the lisinopril vs chlorthalidone comparisons, results were generally consistent. Thus, for the important diabetic population lisinopril appeared to have no specific advantage (and amlodipine no particular detrimental

effect) for most cardiovascular disease outcomes when compared with chlorthalidone (Figure 25.5).

The doxazosin vs chlorthalidone arm had already been stopped in year 2000[44], due to superiority of chlorthalidone in some endpoints, especially chronic heart failure (CHF). CHF risk was doubled (4-year rates, 8.13% vs 4.45%; RR 2.04; p < 0.001). Total mortality did not differ, but the doxazosin arm had a higher risk of stroke (RR 1.19; p = 0.04), and combined CVD (4-year rates, 25.5% vs 21.18%; RR 1.25; p < 0.001) compared with chlorthalidone.

Previous hypertension morbidity/mortality trials using thiazide diuretics or beta-blockers as initial therapy showed a clear reduction in cardiovascular morbidity and mortality rates in nondiabetic as well as in type 2 diabetic patients[45,46]. Their failure to completely reverse the risk of hypertension was thought to be the result of their negative "metabolic effects", such as hyperglycemia, increased cholesterol levels, and hypokalemia. After 4 years' treatment[55] a significantly higher number of the initially non-diabetic patients (p < 0.001) developed a new diabetes (blood glucose > 126 mg dL^{-1}) in the chlorthalidone (11.6%) vs lisinopril (8.1%) arm. In addition, cholesterol levels > 240 mg dL^{-1} and potassium levels < 3.5 m^2 L^{-1} were significantly more often found in the chlorthalidone group, but these metabolic differences did not translate into more CHD events or all-cause mortality compared with the two other groups.

The ALLHAT study did not include young patients, but the equivalence or superiority of diuretics was seen across the entire spectrum of ages represented, in diabetics and in black patients. No data in the study results should discourage clinicians from using ACE inhibitors or calcium antagonists, especially in combination with a diuretic.

The ALLHAT study clearly demonstrates that newer drugs are not necessarily better than older drugs[57]. The results indicate that antihypertensive regimens for almost all patients should begin with a diuretic, unless there is a specific contraindication. For patients currently on regimens that exclude a diuretic, a diuretic may be added or substituted. For example, a diabetic hypertensive on an ACE inhibitor should continue with the drug, but may benefit from the addition of a low-dose diuretic.

PROTECTION OF DIABETIC NEPHROPATHY BY ANTIHYPERTENSIVE THERAPY

A cumulative incidence of diabetic nephropathy of 25–40% has been documented after duration of diabetes of at least 25 years in both type 1 and type 2 diabetic patients[2,4]. Diabetic nephropathy has become the leading cause (25–45%) of end-stage renal disease (ESRD) worldwide. Until the early 1980s, death occurred on average 5–7 years after the onset of persistent proteinuria. The two main treatment strategies for primary prevention of diabetic nephropathy are improved glycemic control and BP lowering, particularly using drugs such as ACE inhibitors. Megatrials and meta-analyses have clearly demonstrated the beneficial effect of both treatment modalities.

Antihypertensive treatment of patients with overt diabetic nephropathy induces a reduction in albuminuria and in the glomerular filtration rate (GFR), it delays development of ESRD and improves survival of patients. These benefits have been demonstrated with a variety of BP lowering agents, including beta-blockers, CCBs, diuretics and ACE inhibitors. A meta-analysis[58] of 100 controlled and uncontrolled trials assessed the relative efficacy of different antihypertensive agents on proteinuria and renal function in patients with diabetes.

Treatment with ACE inhibitors, CCBs and beta-blockers had a similar effect on mean arterial pressure. The greatest reductions in urinary albumin excretion rate (UAER) occurred in diabetic patients treated with ACE inhibitors. ACE inhibitors and CCBs appeared to have a more favorable effect on GFR compared with other antihypertensive agents. Limited information is available on the long-term superiority of ACE inhibitors in comparison with other antihypertensive drugs in the progression of nephropathy.

Lewis and co-workers[29] compared captopril with placebo over 3 years in 409 type 1 diabetic patients with mild renal insufficiency due to diabetic nephropathy (proteinuria > 500 mg 24 h^{-1}, serum creatinine level < 2.5 mg dL^{-1}). Captopril treatment nearly halved the rate of increased serum creatinine levels, and of those requiring dialysis or transplantation, or who died. The difference in the median diastolic BP during the study was < 4 mmHg.

Unfortunately, no long-term study has been published concerning the effects of ACE inhibitors on the progression of diabetic nephropathy in patients with type 2 diabetes. A review[59] of six studies of patients with type 2 diabetes followed for at least 1 year compared the use of ACE inhibitors with non-ACE inhibitors on the GFR. A decline in GFR (typically 10 mL mean^{-1} years^{-1}) was reduced by lowering BP in all but one study. When ACE inhibitors were compared with thiazide diuretics, beta-blockers and CCBs, there was no significant differences in the rate of decline of GFR between the different classes of agents.

RENAL PROTECTION BY ANGIOTENSIN II RECEPTOR BLOCKERS

In the CALM (Candesartan and Lisinopril and Microalbuminuria) study[60], the effects of candesartan or lisinopril on both BP and urinary albumin excretion were studied in patients with microalbuminuria, hypertension and type 2 diabetes. A prospective, randomized double-blind study design was used, whereby 12 weeks monotherapy with candesartan or lisinopril were followed by 12 weeks monotherapy or combination treatment. The authors concluded

that candesartan 16 mg once daily is as effective as lisinopril 20 mg once daily in reducing BP and microalbuminuria in hypertensive patients with type 2 diabetes. Dual blockade of the renin–angiotensin system by ACE inhibitors and angiotensin-receptor blockers is more effective in reducing BP and, to some extent, albuminuria.

The theory that the dual blockade of the RAS I is more effective than single therapy with either ACE or AT1-blockers has recently been supported by Rossing *et al.*[61]. These authors have added either candesartan or placebo to 18 type 2 diabetic patients with diabetic nephropathy resistant to conventional antihypertensive combination therapy, including ACE-inhibitors, diuretics and beta-blockers. Addition of candesartan to usual antihypertensive treatment induced a mean reduction in albuminuria of 25%, a reduction in 24 h systolic BP of 10 mmHg (138 versus 148 mmHg) and a mean reduction in GFR of 5 mL min^{-1}.

Three large long-term intervention studies[40–42] in type 2 diabetic patients with early or advanced diabetic nephropathy (Table 25.4)

Table 25.4 Comparison of major endpoints in the IDNT and RENAAL trials

	RRR (%)			
	RENAAL	**IDNT**		
	Losartan vs control	Irbesartan vs control	Irbesartan vs amlodipine	Amlodipine vs control
Doubling of Creat, ESRD, or death	**16 (P=0.02)**	**20 (P=0.02)**	**23 (P=0.006)**	**–4 (P=0.69)**
Doubling of Creat	25 (P=0.006)	33 (P=0.003)	37 (P<0.001)	–6 (P=0.60)
ESRD	28 (P=0.002)	23 (P=0.07)	23 (P=0.07)	0 (P=0.99)
Death	–2 (P=0.88)	8 (P=0.57)	–4 (P=0.8)	12 (P=0.4)
CV Morbidity & Mortality	10 (P=0.26)	9 (P=0.4)	–3 (P=0.79)	12 (P=0.29)

Lewis EJ et al. *N Engl J Med* 2001;345:851–860.
Brenner B et al. *N Engl J Med* 2001;345:861–869.

have been performed recently with two different angiotensin II receptor-blocker agents (irbesartan and losartan). In IDNT (Irbesartan Diabetic Nephropathy Trial), 1715 patients with hypertension and type 2 diabetic nephropathy were randomized to daily treatment with 300 mg irbesartan, 10 mg amlodipine, or placebo in a prospective double masked trial[40]. BP control was to the same target, < 135/85 mmHg, in all groups. Primary endpoint was a composite of time of doubling of entry serum creatinine, development of ESRD or all cause mortality. Treatment with irbesartan was associated with a 20% risk reduction of the primary composite endpoint events when compared with placebo ($p = 0.024$) and a 23% risk reduction versus amlodipine ($p = 0.006$). There was a 33% RR with respect to doubling of serum creatinine, favoring irbesartan when compared with placebo ($p = 0.003$), and a 37% reduction versus amlodipine ($p = 0.001$). A 23% risk reduction of ESRD for irbesartan relative to both placebo ($p = 0.074$) and to amlodipine ($p = 0.074$) was observed (Table 25.4). Serum creatinine for the entire cohort rose 24% more slowly ($p = 0.008$) in patients assigned to irbesartan than those assigned to placebo, and 21% more slowly than with amlodipine ($p = 0.02$). Proteinuria was significantly reduced in the irbesartan group throughout the study, and not in the amlodipine or placebo groups. Remarkably, there was no significant differences in the risk of all cause mortality, or in the cardiovascular composite endpoint. The investigators concluded, that

- The angiotensin II receptor blocker irbesartan is an effective protective agent against the progression of type 2 diabetic nephropathy
- This reno-protection is independent of BP reduction.

In the IRMA-II (Irbesartan Microalbuminuria Type 2) trial[41], the effect of 300 mg of irbesartan once daily was studied in 590 type 2 diabetic patients with hypertension and microalbuminuria (early stage diabetic nephropathy). Treatment with irbesartan resulted in a 70% relative RR ($p = 0.0004$) for progression from early to a late and more serious stage of kidney disease (Table 25.4) compared with patients who did not receive the angiotensin II receptor antagonist[41].

In the RENAAL (Reduction of Endpoints in Non-Insulin Dependent Diabetes mellitus with the Angiotensin II Antagonist Losartan) Study[42], the potential renal protective effect of losartan (50–100 mg day[-1]) was studied in comparison with placebo in 1513 hypertensive type 2 diabetic patients with proteinuria. In both treatment groups, conventional antihypertensive drugs like calcium antagonists, diuretics, beta-adrenergic blockers and alpha$_1$ specific blockers were used. Other angiotensin-II receptor antagonists and ACE inhibitors were excluded from the study. In comparison with the control group, treatment with losartan[42], reduced the risk (Table 25.4) for progression to ESRD by 28% ($p = 0.002$) and the risk for doubling of serum creatinine by 25% ($p = 0.006$). By contrast, the death risk did not significantly differ between the two groups (21.0 versus 20.3%).

CHOICE OF ANTIHYPERTENSIVE DRUG THERAPY

In type 1 diabetic patients presenting with hypertension the use of ACE-inhibitors is recommended as first-line treatment, since diabetic nephropathy is the underlying cause in most of the cases. The choice of first-line treatment in type 2 diabetic patients is more difficult, since data for the initial treatment of hypertension in newly diagnosed patients are only available for captopril and atenolol (UKPDS study). In the early trials of antihypertensive therapy thiazide diuretics and beta-blocking agents were commonly used. The increased risk of deterioration of metabolic factors, like glycemic control and hypertriglyzeridaemia, associated with relatively high dosages, were thought to be disadvantages for diabetic patients. New evidence has demonstrated that low-dose thiazides (SHEP, STOP 2), beta-blockers (UKPDS, STOP 2), calcium antagonists (HOT, Syst-EUR), ACE inhibitors (UKPDS, CAPPP, HOPE, STOP 2) as well as angiotensin II receptor antagonists (LIFE) are safe and effective with respect to cardiovascular outcome in

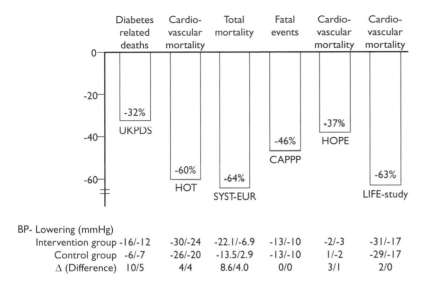

Figure 25.6 Effects of blood pressure lowering on cardiovascular events in diabetic patients.

BP- Lowering (mmHg)	Diabetes related deaths	Cardio-vascular mortality	Total mortality	Fatal events	Cardio-vascular mortality	Cardio-vascular mortality
Intervention group	-16/-12	-30/-24	-22.1/-6.9	-13/-10	-2/-3	-31/-17
Control group	-6/-7	-26/-20	-13.5/2.9	-13/-10	1/-2	-29/-17
Δ (Difference)	10/5	4/4	8.6/4.0	0/0	3/1	2/0

diabetic patients, as has been demonstrated in various studies (Figure 25.6).

The impressive and consistent data on renal and cardiovascular protection afforded by ACE inhibitors resulted in many experts recommending the use of this group of drugs as the preferred first-line therapy in diabetic patients. Since excellent protective effects for cardiovascular morbidity and mortality were also demonstrated for calcium antagonists in the HOT and SYST-EUR trials[37,38] and for beta-blockers in the UKPDS[46,47,50], the preferred use of ACE inhibitors has been questioned and criticized[58]. The choice of a specific antihypertensive class for the treatment of hypertension in diabetic patients is probably of minor relevance, since the majority of diabetic patients with hypertension require at least two antihypertensive drugs to achieve tight BP targets. To achieve a BP of < 130/85 mmHg, > 60% of patients will require combination therapy. In the HOT study, 76% of the patients assigned to the lowest target diastolic BP of ≤ 80 mmHg required combination therapy[37].

In the UKPDS[46], 62% of those who were assigned to intensive BP control required combination therapy at a similar BP level. In the INSIGHT study[62] patients with diabetes

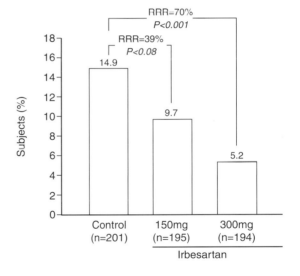

Figure 25.7 Development of overt proteinuria in the IRMA 2 trial. Parving H-H et al. N Engl J Med 2001;345:870–8.

were the most resistant to antihypertensive treatment, requiring second and third drugs 40% and 100% more frequently than nondiabetic patients. Despite the higher use of combination therapy, the diabetic patients achieved the highest final BP for any risk group.

Combination therapy may also be more beneficial than monotherapy in reducing the risk of cardiovascular events. Consequently, anti-hypertensive combination therapy for type 2 diabetic patients is increasingly becoming standard practice.

REFERENCES

1 Bild D, Teutsch SM. The control of hypertension in persons with diabetes: a public health approach. *Publ Health Rep* 1987;102:522–9.

2 Andersen AR, Christiansen JS, Andersen JK *et al.* Diabetic nephropathy in type 1 (insulin-dependent) diabetes: an epidemiological study. *Diabetologia* 1983;25:496–501.

3 Viberti GC, Keen H, Wiseman MJ. Raised arterial pressure in parents of proteinuric insulin-dependent diabetics. *Br Med J* 1987;295:575–7.

4 Ritz E, Orth SR. Nephropathy in patients with type 2 diabetes mellitus. *N Engl J Med* 1999;341:1127–33.

5 Reaven GM, Lithell H, Landsberg L. Hypertension and associated metabolic abnormalities. The role of insulin resistance and the sympathoadrenal system. *N Engl J Med* 1996;334:374–81.

6 DeFronzo RA, Ferrannini E. Insulin resistance—a multifaceted syndrome responsible for NIDDM, obesity, hypertension, dyslipidemia and atherosclerotic disease. *Diabetes Care* 1991;14:173–94.

7 The Hypertension Diabetes Study Group. Hypertension in Diabetes Study (HDS). 1. Prevalence of hypertension in newly presenting type 2 diabetic patients and the association with risk factors for cardiovascular and diabetic complications. *J Hypertens* 1993;11:309–17.

8 Gress TW, Nieto FJ, Shahar E *et al.* Hypertension and antihypertensive therapy as risk factors for type 2 diabetes mellitus. *N Engl J Med* 2000;342: 905–12.

9 Hansson L, Lindholm LH, Niskanen L *et al.* Effect of angiotensin-converting-enzyme inhibition compared with conventional therapy on cardiovascular morbidity and mortality in hypertension: the Captopril Prevention Project (CAPPP) randomised trial. *Lancet* 1999;353: 611–16.

10 Yusuf S, Sleight P, Pogue J, Bosch J, Davies R, Dagenais G. Effects of an angiotensin-converting-enzyme inhibitor, ramipril, on cardiovascular events in high-risk patients. The Heart Outcomes Prevention Evaluation Study Investigators. *N Engl J Med* 2000;342:145–53.

11 Poulsen PL, Beck T, Ebbehoi E *et al.* Ambulatory blood pressure in the transition from normo- to microalbuminuria. A longitudinal study in IDDM patients. *Diabetes* 1994;43:1248–53.

12 Equiluz-Bruck S, Schnack C, Kopp HP, Schernthaner G. Nondipping of nocturnal blood pressure is related to urinary albumin excretion rate in patients with type-2 diabetes mellitus. *Am J Hypertens* 1996;9:1139–43.

13 Chen JW, Jen SL, Lee WL *et al.* Differential glucose tolerance in dipper and nondipper essential hypertension. *Diabetes Care* 1998;21:1743–8.

14 Poulsen PL, Beck T, Ebbehoi E *et al.* 24h ambulatory blood pressure and retinopathy in normo-albuminuric IDDM patients. *Diabetologia* 1998;41:105–10.

15 Nakano S, Fukuda M, Hotta F *et al.* Reversed circadian blood pressure rhythm is associated with occurrences of both fatal and nonfatal vascular evennts in NIDDM subjects. *Diabetes* 1998;47:1501–6.

16 Schernthaner G, Ritz E, Philipp T, Bretzel R. Night time blood pressure in diabetic patients—the submerged portion of the iceberg? *Nephrol Dial Transplant* 1999;14:1061–4.

17 Joint National Committee in Prevention, Detection, Evaluation, and Treatment of Blood Pressure (JNC VI). The Sixth Report of the Joint National Committee on Prevention, Detection, Evaluation, and Treatment of High Blood Pressure. *Arch Intern Med* 1997;157:2414–46.

18 The National High Blood Pressure Education Program Working Group. National high blood pressure education program working group report on hypertension in diabetes. *Hypertension* 1994;23:145–58.

19 Weidmann P, Beretta-Piccoli C, Keusch G *et al.* Sodium-volume factor, cardiovascular reactivity and hypotensive mechanism of diuretic therapy in mild hypertension associated with diabetes mellitus. *Am J Med* 1979;67:779–84.

20 Bengtsson C, Blohmé G, Lapidus L *et al.* Do anti-hypertensive drugs precipitate diabetes? *Br Med J* 1984;289:1495–7.

21 Hunter SJ, Wiggam JI, Ennis CN *et al.* Comparison of effects of captopril used either alone or in combination with a thiazide diuretic on insulin action in hypertensive type 2 diabetic patients: a double-blind crossover study. *Diabet Med* 1999;16:482–7.

22 Klauser R, Prager R, Gaube S *et al.* Metabolic effects of isradipine versus hydrochlorothiazide in diabetes mellitus. *Hypertension* 1991;17:15–21.

23 Parving H-H, Andersen AR, Smidt UM et al. Effect of antihypertensive treatment on kidney function in diabetic nephropathy. *Br Med J* 1987;294:1443–7.

24 Lager I, Blohme G, Smith U. Effect of cardioselective and non selective beta-blockade on the hypoglycaemic response in insulin-dependent diabetics. *Lancet* 1979;i:458–62.

25 Ostman J. Beta-adrenergic blockade and diabetes mellitus. A review. *Acta Med Scand* 1983;672:69–77.

26 Pollare T, Lithell H, Selinus I, Berne C. Sensitivity to insulin during treatment with atenolol and metoprolol: a randomized, double blind study of effects on carbohydrate and lipoprotein metabolism in hypertensive patients. *BMJ* 1989;198:1152–7.

27 Pollare T, Lithell H, Berne C. A comparison of the effects of hydrochlothiazide and captopril on glucose and lipid metabolism in patients with hypertension. *N Engl J Med* 1989;321:868–73.

28 Hommel E, Parving H-H, Mathiesen ER et al. Effect of captopril on kidney function in insulin-dependent diabetic patients with nephropathy. *Br Med J* 1986;293:467–70.

29 Lewis EJ, Hunsickler LG, Bain RP et al. The effect of angiotensin-converting-enzyme inhibition on diabetic nephropathy. *N Engl J Med* 1993;329:1456–62.

30 Marre M, Leblanc H, Suarez L et al. Converting enzyme inhibition and kidney function in normotensive diabetic patients with persistent microalbuminuria. *Br Med J* 1987;294:1448–52.

31 Ravid M, Savin H, Jutrin I et al. Efficacy of captopril in normotensive diabetic patients with microalbuminuria: 8 years follow up [abstract]. *Diabetologia* 1995;38 Suppl.1:A46.

32 Hostetter Th, Tennke HG, Brenner BM. The case for intrarenal hypertension in the initiation and progression of diabetic and other glomerulopathies. *Am J Med* 1982;72:375–80.

33 Chellingsworth MC, Kendall MJ, Wright AD et al. The effects of verapamil, diltiazem, nifedipine and propranolol on metabolic control in hypertensives with non-insulin-dependent diabetes mellitus. *J Hum Hypertens* 1989;3:35–9.

34 Grossmann E, Messerle FH. Calcium antagonists in cardiovascular disease: a necessary controversy but an unnecessary panic. *Am J Med* 1997;102:147–9.

35 Estacio RQ, Jeffers BW, Hiatt WR et al. The effect of nisoldipine as compared with enalapril on cardiovascular outcomes in patients with non-insulin-dependent diabetes and hypertension. *N Engl J Med* 1998;338:645–52.

36 Tatti P, Pahor M, Byington RB et al. Outcome results of the Fosinopril Versus Amlodipine Cardiovascular Events randomized trial (FACET) in patients with hypertension and NIDDM. *Diabetes Care* 1998;21:597–603.

37 Hansson L, Zanchetti A, Carruthers SG et al. for the HOT Study Group. Effects of intensive blood-pressure lowering and low-dose aspirin in patients with hypertension: Principal results of the hypertension optimal treatment (HOT) randomised trial. *Lancet* 1998;351:1755–62.

38 Tuomilehto J, Rastenyte D, Birkenhager WH et al. Systolic Hypertension in Europe Trial Investigators. Effects of calcium-channel blockade in older patients with diabetes and systolic hypertension. *N Engl J Med* 1999;340:677–84.

39 Schnack CH, Schernthaner G. Angiotensin-II Typ-I Rezeptor-Antagonisten und Diabetes mellitus. *Wiener Med Wochenschr* 2001;151:165–8.

40 Lewis EJ, Hunsicker LG, Clarke WR et al. for the Collaborative Study Group: Renoprotective effect of the angiotensin-receptor antagonist Irbesartan in patients with nephropathy due to type 2 diabetes. *N Engl J Med* 2001;345:851–60.

41 Parving H-H, Lehnert H, Bröchner-Mortensen J et al. for the Irbesartan in Patients with Type 2 Diabetes and Microalbuminuria Study Group. The effect of Irbesartan on the development of diabetic nephropathy in patients with type 2 diabetes. *N Engl J Med* 2001;345:870–8.

42 Brenner BM, Cooper ME, De Zeeuw D et al. for the RENAAL Study Investigators. *N Engl J Med* 2001;345:861–9.

43 Giordano M, Matsuda M, Sanders L et al. Effects of angiotensin-converting enzyme inhibitors, Ca^{2+} channel antagonists, and alpha-adrenergic blockers on glucose and lipid metabolism in NIDDM patients with hypertension. *Diabetes* 1995;44:665–71.

44 The Antihypertensive and Lipid-Lowering Treatment to Prevent Heart Attack Trial (ALLHAT): Major cardio-vascular events in hypertensive patients randomized to Doxazosin versus Chlorthalidone. *J Am Med Assoc* 2000;283:1967–75.

45 Curb JD, Pressel SL, Cutler JA et al. Systolic Hypertension in the Elderly Program Cooperative Research Group. Effect of diuretic-based antihypertensive treatment on cardiovascular disease risk in older diabetic patients with isolated systolic hypertension. *J Am Med Assoc* 1996;276:1886–92.

46 UK Prospective Diabetes Study (UKPDS) Group. Tight blood pressure control and risk of macrovascular and microvascular complication in type-2 diabetes: UKPDS 38. *BMJ* 1998;317:703–13.

47 UK Prospective Diabetes Study (UKPDS) Group: Efficacy of atenolol and captopril in reducing risk of macrovascular and microvascular complications in type-2 diabetes: UKPDS 39. *BMJ* 1998; 317:713–20.

48 Brown MJ, Palmer CR, Castaigne A *et al.* Morbidity and mortality in patients randomised to double-blind treatment with a long-acting calcium-channel blocker or diuretic in the International Nifedipine GITS study: Intervention as a goal in hypertension treatment (INSIGHT). *Lancet* 2000;356:366–72.

49 Hansson L, Hedner T, Lund-Johansen P *et al.* Randomised trial of effects of calcium antagonists compared with diuretics and β-blockers on cardiovascular morbidity and mortality. *Lancet* 2000;356:359–65.

50 Adler AI, Stratton M, Neil HAW *et al.* on behalf of the UK Prospective. Association of systolic blood pressure with macrovascular complications of type-2 diabetes (UKPDS 36): prospective observational study. *BMJ* 2000;321:412–19.

51 Heart Outcomes Prevention Evaluation (HOPE) Study Investigators. Effects of ramipril on cardiovascular and microvascular outcomes in people with diabetes mellitus: results of the HOPE study and MICRO-HOPE substudy. *Lancet* 2000;355:253–9.

52 Dahlöf B, Devereux RB, Kjeldsen SE *et al.* Cardiovascular morbidity and mortality in the Losartan Intervention for endpoint reduction in hypertension study (LIFE): a randomised trial against atenolol. *Lancet* 2002;359:995–1003.

53 Lindholm LH, Ibsen H, Dahlöf B *et al.* Cardiovascular morbidity and mortality in patients with diabetes in the Losartan Intervention for endpoint reduction in hypertension study (LIFE): a randomised trial against atenolol. *Lancet* 2002;359:1004–10.

54 Lindholm LH, Hansson L, Ekbom T *et al.* Comparison of antihypertensive treatments in preventing cardiovascular events in elderly diabetic patients: results from the Swedish Trial in Old Patients with Hypertension-2. *J Hypertens* 2000;18:1671–5.

55 The Antihypertensive and Lipid-Lowering Treatment to Prevent Heart Attack Trial (ALLHAT). Major outcomes in high-risk hypertensive patients randomized to angiotensin-converting enzyme inhibitor or calcium channel blocker vs diuretic. *JAMA* 2002;288:2981–97.

56 Cushman WC, Ford CE, Cutler JA *et al.* Success and predictors of blood pressure control in diverse North American settings: the Antihypertensive and Lipid-Lowering Treatment to Prevent Heart Attack Trial (ALLHAT). *J Clin Hypertens (Greenwich)* 2002;4:393–405.

57 Appel LJ. The verdict from ALLHAT – thiazide diuretics are the preferred initial therapy for hypertension. *JAMA* 2002;288:3039–42.

58 Grossmann E, Messerli FH, Goldbourt U. High blood pressure and diabetes mellitus. Are all antihypertensive drugs created equal? *Arch Intern Med* 2000;160:2447–52.

59 Baba T, Neugebauer S, Watanabe T. Diabetic nephropathy. Its relationship to hypertension and means of pharmacological intervention. *Drugs* 1997;54:197–234.

60 Mogensen CE, Neldam S, Tikkanen I *et al.* for the CALM study group. Randomised control trial of dual blockade of renin-angiotensin system in patients with hypertension, microalbuminuria, and non-insulin dependent diabetes: the candesartan and lisinopril microalbuminuria (CALM) study. *BMJ* 2000;321:1440–44.

61 Rossing K, Christensen PK, Jensen BR, Parving HH. Dual blockade of the rennin–angiotensin system in diabetic nephropathy: a randomized double-blind crossover study. *Diabetes Care* 2002;25:95–100.

62 Brown MJ, Castaigne A, De Leeuw PW *et al.* Influence of diabetes and type of hypertension on the response to antihypertensive treatment. *Hypertension* 2000;35:1038–42.

26

Cardiac and peripheral vascular disease evaluation

Ruchira Glaser and Susan E Wiegers

THE IMPACT OF CORONARY ARTERY DISEASE ON THE DIABETIC POPULATION

Cardiovascular disease (CVD) is a leading cause of death in the diabetic population, accounting for close to 80% of the mortality in diabetic patients in North America[1,2]. Patients with diabetes mellitus have a significantly higher risk for and a higher mortality from coronary artery disease (CAD). The diabetic patient has a two- to four-fold increase in the risk for development of CAD[3–6].

Diabetic patients are not only over-represented among those patients with myocardial infarction (MI), but also have a worse prognosis than non-diabetic patients[7–9]. Several large studies, including the Thrombolysis and Angioplasty in Myocardial Infarction (TAMI) trial, have shown that, even in the thrombolytic era, in-hospital mortality rates in diabetic patients remain 1.5–2 times higher than in nondiabetic patients[2,10–15].

In the Finnish Monitoring International Cardiovascular Disease (FINMONICA) trial, the 1-year case fatality rate for a first MI, including prehospital mortality, was 45% in diabetic men and 39% in diabetic women in the population studied. These case fatality rates were significantly higher than those of nondiabetic subjects (38% and 25% for men and women, respectively)[7]. In addition, many studies have demonstrated that, among survivors of MI, diabetic patients have higher late-mortality rates than do nondiabetic patients[9,16–22].

It has recently also been suggested that diabetic patients without a history of MI have as high a risk of MI as do nondiabetic patients with previous MI. In a Finnish population cohort study, the 7-year incidence of MI, both fatal and nonfatal, among over 1000 nondiabetic patients without prior history of MI was 3.5%. In those nondiabetic patients with a prior history of MI, the incidence was 18.8%. This incidence was comparable to that of diabetic patients without any prior history of MI (20%)[23]. Data such as these underscore the need for screening asymptomatic diabetic patients in a manner similar to that for nondiabetic patients with previous infarction.

UNIQUE CHARACTERISTICS OF CAD IN THE DIABETIC POPULATION

Several features distinguish CAD in the diabetic population from the nondiabetic population. Factors such as premature presentation, greater extent of disease, coagulation abnormalities, and autonomic dysfunction may contribute to the higher morbidity and mortality of coronary heart disease in the diabetic patient (Table 26.1).

Premature presentation

Diabetic patients often present with premature CAD. In type 1 diabetes patients, the duration of diabetes is the most important predictor of premature CAD, and CAD may present as early

Table 26.1 Unique characteristics of cardiovascular disease in the diabetic patient

Premature presentation
Extensive disease upon initial presentation
    Multiple coronary arteries diseased
    Distal coronary artery disease
    Small vessel disease
    Impaired autoregulation in vessels
Increased risk of developing heart failure
Acceleration of coronary thrombosis
Autonomic dysfunction
    Impaired vagal activity and increased
    sympathetic tone
      – Increased risk for ischemic events
      – Increased risk for sudden cardiac death
    Impaired pain response to ischemia
      – Atypical symptoms of ischemia
      – Absence of symptoms of ischemia

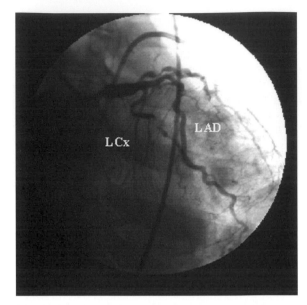

(a)

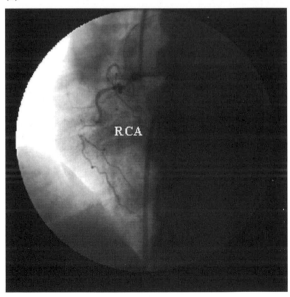

(b)

Figure 26.1 Coronary angiogram of a patient with type 2 diabetes. The left main coronary artery has mild stenosis distally. The left circumflex artery is occluded proximally. The first diagonal branch of the left coronary artery is diffusely and severely diseased, with multiple severe proximal lesions. The right coronary artery is subtotally occluded proximally. Note both the presence of severe obstructive proximal coronary artery disease, as well as the multiple vessels involved and the diffuse distal extent of disease.

as the 3rd or 4th decade of life. These patients often lack other traditional CAD risk factors, such as hypercholesterolemia, hypertension, tobacco use, and family history of premature CAD. In contrast, type 2 diabetes patients typically have several cardiovascular risk factors and present in the 5th or 6th decade of life, or later[24].

Extent of disease

The diabetic patient often has more extensive CAD at the time of diagnosis as well. Multi-vessel CAD is common. Pathological and angiographic evidence indicate that the coronary arteries are more diffusely and distally diseased in diabetic patients[2,24-28]. Recognition of the propensity for severe CAD in patients presenting with MI is especially important because the presence of multivessel coronary disease predicts short-term mortality in patients with acute MI[29,30]. Multivessel disease also contributes significantly to the increased rates of recurrent ischemic episodes and infarction seen in diabetic patients. This is true for severe (> 70% obstruction) and less severe lesions. Plaque disruption leading to infarction most often occurs in vessels with mild to moderate stenoses[31,32]. Thus, recurrent ischemic events are often also the result of the increased number of vessels with mild to moderate disease found in diabetic patients (Figure 26.1).

In addition to a greater extent of epicardial CAD, there may be generalized endothelial dysfunction and abnormalities of small vessels in the diabetic patient. Dilatation of the coronary arteries in response to hypoxia is mainly dependent upon endothelium-relaxing factor[2,33]. Impaired endothelium-dependent relaxation is present in the vascular beds, including coronary arteries, of diabetic patients[34-36]. The autoregulatory responses in the microcirculation also appear to be impaired[2].

Increased risk for the development of congestive heart failure

Diabetic patients, especially women, are at increased risk for developing congestive heart failure[24]. This increase in congestive heart failure causes much of the excess in-hospital mortality of diabetic patients with acute MI[2,10,16,37-45]. The higher incidence of heart failure post-MI in the diabetic patient has been attributed to a higher degree of diffuse atherosclerotic disease. Inadequate tissue perfusion to the noninfarcted myocardium leads not only to greater underlying global systolic dysfunction, but also to the inability of the noninfarcted myocardium to adequately compensate for the dysfunction of the acutely infarcted region[2,24]. In the TAMI trials, ventricular function assessed in the catheterization laboratory by left ventriculography was worse in noninfarcted areas in diabetic patients, compared with nondiabetic patients[46]. There is still controversy about the existence of a specific 'diabetic cardiomyopathy', due to factors other than ischemia, which leads to systolic dysfunction.

Diastolic function is also impaired in diabetic patients in the absence of significant CAD, and is likely an important contributor to worse patient outcomes[24]. On initial presentation with congestive symptoms, diabetic patients often have diminished left ventricular compliance and normal systolic function when compared with nondiabetic patients[2,47-53]. The higher incidence of coexistent hypertension in diabetic patients may account for a large part of the diastolic dysfunction observed, although even patients without hypertension have manifested diastolic impairment[2]. Left ventricular hypertrophy is present in 28% of non-hypertensive type 2 diabetic patients, compared with < 10% of matched patients without diabetes[54].

Coagulation abnormalities

An increase in luminal thrombus formation may contribute to acute coronary syndromes in the diabetic patient. Coagulation abnormalities associated with diabetes include increased platelet aggregation, increased levels of fibrinogen, and increased levels of plasminogen activator inhibitor (PAI-1). Increased platelet aggregation may be related to hyperglycemia, while elevated levels of PAI-1 may be related to the hypertriglyceridemia and hyperlipidemia often seen in diabetes[24].

These coagulation disturbances may also decrease the efficacy of thrombolytic therapy in the treatment of ST-segment elevation MI. The TAMI trials failed to show a difference in angiographic patency rates in diabetic compared with nondiabetic patients[46]. However, noninvasive measures of reperfusion have suggested that reperfusion is achieved less frequently in diabetic patients. In addition, diabetic patients have benefited from aggressive platelet inhibition from platelet glycoprotein IIb/IIIa antagonists in recent trials of acute coronary syndromes and percutaneous coronary intervention[55,56]. Thus, there is evidence that the coagulation disturbances seen in diabetic patients may impair the efficacy of therapy for acute coronary syndromes, including unstable angina and MI.

Autonomic dysfunction

The autonomic innervation of the heart may be affected in diabetic patients. Diminished heart-rate variability and elevation in resting heart-rate are often present in early autonomic neuropathy in diabetic patients[2,24]. Increased sympathetic activity, or decreased vagal activity may contribute to sudden cardiac death. In addition, increased sympathetic activity may facilitate ischemic events.

Autonomic neuropathy may also impair the pain response to ischemia in diabetic patients. This can complicate the detection of CAD, since the diabetic patient may be asymptomatic, or manifest atypical symptoms, such as dyspnea, increased fatigue, or indigestion[24].

INCIDENCE OF ASYMPTOMATIC CAD IN THE DIABETIC PATIENT

It is not surprising that the incidence of asymptomatic coronary disease in the diabetic population is significant. The Milan Study on Atherosclerosis and Diabetes (MiSAD) group found that 12% of the 925 asymptomatic patients with type 2 diabetes had ST depression consistent with ischemia during treadmill stress testing. Approximately half of these patients additionally had nuclear scans consistent with CAD[57,58] (see below). Additional smaller studies have reported asymptomatic CAD by coronary angiography in approximately 8–12% of diabetic patients. However, these studies also demonstrated a fairly low positive predictive value of noninvasive stress testing in the diabetic population, raising concern about the utility of general noninvasive screening of the asymptomatic diabetic population[57,59,60].

BENEFITS OF EARLY DETECTION OF CAD

The benefits of early detection of CAD in the diabetic population include implementation of medical therapy targeted at prevention of further morbidity and mortality from CAD, identification of patients who would gain survival benefits from revascularization, and modification of lifestyle and other factors that may impact on disease progression.

IMPLEMENTATION OF MEDICAL THERAPY

Modification of other cardiovascular risk factors

Modification of cardiovascular risk factors beside diabetes may reduce morbidity and mortality from future events. Perhaps the most striking example is the recent demonstration of mortality reduction in lipid-lowering trials. In the Scandinavian Simvastatin Survival Study, 2200 patients with CAD receiving simvastatin were compared with patients receiving placebo. Lowering cholesterol was associated with a 42% reduction in cardiovascular mortality and a 30% reduction in overall mortality. In the 5% of patients in the trial with diabetes, simvastatin treatment was associated with a 55% reduction in major coronary events[24,61]. In the Cholesterol and Recurrent Events (CARE) trial, in which diabetic patients comprised approximately 14% of the study population, there was a 25% reduction in coronary heart disease events[62]. Based on secondary prevention trials such as these, the present National Cholesterol Education Program guidelines distinguish lipid-lowering therapy goals based upon the presence of coronary disease in the general population[63]. Prospective studies of lipid-lowering specifically in the diabetic population, including primary prevention trials, are presently underway[64].

In addition to patients with hypertension with proteinuria, angiotensin-converting enzyme (ACE) inhibitor therapy is indicated in diabetic patients with CAD and left ventricular dysfunction[24]. Thus, the demonstration of CAD or left ventricular systolic dysfunction may impact upon the ideal antihypertensive regimen in diabetic patients.

Implementation of anti-ischemic therapy

The presence of asymptomatic coronary disease may also prompt more aggressive anti-ischemic therapy. Agents such as ACE inhibitors, beta-blockers and aspirin may reduce adverse cardiovascular outcomes in patients with CAD and diabetes.

Recent evidence suggests further benefit of ACE inhibitor therapy in diabetic patients. The Heart Outcomes Prevention Evaluation (HOPE) study examined over 9000 patients over the age of 55 who had evidence of vascular disease or diabetes plus one other cardiovascular risk factor. Of the study population, 38% had diabetes. Treatment with the ACE inhibitor ramipril reduced the composite endpoint of MI, stroke or death from cardiovascular causes at mean follow-up of 5 years by 22% compared with placebo. In addition, the rates of cardiovascular death and MI were reduced by 26% and 20%, respectively. In a subgroup analysis, the incidence of other complications related to diabetes, such as diabetic nephropathy (defined as urinary albumin excretion of at least 300 mg per day or urinary protein excretion of 500 mg per day), the need for renal dialysis, and the need for laser therapy for diabetic retinopathy, was also significantly decreased in those diabetic patients receiving ramipril[65].

Beta-blocker therapy effectively reduces reinfarction and sudden death in diabetic patients post MI[2,66–69]. In the Bezafibrate Infarction Prevention Study, Type 2 diabetes patients treated with beta-blocker therapy had close to a 50% reduction in mortality compared with those patients not receiving beta-blocker therapy[24,70]. Thus, knowledge of prior silent MI may impact upon the decision to use beta-blocker therapy in the diabetic patient.

Aspirin therapy for secondary prevention of CAD in diabetics and nondiabetics is also beneficial. In a meta-analysis of 145 prospective studies of the use of aspirin compared with placebo, diabetics and nondiabetics had similar reductions in MI, stroke, transient ischemic attacks, or signs of CAD[71]. In addition to secondary prevention for large vessel disease, the American Diabetes Association has recommended consideration of aspirin therapy for primary prevention in high-risk men and women[24,72]. The early detection of coronary disease in diabetic patients may therefore significantly influence medication use targeted at both modification of cardiovascular risk factors and prevention of further ischemic events.

Referral for revascularization

The Bypass Angioplasty Revascularization Investigation (BARI) trial showed improved 5-year survival in symptomatic diabetic patients with multivessel CAD who underwent coronary artery bypass grafting (CABG) compared with medical management[73]. The outcome in patients who underwent surgical revascularization was superior to that of diabetic patients who had multivessel percutaneous transluminal coronary angioplasty (PTCA)[73,74]. The 8-year follow up analysis of the Emory Angioplasty versus Surgery Trial (EAST) had similar findings[75]. In addition, a recent subgroup analysis of the diabetic population in the Arterial Revascularization Therapy Study confirmed that those patients who underwent multivessel coronary stenting had lower event-free survival rates at 1 year compared with those patients receiving CABG[76]. Thus, identification of severe multivessel coronary disease is paramount, because surgical revascularization may significantly improve a diabetic patient's mortality and event-free survival.

The Asymptomatic Cardiac Ischemia Pilot (ACIP) study addressed broader indications for surgical revascularization in asymptomatic CAD. In each treatment strategy, 13–19% of patients had diabetes. Five hundred and fifty-eight patients with ischemia during stress testing and ambulatory ECG monitoring, and who had coronary anatomy suitable for revascularization, were randomized to angina-guided drug therapy, angina plus ischemia guided drug therapy, or revascularization by angioplasty or bypass surgery. Two years after randomization, the total mortality was 6.6% in the angina-guided group, compared with 4.4% in the ischemia-guided group, and 1.1% in the revascularization group[77]. Although further data are needed to confirm whether more liberal indications for revascularization are warranted, these pilot data further support a role for revascularization of asymptomatic patients.

Lifestyle and other risk modification

Finally, there may be some benefit in more aggressive nutrition control and exercise in diabetic patients with CVD. Although they may already be counseled on proper nutrition and exercise, the added concern about known coronary heart disease may further motivate these patients.

While microvascular complications are reduced with strict glycemic control in type I diabetic patients, the high-dose exogenous insulin and insulin resistance syndromes (IRS) characteristic of type 2 diabetes may have differential effects on the macrovasculature. There are no well-controlled studies demonstrating reduced CVD in patients with improved glucose control. However, the Diabetes Mellitus Insulin-Glucose Infusion Acute Myocardial Infarction (DIGAMI) study found that hospital use of insulin glucose infusion, followed by 3 months of intensive insulin therapy in patients with acute MI, reduced cardiovascular mortality by 29% at 1 year in type 2 diabetic patients. Planned prospective trials in diabetic patients with coronary disease should further define the utility of improved glycemic control in reducing disease progression[78].

TARGET SUBGROUPS FOR SCREENING

One of the challenges facing the clinician caring for the diabetic patient is the determination of if, and when, testing for CAD is warranted (Table 26.2). Given the high incidence and impact of CVD in diabetic patients, it is clear that patients with symptoms, either typical or atypical, should undergo a noninvasive evaluation. It should be emphasized, however, that patients presenting with symptoms consistent with unstable angina should be referred urgently to cardiology care for a potential invasive evaluation. In addition, previously sedentary diabetic patients who are now initiating an exercise program should undergo a noninvasive evaluation, in order to identify those patients at high risk of an acute ischemic event while beginning the new exercise regimen.

Diabetic patients undergoing procedures with high cardiovascular risk benefit from preoperative evaluation for ischemia (Table 26.3). Those patients with reduced functional capacity undergoing intermediate risk procedures should undergo preoperative stress testing[79]. Those patients undergoing renal transplantation especially benefit from perioperative stress testing, because of the high likelihood of concomitant coronary atherosclerosis. In fact, the American Diabetes Association recommends that all patients with type 2 diabetes, and those with type 1 diabetes over the age of 35, with either

Table 26.2 Indications for noninvasive screening for coronary artery disease in the diabetic patient

Symptomatic

1 Presence of typical or atypical symptoms of stable angina

Asymptomatic

2 Age > 35 years and initiation of a new exercise program in a previously sedentary lifestyle

3 Preoperative evaluation prior to high or intermediate risk surgery in a patient with decreased functional capacity

4 Evidence of myocardial infarction or ischemia on baseline electrocardiogram

5 The presence of 2 or more of the following concomitant risk factors:[a]

    a Total cholesterol > 240 mg dL^{-1}, LDL cholesterol > 160 mg dL^{-1}, or HDL cholesterol < 35 mg dL^{-1}

    b Blood pressure > 140/90 mmHg

    c Smoking

    d Family history of premature coronary artery disease

    e Positive micro/macroalbuminuria test

[a]According to American Diabetes Association guidelines.

persistent microalbuminuria or overt nephropathy undergo cardiac testing[24]. However, the indications for testing are less clear in patients who do not complain of symptoms, and are not about to undergo surgery or changes in exertion.

In their guidelines regarding exercise testing, the American College of Cardiology (ACC) has stated that, in asymptomatic people without known CAD, there is no Class I indication for routine stress testing. However, the ACC notes that, given data from trials such as the ACIP study and the Coronary Artery Surgery Study, a subgroup of asymptomatic patients with multiple risk factors may benefit from stress testing[80]. In contrast, the American Diabetes Association

Table 26.3 Cardiac risk[a] stratification for noncardiac surgical procedures

High (Reported cardiac risk often > 5%)

Emergent major operations, particularly in the elderly

Aortic and other major vascular

Peripheral vascular

Anticipated prolonged surgical procedures associated with large fluid shifts and/or blood loss

Intermediate (Reported cardiac risk generally < 5%)

Carotid endarterectomy

Head and neck

Intraperitoneal and intrathoracic

Orthopedic

Prostate

Low[b] (Reported cardiac risk generally < 1%)

Endoscopic procedures

Superficial procedure

Cataract

Breast

[a]Combined incidence of cardiac death and nonfatal MI.

[b]Do not generally require further preoperative cardiac testing.

Reprinted with permission from Eagle et al.[79].

has recommended that those asymptomatic diabetic patients with two or more of the following risk factors be tested:

- Total cholesterol $\geq$ 240 mg dL^{-1}
- LDL cholesterol $\geq$ 160 mg dL^{-1} or HDL cholesterol < 35 mg dL^{-1}
- Blood pressure > 140/90 mmHg
- Smoking
- Family history of premature CAD
- Positive micro/macroalbuminuria test.

In addition, they recommend stress testing for patients with resting electrocardiograph suggesting ischemia or infarction, or patients with evidence of peripheral or carotid arterial occlusive disease. It has been reported that most diabetic patients with lower-extremity occlusive arterial disease die from CVD[24].

METHODS OF DETECTION OF CAD

Several modalities may be used for detection of CAD once the decision to screen a patient has been made. Stress testing, either exercise or pharmacologic, and either with or without perfusion imaging techniques, ambulatory electrocardiography, and electron beam computed tomography (EBCT) may be used.

Stress testing

The choice of initial stress test modality should be based on several factors, including the resting electrocardiogram, ability of the patient to exercise, and local expertise and availability. In general, patients should exercise when able. Knowledge of the patient's exercise capacity provides an independent assessment of prognosis. The results of a patient's stress test should be interpreted in light of the exercise capacity. Measures of exercise capacity include maximal exercise duration, maximal metabolic equivalent (MET) level achieved, maximum workload achieved, and maximum heart rate and heart rate–blood pressure product[80].

Exercise electrocardiography, the least expensive noninvasive test for myocardial ischemia, is two times less expensive than stress echocardiography and five times less expensive than stress single-photon-emission computed tomography (SPECT). Drugs such as digoxin may cause false positive results in the exercise electrocardiogram[81]. Data pooled from 132 studies show that the sensitivity and specificity of routine exercise electrocardiography are 68% and 77%, respectively[82,83]. However, there is wide variability in studies, depending upon the diagnostic criteria used, and the patient population. For example, women have increased false positive rates on routine treadmill testing compared with men. Inability to achieve 85% of maximum predicted heart rate may influence the results of the test.

Negative inotropic medications, such as beta-blockers and calcium-channel blockers may decrease the sensitivity of the test, resulting in false negative tests.

When patients have preexcitation (Wolff–Parkinson–White), ventricular paced rhythm, significant ST-segment depressions, and left bundle branch block on the baseline electrocardiogram, they require additional nuclear imaging or echocardiography to detect ischemia. The American Diabetes Association additionally recommends that those diabetic patients with typical anginal symptoms or resting q waves on electrocardiogram undergo a stress perfusion study. In either case, the exercise portion of the test remains a valuable component.

If patients are unable to exercise because of other limitations, such as arthritis, amputations, other orthopaedic problems, symptomatic peripheral vascular disease, or severe pulmonary disease, they should undergo pharmacologic testing with nuclear imaging or echocardiography. Dobutamine is a positive ionotropic agent that provokes ischemia by increasing myocardial work and thus oxygen demand. Adenosine and dipyridamole are vasodilators that cause relative increases in flow in non-diseased coronary arteries compared with arteries with significant stenoses.

SPECT has a higher sensitivity for the detection of CAD than does exercise electrocardiography alone[81]. However, estimates of the perfusion imaging performance, in terms of sensitivity and specificity, are highly variable. The sensitivity of stress echocardiography is likely in the same range or slightly lower than that of radionuclide perfusion imaging[81]. This technique's success is also highly dependent upon the experience of the operator and center. Special technique considerations may be needed in women, obese patients, or patients with emphysema; they may require attenuation correction during SPECT to accommodate artifactual defects from diaphragmatic or breast and tissue attenuation. Similarly, the potentially limited echocardiographic image quality in obese patients, or patients with severe pulmonary disease, may preclude the use of stress echocardiography in certain patients.

As previously discussed, some small studies suggest decreased positive predictive value of the routine exercise test, as well as nuclear imaging testing, in the diabetic population[57,59,60]. Again, the data on patients with diabetes specifically within these modalities are not well-established, and require further specific investigation in larger series of patients. It is for these reasons that, in its guidelines, the American College of Cardiology presently recommends that, in most cases, initial screening of the asymptomatic patient be done with routine exercise electrocardiography, if possible[80]. The American Diabetes Association does make the distinction that, in certain high risk diabetic patients, as already outlined, perfusion imaging or stress echocardiography is warranted as the initial screening test[24].

Ambulatory electrocardiogram

The data on ambulatory electrocardiogram are at present insufficient to justify the routine use of this modality to detect CAD in the asymptomatic diabetic patient[24]. In the ACIP trial, those patients with diabetes had less demonstrable ischemia on ambulatory electrocardiography than nondiabetic patients. This was despite more extensive CAD in that population[84].

Electron beam computed tomography

Coronary artery calcification has been correlated with coronary artery atherosclerosis, but also increases with age. Proponents have advocated this method to detect 'subclinical' disease in asymptomatic patients. However, data at this point are insufficient to justify the use of EBCT as a general screening modality.

MANAGEMENT OF A POSITIVE SCREENING TEST

The outcome of an indeterminate, submaximal stress test in the diabetic patient should prompt repetition of the test with pharmacologic stress and perfusion imaging. Many diabetic patients may not experience typical chest pain during exercise, for the reasons previously discussed.

Pre-test risk	ETT results			
	Normal	Mildly positive	Moderately positive	Markedly positive
High 4-5 risk factors**	√√	√√√	√√√√	√√√√
Moderate 2-3 risk factors	√	√√√	√√√	√√√√
Low 0-1 risk factors	√	√√√	√√√	√√√√

√ Routine follow-up
√√ Close follow-up
√√√ Imaging
√√√√ Cardiology referral/possible catheterization

Figure 26.2 Appropriate follow-up after screening exercise treadmill test (ETT). After initial exercise stress testing of asymptomatic diabetic patients, the type of follow-up depends on the pretest risk and the degree of abnormality on the stress test. Normal follow-up indicates annual reevaluation of symptoms and signs of CHD and electrocardiogram (ECG). A repeat ETT should be considered in 3–5 years if clinical status is unchanged. Close follow-up means shorter intervals between evaluation and follow-up ETT, i.e., 1–2 years. Pretest risk is assigned based on the presence of other vascular disease and risk factors. Reprinted, with permission, from: *Diabetes Care*, 1998;21:1551–9.

Autonomic dysfunction may affect their ability to achieve an adequate heart rate as well (Figure 26.2).

On the other hand, a negative exercise electrocardiographic test at a high workload provides reassurance that the likelihood of advanced CAD is extremely low. It is important to interpret the findings of stress testing in light of the clinical pre-test probability of disease, as well as the extent of disease found on testing. The maximal value of stress testing is in those patients with an intermediate pre-test suspicion for disease.

A positive exercise electrocardiographic test should prompt either repetition with perfusion imaging or direct cardiac catheterization if the patient has high-risk clinical features, such as hypotension, bradycardia, ventricular dysrhythmias or pulmonary edema, on the initial test.

Patients should also be referred directly for cardiac catheterization if ischemia is induced by low-level exercise (< 4 METs or heart rate < 100 beats per min or < 70% age predicted) and manifested by one or more of the following:

- Horizontal or downsloping ST depression > 0.1 mV
- ST-segment elevation > 0.1 mV in a noninfarct lead
- Five or more abnormal leads
- Persistent ischemic response > 3 min after exertion
- Typical angina[79].

If there are moderate or large perfusion defects on imaging, or defects representative of multiple vascular territories, there should be referral for cardiac catheterization in almost all circumstances. The identification of left main coronary disease, proximal left anterior descending artery disease, and multivessel disease is especially important, given the proven added benefits of revascularization in diabetic patients with severe anatomy[25,73]. Conversely, in a patient with low suspicion for disease and relatively small, distal perfusion defects suggestive of distal CAD, it is often reasonable to medically manage the patient with close follow-up.

PERIPHERAL VASCULAR DISEASE

Peripheral vascular disease (PVD) is a common clinical feature that impacts significantly on prognosis and healthcare costs in the diabetic patient. Diabetic patients comprise a significant proportion of those patients hospitalized with PVD. In the UK, of all admissions for PVD during the 4-year period 1991–1995, 15.4% of patients were diabetic. This represents an age-standardized relative risk (RR) of admission of 7.6 and 6.9 for diabetic men and women, respectively, when compared with nondiabetic patients. Furthermore, the RR of hospital mortality was 2.8 compared with nondiabetics, and the RR of surgery was 31.1 compared with nondiabetics. Eighty-seven per cent of the cost of hospitalization was attributable to the diabetic state[85].

Among diabetic patients, peripheral vascular disease is common. In a study by Kreins *et al.*, at 13 year follow-up, the actuarially determined cumulative risks for intermittent claudication, nonpalpable dorsalis pedis pulse, and arterial calcification were, respectively, 37.9%, 34.5%, and 60.9% for men and 24.3%, 37.6%, and 32.2% for women[86]. Other studies of diabetic patients have reported prevalence rates of peripheral vascular disease as high as 22%[87].

Features of PVD in diabetic patients

Diabetic patients with PVD have several distinct features when compared with nondiabetic patients. A greater proportion of diabetic patients with PVD have concomitant hypertension[88]. In addition, diabetic patients have more distal disease[88,89]. Diabetic patients with PVD have more progressive and severe disease, and are more likely to undergo surgery and amputation[85,88,89]. Rates of gangrene or amputation of lower limbs as much as 10–20 times more frequent in diabetic than in control subjects have been reported[90,91], and among diabetic patients, the risk of amputation increases with age. The annual amputation rates in patients < 45 was 14 per 10 000, versus 45 per 10 000 in diabetics aged 45–64, versus 101 per 10 000 in those > 65. Not surprisingly, duration of diabetes has been found to be a strong risk factor for amputation[91].

The risks of fatal and non-fatal MI and stroke are also increased in both diabetic and nondiabetic PVD subjects[85,88,92,93]. Cirqui *et al.*, found vascular mortality five times higher in patients with claudication over a period of 10 years. Another group reported an annual rate of fatal and non-fatal cardiovascular events in the range 3.5–8% per year[94,95]. One study found that 67% of diabetic patients dying from cardiovascular causes within the 5-year observation had PVD at baseline, compared with 15% of those who survived[96]. Diabetic patients with claudication are therefore at high risk of future stroke, MI and premature death.

Evaluation in the primary care setting

All diabetic patients should be screened for PVD by including components targeted toward detection of signs and symptoms in the routine history and physical exam. In a workshop examining PVD in diabetes, the American Diabetes Association and American Heart Association made the following joint recommendations for annual screening[97]:

- The history should include questions about the presence and degree of claudication or ischemic rest pain.
- The physical exam should include inspection of the legs and feet for ulcers and skin changes.
- The tibialis posterior and the dorsalis pedis pulses should be examined and the femoral pulse auscultated for bruits.

Claudication

Diabetic patients should be asked annually about the presence of exercise-induced calf leg pain. Although the most common site for exercise-induced pain is the calf, it can also develop in the thigh, hip, or buttock when the disease is localized above the inguinal ligament. Often the pain will start in the calf and then progress to the thigh and/or buttock if exercise is continued despite the onset of pain. The Rose intermittent claudication questionnaire, allowed for standardization of many of these features of claudication. Severe claudication most often results from multilevel arterial disease, which can be evaluated in the noninvasive laboratory. Patients with lifestyle-limiting exercise-induced calf pain should be referred for specialist vascular assessment. Measurement of an ankle brachial index (ABI), or referral for specialist vascular assessment should also be considered for patients with any leg pain not clearly ascribed to a nonvascular cause.

Signs of critical ischemia

Critical ischemia is defined as clinical presentation that, if not reversed, is likely to result in an amputation either at the level of the foot or below the knee. Ischemic rest pain occurs in the toes and forefoot, and will, during its early phases, be relieved by dependency. If it does not improve with development of collateral circulation, amputation will be necessary unless some form of intervention, either surgical or endovascular, is performed. When a break in the skin occurs at any location in the foot or lower leg, healing of the ulceration may not occur unless some form of intervention is carried out. The single exception may be for a patient who has an ulcer over a pressure-point or at a site of direct injury that is secondary to neuropathy. However, ischemia and neuropathy may coexist, making patients in this subset candidates for amputation unless the occlusion is either bypassed or eliminated by transluminal angioplasty. Tissue death, when it involves one or more toes or the forefoot, will require amputation that may be limited to the involved areas if direct intervention can bring more blood to the ischemic area. Although not as definitive as ischemic rest pain, ulceration and gangrene, skin atrophy, nail changes, and dependent rubor in some patients may require further evaluation. This is particularly true if the ABI is found to be abnormal.

Palpation of peripheral pulses

Palpation of leg pulses should be performed on an annual basis for all adult patients with diabetes. An absent or decreased tibialis posterior pulse is an indication for performing an ABI. Since the sensitivity and positive predictive value are moderate for detection, a significant number of cases will be identified by detection of a reduction or absence of these pulses. Furthermore, the presence of these pulses in low-risk diabetic subjects helps to confirm the absence of significant disease. It should be remembered that the dorsalis pedis pulse is congenitally absent in up to 12% of normal subjects[98].

Femoral bruits

The detection of femoral bruits is an indication for performing an ABI. Although auscultation for femoral bruits has similar difficulties to those described for pulse palpation, it nonetheless has sufficient sensitivity to merit annual performance.

Screening methods

The clinical exam and Rose questionnaire are useful, although unfortunately fairly insensitive

tools for the diagnosis of lower extremity vascular disease[99]. Ancillary modalities include the ABI, toe systolic blood pressure, ultrasound duplex scanning, tissue PO_2 measurement, and arteriography.

Ankle brachial index

The ABI is a ratio of Doppler recorded systolic arterial blood pressures in the lower and upper extremities[98]. ABI measurement is recommended for the following situations:

- Any diabetic patient newly detected to have decreased pulses, femoral bruits, or a foot ulcer
- Any diabetic patient with leg pain of unknown etiology
- All patients with insulin-dependent diabetes mellitus aged ≥ 35 years, or with 20 or more years' duration of diabetes, undergoing baseline examination
- All patients with non-insulin-dependent diabetes mellitus aged ≥ 40 years undergoing baseline examination.

The potential for medial wall calcification to raise systolic ankle pressure above the normal range, even in the presence of occlusive disease, means that the ABI alone may not be sufficient to detect vascular insufficiency, and thus further testing may be indicated. This medial calcinosis is more common in the diabetic patient[100].

The results of ABI measurements help to guide further management. An ABI < 0.50 in any vessel should prompt expeditious referral for specialist vascular assessment, since these patients almost certainly have severe PVD. An ABI of 0.50–0.90 warrants a follow-up evaluation within 3 months, because these patients are likely to have mild to moderate PVD. If the subsequent ABI is < 0.90, intensive risk factor modification and annual ABI follow-up is recommended. If the repeat ABI is > 0.90, further follow-up ABI may be performed every 2 or 3 years. Similarly, if an initial ABI is > 0.90, repeat testing need only be done every 2 to 3 years since these patients are unlikely to have PVD.

Any incompressible ankle artery (systolic ankle pressure > 300 mmHg) or ankle pressure 275 mmHg above arm pressure, should prompt follow-up measurements within 3 months. If confirmed, these patients should be referred for specialist vascular assessment because they almost certainly have significant medial wall calcification, and measurement of ankle pressure to determine lower extremity disease is therefore compromised. These patients are also at high risk for both macrovascular and microvascular complications, and should be entered into an intensive risk-factor modification program[97].

Toe systolic blood pressure

The toe systolic blood pressure (TSBP) overcomes the false elevation of ankle pressures from calcification and has a similar repeatability to the ABI. TSBP also enables pressure to be assessed in patients with leg ulcers, where the use of an ankle cuff is not possible[97].

Ultrasonic duplex scanning

Although the technology is evolving, ultrasound duplex scanning plays an increasingly important role in vascular testing. It can provide information about the exact location of arterial disease, though it cannot be used as an index of severity.

Tissue PO$_2$

The likelihood of healing of ischemic skin lesions may be assessed by the measurement of tissue PO$_2$. It is generally believed that values < 20 mmHg indicate questionable capacity for healing and those < 10 mmHg are not compatible with healing. The PO$_2$, is also a sensitive indicator of improvement in blood flow resulting from either collateral flow development or surgical treatment. It may also be used to determine the level of amputation when this becomes necessary.

Arteriography

Though invasive, arteriography remains the definitive diagnostic procedure prior to any form of surgical intervention. It should not be used as a diagnostic procedure to establish the presence of arterial disease.

Therapy after positive screening

Intensive risk factor modification

As previously discussed, all patients with a confirmed ABI of < 0.90, and/or ankle systolic pressure > 300 mmHg, and/or ankle blood pressure 275 mmHg above arm pressure and/or exercise-induced calf pain not present at rest, should be carefully screened for cardiovascular risk factors. The American Diabetes Association recommends that patients with diabetes who have PVD be treated as if they had coronary heart disease for the purposes of cholesterol-lowering therapies[101,102]. Blood pressure should also be carefully monitored and managed. In a study of 4801 white, Asian Indian, and African–Caribbean UK diabetes patients, each 10 mm Hg decrease in updated mean systolic blood pressure was associated with reductions in risk of 12% for any complication related to diabetes, 15% for deaths related to diabetes, 11% for MI, and 13% for microvascular complications[103]. In the same patient population, each 1% reduction in updated mean glycosylated hemoglobin (HbA1c) was associated with reductions in risk of 21% for any endpoint related to diabetes, 21% for deaths related to diabetes, 14% for MI, and 37% for microvascular complications[104]. Cessation of smoking is also of paramount importance as well.

Aspirin

As previously discussed, data from secondary prevention trials in nondiabetic subjects indicate that aspirin has a protective effect on subsequent cardiovascular mortality and morbidity[71]. However, the only prospective study so far reported that evaluates the efficacy of 5 years of aspirin treatment in diabetic patients with PVD is the Veterans Administration Cooperative Study, which assessed the efficacy of aspirin (650 mg day^{-1}) and dipyridamole in preventing the progression of cardiovascular and PVD in 231 diabetic men with limb gangrene or recent amputation for ischemia. There were no differences in major endpoints, such as atherosclerotic vascular death (22% versus 19%, respectively, in treated and control subjects), or amputation of the opposite extremity (20%

versus 24% in treatment and control subjects)[105]. A large secondary prevention trial of aspirin and/or other antiplatelet drugs in diabetic subjects with PVD is therefore needed[106].

Other pharmacologic therapy

Pentoxifylline, a hemorrheologic agent, is approved for the symptomatic treatment of intermittent claudication. It is reported to improve the microcirculation and tissue perfusion, although not all investigators agree that it provides symptomatic relief[100,107,108].

Percutaneous and surgical therapy

Percutaneous revascularization has significantly improved the prospects for patients with peripheral arterial disease. It does carry increased complications of angiography in diabetic patients, many of whom have concomitant renal disease and may experience contrast nephropathy. However, despite this risk, percutaneous revascularization is a lower risk procedure that provides an excellent alternative to surgery in select patients[109]. Surgical therapy remains the definitive therapeutic option in many patients. In the 1990s, however, despite increasing rates of surgical and percutaneous revascularization, including thrombolytic therapy and endovascular stents, there was no decrease in the rates of major amputation in the general population[110].

FUTURE GOALS

Given the unique characteristics and tremendous impact of cardiovascular and peripheral vascular disease in the diabetic population, large prospective studies specifically examining pathophysiology, screening, and efficacy of therapy in this population are warranted. The BARI 2 trial will be a prospective randomized trial of diabetic patients that compares medical therapy, percutaneous coronary intervention, and CABG in the setting of strict blood glucose control. In addition, trials examining the role of HMG-CoA reductase inhibitors, as well as gemfibrozil and other fibrate drugs, specifically in the diabetic population, have been proposed or are ongoing. Studies such as these should provide further insight to guide prevention strategies in this high-risk population.

In the meantime, it is important to recognize both the considerable potential for, and serious adverse effects of cardiovascular and peripheral vascular disease in the diabetic population. There is justification to have a lower threshold to screen for CVD, and to aggressively modify other cardiovascular risk factors when faced with the challenges of managing the diabetic patient.

REFERENCES

1 American Diabetes Association. Consensus statement: role of cardiovascular risk factors in prevention and treatment of macrovascular disease in diabetes. *Diabetes Care* 1993;16(Suppl 2):72–8.

2 Aronson D, Rayfield EJ, Chesebro JH. Mechanisms determining course and outcome of diabetic patients who have had acute myocardial infarction. *Ann Intern Med* 1997;126:296–306.

3 Kannel WB, McGee DL. Diabetes and glucose tolerance as risk factors for cardiovascular disease: the Framingham Study. *Diabetes Care* 1979;2:120–6.

4 Pyorala K, Laasko M, Uusitupa M. Diabetes and atherosclerosis: an epidemiologic view. *Diabetes Metabol Rev* 1987;3:463–524.

5 Stamler J, Vaccaro O, Neaton JD *et al.* Diabetes, other risk factors, and 12-year cardiovascular mortality for men screened in the Multiple Risk Factor Intervention Trial. *Diabetes Care* 1993;16:434–44.

6 Winngard DL, Barrett-Connor E. Heart disease and diabetes. In: Group NDD, editor. *Diabetes in America*. 2nd edn. Washington, DC; Government Printing Office, 1995: 429–48.

7 Miettinen H, Lehto S, Salomaa VV. Impact of diabetes on mortality after the first myocardial infarction. *Diabetes Care* 1998;21:69–75.

8 Abbott RD, Donahue RP, Kannel WB *et al.* The impact of diabetes on survival following myocardial infarction in men vs. women: the Framingham Study. *J Am Med Assoc* 1988;260:3456–60.

9 Herliz J, Karlson BW, Edvardsson N *et al.* Prognosis in diabetics with chest pain or other

symptoms suggestive of acute myocardial infarction. *Cardiology* 1992;80:237–45.

10 Granger CB, Califf RM, Young S *et al.* Outcome of patients with diabetes mellitus and acute myocardial infarction treated with thrombolytic agents. The Thrombolysis and Angioplasty in Myocardial Infarction (TAMI) Study Group. *J Am Coll Cardiol* 1993;21:920–5.

11 Mueller HS, Cohen LS, Braunwald E *et al.* Predictors of early mortality and morbidity after thrombolytic therapy of acute myocardial infarction. Analyses of patient subgroups in the Thrombolysis in Myocardial Infarction (TIMI) trial, Phase II. *Circulation* 1992; 85:1254–64.

12 Barbash GI, White HD, Modan M *et al.* Significance of diabetes mellitus in patients with acute myocardial infarction receiving thrombolytic therapy. Investigators of the International Tissue Plasminogen Activator/Streptokinase Mortality Trial. *J Am Coll Cardiol* 1993;22:707–13.

13 Hillis LD, Forman S, Braunwald E. Risk stratification before thrombolytic therapy in patients with acute myocardial infarction. The Thrombolysis in Myocardial Infarction (TIMI) Phase II Co-Investigators. *J Am Coll Cardiol* 1990;16:313–5.

14 Murphy JF, Kahn MG, Krone RJ. Prethrombolytic versus thrombolytic era risk stratification of patients with acute myocardial infarction. *Am J Cardiol* 1995;76:827–9.

15 Klein HH, Hengstenberg C, Peuckert M *et al.* Comparison of death rates from acute myocardial infarction in a single hospital in two different periods (1977–1978 versus 1988–1989). *Am J Cardiol* 1993;71:518–23.

16 Stone PH, Muller JE, Hartwell T *et al.* The effect of diabetes mellitus on prognosis and serial left ventricular function after acute myocardial infarction: contribution of both coronary disease and diastolic left ventricular dysfunction to the adverse prognosis. The MILIS Study Group. *J Am Coll Cardiol* 1989;14:49–57.

17 Smith JW, Marcus FI, Serokman R. Prognosis of patients with diabetes mellitus after acute myocardial infarction. *Am J Cardiol* 1984;54:718–21.

18 Herlitz J, Malmberg K, Karlson BW *et al.* Mortality and morbidity during a five-year follow-up of diabetics with myocardial infarction. *Acta Med Scand* 1988;224:31–8.

19 Ulvenstam G, Aberg A, Bergstrand R *et al.* Long-term prognosis after myocardial infarction in men with diabetes. *Diabetes* 1985;34:787–92.

20 Karlson BW, Herlitz J, Hjalmarson A. Prognosis of acute myocardial infarction in diabetic and non-diabetic patients. *Diabet Med* 1993;10:449–54.

21 Abbott RD, Donahue RP, Kannel WB *et al.* The impact of diabetes on survival following myocardial infarction in men vs women. The Framingham Study. *J Am Med Assoc* 1988;260:3456–60.

22 Jacoby RM, Nesto RW. Acute myocardial infarction in the diabetic patient: pathophysiology, clinical course and prognosis. *J Am Coll Cardiol* 1992;20:736–44.

23 Haffner SM, Lehto S, Ronnemaa T *et al.* Mortality from coronary heart disease in subjects with type 2 diabetes and in nondiabetic subjects with and without prior myocardial infarction. *N Engl J Med* 1998;339:229–34.

24 Consensus development conference on the diagnosis of coronary heart disease in people with diabetes: 10–11 February 1998, Miami, Florida. American Diabetes Association. *Diabetes Care* 1998;21:1551–9.

25 Barzilay JI, Kronmal RA, Bittner V *et al.* Coronary artery disease and coronary artery bypass grafting in diabetic patients aged >65 years (report from the coronary artery surgery study [CASS] registry). *Am J Cardiol* 1994;74:334–9.

26 Waller BF, Palumbo PJ, Lie JT *et al.* Status of coronary arteries at necropsy in diabetes mellitus with onset after age 30 years. Analysis of 229 diabetic patients with and without evidence of coronary heart disease and comparison to 183 control subjects. *Am J Med* 1980;69:498–506.

27 Stein B, Weintraub WS, Gebhart SP *et al.* Influence of diabetes mellitus on early and late outcome after percutaneous transluminal coronary angioplasty. *Circulation* 1992;91:979–89.

28 Vigorito C, Betocchi S, Bonanzi G *et al.* Severity of coronary artery disease in diabetic patients. Angiographic study of 34 diabetic and 120 nondiabetic patients. *Am Heart J* 1980;100 (6 Pt 1):782–7.

29 The effects of tissue plasminogen activator, streptokinase, or both on coronary artery patency, ventricular function, and survival after acute myocardial infarction. The GUSTO Angiographic Investigators. *N Engl J Med* 1993;329:1615–22.

30 Muller DW, Topol EJ, Ellis SG *et al.* Multivessel coronary artery disease: a key predictor of short-term prognosis after reperfusion therapy for acute myocardial infarction. Thrombolysis and Angioplasty in Acute Myocardial Infarction (TAMI) Study Group. *Am Heart J* 1991;121 (4 Pt 1):1042–9.

31 Fuster V, Badimon L, Badimon JJ *et al.* The patho-genesis of coronary artery disease and the acute coronary syndromes (2). *N Engl J Med* 1992;326:310–8.

32 Libby P. Molecular bases of the acute coronary syndromes. *Circulation* 1995;91:2844–50.

33 Umans JG, Levi R. Nitric oxide in the regulation of blood flow and arterial pressure. *Annu Rev Physiol* 1995;57:771–90.

34 Johnstone MT, Creager SJ, Scales KM *et al.* Impaired endothelium-dependent vasodilation in patients with insulin dependent diabetes mellitus. *Circulation* 1993;88:2510–6.

35 Cohen RA. Dysfunction of vascular endothelium in diabetes mellitus. *Circulation* 1993;87 (Suppl 5):67–76.

36 Tesfamariam B. Free radicals in diabetic endothe-lial cell dysfunction. *Free Radical Biol Med* 1994;16:383–91.

37 Jaffe AS, Spadaro JJ, Schechtman K *et al.* Increased congestive heart failure after myocar-dial infarction of modest extent in patients with diabetes mellitus. *Am Heart J* 1984;108:31–7.

38 Savage MP, Krolewski AS, Kenien GG *et al.* Acute myocardial infarction in diabetes mellitus and significance of congestive heart failure as a prog-nostic factor. *Am J Cardiol* 1988;62:665–9.

39 Rytter L, Troelsen S, Beck-Nielsen H. Prevalence and mortality of acute myocardial infarction in patients with diabetes. *Diabetes Care* 1985;8:230–4.

40 Czyzk A, Krolewski AS, Szablowska S *et al.* Clinical course of myocardial infarction among diabetic patients. *Diabetes Care* 1980;3:526–9.

41 Tansey MJ, Opic LH, Kennelly BM. High mortal-ity in obese women diabetics with acute myocar-dial infarction. *Br Med J* 1977;1:1624–6.

42 Kouvaras G, Cokkinos D, Spyropoulou M. Increased mortality of diabetics after acute myocardial infarction attributed to diffusely impaired left ventricular performance as assessed by echocardiography. *Jpn Heart J* 1988;29:1–9.

43 Malmberg K, Ryden L. Myocardial infarction in patients with diabetes mellitus. *Eur Heart J* 1988;9:259–64.

44 Lomuscio A, Castagnone M, Vergani D *et al.* Clinical correlation between diabetic and non diabetic patients with myocardial infarction. *Acta Cardiol* 1991;46:543–54.

45 Yudkin JS, Oswald GA. Determinants of hospital admission and case fatality in diabetic patients with myocardial infarction. *Diabetes Care* 1988; 11:351–8.

46 Granger CB, Califf RM, Young S *et al.* Outcome of patients with diabetes mellitus and acute myocardial infarction treated with thrombolytic agents. The Thrombolysis and Angioplasty in Myocardial Infarction (TAMI) Study Group. *J Am Coll Cardiol* 1993;21:920–5.

47 Raev DC. Which left ventricular function is impaired earlier in the evolution of diabetic cardiomyopathy? An echocardiographic study of young type I diabetic patients. *Diabetes Care* 1994;17:633–9.

48 Riggs TW, Transue D. Doppler echocardio-graphic evaluation of left ventricular diastolic function in adolescents with diabetes mellitus. *Am J Cardiol* 1990;65:899–902.

49 Paillole C, Dahan M, Paycha F *et al.* Prevalence and significance of left ventricular filling abnor-malities determined by Doppler echocardiogra-phy in young type I (insulin-dependent) diabetic patients. *Am J Cardiol* 1989;64:1010–6.

50 Uusitupa M, Mustonen J, Laakso M *et al.* Impairment of diastolic function in middle-aged type 1 (insulin-dependent) and type 2 (non-insulin-dependent) diabetic patients free of cardiovascular disease. *Diabetologia* 1988;31:783–91.

51 Zarich SW, Arbuckle BE, Cohen LR *et al.* Diastolic abnormalities in young asymptomatic diabetic patients assessed by pulsed Doppler echocardio-graphy. *J Am Coll Cardiol* 1988;12:114–20.

52 Mildenberger RR, Bar-Shlomo B, Druck MN *et al.* Clinically unrecognized ventricular dysfunction in young diabetic patients. *J Am Coll Cardiol* 1984;4:234–8.

53 Shapiro LM, Leatherdale BA, Mackinnon J *et al.* Left ventricular function in diabetes mellitus. II: Relation between clinical features and left ventricular function. *Br Heart J* 1981;45:129–32.

54 Bloomgarden ZT. The European Association for the Study of Diabetes Annual Meeting, 1998: Complications of diabetes. *Diabetes Care* 1999;22:1364–70.

55 Bhatt DL, Marso SP, Lincoff AM *et al.* Abciximab reduces mortality in diabetics following percuta-neous coronary intervention. *J Am Coll Cardiol* 2000;35:922–8.

56 Theroux P, Alexander J, Jr., Pharand C *et al.* Glycoprotein IIb/IIIa receptor blockade im-proves outcomes in diabetic patients presenting with unstable angina/non-ST-elevation myocar-dial infarction: results from the Platelet Receptor Inhibition in Ischemic Syndrome Management in Patients Limited by Unstable Signs and

Symptoms (PRISM-PLUS) study. *Circulation* 2000;102:2466–72.

57 Nesto RW. Screening for asymptomatic coronary artery disease in diabetes. *Diabetes Care* 1999;22:1393–5.

58 Anonymous. Prevalence of unrecognized silent myocardial ischemia and its association with atherosclerotic risk factors in noninsulin-dependent diabetes mellitus. Milan Study on Atherosclerosis and Diabetes (MiSAD) Group. *Am J Cardiol* 1997;79:134–9.

59 Naka M, Hiramatsu K, Aizawa T *et al.* Silent myocardial ischemia in patients with non-insulin dependent diabetes mellitus as judged by treadmill exercise testing and coronary angiography. *Am Heart J* 1992;123:46–53.

60 Koistinen MJ. Prevalence of asymptomatic myocardial ischaemia in diabetic subjects. *Br Med J* 1990;301:92–5.

61 Pyorala K, Pedersen TR, Kjekshus J *et al.* Cholesterol lowering with simvastatin improves prognosis of diabetic patients with coronary heart disease. A subgroup analysis of the Scandinavian Simvastatin Survival Study (4S). *Diabetes Care* 1997;20:614–20.

62 Sacks FM, Pfeffer MA, Moye LA *et al.* The effect of pravastatin on coronary events after myocardial infarction in patients with average cholesterol levels. Cholesterol and Recurrent Events Trial investigators. *N Engl J Med* 1996;335:1001–9.

63 Expert Panel on Detection, Evaluation and Treatment of High Blood Cholesterol in Adults. Executive Summary of The Third Report of The National Cholesterol Education Program (NCEP) Expert Panel on Detection, Evaluation, And Treatment of High Blood Cholesterol In Adults (Adult Treatment Panel III). *J Am Med Assoc* 2001;285:2486–97.

64 Steiner G. Lipid intervention trials in diabetes. *Diabetes Care* 2000;23 Suppl 2:B49–B53.

65 The Heart Outcomes Prevention Evaluation Study Investigators. Effects of an angiotensin-converting-enzyme inhibitor, ramipril, on cardiovascular events in high-risk patients. *N Engl J Med* 2000;342:145–53.

66 Kjekshus J, Gilpin E, Cali G *et al.* Diabetic patients and beta-blockers after acute myocardial infarction. *Eur Heart J* 1990;11:43–50.

67 Kendall MJ, Lynch KP, Hjalmarson A *et al.* Beta-blockers and sudden cardiac death. *Ann Intern Med* 1995;123:358–67.

68 Malmberg K, Herlitz J, Hjalmarson A *et al.* Effects of metoprolol on mortality and late infarction in diabetics with suspected acute myocardial infarction. Retrospective data from two large studies. *Eur Heart J* 1989;10:423–8.

69 Gundersen T, Kjekshus J. Timolol treatment after myocardial infarction in diabetic patients. *Diabetes Care* 1983;6:285–90.

70 Jonas M, Reicher-Reiss H, Boyko V *et al.* Usefulness of beta-blocker therapy in patients with non-insulin dependent diabetes mellitus and coronary artery disease. *Am J Cardiol* 1996;77:1273–7.

71 Anonymous. Collaborative overview of randomised trials of antiplatelet therapy—I: Prevention of death, myocardial infarction, and stroke by prolonged antiplatelet therapy in various categories of patients. Antiplatelet Trialists' Collaboration. *Br Med J* 1994;308:81–106.

72 Anonymous. Aspirin therapy in diabetes. American Diabetes Association. *Diabetes Care* 1997;20:1772–3.

73 Anonymous. Influence of diabetes on 5-year mortality and morbidity in a randomized trial comparing CABG and PTCA in patients with multivessel disease: the Bypass Angioplasty Revascularization Investigation (BARI). *Circulation* 1997;96:1761–9.

74 Chaitman BR, Rosen AD, Williams DO *et al.* Myocardial infarction and cardiac mortality in the Bypass Angioplasty Revascularization Investigation (BARI) randomized trial. *Circulation* 1997;96:2162–70.

75 King SB, 3rd, Kosinski AS, Guyton RA *et al.* Eight-year mortality in the Emory Angioplasty versus Surgery Trial (EAST). *J Am Coll Cardiol* 2000;35:1116–21.

76 Abizaid A, Costa MA, Centemero M *et al.* Clinical and economic impact of diabetes mellitus on percutaneous and surgical treatment of multivessel coronary disease patients: insights from the Arterial Revascularization Therapy Study (ARTS) trial. *Circulation* 2001;104:533–8.

77 Davies RF, Goldberg AD, Forman S *et al.* Asymptomatic Cardiac Ischemia Pilot (ACIP) study two-year follow-up: outcomes of patients randomized to initial strategies of medical therapy versus revascularization. *Circulation* 1997;95:2037–43.

78 Malmberg K, Ryden L, Efendic S *et al.* Randomized trial of insulin-glucose infusion followed by subcutaneous insulin treatment in diabetic patients with acute myocardial infarction (DIGAMI study): effects on mortality at 1 year. *J Am Coll Cardiol* 1995;26:57–65.

79 Eagle KA, Brundage BH, Chaitman BR *et al.* Guidelines for perioperative cardiovascular evaluation for noncardiac surgery. Report of the American College of Cardiology/ American Heart Association Task Force on Practice Guidelines. Committee on Perioperative Cardiovascular Evaluation for Noncardiac Surgery. *Circulation* 1996;93:1278–317.

80 Gibbons RJ, Balady GJ, Beasley JW *et al.* ACC/AHA Guidelines for Exercise Testing: Executive Summary: A Report of the American College of Cardiology/American Heart Association Task Force on Practice Guidelines (Committee on Exercise Testing). *Circulation* 1997;96:345–54.

81 Lee TH, Boucher CA. Clinical practice. Noninvasive tests in patients with stable coronary artery disease. *N Engl J Med* 2001;344:1840–5.

82 Garber AM, Solomon NA. Cost-effectiveness of alternative test strategies for the diagnosis of coronary artery disease. *Ann Intern Med* 1999;130:719–28.

83 Gianrossi R, Detrano R, Mulvihill D *et al.* Exercise-induced ST depression in the diagnosis of coronary artery disease. A meta-analysis. *Circulation* 1989;80:87–98.

84 Caracciolo EA, Chaitman BR, Forman SA *et al.* Diabetics with coronary disease have a prevalence of asymptomatic ischemia during exercise treadmill testing and ambulatory ischemia monitoring similar to that of nondiabetic patients. An ACIP database study. ACIP Investigators. Asymptomatic Cardiac Ischemia Pilot Investigators. *Circulation* 1996;93:2097–105.

85 Currie CJ, Morgan CL, Peters JR. The epidemiology and cost of inpatient care for peripheral vascular disease, infection, neuropathy, and ulceration in diabetes. *Diabetes Care* 1998;21:42–8.

86 Kreines K, Johnson E, Albrink M *et al.* The course of peripheral vascular disease in non-insulin-dependent diabetes. *Diabetes Care* 1985;8:235–43.

87 Vigilance JE, Reid HL, Richards-George P. Peripheral occlusive arterial disease in diabetic clinic attendees. *West Ind Med J* 1999;48:143–6.

88 Jude EB, Oyibo SO, Chalmers N *et al.* Peripheral arterial disease in diabetic and nondiabetic patients: a comparison of severity and outcome. *Diabetes Care* 2001;24:1433–7.

89 Calle-Pascual AL, Duran A, Diaz A *et al.* Comparison of peripheral arterial reconstruction in diabetic and non-diabetic patients: a prospective clinic-based study. *Diabetes Res Clin Pract* 2001;53(Suppl):129–36.

90 Hughson WG, Mann JI, Tibbs DJ *et al.* Intermittent claudication: factors determining outcome. *Br Med J* 1978;1:1377–9.

91 Bild DE, Selby JV, Sinnock P *et al.* Lower-extremity amputation in people with diabetes. *Diabetes Care* 1989;12:24–31.

92 Dormandy JA, Murray GD. The fate of the claudicant—a prospective study of 1969 claudicants. *Eur J Vasc Surg* 1991;5:131–3.

93 Coffman JD. Intermittent claudication and rest pain: physiologic concepts and therapeutic approaches. *Prog Cardiovasc Dis* 1979;22:53–72.

94 Criqui MH, Langer RD, Fronek A *et al.* Mortality over a period of 10 years in patients with peripheral arterial disease. *N Engl J Med* 1992;326:381–6.

95 Anonymous. Prevention of atherosclerotic complications: controlled trial of ketanserin. Prevention of Atherosclerotic Complications with Ketanserin Trial Group. *Br Med J* 1989;298:424–30.

96 Janka HU, Standl E, Mehnert H. Peripheral vascular disease in diabetes mellitus and its relation to cardiovascular risk factors: screening with the Doppler ultrasonic technique. *Diabetes Care* 1980;3:207–13.

97 Orchard TJ, Strandness DE, Jr. Assessment of peripheral vascular disease in diabetes. Report and recommendations of an international workshop sponsored by the American Diabetes Association and the American Heart Association September 18–20, 1992 New Orleans, Louisiana. *Circulation* 1993;88:819–28.

98 McDermott MM. Ankle brachial index as apredictor of outcomes in peripheral arterial disease. *J Lab Clin Med* 1999;133:33–40.

99 Criqui MH, Fronek A, Klauber MR *et al.* The sensitivity, specificity, and predictive value of traditional clinical evaluation of perpheral arterial disease: results from non-invasive testing in a defined population. *Circulation* 1985;71:516–21.

100 Spitell JA. Peripheral arterial disease. *Dis Mon* 1994;40:645–99.

101 Anonymous. Role of cardiovascular risk factors in prevention and treatment of macrovascular disease in diabetes. American Diabetes Association. *Diabetes Care* 1989;12:573–9.

102 Anonymous. Detection and management of lipid disorders in diabetes. American Diabetes Association. *Diabetes Care* 1993;16:828–34.

103 Adler AI, Stratton IM, Neil HA *et al.* Association of systolic blood pressure with macrovascular and microvascular complications of type 2 diabetes (UKPDS 36): prospective observational study. *Br Med J* 2000;321:412–9.

104 Stratton IM, Adler AI, Neil HA *et al.* Association of glycaemia with macrovascular and microvascular complications of type 2 diabetes (UKPDS 35): prospective observational study. *Br Med J* 2000;321:405–12.

105 Colwell JA, Bingham SF, Abraira C *et al.* Veterans Administration Cooperative Study on antiplatelet agents in diabetic patients after amputation for gangrene: II. Effects of aspirin and dipyridamole on atherosclerotic vascular disease rates. *Diabetes Care* 1986;9:140–8.

106 Cimminiello C, Milani M. Diabetes mellitus and peripheral vascular disease: is aspirin effective in preventing vascular events? [see comments]. *Diabetologia* 1996;39:1402–4.

107 Lindgaarde F, Jelnes R, Bjorkman H *et al.* Conservative drug treatment in patients with moderately severe chronic occlusive peripheral arterial disease. *Circulation* 1989;80:1549–56.

108 Spitell JA. Pentoxifylline and intermittent claudication. *Ann Intern Med* 1985;102:126–7.

109 Isner JM, Rosenfield K. Angioplasty/coronary heart disease: redefining the treatment of peripheral artery disease: role of percutaneous revascularization. *Circulation* 1993;88:1534–57.

110 Feinglass J, Brown JL, LoSasso A *et al.* Rates of lower extremity amputation and arterial reconstruction in the United States, 1979 to 1996. *Am J Publ Health* 1999;89:1222–7.

27

Anesthesia and surgery in the diabetic patient

Jeffrey I Joseph

PERIOPERATIVE APPROACH TO THE SURGICAL PATIENT WITH DIABETES

Hyperglycemia is common in surgical patients, even if they have not previously had diabetes[1]. Hyperglycemia or relative insulin deficiency (or both), during major surgery and critical illness, may directly (or indirectly) confer a predisposition to complications[1-5]. Intensive insulin therapy and tight glucose control have been shown to decrease the incidence of postoperative complications and improve long-term outcome[5-7].

The optimal range of blood glucose control in the perioperative setting remains controversial. Current therapeutic methods often fail to achieve the desired degree of blood glucose control[8]. Methods that attempt to maintain tight control (90–120 mg dL^{-1}) are associated with fluctuations in blood glucose levels beyond the desired range, and a high incidence of hypoglycemia[5]. The blood glucose range 100–180 mg dL^{-1} has traditionally been recommended to minimize the risk of hypoglycemia and its sequelae. Levels > 180 mg dL^{-1} exceed the renal threshold for glucose and increase the risk of dehydration and electrolyte imbalance[9,10]. Levels > 200 mg dL^{-1} increase the risk of infection and cerebral and myocardial ischemia. Even brief periods of hyperglycemia adversely affect cellular and humoral immunity[11]. Acute hyperglycemia delays gastric emptying and may increase the risk of aspiration pneumonia. The fear of neuro

glycopenia (seizure, coma, and death) dictates the psychology of diabetes management in the hospital setting. Nurses and physicians err on the side of moderate hyperglycemia to avoid the consequences of low blood glucose levels[10,12]. Recent prospective controlled studies have demonstrated decreased complications and improved long-term survival with tight blood glucose control[2,5-7].

Van den Berghe *et al.*[5] recently studied a mixed intensive care unit (ICU) population of medical and postoperative surgical patients. End-organ complications were decreased and long-term survival increased, when blood glucose levels were controlled in the near-normal range using intensive insulin therapy. Mortality in the group of patients who required ICU care for > 5 days decreased from 20.2% in the conventional-treatment group (~180–200 mg dL^{-1} range) to 10.6% in the intensive-treatment group (~90–110 mg dL^{-1} range) at 12 months post-discharge. Intensive insulin therapy and tight glucose control provided the greatest protection from death, by decreasing the incidence and severity of systemic infection (multiple-organ failure with a proven septic focus). The intensive-treatment group had an overall 34% reduction in (in-hospital) mortality, 46% reduction in bloodstream infections, 41% reduction in renal failure requiring dialysis, 50% reduction in the median number of red blood cell transfusions, and a reduction in the need for prolonged mechanical ventilation. Hypo-glycemia (blood glucose level ≤ 40 mg dL⁻¹) occurred in 39 patients in the intensive-treatment group (n = 765) and six patients in the conventional-treatment group (n = 783)[5].

Tight glucose control has been achieved with a variety of regimens. A variable-rate intra-venous infusion of regular insulin has been shown to be the most effective method of providing blood glucose control in surgical patients with diabetes and stress-induced hyper-glycemia[9,10]. Insulin dose algorithms are based upon physiological principles and the pharma-cokinetic–dynamic profiles of intravenous insulin. The risk:benefit ratio of tight blood glucose control should be determined on an individual patient basis. An accurate bedside glucose meter, properly trained nurses, and frequent glucose monitoring are mandatory for the safe and effective application of intensive-insulin therapy. Higher glycemic goals are required in patients who experience hypo-glycemia unawareness and when nursing issues prevent an adequate frequency of blood glucose monitoring and bedside vigilance. Tight blood glucose control is often difficult to achieve with current methods of subcutaneous insulin injec-tion because insulin absorption is variable and blood glucose levels are not measured with sufficient frequency[10,13,14].

THE DIABETIC SURGICAL POPULATION

Approximately 4.0 million individuals with diabetes are admitted to US hospitals each year. The majority of hospitalizations are related to the micro- and macrovascular complications of diabetes, rather than the acute control of blood glucose[15]. Diabetic patients require surgical procedures on the eye (laser retina), heart (coro-nary artery bypass surgery, percutaneous trans-luminal coronary angioplasty), and major blood vessels (carotid endarterectomy, peripheral artery bypass surgery) more frequently than the non-diabetic population. Procedures related to the management of chronic renal failure (kidney transplantation, hemodialysis/peritoneal dialy-sis access formation) and other microvascular complications (limb amputation, incision and drainage of an abscess, penile prosthesis) are also required more frequently as a consequence of long-term hyperglycemia[15,16].

It is estimated that 6.0 million patients develop significant hyperglycemia each year while in the hospital. Many of these patients will have a prior diagnosis of type 1, type 2, gestational, or secondary diabetes. Approximately half of the hyperglycemic patients will have previously undiagnosed diabetes, and will require insulin or oral hypoglycemic therapy following discharge from the hospital[2,15,16]. A significant number of non-diabetic patients will develop hyperglycemia due to the metabolic stress of anesthesia, surgery, pain, and systemic illness[1,17]. Although insulin is often required during the stressful event, medica-tion is often not required following hospital discharge. The number of surgical patients with diabetes and impaired glucose tolerance (IGT) is expected to increase over the next 15 years, due to the aging baby-boom population, the sedentary lifestyle of the US population, and the increasing incidence of obesity[16].

It is important to identify patients who do not produce endogenous insulin (type 1 diabetes, ketosis prone) and those with insulin resistance and limited endogenous insulin production (type 2 diabetes with severely impaired beta-cell function). This group of patients has the poten-tial to develop clinically significant ketosis, acidosis, and unstable glucose metabolism following the stress of surgery. Type 2 diabetics previously treated by diet, exercise, and oral hypoglycemic agents should not develop keto-sis, because sufficient endogenous insulin is produced to inhibit lipolysis and partial oxida-tion of free fatty acids[1,4,10].

THE METABOLIC STRESS RESPONSE

The clinical course of the surgical patient can be characterized by predictable physiological changes (hormonal, metabolic, and hemody-namic) that occur along a continuum (Table 27.1). Perioperative complications can be avoided with timely recognition of an inade-quate compensatory response (deviations from the expected pattern) followed by appropriate supportive care.

Table 27.1 The metabolic stress response to anesthesia and major surgery in patients with type 2 diabetes

	Preop fasting	Anesthesia	Evening surgery	Postoperative Day 1	Postoperative Day 3
Insulin secretion	– –	–	±	±	±
Insulin sensitivity	–	– – –	– – –	– – –	– –
Glucagon	+	–	–	±	±
Epinephrine	+	+ +	+ + +	+ +	+
Norepinephrine	+	+ +	+ + +	+ + +	+ +
Cortisol	+	+ +	+ + +	+ +	+ +
Growth hormone	–	+	+	+	+
Glycogenolysis	+ + +	+ +	+ +	+	+
Gluconeogenesis	+ +	+ +	+ + +	+ + +	+ +
Proteolysis	+	+	+ +	+ +	+
Lipolysis	+	±	±	±	±
Ketogenesis	+ +	+	±	±	±
Heart rate	±	±	+ + +	+ +	+ +
Respiratory rate	±	–	+ +	+ +	+ +
Cardiac contractility	±	–	+ +	+ +	+ +

+ increased effect , – decreased effect , ± variable effect. Effects may be attenuated by anaesthetic/analgesic techniques and cardiovascular medications.

Cellular metabolism, core temperature, and peripheral blood flow decrease during anesthesia, and remain low in the immediate postoperative period. Processes not essential to the immediate survival of the patient decrease to basal levels. Blood flow is preferentially diverted to the vital organs and wound. The disruption of capillaries and tissue edema within the surgical wound require increased blood flow for the delivery of essential cellular nutrients. The wound requires elevated levels of oxygen, glucose, free fatty acids, amino acids, lactic acid, and ketone bodies to satisfy the nutritional needs of neutrophils, macrophages, and fibroblasts. Blood levels of catecholamines (epinephrine, norepinephrine), catabolic hormones (glucagon, cortisol, growth hormone), and cytokines (interleukin-1, tumor necrosis factor) increase in proportion to the degree of tissue injury and the number of white blood cells invading the surgical wound[1,4,18]. Insulin resistance and enhanced hepatic/renal gluconeogenesis are most pronounced during the acute phase of surgical stress. The hyperdynamic and catabolic responses (proteolysis, lipolysis, gluconeogenesis) slowly resolve once new capillaries form within the healing wound. A prolonged stress response suggests inadequate nutrient delivery to the wound, or infection[19]. Still unanswered is whether hyperglycemia is a mechanism to optimize wound homeostasis, or an unwanted side effect of the stress response.

PREOPERATIVE EVALUATION OF THE DIABETIC PATIENT

A surgical procedure cannot be considered successful unless the patient recovers with an equal or improved quality of life and long-term survival. Patients with long-standing diabetes are at increased risk of developing complications. The goal of preoperative assessment is to identify patient risk factors and quantify risk, in order to decide the appropriateness of the planned surgical procedure and the timing of surgery. History, physical and selective tests are used to identify the presence and severity of co-existing disease. The patient's condition can then be optimized prior to anesthesia and surgery. Procedures of short duration with minimal tissue trauma, blood loss and fluid shifts are usually well tolerated (even by the high-risk patient). Elderly patients requiring emergency surgery (especially on the heart and great vessels) experience the highest risk. Successful outcomes require surgical skill and close communication between the physicians, nurses, and patient. A well-developed and implemented treatment plan remains the key to avoiding complications that may lead to decreased quality of life and premature death.

Patients with diabetes are at increased risk of developing chronic renal failure. Diabetic nephropathy progresses to renal insufficiency/failure in 35% of type 1 and 10% of type 2 diabetics. The duration of diabetes, degree of glycemic control, and level of proteinuria are useful to estimate the severity of pre-existing nephropathy. The highest incidence of perioperative renal failure has been documented in older diabetics following cardiac and vascular surgery. Renal parenchyma may be injured by decreased renal blood flow (low cardiac output, prolonged hypotension, or surgical clamp), atherosclerotic emboli, free hemoglobin, nephrotoxic antibiotics, radiographic contrast agents, and sepsis. Chronic use of angiotensin converting enzyme (ACE) inhibitors has been associated with an increased risk of perioperative renal insufficiency. Modern anesthetic agents rarely cause direct renal tissue damage. Adequate hydration (optimal renal blood flow) is mandatory to decrease the risk of acute renal failure[20,21].

Patients with diabetic neuropathy may be at increased risk for developing a peripheral nerve injury during surgery. Diabetic nerves may be more susceptible to ischemia from stretch and compression, leading to permanent disability. The brachial plexus, ulnar nerve, and sciatic nerve are most commonly affected. It is unknown whether transient hyperglycemia increases the incidence of perioperative nerve injury.

Although uncommon, aspiration pneumonia may lead to prolonged mechanical ventilation and death. The risk of aspiration may be increased in the diabetic patient due to gastroparesis (solid food remains in stomach > 12 h) and increased difficulty in placing an endotracheal tube (obesity and stiff cervical spine). Transient hyperglycemia is known to reduce gastric motility and delay gastric emptying. Promotility agents and proton pump inhibitors may be indicated in some diabetics[21,22]. Patients should be weaned as quickly as possible from mechanical ventilation to minimize the risk of nosocomial pneumonia.

The risk of infection is increased in diabetic surgical patients[6,7]. Proven methods of decreasing the risk of infection include maintaining normal body temperature, normal nutritional status, and near-normal blood glucose control. Intravenous and urinary catheters should be inserted using strict aseptic technique and removed as quickly as possible[23].

Diabetes and IGT are major risk factors for the development of atherosclerotic vascular disease[24]. Diabetics have a nearly six-fold greater risk of developing a first-time myocardial infarction (MI) (20.2% versus 3.5%) and a higher rate of re-infarction (45% versus 18.8%) when compared with non-diabetics[25]. Associated risk factors (hypertension, dyslipidemia, family history, central obesity, and smoking) greatly increase the risk of a diabetic dying from cardiovascular disease[24,26]. MI continues to be the leading cause of mortality in hospitalized patients with diabetes. The incidence of perioperative MI (< 7 days after non-cardiac surgery) in patients without a history of previous MI has been reported to be in the range of 0.13–0.66%. A higher incidence has been confirmed in patients with diabetes. Patients who have experienced a previous MI have an increased risk of acute MI in the perioperative period (4.3–15.9%). The incidence of MI peaks during the first 24 h after surgery, with most occurring on the first night. The risk of perioperative MI increases significantly for 3–6 months following an acute MI (range 6–54% risk). After 6 months, the risk of perioperative MI decreases to approximately 4–6%. Elective surgery should be delayed 6 months following an acute MI, especially if non-invasive testing reveals significant myocardium at risk[21,22].

Perioperative MI is associated with a high mortality (27–69%) compared with acute MI not associated with surgery (15–20%)[27]. The greatest mortality occurs in diabetic patients who develop congestive heart failure (CHF). Diabetic hearts have decreased coronary flow reserve, decreased contractile reserve, and decreased compensatory response of the non-infarcted myocardial segments[28]. The pathophysiology of perioperative MI is the same as for acute MI in the non-surgical setting[29]. In addition, surgery and diabetes produce a hyperdynamic and mildly prothrombotic state, making the diabetic coronary artery more prone to fissure and thrombosis. Myocardial ischemia and infarction are almost always silent in the perioperative period, and may not be associated with Q-waves or ST-segment elevation.

A number of clinical scoring systems have been developed to more accurately define cardiovascular risk in the perioperative setting[30,31]. Recent scoring systems place more emphasis on active co-existing conditions and the location/complexity of the proposed surgical procedure[32]. The American Heart Association's Task Force on Practice Guidelines has defined perioperative risk based upon end-organ pathology and whether the disease process is stable or unstable. Long-standing diabetes was judged an intermediate predictor of cardiovascular risk. Coronary angiography may be useful to define therapy in high-risk patients, or intermediate-risk patients about to undergo a high-risk surgical procedure[33]. The benefit of preoperative angioplasty with stent placement has not been evaluated in a controlled trial. Successful coronary artery bypass graft (CABG) surgery has been shown to decrease the risk of MI following subsequent non-cardiac surgery[22]. Emergent CABG surgery prior to urgent non-cardiac surgery cannot be recommended due to excessive risk.

Intra- and post-operative beta-blockade have been shown to protect the myocardium from ischemia/infarction and improve long-term outcome. Beta-blockade has been used in many surgical patients with diabetes and heart failure without adverse effect.

Diabetic patients with a prior stroke are at increased risk of stroke in the perioperative period. The highest incidence of cerebral ischemia and stroke follows cardiac and vascular surgery. Focal ischemia occurs when athero-sclerotic emboli travel from the thoracic and cerebral arteries to the brain[34]. The area of cerebral ischemia at risk of infarction may increase due to enhanced coagulation, decreased fibrinolysis and altered cellular metabolism. Hemodynamic instability due to autonomic neuropathy, dehydration, cardiopulmonary bypass, heart failure, and anesthetics may increase the risk of global cerebral ischemia[21,22,28].

RATIONALE FOR CONTROL OF BLOOD GLUCOSE

Normal metabolism should be mimicked as closely as possible. Therapeutic goals include the avoidance of hypoglycemia, hyperglycemia, lipolysis, ketogenesis, proteolysis, dehydration, and electrolyte imbalance. Adequate insulin levels must be provided to counterbalance the catabolic hormones and stress response[1,5]. Aggressive glucose control using intensive insulin therapy should be considered for all patients, to decrease morbidity and improve long-term outcome[2,5–7].

Hypoglycemia

Factors that predispose the surgical patient to hypoglycemia include prolonged fasting, inadequate/delayed food intake, changing insulin sensitivity, variability in subcutaneous insulin absorption, and changing renal function[2,5,10,13,14]. The danger of hypoglycemia may be increased because the signs and symptoms of neuroglycopenia are masked by sedatives, anesthetics, and cardiovascular medications[10]. Signs of hypoglycemia (diaphoresis, tachycardia, hypertension) may be mistaken for inadequate levels of general anesthesia[21]. Changes in mental status, including focal neurological symptoms, may persist for hours to days following even a single episode of severe neuroglycopenia.

Frequent blood glucose monitoring is the key to avoiding hypoglycemia. Although the optimal frequency of monitoring has not been determined, many experts recommend hourly blood glucose measurements during and immediately following major surgery[2,10]. Less frequent monitoring (every 2–6 h) has been recommended following the return of metabolic stability[35]. Diabetics with high insulin sensitivity and hypoglycemia unawareness should be monitored more closely. Unfortunately, many clinicians do not monitor glucose levels with the recommended frequency. Golden *et al.* studied 411 adult diabetics undergoing CABG surgery. Only six capillary blood glucose measurements were taken during the 36 h period following surgery. The mean blood glucose level exceeded 200 mg dL^{-1} in > 75% of the patients, and one patient experienced severe hypoglycemia[8]. Other reports document a low frequency of blood glucose monitoring in the perioperative period[36].

Many experts recommend an infusion of glucose to minimize the risk of hypoglycemia[2,9]. Approximately 100–125 g of exogenous glucose per day are required to meet the basal caloric needs of the surgical patient, and to prevent ketosis and excessive protein breakdown. The additional calories required in the postoperative period can be provided with an infusion of glucose averaging 1.2–2.4 mg kg^{-1} min^{-1} (5–15 g h^{-1} for an adult)[12,13,37]. Higher rates of glucose infusion often cause hyperglycemia in diabetic and non-diabetic surgical patients. Non-glucose-containing fluids are commonly infused during surgery to avoid hyperglycemia. Withholding glucose has been justified by the low incidence of hypoglycemia[21]. Controlled studies are needed to more clearly define the importance of exogenous glucose (and other nutrients) during and after major surgery.

Diabetic ketoacidosis

Increased catecholamine and catabolic hormone levels combine with an absolute or relative insulin deficiency to cause lipolysis and ketoacidosis (DKA). Clinically significant ketosis and acidosis can occur even when blood glucose levels are only modestly elevated. Many cases of DKA occur in patients with plasma glucose concentrations < 300 mg dL^{-1}. Euglycemic DKA (100 mg dL^{-1} glucose range) has been reported in surgical patients[4]. Patients with DKA caused by a medical etiology often present with symptoms resembling an acute surgical abdomen. Surgery should be delayed until the underlying cause is identified, because abdominal symptoms often resolve following hydration and improved metabolic control[21]. Although much more common in patients with type 1 diabetes, DKA can occur in type 2 diabetics with insulin resistance and limited endogenous insulin production[2,9,10,12].

Hyperosmolar nonketotic syndrome

Surgical patients with diabetes and IGT are susceptible to volume depletion and electrolyte imbalance leading to the hyperosmolar non-ketotic syndrome. Intravenous fluids are required to replace the pre-existing volume deficient, hemorrhage, third-space losses, gastrointestinal losses, and the ongoing osmotic diuresis. Appropriate attention to intravascular volume will facilitate hepatic-renal blood flow and correction of the hyperosmolar condition. Placement of a pulmonary artery catheter and/or trans-oesophageal endoscope (TEE) may provide useful data to guide fluid management, especially in the diabetic with renal insufficiency or decreased cardiac reserve[21].

Nosocomial infection

Hyperglycemia has been firmly established as an independent risk factor for the development of infection. In animal and human studies, even brief periods of hyperglycemia interfere with leukocyte chemotaxis, opsinization, and phagocytosis[11]. Furnary *et al.* demonstrated in a prospective, controlled study of coronary artery bypass patients that tight glucose control (below 220 mg dL^{-1}) can decrease the incidence of deep sternal wound infection (2.0–0.8%)[7]. Other perioperative studies have demonstrated an association between tight blood glucose control and decreased risk of bacteremia, pneumonia, sepsis, cystitis, and wound infection[6,38].

Wound strength

Hyperglycemia may affect fibroblast function during the period of granulation tissue formation and maturation. Decreased levels and cross-linking of collagen may impair wound healing and wound strength. Animal and human studies have demonstrated impaired wound healing/strength when blood glucose levels exceed 200 mg dL^{-1} in the days following surgery.

Perioperative MI, CHF, stroke

Controlled studies have tried to define whether tight glucose control using intensive insulin therapy can improve long-term outcome following acute MI. The Diabetes Insulin Glucose in Acute Myocardial Infarction (DIGAMI) study randomized acute MI patients to receive either conventional diabetes care or tight glucose control using an intravenous infusion of glucose–insulin–potassium (GIK) followed by multiple daily subcutaneous insulin injections. In-hospital mortality decreased 58%, 1-year mortality decreased 52%, and 3-year mortality decreased 25% in diabetics managed with intensive therapy[39]. Capes et al. performed a retrospective meta-analysis of 15 clinical studies. Non-diabetics with stress hyperglycemia following an acute MI (above 109–124 mg dL^{-1}) had a four-fold increased rate of in-hospital mortality. Diabetic patients with hyperglycemia (above 124–180 mg dL^{-1} range) had a two-fold increased rate of in-hospital mortality. Hyperglycemia was also associated with an increased incidence of post MI CHF and cardiogenic shock[40]. Kalin et al. provided tight blood glucose control (< 200 mg dL^{-1}) in 400 diabetic CABG patients. In-hospital mortality in the intensively managed group was similar to the mortality rate in a matched group of 876 patients without diabetes (1.75% versus 1.71%). In the same time period, the National Cardiac Surgery Database reported 50% higher in-hospital mortality[41]. GIK infu-

sions have been recommended to promote myocardial utilization of glucose for energy production[13,37]. Fatty acids are preferentially utilized by the myocardium when insulin levels are deficient, leading to enhanced oxygen consumption, and an increased incidence of myocardial ischemia, arrythmias, and contractile dysfunction[1,4].

Hyperglycemia is associated with increased infarct size and worsened long-term outcome following cerebral ischemia. Elevated glycosylated hemoglobin (HbA1C) and blood glucose levels at the time of hospital admission have been shown to correlate with cerebral infarct size and long-term prognosis[34]. Controlled trials are required to determine whether tight glucose control can improve outcome following cerebral ischemia, stroke, or spinal cord injury.

Glycemic goals

Glycemic goals in the perioperative period remain controversial[2,5–7,10,12]. Previous reviews recommended target glucose levels in the 100–180 mg dL^{-1} range. This level of glycemia was selected to prevent dehydration (osmotic diuresis) and infection, and to minimize the risk of hypoglycemia[7,9,10]. Recent outcome studies have advocated tighter glucose control. The prospective, controlled ICU study by Van den Berge et al. demonstrated reduced morbidity and mortality in a group of critically ill patients (mostly surgical) managed with near-normal glucose control (90 and 110 mg dL^{-1}). Unfortunately, tight glucose control was associated with a high incidence of hypoglycemia[5]. Most experts agree that glucose levels should be controlled in all hyperglycemic patients, regardless of previous diabetes status[2,10,12].

METHODS OF ACHIEVING NEAR-NORMAL GLUCOSE CONTROL

Treatment regimens should focus on safety and simplicity to minimize the risk of errors that may cause hypoglycemia. A recent program established by the US Pharmacopoeia to track hospital drug errors reported that errors involving insulin delivery ranked second in number,

Table 27.2 Variable-rate, intravenous infusion of regular insulin

☐ Replace chlorpropamide 5 days before surgery with short-acting sulphonylurea

☐ Discontinue metformin 48 h before procedures associated with renal dysfunction (risk for lactic acidosis)

☐ Withhold oral hypoglycemic agent(s) on the morning of surgery

☐ If non-emergent surgery, control blood glucose prior to procedure (90–180 mg dL^{-1})

☐ Hold solid food for > 8 h (longer with history of gastroparesis). Clear liquids permitted until 2 h before surgery

☐ Antihypertensive and antianginal medication taken with water

☐ Measure fasting blood glucose level using calibrated bedside glucose monitor

☐ Provide usual dose of intermediate-acting insulin at bedtime the evening before surgery

☐ Insist upon early admission to hospital. Start intravenous infusion of 10% glucose in water or 0.45% saline (10 g h^{-1}) around 7:00 am. Infuse isotonic saline solution if dehydrated due to bowel prep, prolonged fast, or osmotic diuresis.

☐ Prepare an insulin solution that contains 250 U short-acting (regular) insulin in 250 mL 0.9% saline (1U mL^{-1}). Flush tubing with 50 mL insulin solution to minimize the effects of surface binding on insulin delivery

☐ Start intravenous infusion of insulin around 7:00 am using a separate calibrated pump. Choose an initial insulin infusion rate, typically 1.0 U h^{-1}.

☐ Insulin and glucose infusions may be piggy-backed into the same intravenous catheter

☐ Measure blood glucose at least once every hour during and following major surgery

☐ Titrate variable-rate insulin infusion to hourly blood glucose measurements, intravenous glucose infusion rate, and anticipated level of metabolic stress (Table 27.3)

☐ Determine optimal glycemic range for individual patient. Maintain blood glucose levels in 90–180 mg dL^{-1} range for average control, and 90–120 mg dL^{-1} for tight control. Frequent blood glucose monitoring and aggressive insulin titration are required to avoid hypoglycemia

☐ Inject 15–25 mL 50% glucose solution for symptomatic hypoglycemia

☐ Measure electrolytes daily. Hyponatremia and hypokalemia are common in the postoperative period

☐ Measure urine for glucose and ketones when blood glucose > 250 mg dL^{-1}

☐ Convert variable-rate intravenous insulin regimen to a subcutaneous insulin regimen once the patient is tolerating solid food. Discontinue insulin infusion 30–60 min after injecting subcutaneous insulin (Table 27.6)

☐ Adjust subcutaneous insulin-dosage schedule and re-institute oral hypoglycemic agent(s) doses prior to hospital discharge

and first as the leading cause of patient morbidity[42]. Simplicity is also required because overworked nurses and junior physicians often undertake bedside management. A variety of insulin delivery algorithms are currently used to manage blood glucose levels in the perioperative setting.

Variable-rate intravenous insulin infusion regimen

A variable-rate intravenous infusion of regular insulin is the safest and most versatile method of managing blood glucose levels during and after major surgery (Table 27.2). The safety of an intravenous infusion regimen has been demonstrated in the operating room, intensive care unit, and on the general surgical floor[2,10,12,43]. The usual starting dose for the variable-rate insulin infusion is 1.0 U h^{-1}, with smaller starting doses recommended for patients with high insulin sensitivity (athletes and thin women). Higher doses of insulin (2.0–4.0 U h^{-1}) are recommended by some experts to increase the time to metabolic decompensation, should there be an interruption of insulin delivery[44]. The majority of clinicians use a

Table 27.3 Variable-rate insulin infusion regimen for tight blood glucose control (fixed-rate glucose infusion)

Blood glucose measurement (mg dL^{-1})	Intravenous insulin dose
< 80	Discontinue infusion for 30 min
	Administer 20–30 mL 50% dextrose
	Re-measure blood glucose in 30 min
	Restart insulin infusion at 0.5 U h^{-1} after blood glucose > 100 mg dL^{-1}
81–120	No change in insulin infusion rate
121–180	Decrease rate by 0.2 U h^{-1}
181–240	Increase by 0.4 U h^{-1}
241–300	Increase by 0.6 U h^{-1}
> 300 mg dL^{-1}	Increase by 1 U h^{-1}

Typical initial infusion rate 0.02 U kg^{-1} h^{-1} (~1.0–1.5 U h^{-1}) may be adjusted higher for patients with insulin resistance, and lower for insulin-sensitive patients. Surgical patients generally require 0.3–0.4 U of insulin per gram of glucose infused per hour. Higher infusion rates are required in some patients with liver disease (0.5–0.6 U g^{-1} h^{-1}), sepsis (0.6–0.8 U g^{-1} h^{-1}), obesity (0.4–0.6 U g^{-1} h^{-1}), and those receiving catecholamine or glucocorticoid therapy (0.5–0.8 U g^{-1} h^{-1}). Lower infusion rates may be required with hepatic and renal failure, or CHF. Large doses of insulin are often required during anesthesia and surgery (especially hypothermic cardiopulmonary bypass) to counter the effects of insulin resistance. Frequent blood glucose monitoring is required in the immediate postoperative period to avoid hypoglycemia following the resolution of insulin resistance.

(Modified from References 2, 9, 10, 12, 39 and 49).

variable-rate insulin infusion and a fixed-rate glucose infusion. The rate of insulin delivery is typically adjusted once hourly (0.5–5.0 U h^{-1}), based upon frequent blood glucose measurements. An algorithm is used to recommend the subsequent hour's dose of insulin (Table 27.3). An algorithm using a variable-rate glucose infusion has also been described (Table 27.4).

Watts *et al.* were able to achieve tight glucose control (mean glucose 136 ± 15 mg dL^{-1}) and a low incidence of hypoglycemia using separate infusions of insulin and glucose. Patients managed with conventional therapy (subcutaneous sliding-scale insulin or fixed-rate insulin infusion) were not able to achieve tight glucose control (mean glucose 208 ± 20 mg dL^{-1}, 30–306 mg dL^{-1} range)[37].

In general, diabetic surgical patients require 0.3–0.4 U of insulin per gram of infused glucose per hour (0.3–0.4 U g^{-1} h^{-1})[2,9,10,12]. Higher doses of insulin are required for patients with pre-existing or acquired insulin resistance due to obesity, systemic infection, hypothermic cardiopulmonary bypass, certain anesthetics, elevated catecholamine levels, and steroid therapy[46]. Patients with renal, hepatic, and heart failure may require decreased insulin doses.

GIK intravenous infusion regimen

An alternative intravenous insulin regimen contains a fixed concentration of glucose, potassium, and regular insulin in one solution bag. The 'GIK regimen' gained widespread clinical acceptance in the 1970s because of its simplicity and safety. Insulin and glucose are delivered in balanced proportions at a constant rate (100 mL h^{-1}) without the need for an electronic pump. Unfortunately, this method lacks flexibility and often fails to achieve desired glucose control

Table 27.4 Variable-rate insulin/variable rate glucose infusion regimen for tight blood glucose control

Blood glucose (mg dL^{-1})	Intravenous insulin dose (U h^{-1})	10% glucose infusion rate (mL h^{-1})
< 70	Discontinue infusion[1]	75
71–100	1.0	65
101–150	1.5	50
151–200	2.0	50
201–250	3.0	50
251–300	4.0	40
> 300	12.0	25

[1]Discontinue insulin infusion for 30 min; administer 10–20 mL 50% dextrose; re-measure blood glucose in 30 min, and restart insulin infusion after blood glucose > 100 mg dL^{-1}.

Although this regimen is more difficult to implement in the clinical setting (two variables are changed simultaneously), it has the potential to provide superior glycemic control with less risk of hypoglycemia. (Modified from Reference 44)

compared with the variable-rate method. Any significant change in the requirement for insulin, glucose, or potassium would necessitate a change from the original mixture to a new solution bag with the appropriate proportions (Table 27.5)[13,46].

Intermittent intravenous bolus injection regimen

The bolus intravenous injection of regular insulin is the most common method used by anesthesiologists to control blood glucose levels[36]. This method is without physiological basis and cannot be recommended. The short pharmacokinetic (4–7 min) and biological half-life (< 20 min) of an intravenous insulin bolus produces extremely high (but short-lived) plasma and tissue insulin levels[10]. Rapid changes in substrate availability may lead to lactic and ketoacidosis[1,2,4,9]. Insulin receptors may become saturated and cause a prolonged hypoglycemic effect.

Subcutaneous injections of insulin regimen

Subcutaneous administration continues to be the most common route for insulin delivery in the pre- and post-operative period. Absorption of regular insulin from the subcutaneous tissue is often slow and variable. The coefficient of variation between patients has been shown to exceed 50%. Intra-individual coefficient of variation exceeds 25%[14]. Greater variability of absorption should be expected in the surgical patient.

Sliding-scale insulin regimens based upon retrospective hyperglycemia often fail to achieve the desired degree of glycemic control[6,8,10]. This technique does not consider events that produce an increase in metabolic stress, the timing of meals, and the differences in insulin requirements at different times of the day[9]. Despite its lack of recommendation in recent medical literature, the sliding-scale method remains the most common technique for managing blood glucose levels in the perioperative period[47].

In contrast, insulin algorithms take into account patient- and surgery-specific information. Short-acting (regular) insulin is typically given prior to a meal or snack and combined with a morning and/or evening dose of intermediate-acting insulin. Algorithms direct the supplemental dose of regular insulin based upon the previous 24 h insulin dose (insulin sensitivity), carbohydrate load, lag-time before

Table 27.5 Fixed-rate GIK infusion regimen

☐ Replace chlorpropamide 5 days before surgery with short-acting sulphonylurea. Discontinue metformin 48 h before procedures associated with renal dysfunction (risk for lactic acidosis)

☐ Withhold oral hypoglycemic agent(s) the morning of surgery

☐ If non-emergent surgery, control blood glucose prior to procedure (90–180 mg dL^{-1}).

☐ Hold solid food for > 8 h (longer with patient history of gastroparesis). Clear liquids permitted until 2 h before surgery

☐ Antihypertensive and antianginal medication taken with water

☐ Measure fasting blood glucose level with calibrated bedside glucose monitor

☐ Inject one-half usual morning dose of intermediate-acting insulin upon awakening. Inject one-half of usual morning dose of short-acting insulin if fasting blood glucose level exceeds 200 mg dL^{-1}. Hold insulin for fasting blood glucose levels < 100 mg dL^{-1}

☐ Insist upon early admission to hospital. Start intravenous infusion of 10% glucose in water or 0.45% saline (5–10 g h^{-1}) around 7:00 am. Infuse isotonic saline solution if dehydrated due to bowel prep, prolonged fast, or osmotic diuresis.

☐ Monitor blood glucose hourly until the induction of anaesthesia and surgery.

☐ Replace glucose infusion with 'GIK' solution, 2 h prior to surgery. Mix glucose (5000 mg), regular insulin (15 U), and potassium (10 mmol KCl) in 500 mL water to form a 10% dextrose 'GIK' solution. Infuse at 100 mL h^{-1} through a peripheral vein.

☐ Measure blood glucose once-hourly during and immediately following major surgery. Frequency of blood glucose monitoring may be decreased to every 2–4 h in fasting patients with residual endogenous insulin production, average insulin sensitivity, and no history of hypoglycemia unawareness.

☐ Determine optimal glycemic range for individual patient. Maintain blood glucose levels within 100–200 mg dL^{-1} range. Tight blood glucose control (90–120 mg dL^{-1}) may be difficult to achieve with this regimen.

☐ If blood glucose > 200 mg dL^{-1}, change GIK solution to 20 U insulin per 500 mL.

☐ If blood glucose < 90 mg dL^{-1}, change GIK solution to 5 U insulin per 500 mL.

☐ Inject 25–50 mL 50% glucose solution for symptomatic hypoglycemia.

☐ Measure electrolytes daily and change GIK solution as necessary. Hyponatremia and hypokalemia are common in the postoperative period.

☐ Measure urine for glucose and ketones when blood glucose > 250 mg dL^{-1}.

☐ Convert GIK to a subcutaneous insulin regimen once the patient is able to tolerate solid food. Discontinue GIK infusion 30–60 min after injecting subcutaneous insulin (Table 27.6).

☐ Adjust subcutaneous insulin-dosage schedule and re-institute oral hypoglycemic agent(s) prior to hospital discharge.

meals, degree of surgical stress, and level of patient activity[2,9,10]. Regular insulin should be used with caution (or avoided) at bedtime to decrease the risk of early morning hypoglycemia (Table 27.6). Rapid-acting insulin injected immediately prior to a meal may provide improved glycemic control.

In-hospital artificial endocrine pancreas

An artificial endocrine pancreas (AP) was commercialized in the 1970s (Biostator, Miles Laboratory, Frankfurt, Germany) to automate the process of blood glucose monitoring and insulin delivery. The device contained a

Table 27.6 Postoperative blood glucose management when patient tolerates solid food (algorithm for variable subcutaneous insulin injections)

Subcutaneous dose of short-acting insulin (U)

Blood glucose (mg dL^{-1})	Breakfast	Lunch	Dinner	2200h
< 70	3	2	2	0
71–100	4	3	3	0
101–150	6	4	4	0
151–200	8	6	6	0
201–250	10	8	8	1
251–300	12	10	10	2
> 300	14	12	12	3

Administer 10–15 U intermediate-acting insulin at bedtime (NPH at 2200 h).

Reduce NPH dose if hypoglycemia present at 0300 h.

Administer oral glucose or 20–40 mL 50% glucose solution (intravenous) for hypoglycemia.

Continue glucose/insulin infusions until the patient is metabolically stable and tolerates solid food. Discontinue insulin/glucose infusions 30–60 min after the administration of subcutaneous insulin. Measure blood glucose level before each meal, at 2200 h, and at 0300 h. Provide three meals and three small snacks per day (20–30 kcal kg^{-1} day^{-1}). Administer short-acting insulin 30 min before each meal. Make sure meal is provided at appropriate time interval. Rapid-acting insulin may be given immediately prior to the meal. Dose insulin according to the above schedule. (Modified from Reference 44.)

flow-through glucose sensor connected to an intravenous catheter. Glucose was measured every few minutes with accuracy similar to a laboratory glucometer. Insulin and glucose were infused according to a preprogrammed computer algorithm. The subsequent dose of insulin (or glucose) was based upon the absolute glucose concentration and the rate of change of blood glucose over time. Tight glucose control could be achieved without hypoglycemia in the majority of clinical situations. Unfortunately, the device was too large and complex for routine clinical application. The sensor required frequent manual re-calibration and > 200 mL blood loss per day[48]. Several groups are attempting to develop a modern version of the bedside AP that overcomes the limitations of prior devices (Figure 27.1).

PERIOPERATIVE MANAGEMENT OF THE TYPE 2 DIABETIC: MAJOR SURGERY

Type 2 diabetics unable to increase endogenous insulin secretion may behave metabolically in the perioperative period similar to the classic patient with type 1 diabetes[1,2,4]. Intensive insulin therapy and frequent blood glucose monitoring are required to control blood glucose levels and minimize the risk of ketoacidosis and hypoglycemia[9,12]. A variable-rate insulin infusion/fixed-rate glucose infusion method provides the greatest flexibility, safety, and degree of glycemic control. Infusions can be discontinued once the patient is able to tolerate solid food, or restarted if the patient experiences prolonged nausea and emesis[10]. Following satisfactory

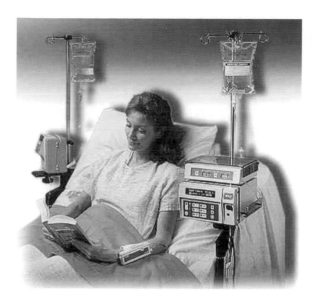

Figure 27.1 VIA-GLU continuous blood glucose monitoring system developed by Metracor Technologies (San Diego, CA) demonstrating patient-worn glucose sensor, bedside monitor, and calibration solution (www.metracor.com, visited 5 November 2002).

return of gastrointenstinal function, subcutaneous regular insulin can be carefully titrated according to meals and the clinical situation (Table 27.6).

Patients with type 2 diabetes previously managed by diet, exercise, and oral hypoglycemic agents should have sufficient endogenous insulin production to avoid ketosis and excessive hyperglycemia. Many patients, however, will require insulin therapy to counter the hyperglycemic effects of adrenaline and the catabolic hormones. A continuous insulin infusion is recommended for all patients requiring major surgery. Subcutaneous insulin regimens should be considered when the clinician anticipates a brief period of fasting in a patient with well-controlled blood glucose levels[2,9,10].

Surgery should be scheduled as early in the morning as possible. A solution of glucose should be started around 7:00 am and infused at a rate of 5–10 g h[-1]. Patients who normally take NPH and regular insulin before breakfast may take one-half to two-thirds of their usual dose (of

each type of insulin) on the morning of surgery. Regular insulin should be withheld if the fasting glucose measurement detects hypoglycemia. The dose should be increased if fasting glucose exceeds 200 mg dL[-1]. Alternatively, patients may be given NPH insulin at bedtime the night before surgery. Upon awakening, the patient can receive one-half to two-thirds of their usual morning dose of NPH insulin (with little or no regular insulin). The NPH insulin dose from the evening before will peak around 6:00 to 9:00 am and the morning dose will attenuate postoperative hyperglycemia[2,35]. A reduced dose of Ultralente can be given before surgery without undue risk of hypoglycemia. When early morning surgery is not feasible, the morning dose of subcutaneous insulin should be withheld. Intravenous infusions of insulin and glucose should be started around 7:00 am and titrated to hourly glucose measurements[9,10].

Patients using an external insulin pump with rapid-acting insulin (CSII) should continue basal rate therapy until the time of surgery. The pump should be removed prior to surgery, followed immediately by an intravenous infusion of regular insulin. Insulin should never be withheld from patients with suspected type 1 diabetes because ketoacidosis can develop while the patient is waiting for surgery. Oral hypoglycemic agents are typically withheld the morning of surgery. Glucose levels must be monitored frequently if long-acting oral agents are continued until the day before surgery[2,9,49].

PERIOPERATIVE MANAGEMENT OF THE TYPE 2 DIABETIC: OUTPATIENT SURGERY

Type 2 diabetic patients who are well controlled by diet and exercise can be managed without insulin in the ambulatory surgical setting[50]. Patients treated with oral hypoglycemic agents should be started on an intravenous glucose infusion and given their medication preoperatively. Alternatively, the oral hypoglycemic agent can be withheld prior to a brief surgical procedure and given with the first postoperative meal. The oral hypoglycemic agent should be withheld for fasting hypoglycemia, followed by an intravenous infusion of glucose. Post-operative glucose levels are often increased above 250 mg dL^{-1} when insulin or oral agents are withheld from type 2 diabetics undergoing outpatient surgery[51]. These data have led to the recommendation that insulin therapy should be considered for all type 2 diabetics managed with an oral hypoglycemic agent. Patients previously treated with insulin should receive subcutaneous insulin or an intravenous infusion of insulin during the perioperative period. Patients who experience postoperative nausea and emesis are at increased risk for hypoglycemia and metabolic decompensation: admission to the hospital may therefore be required[10].

REFERENCES

1 McCowen KC, Malhotra A, Bistian BR. Endocrine and metabolic dysfunction syndromes in the critically ill: stress-induced hyperglycemia. *Crit Care Clin* 2001;17:793–894.

2 Jacober SJ, Sowers JR. An update on perioperative management of diabetes. *Arch Intern Med* 1999;159:2405–11.

3 Liu SS, Carpenter RL, Mackey DC *et al.* Effects of perioperative analgesic technique on rate of recovery after colon surgery. *Anesthesiology* 1995;83:757–65.

4 Foster K, Alberti K, Binder C *et al.* Lipid metabolism and nitrogen balance after abdominal surgery in man. *Br J Surg* 1979;66:242–5.

5 Van den Berghe G, Wouters P, Weekers F *et al.* Intensive insulin therapy in critical ill patients. *N Engl J Med* 2001;345:1359–67.

6 Golden SH, Peart-Vigilance C, Kao WH, Brancati FL. Perioperative glycemiac control and the risk of infectious complications in a cohort of adults with diabetes. *Diabetes Care* 1999;22:1408–14.

7 Furnary AP, Zerr KJ, Grunkemeier GL, Starr A. Continuous intravenous insulin infusion reduces the incidence of deep sternal wound infection in diabetic patients after cardiac surgical procedures. *Ann Thorac Surg* 1999;67:352–60.

8 Golden SH, Peart-Vigilance C, Kao WH, Brancati FL. Perioperative glycemic control and the risk of infectious complications in a cohort of adults with diabetes. *Diabetes Care* 1999;22:1408–14.

9 Hirsch IB, McGill JB. Role of insulin in management of surgical patients with diabetes mellitus. *Diabetes Care* 1990;13:980–91.

10 Hirsch IB, McGill JB, Cryer PE, White PF. Perioperative management of surgical patients with diabetes mellitus. *Anesthesiology* 1991;74:346–59.

11 Rassias AJ, Marrin CA, Arruda J *et al.* Insulin infusion improves neutrophil function in diabetic cardiac surgery patients. *Anesth Analg* 1999;88:1011–16.

12 Levetan CS, Magee MF. Hospital management of diabetes. *Endocrinol Clin N Am* 2000;29:745–70.

13 Pezzarossa A, Taddei F, Cimicchi MG *et al.* Perioperative management of diabetic subjects: subcutaneous versus intravenous insulin administration during glucose-potassium infusion. *Diabetes Care* 1988;11:52–8.

14 Galloway JA, Spradlin CT, Howey DC, Dupre J. Intrasubject differences in pharmacokinetics and pharmacodynamic responses: the immutable problem of present-day treatment? *Diabetes* 1986; Excerpta Medica: 877–86.

15 American Diabetes Association. Direct and indirect costs of diabetes in the United States. American Diabetes Association www. diabetes.org/main

16 National Center for Health Statistics. Center for Disease Control, US Department of Health and Human Services. www.cdc.gov, visited 5 November 2002.

17 Levetan CS, Passaro M, Jablonski K. Unrecognized diabetes among hospitalized patients. *Diabetes Care* 1998;21:246–9.

18 Clarke RSJ, Johnston H, Sheridan N. The influence of anesthesia and surgery on plasma cortisol, insulin and free fatty acids. *Br J Anaesth* 1970;42:295–9.

19 McCowen KC, Malhotra A, Bistrian BR. Stress-induced hyperglycemia. *Crit Care Clin* 2001;17:107–24.

20 Mangano CM, Diamondstone LS, Ramsay JG *et al.* Renal dysfunction after myocardial revascularization: risk factors, adverse outcomes, and hospital resource utilization. The Multicenter Study of Perioperative Ischemia Research Group. *Ann Intern Med* 1998;128:194–203.

21 Barash PG, Cullen BF, Stoelting RK. *Clinical anesthesia.* 3rd edition. Philadelphia: Lippincott-Raven, 1997.

22 Mangano DT. Perioperative cardiac morbidity. *Anesthesiology* 1990;72:153–84.

23 Hjortrup A, Sorensen C, Dyremose E *et al.* Influence of diabetes on operative risk. *Br J Surg* 1985;72:785–7.

24 Harris MI. Health care and health status and outcomes for patients with type 2 diabetes. *Diabetes Care* 2000;23:754–8.

25 Haffner SM, Lehto S, Ronnemaa T *et al.* Mortality from coronary heart disease in subjects with type 2 diabetes and in nondiabetic subjects with and without prior myocardial infarction. *N Engl J Med* 1998;339:1714–5.

26 Daviglus ML, Stamler J. Major risk factors and coronary heart disease: much has been achieved but crucial challenges remain. *J Am Coll Cardiol* 2001;38:1012–7.

27 Steen PA, Tinker JH, Tarhan S. Myocardial reinfarction after anesthesia and surgery. *J Am Med Assoc* 1978;239:256.

28 Roghi A, Palmieri B, Crivellaro W *et al.* Relationship of unrecognized myocardial infarction, diabetes mellitus and type of surgery to postoperative cardiac outcomes in vascular surgery. *Eur J Vasc Endovasc Surg* 2001;21:9–16.

29 Dawood MM, Gutpa DK, Southern J *et al.* Pathology of fatal perioperative myocardial infarction: implications regarding pathophysiology and prevention. *Int J Cardiol* 1996;57:37–44.

30 Goldman L. Assessing and reducing cardiac risks of non-cardiac surgery. *Am J Med* 2001;110:260–6.

31 Cooperman M, Pflug B, Martin EW Jr, Evans WE. Cardiovascular risk factors in patients with peripheral vascular disease. *Surgery* 1978;84: 505–9.

32 Ashton CM, Wray NP. Preoperative assessment of patients with coronary disease. *N Engl J Med* 1996;334:1064–5.

33 Scanlon PJ, Faxon DP, Audet AM *et al.* ACC/AHA guidelines for coronary angiography. A report of the American College of Cardiology/American Heart Association Task Force on practice guidelines (Committee on Coronary Angiography). *J Am Coll Cardiol* 1999;33:1756–824.

34 Kiers L, Davis S, Larkins R. Stroke topography and outcome in relation to hyperglycemia and diabetes. *J Neurol Neurosurg Psychiatry* 1992;55: 263–70.

35 Schade DS. Surgery and diabetes. *Med Clin N Am* 1988;72:1531–43.

36 Farkas-Hirsch R, Boyle PJ, Hirsch IB. Glycemic control of the surgical patient with IDDM. *Diabetes* 1989;(Suppl 2); 39A.

37 Watts NB, Gebhart SP, Clark RV, Phillips RS. Perioperative management of diabetes mellitus: steady-state glucose control with bedside algorithm for insulin adjustment. *Diabetes Care* 1987;10:722–8.

38 Pomposelli JJ, Baxter JK 3rd, Babineau TJ *et al.* Early postoperative glucose control predicts nosocomial infection rate in diabetic patients. *J Parenteral Enteral Nutr* 1998;22:77–81.

39 Malmberg K, Ryden L, Efendic S. Randomized trial of insulin-glucose infusion followed by subcutaneous insulin treatment in diabetic patients with acute myocardial infarction (DIGAMI study): effects on mortality at 1 year. *J Am Coll Cardiol* 1995;26:57–65.

40 Capes SE, Hunt D, Malmberg K, Gerstein HC. Stress hyperglycaemia and increased risk of death after myocardial infarction in patients with and without diabetes: a systematic overview. *Lancet* 2000;355:773–8.

41 Kalin MF, Tranbaugh RF, Salas J. Intensive intervention by a diabetes team diminishes excess hospital mortality in patients with diabetes who undergo coronary artery bypass graft. *Diabetes* 1998;47:A87.

42 US Pharmacopoeia report. Summary of 1999 information submitted to MedMARx: A national database for hospital medication error reporting. www.usp.org

43 Dunnet JM, Holman RR, Turner RC, Sear JW. Diabetes mellitus and anesthesia: a summary of perioperative management of the patient with diabetes mellitus. *Anaesthesia* 1988;43:533–7.

44 Gill GV. Surgery in patients with diabetes mellitus. In: Pickup J, Williams G (ed). *Textbook of diabetes*. Oxford: Blackwell Science 1997:1–71.7.

45 Rosenstock J, Raskin P. Surgery: practical guidelines for diabetes management. *Clin Diabetes* 1987;5:49–61

46 Alberti KG, Gill GV, Elliott MJ. Insulin delivery during surgery in the diabetic patient. *Diabetes Care* 1982;5(Suppl 5):65–77.

47 Genuth SM. The automatic (regular insulin) sliding scale or 2, 4, 6, 8– call HO. *Clin Diabetes* 1994;12:40–2.

48 Albisser AM, Leibel BS, Ewart TG *et al.* An artificial endocrine pancreas. *Diabetes* 1974;23:389–96.

49 Alberti kgMM, Thomas DJB. The management of diabetes during surgery. *Br J Anaesth* 1979;51: 693–710.

50 Husband DJ, Tahi AC, Alberti KG. Management of diabetes during surgery with glucose-insulin-potassium infusion. *Diabetic Med* 1986;3:69–74.

51 Malling B, Knudsen L, Christiansen BA *et al.* Insulin treatment in non-insulin-dependent diabetic patients undergoing minor surgery. *Diabetes Nutr Metab* 1989;2:125–31.

28

Type 2 diabetes: geriatric considerations

Serge A Jabbour and Barry J Goldstein

INTRODUCTION

During the past decade, diabetes mellitus has received growing recognition as an important clinical and public health problem throughout the world. Recent surveys indicate that more than 16 million Americans (6% of the US population) have type 2 diabetes. Perhaps even more important is the finding that up to ~40% of affected individuals are unaware that they have the disease, even though they may have marked hyperglycemia and are at risk of developing the long-term complications of diabetes.

With advancing age, there is a tendency towards worsening glucose tolerance and a concomitant increased incidence of diabetes. The prevalence of known cases of diabetes increases from 6% for persons aged 45–64 years to 12% for those aged ≥ 65 years. Most patients with diabetes have type 2 diabetes, and nearly half of all persons known to have type 2 diabetes are older than 65 years[1]. Medical care for diabetic patients is extraordinarily costly; approximately two-thirds of all medical costs related to diabetes are attributable to the elderly. Expenses related to diabetes care have been estimated at $100 billion per year, accounting for 10–15% of all healthcare costs in the USA and 25% of all Medicare costs[2]. As the population ages, it is essential that all healthcare providers pay appropriate attention to the growing burden of this chronic disorder.

Diagnostic criteria

An expert panel established new criteria for the diagnosis of diabetes in June of 1997 (Table 28.1). These changes were made in response to updated epidemiological data showing that a fasting glucose value of ≥ 126 mg dL⁻¹ (compared with the previous value of 140 mg dL⁻¹) was a more accurate predictor of the glucose level that

---

Table 28.1 Diagnostic criteria for type 2 diabetes

Symptoms of diabetes (polyuria, polydipsia, unexplained weight loss) plus plasma glucose concentration ≥ 200 mg dL⁻¹ (11.1 mmol L⁻¹) at any time of day, without regard to time since last meal

Fasting plasma glucose level ≥ 126 mg dL⁻¹ (7.0 mmol L⁻¹)

2 h plasma glucose ≥ 200 mg dL⁻¹ during an oral glucose tolerance test (OGTT; 75 g oral glucose load)

In the absence of unequivocal hyperglycemia with acute metabolic decompensation, these criteria should be confirmed by repeat testing on a different day

The OGTT is not recommended for routine clinical use

has been closely associated with chronic microvascular complications (nephropathy and retinopathy) of diabetes[3]. The new fasting threshold glucose level was a better predictor of the 2 h value of 200 mg dL^{-1} obtained after the ingestion of 75 g of oral glucose during a standard glucose tolerance test (GTT), which has been the 'gold standard' for the diagnosis of diabetes for many years. The new criteria place a special emphasis on measuring the *fasting* glucose level, a more practical, efficient and less expensive alternative to the GTT, which, it turns out, rarely needs to be done in clinical practice.

Screening for diabetes

Since many individuals with blood glucose levels elevated into the diabetic range are undiagnosed, screening guidelines have been developed by the American Diabetes Association to assist practitioners with the clinical identification of patients that have asymptomatic disease (Table 28.2). As the prevalence of diabetes increases with age, all people over 45 years of age should be screened. Obese and ethnic

minority populations are at higher risk and should be especially targeted[4].

PATHOPHYSIOLOGY OF DIABETES

In order to maintain normal glucose levels in the blood circulation, insulin must be available and capable, through its cellular action, of promoting the uptake and metabolism (disposal) of glucose into skeletal muscle and adipose tissue. In addition, sufficient insulin action must occur in the liver to suppress hepatic glucose production, the major source of circulating glucose in the fasting state. Several pathophysiologic changes have been shown to precede the development of the hyperglycemia of type 2 diabetes[5,6]. One essential factor is the appearance of insulin resistance, a tissue abnormality characterized by defects in insulin action. Insulin resistance exists whenever insulin elicits less than the expected biological effect, and involves suppression of glucose production by the liver, as well as glucose disposal into muscle and fat tissue. Insulin resistance can be worsened by a variety of factors, most notably increases in the relative percentage of body adiposity and a sedentary lifestyle. In the elderly, the gradual loss of skeletal muscle mass with aging contributes to deficiencies in glucose disposal. Insulin resistance leads to a compensatory increase in the circulating insulin level, which overcomes the relative block in insulin action and prevents an increase in glucose levels.

Eventually, a defect affecting the secretion of insulin by the beta-cell impairs its ability to sustain the heightened level of insulin output required to balance tissue insulin resistance. When this occurs, the level of glucose begins to rise into the diabetic range. Initially, the lack of sufficient insulin in the bloodstream leads to an increase in post-meal glucose levels, due to a reduction in tissue glucose metabolism. A later effect is an increase in glucose production by the liver, especially in the fasting state, which is due to insufficient insulin action in this tissue. Thus, type 2 diabetics have three major pathophysiological features that provide a useful framework which allows us to design a 'stepped' therapeutic approach:

Table 28.2 Guidelines for screening of asymptomatic subjects for type 2 diabetes

All individuals ≥ 45 years of age; if normal, repeat every 3 years

Consider testing at a younger age or more frequently for high-risk individuals:

Obese (body mass index ≥ 27 kg m^{-2})

First-degree relative with diabetes

High-risk ethnic population (e.g., African–American, Asian, Hispanic, Native American)

Delivered a baby weighing > 9 lb or have had gestational diabetes

Hypertensive (≥ 140/90 mm Hg)

HDL-C level ≤ 35 mg dL^{-1} and/or a triglyceride level ≥ 250 mg dL^{-1}

Impaired glucose tolerance or impaired fasting glucose (110–126 mg dL^{-1}) on previous testing

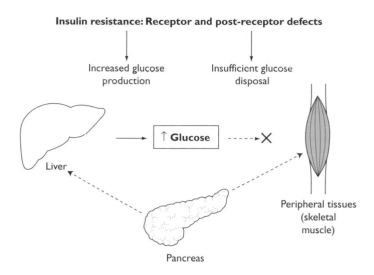

Insulin resistance: Receptor and post-receptor defects

Increased glucose production

Insufficient glucose disposal

↑ Glucose ----→ X

Liver

Pancreas

Impaired insulin secretion

Peripheral tissues (skeletal muscle)

Figure 28.1 Sites of the three major pathogenic defects that lead to type 2 diabetes. Insulin resistance in muscle causes reduced glucose disposal from the bloodstream and insulin resistance in liver causes increased glucose production. Impaired insulin secretion by the pancreatic beta cells is a critical feature that leads to hyperglycemia when the amount of insulin secreted and the timing of the insulin response to glucose are defective.

- Impaired beta-cell function
- Insulin resistance with increased glucose output by the liver
- Insulin resistance with defective glucose disposal after meals in muscle and fat tissue (Figure 28.1).

CLINICAL PRESENTATION OF TYPE 2 DIABETES IN THE ELDERLY

The clinical presentation of diabetes mellitus in the elderly can sometimes be confounded[7,8]. At one extreme, patients may be completely asymptomatic, while at the other extreme they may present with hyperosmolar coma, because thirst perception is decreased and dehydration can occur rapidly with rising hyperglycemia. Thus, attention should be paid to screening older individuals at risk for diabetes, as mentioned above, in order to detect diabetes at an earlier, less symptomatic stage. When symptomatic, elderly patients may not present with the classic symptoms of polyuria, polydipsia and polyphagia, but rather with more generalized symptoms, such as weight loss or fatigue associated with increasing nocturia. Presentation with bacterial or fungal infections of the skin or genitourinary tract that are mild but slow to heal may provide a clinical clue to a hyperglycemic state[9]. Diabetes in older people is insidious and patients may therefore present with an established complication that may have developed over many years.

COMPLICATIONS OF TYPE 2 DIABETES IN THE ELDERLY

Complications of type 2 diabetes in the elderly can involve macrovascular disease (cardiovascular, cerebrovascular or peripheral vascular disease) or microvascular processes, such as retinopathy, nephropathy and neuropathy. Atherosclerosis in patients with diabetes is closely linked to insulin resistance, which is accompanied by a constellation of cardiovascular risk factors that comprise the 'insulin resistance' (IRS) or 'metabolic' syndrome (Table 28.3). The underlying basis of these diverse signs and laboratory findings is not well understood, but they have in common their propensity to enhance large vessel atherosclerosis, leading to coronary artery disease and stroke[10].

Since patients with diabetes frequently also harbor many additional risk factors, the overall approach to patient management must include adequate attention to the control of these clinical variables, such as obesity, smoking, hypertension, dyslipidemia and physical inactivity.

Table 28.3 Clinical features of IRS ('Syndrome X')

Abdominal obesity

Acanthosis nigricans

Hypertension

Dyslipidemia (small, dense LDL, high triglycerides, low HDL)

Hyperuricemia

Coagulation system abnormalities (high PAI-1 levels)

Impaired glucose tolerance

Hyperinsulinemia

Aggressive treatment of hyperlipidemia in the elderly diabetic is no longer controversial; in the Cholesterol and Recurrent Events (CARE) trial, aggressive cholesterol lowering with statin therapy significantly reduced the risk of major coronary events, coronary death and stroke over a 5-year period in patients ≥ 65 years who had a previous myocardial infarction but average blood cholesterol levels[11].

Diabetic nephropathy and neuropathy both develop more frequently in older patients with type 2 diabetes. As in younger patients, microalbuminuria is the first indication of nephropathy and is followed by proteinuria. Early intervention with ACE inhibitors, as well as improved blood pressure and glycemic control, can significantly slow the rate of decline in renal function[12]. Elderly patients with compromised renal function should be evaluated for other renal abnormalities, including genitourinary tract obstructions and infections, which are more common in this population[9].

Diabetic neuropathy is also common in elderly patients with type 2 diabetes. The most common manifestations are paresthesias, tingling, burning, and diminished pain sensation, primarily in the feet, which may lead to ulceration, infection and, eventually, gangrene and ultimately amputation if significant peripheral vascular disease is present[9].

Diabetic retinopathy is the leading cause of blindness in patients with type 2 diabetes in the USA[2,9]. Older patients with diabetes are also at increased risk of blindness as a result of glaucoma, cataracts and macular degeneration. Regular ophthalmological evaluation, at least once per year, is essential.

Elderly patients with diabetes often experience gastroparesis, a reduction in gastric motility with delayed emptying[13]. Gastroparesis may cause unexpected postprandial hyperglycemia and changes in insulin requirements.

APPROACH TO DIABETES CONTROL

The principles of treatment for diabetes in elderly patients are similar to those in younger patients; however, modifications according to comorbidities associated with aging are often necessary. The general principles of diabetes disease management are to normalize the derangements in glucose metabolism and other cardiovascular risk factors as much as possible. The American Diabetes Association has provided a consensus of treatment goals for all patients with diabetes (Table 28.4). Aggressive control of blood glucose has been repeatedly shown in a variety of clinical studies to significantly delay the onset, or slow the progression of the microvascular complications of both type 1 and type 2 diabetes[15,16]. Some of the most relevant data for type 2 diabetes come from the UK Prospective Diabetes Study (UKPDS), which studied more than 5000 patients with type 2 diabetes, some for over 10 years of follow-up. This study demonstrated that even an apparently modest lowering of the glycosylated hemoglobin (HbA1c) (from 7.9% to 7.0%) using intensive glucose management had a beneficial effect in reducing the risk of diabetes-related microvascular complications, as well as a strong tendency towards reducing the risk of cardiovascular events. This study also provided important insight into the natural history of the progression of type 2 diabetes over time.

The UKPDS also demonstrated that most patients experience a gradual failure of beta-cell insulin secretion over time. This defect results in the need to use progressively more potent

Table 28.4 Treatment goals for type 2 diabetes	
Parameter	**Therapeutic goal**[a]
Body mass index	< 25 kg m^{-2}
Blood pressure	< 130/80–85
Plasma glucose	
Fasting	80–120 mg dL^{-1}
Postprandial (2 h)	< 160 mg dL^{-1}
HbA1c	< 7%
Total cholesterol	< 200
HDL-C	> 45
LDL-C	< 100–130[a]
Triglycerides	< 150–200[a]

[a] Target may be adjusted based on the presence of additional cardiovascular risk factors, especially in elderly subjects[14].

combinations of oral medications, and in the eventual requirement for insulin injections in many patients to maintain glucose control[17]. This 'stepped' approach to diabetes therapy to maintain control has been the experience of many practitioners, although the understanding that it is caused by beta-cell failure in the pancreas has only recently been widely appreciated.

Diet and weight reduction

Any treatment plan should begin with non-pharmacologic measures that also help to reduce insulin resistance: caloric restriction, weight reduction if necessary and aerobic exercise. Dietary modification can improve many aspects of type 2 diabetes, including obesity, hypertension, and insulin resistance. The improvement in glycemic control is related to the degree of both caloric restriction and weight reduction[18,19]. A low caloric diet can lead to a substantial reduction in fasting blood glucose and improved sensitivity within as little as 5 days, well before significant weight reduction occurs[18]. However,

this benefit will persist only if negative caloric balance leads to weight reduction.

Patients and practitioners should recognize that weight loss of ~7–10% of initial body weight will result in significant improvement in insulin resistance and enhancement of beta-cell sensitivity to the glucose stimulation of insulin release[18]. Many other related clinical abnormalities will also improve at this level of weight reduction, such as blood pressure and lipid abnormalities. The practical importance of these observations is the realization that extensive weight loss, towards an 'ideal body weight', is difficult or impossible to achieve in most cases and should not be regarded as an essential management goal. A weight reduction of 10 or 15 pounds is a reasonable goal for weight loss that will yield substantial clinical benefits[18,20]. However, it is important to remember that in elderly patients, swallowing difficulties, poor dentition, or ill-fitting dentures that cause discomfort when eating may restrict the diet.

Exercise

Exercise enhances insulin sensitivity and promotes the non-insulin-mediated uptake of glucose into muscle tissue. In the elderly, exercise also helps to maintain overall muscle mass. These beneficial effects can help to control blood glucose in diabetes, as well as delay the progression of impaired glucose tolerance to overt diabetes[21].

When recommending an exercise program to elderly patients, clinicians need to be cautious in evaluating the possibility that patients who have been sedentary may have underlying cardiovascular disease. Patients with the following risk factors should be considered for a cardiac evaluation: age > 35 years, type 2 diabetes of > 10 years' duration, presence of any traditional risk factors for coronary artery disease, presence of microvascular disease (retinopathy or nephropathy, including microalbuminuria), peripheral vascular disease, or autonomic neuropathy[22]. A useful test for cardiac evaluation is a treadmill stress test, with a simultaneous echocardiographic study to determine the presence of ECG abnormalities, as well as potential cardiac-wall motion defects.

Pharmacologic measures

Many oral agents are currently available for treating diabetics (Figure 28.2). The utility of these classes of anti-diabetic agents is enhanced by their different mechanisms of action, which target specific underlying defects in the patho-physiology of type 2 diabetes. These comple-mentary mechanisms allow treatments to be used strategically in various combinations, many of which have been studied in well-designed clinical trials.

Sulfonylureas

Sulfonylureas are still the most widely used drugs for the treatment of type 2 diabetes[23]. The binding of a sulfonylurea drug to a specific protein in the pancreatic beta-cells leads to changes in the fluxes of specific ions and a stim-ulation of insulin secretion at all blood glucose concentrations[24]. Sulfonylureas work best early in the course of diabetes, when sufficient beta-cell function is still present to respond to the stimulation of insulin secretion promoted by these drugs. Approximately 15–20% of patients started on therapy with a sulfonylurea will not have an adequate initial therapeutic response. The rate of secondary failure is approximately 5–10% per year among people who respond initially. The secondary failure rate may reflect

the natural history of type 2 diabetes, with beta-cell function diminishing; sulfonylureas act primarily on beta-cell function[25].

Sulfonylureas do not alleviate the block to insulin action characteristic of the underlying insulin resistance in type 2 diabetes, and evidence is scant to support claims that sulfony-lureas have any clinical extrapancreatic effects. They generally lower blood glucose concentra-tion by about 20%[23,26]. The dose–response of any sulfonylurea agent levels off at or below the middle of the approved dose range. Increasing the dose further simply prolongs the duration of the drug in the circulation, which may be hazardous in the elderly, potentially worsening the possibility of hypoglycemia[27]. One of the major advantages of the sulfonylureas is their capacity to act quickly in responsive patients, generally within a few days of initiating therapy. This is in contrast to the clinical use of metformin, alpha-glucosidase inhibitors, and thiazolidinediones, which may take from a few weeks to several months for a full therapeutic response.

Sulfonylureas are usually well-tolerated, with the exception of hypoglycemia, which occurs more frequently with the longer-acting drugs in the elderly population. However, a 4-year retrospec-tive study of 14 000 patients ≥ 65 years with type 2 diabetes treated with different sulfonylureas

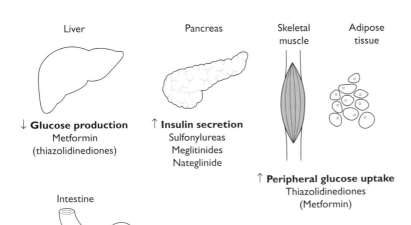

Figure 28.2 Site of action of available oral agents to treat type 2 diabetes. As shown in parentheses, secondary sites of action exist for thiazolidinediones (liver glucose production) and for metformin (peripheral glucose uptake).

showed that episodes of serious hypoglycemia (associated with stroke, myocardial infarction, or death) were rare[28]. The incidence was highest in those patients taking glyburide or chlorpropamide, with fewer episodes in patients taking glipizide GITS or glimepiride[26]. Hypoglycemia in the elderly population can cause dizziness, or mental status changes leading to an accident or fall, with potentially serious consequences. Hypoglycemia with release of adrenaline can also contribute to myocardial ischemia or infarction. Factors that can increase the risk of hypoglycemia include: missed meals, exercise, advanced age, poor nutrition, alcohol abuse, impaired renal or liver function, and concurrent therapy with specific drugs, such as salicylates, sulfonamides, fibrates, and warfarin[29].

In elderly patients with diabetes, it is prudent to increase the dosage of sulfonylurea slowly, using preferably the newer agents, glipizide GITS or glimepiride. Chlorpropamide should especially be avoided because of its prolonged half-life (~36 h), as well as the unique side effects of alcohol-related flushing and the potential for hyponatremia by its effect on the action of antidiuretic hormone[30,31].

Repaglinide

Repaglinide is the first agent from a new class of oral agents called meglitinides. Repaglinide is a benzoic acid derivative that is chemically unrelated to sulfonylureas but acts in a similar way, by enhancing the secretion of insulin from the pancreatic beta-cells. Studies have suggested that the amount of insulin release elicited by repaglinide is reduced at lower glucose concentrations, which may offer some relative protection against hypoglycemia. The major clinical advantage of repaglinide is its rapid onset and short duration of action, which necessitates it being taken 30 min before each meal. The limited duration of action (3–4 h) results in less hypoglycemia between meals. The practical clinical benefit is in patients who require additional insulin secretion, but who would like to avoid hypoglycemia when they choose to skip a meal[32]. This is helpful with patients who have erratic schedules, as well as for those who are trying to reduce their daily caloric intake.

Repaglinide is indicated for monotherapy, or in combination with metformin. Repaglinide should not be taken with sulfonylureas as it has a similar mechanism of action. The recommended dose range is 0.5–4 mg prior to each meal, up to a maximum of 16 mg per day. It should be used cautiously in patients with hepatic or renal dysfunction, and the lower dose range is more appropriate for initiation of therapy in the elderly[33].

Nateglinide

Nateglinide is another new insulin secretion enhancer that is structurally different from repaglinide and the sulfonylureas, and has an additional beneficial effect on the rapid first phase of insulin secretion. Like repaglinide, it is rapidly absorbed and works quickly, so it needs to be taken prior to each meal at doses of 60–120 mg three times a day. No dosage adjustment is necessary in patients with mild-to-severe renal insufficiency, or in patients with mild hepatic insufficiency. Dosing in patients with moderate-to-severe liver disease has not been studied; nateglinide should therefore be used with caution in these patients[34].

Metformin

Metformin has been used worldwide for decades and is a mainstay of therapy for type 2 diabetes[35,36]. The major clinical benefit of metformin is derived from its hepatic effect, which lowers blood glucose production. Secondarily, this leads to a reduced demand for insulin secretion by the pancreas, and a lowering of circulating insulin levels. Since metformin works independently of the pancreas, when used as monotherapy it does not cause hypoglycemia. When used in combination with drugs that increase blood insulin levels, however, including sulfonylureas, repaglinide or insulin, the addition of metformin can lead to hypoglycemia.

Metformin promotes modest weight reduction, or at least weight stabilization, providing an additional rationale for its use in obese type 2 diabetes[25,36,37]. This is in contrast to the weight gain seen in patients taking insulin, some sulfonylureas, or thiazolidinediones[10,15,38]. Metformin typically lowers blood glucose concentrations by approximately 20%, a response similar to that achieved with a sulfonylurea[25,36]. Given in combination with a sulfonylurea, metformin lowers blood glucose concentrations more than either drug alone[25]. Another advantage of metformin over the sulfonylureas is that some studies have shown a beneficial lipid-lowering activity, with reduction in triglyceride and free fatty acid (FFA) concentrations, a small reduction in serum low-density lipoprotein (LDL) cholesterol and a slight elevation in serum high-density lipoprotein (HDL) cholesterol[39].

Metformin should be started at a dose of 500 mg taken with dinner, and increased to twice a day, taken with meals, after a period of 5–7 days. After several weeks, the clinical response can be assessed before implementing a further increase in the dose. The dose of 1 g metformin taken twice a day has been shown to provide maximal clinical benefit[40].

The most common side effects that can limit the clinical use of metformin involve the gastrointestinal tract. These occur in 30% of patients, and lead to discontinuation of therapy in 4%. Diarrhea is most common, and some patients have nausea, vomiting, bloating, flatulence and anorexia. In most cases, these effects are mild to moderate and self-limited. They can be minimized by slow titration of the drug, dosing with meals, or with dose reduction if necessary.

The major contraindication for metformin use is renal dysfunction: serum creatinine ≥ 1.5 mg dL^{-1} in males or ≥ 1.4 mg dL^{-1} in females. A creatinine clearance of at least 60 mL min^{-1} should be documented in an elderly patient before initiating metformin therapy. However, blood creatinine levels may be an unreliable indicator of the creatinine clearance in the elderly because of their decreased lean body (skeletal muscle) mass. Other absolute or relative contraindications include: congestive heart failure requiring pharmacologic treatment because of reduced renal excretion; current liver disease or alcohol abuse; severe infection with decreased tissue perfusion; hypoxic states; serious acute illness; or hemodynamic instability. Metformin should be withheld up to 48 h after use of iodinated contrast material for radiologic studies, and until a normal blood creatinine level is documented[36,41].

Metformin should be used with caution in patients > 75 years, because of the physiologic decline in creatinine clearance with aging. If allowed to accumulate, metformin affects mitochondrial energy metabolism, which can lead to lactic acidosis. When metformin is used properly, this complication is extraordinarily rare, with an incidence of 0.03 cases per 1000 patient-years, but it can be quite serious, leading to death in ~50% of cases. A lower maximal dose, of 500 mg twice a day, or 850 mg once per day, should be considered in elderly patients because of the expected decline in renal function and loss of lean body mass with aging. Patients on metformin should have regular monitoring of blood creatinine levels indicating renal function; however, monitoring of blood lactate levels is not useful. A potential drug interaction exists between metformin and cimetidine, which can lower the renal clearance of metformin by ~27%, due to inhibition of the renal tubular secretion of metformin[42]. This interaction could increase the risk of hypoglycemia in patients taking metformin plus a sulfonylurea or insulin, and could increase the risk of lactic acidosis in those with impaired renal function.

Thiazolidinediones

The thiazolidinediones are true insulin sensitizers that act primarily by augmenting the effects of insulin in peripheral tissues[38,43]. They do not work in the absence of insulin and bind specifically to a class of receptors in the cell nucleus called peroxisome proliferator-activated receptor gamma (PPAR-gamma)[44]. This interaction generates a signal that leads to a change in the expression of a number of gene products which affect fat and muscle cell function. The clinical effect of the thiazolidinediones requires alterations in the complex relationship between lipid and glucose metabolism, especially the effects of FFA on liver glucose production and insulin action in muscle cells. The clinical effectiveness of these compounds may be delayed for a period of up to 4–6 weeks, and may not fully manifest for up to 12 weeks[45].

As expected from their mechanism of action, the thiazolidinediones enhance glucose control, while at the same time actually lowering circulating insulin levels. Since their effects are independent of the pancreas, hypoglycemia is unlikely when thiazolidinediones are used as monotherapy or in combination with metformin, since they also lower circulating insulin levels. In combination with insulin, sulfonylureas or meglitinides—drugs that will increase insulin levels in the bloodstream—the use of thiazolidinediones and metformin can cause low blood glucose reactions.

Two thiazolidinediones, rosiglitazone and pioglitazone, are currently available in much of the world. Clinical doses range from 4–8 mg day^{-1} for rosiglitazone and 15–45 mg day^{-1} for pioglitazone. Although controlled clinical trials and worldwide use of these thiazolidinediones has not demonstrated any evidence of hepatic toxicity, it remains the FDA recommendation that alanine aminotransferase (ALT) testing be performed at baseline, followed by repeated tests every other month for the first year, and then periodically thereafter. These recommendations are based on experience with troglitazone, the first clinically available thiazolidinedione, which had significant adverse hepatic effects and has now been removed from the market. Nevertheless, because of their hepatic metabolism, thiazolidinediones should not be given to patients with known liver disease or alcoholics, and they should not be initiated if the baseline ALT is elevated to > 2.5 times the upper limit of normal. There are no concerns regarding their use in patients with renal insufficiency.

Rosiglitazone has been carefully studied in a population of elderly patients with type 2 diabetes in two randomized, double-blind, placebo-controlled trials, demonstrating that the drug was effective and well-tolerated[46]. In these two 26-week trials, rosiglitazone produced similar treatment effects on lowering fasting plasma glucose and HbA1c in patients aged ≥ 65 years when compared with those younger than 65 years. Therapeutic responses of up to a 79 mg dL^{-1} decrease in fasting glucose and up to 1.6 percentage points drop in HbA1c were observed in patients taking the higher daily dose. This study tracked data on 2526 patients who received rosiglitazone monotherapy in double-blind studies, of which 33% were ≥ 65

years. The incidence of adverse events was similar in patients older or younger than 65 years; however, dependent edema was twice as common in the older age group.

Use of all thiazolidinediones can lead to fluid retention in susceptible patients and therefore they should be used with caution—if at all—in patients with moderate to severe (NYHA Class III–IV) heart failure. Pioglitazone may also have drug interactions with compounds metabolized by the 3A4 P450 system, which may enhance the metabolism of statins and other drugs. Rosiglitazone does not affect the function of the 3A4 system and does not influence the metabolism of these and related compounds.

Since rosiglitazone and pioglitazone can be used as monotherapy, they might be the treatment of choice in older diabetics with mild hyperglycemia, because of the lack of hypoglycemic effect. Advantages of the thiazolidinediones, when compared with metformin, include the lack of gastrointestinal side effects and no restrictions on the use of these drugs in patients with renal insufficiency. The role of thiazolidinediones as insulin sensitizers also has advantages; their effects in reversing a number of the features of the insulin resistance syndrome may eventually be shown in clinical trials to improve cardiovascular outcomes in patients with type 2 diabetes.

Alpha-glucosidase inhibitors
These drugs inhibit gastrointestinal enzymes that convert dietary complex carbohydrates into monosaccharides. In this way, the alpha-glucosidase inhibitors slow the absorption of glucose and delay the appearance of postprandial glucose in the bloodstream. They can be effective in patients with type 2 diabetes treated with diet, or in combination with any other drug modality used for diabetes management[47].

Two drugs are available: acarbose and miglitol. In the UKPDS and other trials, the addition of acarbose elicited only a modest fall in the HbA1c, of 0.5%. There is no risk of hypoglycemia when acarbose or miglitol are used alone[48], which makes them suitable for use in older diabetics. The main disadvantages of these drugs are gastrointestinal side effects, including flatulence, abdominal cramping, diarrhea and, rarely, nausea or vomiting. As the drug delays the absorption of complex carbohydrates, these dietary components can appear in the colon, where enteric bacteria use the carbohydrates as metabolic fuel with gaseous by-products. In some patients, these side effects are mild and can, in general, be minimized if the drug is slowly titrated by increasing the dose slowly over several weeks. They should be used cautiously for patients with a history of gastrointestinal illness, and not at all in patients with active gastrointestinal disease. Rare cases of transaminase elevation have been documented, especially with doses > 300 mg day^{-1}. The liver-enzyme changes are reversible on withdrawal of the drug[47]. ALT should be measured every 3 months during the first year of therapy.

These drugs are given three times a day, at the start of each main meal, starting at a dose of 25 mg day^{-1}, gradually increasing to the maintenance dose in the range of 50–100 mg three times a day.

Insulin therapy in type 2 diabetes

The best approach to the underlying disorder in most patients with type 2 diabetes, who are obese and insulin resistant, is to enhance their insulin sensitivity, encouraging lifestyle changes and the use of insulin-sparing drugs (thiazolidinediones and metformin) whenever possible. This strategy is usually also helpful in the elderly. Patients who are not overweight, or who have recently involuntarily lost weight, may be relatively insulin deficient and could benefit from sulfonylureas as initial therapy. Insulin as the initial therapy is generally reserved for unusual patients with marked, symptomatic hyperglycemia at presentation (> 300 mg dL^{-1}), accompanied by other catabolic features such as marked weight loss, polyuria and polydipsia. Insulin is also indicated in combination with oral agents when these drugs appear to lose their potency over time, primarily because of failure of beta-cell insulin secretion[49].

Transient insulin therapy is also important to consider in patients who have experienced an acute deterioration of glycemic control due to injury, stress or infection. Such patients may present with severe hyperglycemia, dehydration, and uncontrolled weight loss. Ketonuria may be present, but usually there is no anion gap acidosis or significant ketone levels in the blood. Insulin should also be considered in the management of patients with type 2 diabetes during surgery or pregnancy, or for patients with significant liver or kidney disease, where it may not be safe to use certain oral agents.

Patients already on multiple oral agents who require more stringent glycemic control can often benefit from the addition of bedtime intermediate-acting insulin (NPH or Lente) at an approximate dose of 0.25 units kg^{-1}, or preferably glargine at a starting dose of 10 U at bedtime. If this is not sufficiently effective, patients can be switched to two injections of premixed insulin a day (70% NPH/30% regular, or preferably 75% NPL/25% lispro) at a dose of 0.5 U kg^{-1} per day, divided into two-thirds in the morning (30 min before breakfast with 70/30 and within 15 min before breakfast with 75/25), and one-third in the evening (30 min before dinner with 70/30 and within 15 min before dinner with 75/25). Metformin, or especially thiazolidinediones, are added to the regimen (or kept if the patient is already taking these drugs) to enhance glycemic control. They are preferred over sulfonylureas in combination with insulin.

SPECIAL CONSIDERATIONS

Several additional aspects of the management of the older patient with diabetes deserve special consideration. An increased frequency of depression, anxiety, and cognitive dysfunction has been reported in older patients with diabetes[7]. Depression needs to be recognized and treated aggressively, not only to improve compliance but also to reduce the risk of suicide. Antidepressants with increased anticholinergic activity, e.g. imipramine, amitriptyline and paroxetine, should be avoided because they may interact with autonomic dysfunction already present in many older diabetic patients, to cause orthostatic hypotension and urinary retention. In diabetes, desipramine, nortriptyline and sertraline appear to be the most appropriate antidepressants to use[8].

Elevated glucose levels result in osmotic diuresis, which can be associated with the development of incontinence. Hyperglycemia and glycosuria can also lead to nocturia and disturbed sleep. Pressure ulcers, foot lesions, painful shoulder periarthrosis and diabetic amyotrophy are seen with increased frequency in older diabetics, and should be sought on physical examinations[7]. Older patients with diabetes are also at increased risk of developing atypical infections, especially tuberculosis.

SUMMARY

While the basic principles of diabetes management used for the general population also apply to the treatment of this disease in the elderly, a number of special considerations should be taken into account (Table 28.5). Since the justification for tight glucose goals are based on the concern in most patients for the development of complications over many years and decades, these guidelines may be raised somewhat in elderly patients who may not have had diabetes for many years. Thus, the long-term benefit of aggressive diabetes control in an elderly patient with well-documented, new onset diabetes with no early signs of complications, including retinopathy and microalbuminuria, may be questioned, especially if that patient has a limited life expectancy.

In diabetes management, basic non-pharmacological principles should always be emphasized, with diet playing an important role. Exercise, to the safest extent possible, should also be encouraged to build and maintain skeletal muscle mass, which is a crucial aspect of glucose metabolism and disposal. Unfortunately, in many patients, the ability to exercise is hindered by loss of mobility due to osteoarthritis, as well as a long list of other co-morbidities affecting neurological and cardiovascular function. With drug therapy or exercise, hypoglycemia should be carefully avoided in the elderly because of the propensity for low blood glucose to cause mental status changes or dizziness, leading to falls or even myocardial ischemia if adrenergic counter-regulation is activated. The initial choice of drugs should employ agents that do not cause hypoglycemia, such as thiazolidinediones, which are well-tolerated and effective in the elderly, and metformin, which may be limited where patients have renal insufficiency.

Since the insulin-sparing agents work only with sufficient insulin being supplied from the pancreas, there may be a gradual decline in their effectiveness, as relative insulin deficiency sets in over time. In patients with overt hyperglycemia, especially when accompanied by weight loss, the appropriate use of insulin should not be delayed.

Table 28.5 Special considerations for diabetes management in the elderly

Diagnosis	Recognition of worsening glucose tolerance with aging that contributes to the increasing incidence of type 2 diabetes in the elderly population
	Use of screening guidelines to help uncover diabetes at its earliest, asymptomatic stages
Treatment	Use of diet and exercise to help improve insulin resistance and maintain lean body mass
	Avoidance of hypoglycemia when choosing drug therapy
	Prevent mental status change and adrenergic discharge during low blood glucose
	Thiazolidinediones are safe and well-tolerated in the elderly
	Alpha-glucosidase inhibitors are safe but limited by potential gastrointestinal side-effects
	Use of metformin will also avoid hypoglycemia, however, loss of glomerular filtration with aging and decline in renal function needs to be considered
	If employed, short-acting insulin secretagogues and newer agents (repaglinide, glipizide GITS, glimepiride) are safest; avoid chlorpropamide and other insulin secretagogues with long half-lives

REFERENCES

1 Gossain VV, Carella MJ, Rovner DR. Management of diabetes in the elderly: a clinical perspective. *J Assoc Acad Minority Phys* 1994;5:22–31.

2 Roman SH, Harris MI. Management of diabetes mellitus from a public health perspective. *Endocrinol Clin N Am* 1997;26:443–74.

3 American Diabetes Association: Report of the Expert Committee on the Diagnosis and Classification of Diabetes Mellitus. *Diabetes Care* 1997;20:1183–97.

4 American Diabetes Association: Screening for type 2 diabetes. *Diabetes Care* 1999;22(Suppl 1):20–3.

5 Kruszynska YT, Olefsky JM. Cellular and molecular mechanisms of non-insulin dependent diabetes mellitus. *J Invest Med* 1996;44:413–28.

6 Polonsky KS, Sturis J, Bell GI. Non-insulin dependent diabetes mellitus—a genetically programmed failure of the beta cell to compensate for insulin resistance. *N Engl J Med* 1996;334:777–83.

7 Samos FL, Roos BA. Diabetes mellitus in older persons. *Med Clin N Am* 1998;82:791–803.

8 Morley JE. The elderly type 2 diabetic patient: special considerations. *Diabet Med* 1998;15(Suppl 4): 41–6.

9 Rosenstock J. Management of type 2 diabetes mellitus in the elderly. *Drugs Aging* 2001;18:31–44.

10 Reaven GM. Insulin resistance and human disease. *J Basic Clin Physiol Pharmacol* 1998; 9:387–406.

11 Lewis SJ, Moye LA, Sacks FM *et al.* Effect of pravastatin on cardiovascular events in older patients with myocardial infarction and cholesterol levels in the average range: results of the Cholesterol and Recurrent Events (CARE) trial. *Ann Intern Med* 1998;129:681–9.

12 Heart Outcomes Prevention Evaluation Study Investigators. Effects of ramipril on cardiovascular and microvascular outcomes in people with diabetes mellitus: results of the HOPE study and MICRO-HOPE substudy. *Lancet* 2000;22:253–9.

13 Singh I, Marshall Jr MC. Diabetes mellitus in the elderly. *Endocrinol Metab Clin N Am* 1995;24:255–72.

14 American Diabetes Association. Clinical practice recommendations 1996. *Diabetes Care* 1996;19 (Suppl 1):S1–118.

15 DCCT Study Group: The effect of intensive treatment of diabetes on the development and progression of long-term complications in insulin-dependent diabetes mellitus. *N Engl J Med* 1993;329:977–86.

16 UK Prospective Diabetes Study (UKPDS) Group. Intensive blood-glucose control with sulphonylureas or insulin compared with conventional treatment and risk of complications in patients with type 2 diabetes. *Lancet* 1998;352:837–53.

17 American Diabetes Association. Implications of the United Kingdom prospective diabetes study. *Diabetes Care* 1999;22:S27–S31.

18 Henry RR, Schaeffer L, Olefsky JM. Glycemic effects of intensive caloric restriction and isocaloric refeeding in non-insulin-dependent diabetes mellitus. *J Clin Endocrinol Metab* 1985;61:917–25.

19 Wing RR, Blair EH, Bononi P *et al.* Caloric restriction *per se* is a significant factor in improvements in glycemic control and insulin sensitivity during weight loss in obese NIDDM patients. *Diabetes Care* 1994;17:30–6.

20 Niskanen LK, Uusitupa MI, Sarlund H *et al.* Five-year follow-up study on plasma insulin levels in newly diagnosed NIDDM patients and non-diabetic subjects. *Diabetes Care* 1990;13:41–8.

21 Diabetes Prevention Program Research Group. Reduction in the incidence of type 2 diabetes with lifestyle intervention or metformin. *N Engl J Med* 2002;346:393–403.

22 American Diabetes Association. Diabetes mellitus and exercise. *Diabetes Care* 1999;22:S49–S53.

23 Bressler R, Johnson DG. Pharmacological regulation of blood glucose levels in non-insulin-dependent diabetes mellitus. *Arch Intern Med* 1997;157:836–48.

24 Zimmerman BR. Sulfonylureas. *Endocrin Clin N Am* 1997;26:511–22.

25 Hermann LS, Schersten B, Bitzen PO *et al.* Therapeutic comparison of metformin and sulfonylurea, alone and in various combinations. A double-blind controlled study. *Diabetes Care* 1994;17:1100–9.

26 Shorr RI, Ray WA, Daugherty JR *et al.* Individual sulfonylureas and serious hypoglycemia in older people. *J Am Geriat Soc* 1996;44:751–5.

27 Stenman S, Melander A, Groop PH, Groop LC. What is the benefit of increasing the sulfonylurea dose? *Ann Intern Med* 1993;118:169–72.

28 Shorr RI, Ray WA, Daugherty JR *et al.* Incidence and risk factors for serious hypoglycemia in older persons using insulin or sulfonylureas. *Arch Intern Med* 1997;157:1681–6.

29 Bressler P, DeFronzo RA. Drugs and diabetes. *Diabetes Rev* 1994;2:53.

30 Groop L, Eriksson CJ, Huupponen R *et al.* Roles of chlorpropamide, alcohol and acetaldehyde in determining the chlorpropamide-alcohol flush. *Diabetologia* 1984;26:34–8.

31 Kadowaki T, Hagura R, Kajinuma H *et al.* Chlorpropamide-induced hyponatremia. Incidence and risk factors. *Diabetes Care* 1983;6: 468–71.

32 Owens DR. Repaglinide: a new short-acting insulinotropic agent for the treatment of type 2 diabetes. *Eur J Clin Invest* 1999;29(Suppl.2):30–37.

33 Goldberg RB, Einhorn D, Lucas CF *et al.* A randomized placebo-controlled trial of repaglinide in the treatment of type 2 diabetes. *Diabetes Care* 1998;21:1897–903.

34 Hollander PA, Schwartz SL, Gatlin MR *et al.* Importance of early insulin secretion: Comparison of nateglinide and glyburide in previously diet-treated patients with type 2 diabetes. *Diabetes Care* 2001;24: 983–8.

35 Bell PM, Hadden DR. Metformin. *Endocrinol Clin N Am* 1997;26:523–37.

36 Bailey CJ, Turner RC. Drug therapy: metformin. *N Engl J Med* 1996;334:574–9.

37 United Kingdom Prospective Diabetes Study Group. UKPDS 13: relative efficacy of randomly allocated diet, sulphonylureas, insulin, or metformin in patients with newly diagnosed non-insulin-dependent diabetes followed for three years. *Br Med J* 1995;310:83–8.

38 Henry RR. Thiazolidinediones. *Endocrinol Clin N Am* 1997;26:553–73.

39 DeFronzo RA, Goodman AM, and the Multicenter Metformin Study Group. Efficacy of metformin in patients with non-insulin-dependent diabetes mellitus. *N Engl J Med* 1995;333:541–9.

40 Garber AJ, Duncan TG, Goodman AM *et al.* Efficacy of metformin in type 2 diabetes—results of a double-blind, placebo-controlled, dose-response trial. *Am J Med* 1997;103:491–7.

41 Gan SC, Barr J, Arieff AI, Pearl RG. Biguanide-associated lactic acidosis: case report and review of the literature. *Arch Intern Med* 1992;152:2333–6.

42 Somogyi A, Stockley C, Keal J *et al.* Reduction of metformin renal tubular secretion by cimetidine in man. *Br J Clin Pharmacol* 1987;23:545–51.

43 Maggs DG, Buchanan TA, Burant CF *et al.* Metabolic effects of troglitazone monotherapy in type 2 diabetes mellitus—a randomized, double-blind, placebo-controlled trial. *Ann Intern Med* 1998;128:176–85.

44 Spiegelman BM. PPAR-gamma: adipogenic regulator and thiazolidinedione receptor. *Diabetes* 1998;47:507–14.

45 Goldstein BJ. Current views on the mechanism of action of thiazolidinedione insulin sensitizers. *Diabetes Technol Ther* 1999;1:267–75.

46 Kreider M. Rosiglitazone is effective and well tolerated in patients (≥ 65 years with type 2 diabetes [abstract]. 35th Annual Meeting of the European Association for the Study of Diabetes Scientific Sessions, Brussels, Belgium, September, 1999, abstract 854.

47 Lebovitz HE. Alpha-glucosidase inhibitors. *Endocrinol Clin N Am* 1997;26:539–51.

48 Goldberg JL, Josse RG, Hunt JA *et al.* The efficacy of acarbose in the treatment of patients with non-insulin-dependent diabetes mellitus. A multicenter controlled clinical trial. *Ann Intern Med* 1994;121:928–35.

49 Matthews DR, Cull CA, Stratton IM *et al.* UK Prospective Diabetes Study (UKPDS) Group: sulphonylurea failure in non-insulin-dependent diabetic patients over six years. *Diabet Med* 1998;15:297–303.

29

Diabetes in high-risk ethnic populations

Jaime A Davidson

OVERVIEW

Diabetes has reached epidemic proportions in the USA, with almost 17 million Americans being afflicted with the disease[1] (Figure 29.1). The scope of the diabetes epidemic becomes even more significant with the recent classification of 'pre-diabetes', which affects an additional 16 million Americans – most of whom are likely to develop diabetes within the next 10 years[1]. The rest of the world is experiencing similar problems (Figures 29.2 and 29.3); for example in Latin America the growth in the number of those with diabetes (Figure 29.4) will be such that by 2010 the number of diabetic patients is projected to be 20.3 million; by the same date there are projected to be 19 million diabetic patients in North America (Figure 29.5). Similar skyrocket-

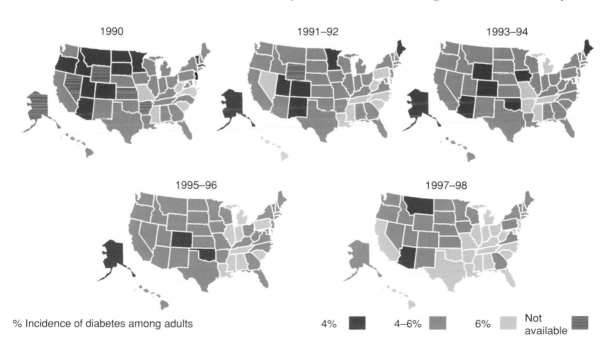

Figure 29.1 Diabetes trends in the USA: 1990–98[2].

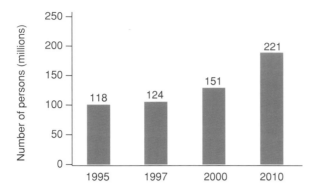

Figure 29.2 Type 2 diabetes: worldwide estimates and projections[3].

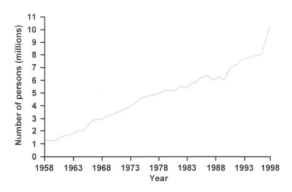

Figure 29.3 Number of persons diagnosed with diabetes 1958–98[4].

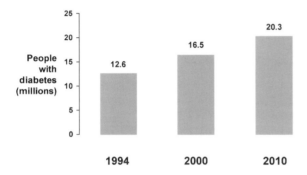

Figure 29.4 Latin America – estimates of diabetes

ing numbers are expected in China and India, the two countries with the largest number of inhabitants in the world, and type 2 diabetes is increasing not only in older populations, but also among younger people[5].

Among Latino, African-American and Native-American populations in North America, the problem of diabetes is even greater, with the prevalence of diabetes being 2–3 times higher than among Caucasians, even after adjustment for the greater overall and more centralized obesity[6,7]. Beginning in 1996, these minority ethnic groups added more patients with type 2 diabetes to the US total than the majority white or Caucasian population[8]. The increasing prevalence of diabetes within high-risk ethnic populations becomes even more significant when considering the tremendous growth of these populations, especially the Latino populations. Among the Latino populations the occurrence of diabetes follows a particular pattern:

- Mainly type 2 diabetes (Figure 29.6)

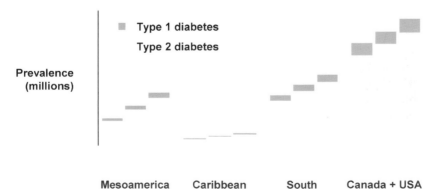

Figure 295 Estimates of increase in diabetes in the Americas[4].

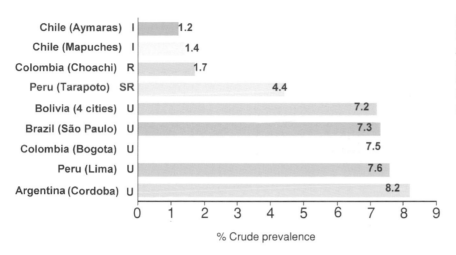

Figure 29.6 Type 2 diabetes is prevalent in Latino America (adapted from data provided by L. De Loreda, S Seclen, P Aschner et al.). U = urban, SR = semi-rural, R = rural, I = indigenous.

- Diabetes is increasing faster in this group than in other groups
- There is also more gestational diabetes
- Type 2 diabetes is occurring among children and adolescents.

For many years, the African-American population was the largest ethnic minority group in the USA. However, from the start of the new millennium, it appears that the Latinos have become the largest ethnic or minority group. Mexican-Americans make up 60% of the Latino population within the USA, followed by Puerto Ricans (10%) and Cuban Americans (3.5%). The remaining 25–30% are from Central and South America, the Caribbean and Spain[9]. However, from small sampling this latter group appears very similar to the otherwise larger groups[9,10].

By the end of 2001, it was estimated that the number of Latinos living in the USA as legal citizens was approximately 39–40 million[11]. When the ~15 million temporary workers of Mexican origin are factored into the calculation, along with those individuals who lack proper documentation (individuals who are both consumers, as well as workers, and recipients of public healthcare services), the true number of Latinos in the USA could be as high as 75 million[11]. This would make the USA one of the largest Latino countries in the world, third only to Brazil and Mexico.

INCIDENCE AND PREVALENCE

Native Americans

Native Americans have one of the highest incidence and prevalence of type 2 diabetes. Approximately 12% of Native Americans over the age of 19 have diabetes. By age 40, approximately 50% have diabetes[11]. One of the reasons for these high numbers of Native Americans with diabetes, mainly from among the Pima tribe, is that undiagnosed type 2 diabetes is virtually nonexistent due to extensive screening within this population[12].

African–Americans

Approximately 2.3 million (10.8%) of all African–Americans have diabetes; approximately one-third of these individuals have not been diagnosed with the disease[13]. It is estimated that African–Americans are 1.7 times more likely to have diabetes than non-Latino whites, with diabetes occurring in approximately 25% of African–Americans between the ages of 65 and 74 years[13].

Latinos

Latinos tend to develop diabetes at an earlier average age than Caucasians. Approximately 25% have diabetes by the age of 45[13]. However, within the various Latino populations there are subtle differences in prevalence. For example, among the three largest Latino groups, the Mexicans and Puerto Ricans show similar prevalences of diabetes at various ages. Cuban Americans have less diabetes early in life, but appear to catch up with Mexicans and Puerto Ricans by age 65, with a similar prevalence of 33–35%[14]. The prevalence of diagnosed diabetes in Puerto Rican populations by age groups was similar in Puerto Rico to Puerto Ricans in New York City; there was also no variation between rural and urban residents[15].

One of the key concerns among healthcare providers is the significant increase in diagnosed cases of type 2 diabetes in children, specifically among children of ethnic backgrounds. Once considered a disease of mature people, over the age of 45[16], type 2 diabetes is now being diagnosed in adolescents and children as young as 5 years of age. Health workers in minority communities attribute this emerging epidemic of type 2 diabetes among ethnic youth to the growing incidence of obesity in children[17,18]. It is important to recognize that these new cases of type 2 diabetes in children are distinctly different from mature onset diabetes of the young (MODY syndrome). While researchers are still somewhat unclear about the cause and etiology of the MODY syndrome, it is clear that MODY is an uncommon, autoimmune dominant syndrome of early onset non-ketosis-prone diabetes that is unrelated to obesity and insulin resistance[19].

The control of diabetes and occurrence of complications have also become a cause of concern. Among US Latinos:

- End-stage renal disease (ESRD) is 6–7 times higher
- There is more retinopathy
- There are more amputations
- Recently, more cardiovascular complications have been seen in this group.

PATHOPHYSIOLOGY

Although a more comprehensive discussion of the pathophysiology of diabetes is presented in Chapter 2, a brief overview is beneficial in order to adequately discuss the differences and similarities of diabetes pathophysiology within high-risk ethnic populations compared with Caucasians.

Diabetes mellitus is a chronic disease with multiple metabolic defects that result in hyperglycemia arising from inadequate insulin activity[20]. Researchers believe that the major cause of inadequate insulin activity is a condition termed insulin resistance, which is defined as an impaired response to the physiological effects of insulin on glucose, lipid, protein metabolism and vascular endothelial function[21]. Approximately 92% of individuals with type 2 diabetes are insulin resistant[22].

Insulin resistance is linked with a cluster of metabolic abnormalities that predispose cardiovascular disease, including: hypertension, obesity, hypertriglyceridemia, reduced plasma high-density lipoproteins (HDL) and increased plasma low-density-lipoproteins (LDL)[23]. Insulin resistance often begins several years before diabetes is diagnosed. During this 'pre-diabetes' phase, insulin production gradually increases in order to compensate for decreasing sensitivity to insulin in muscle and adipose tissues. During this time, the body begins to lose its first-phase insulin response to nutrient intake, resulting in elevated postprandial glucose levels. However, because the pancreas is still able to produce enough insulin to facilitate glucose metabolism (albeit delayed), fasting blood-glucose levels often remain normal in pre-diabetic individuals. Eventually, beta-cell function begins to deteriorate, resulting in insulin deficiency and elevated fasting glucose. Many clinicians now believe that insulin resistance itself is an independent risk factor for cardiovascular disease[24].

There are considerable data showing that some Latino groups, mainly Mexican-Americans, have clear signs of increased peripheral resistance to insulin. In both San Antonio and San Luis Valley, mean insulin levels were higher in Mexican–Americans than in non-Hispanic Caucasians[4]. Further, among non-diabetic Latino children who are obese, with a positive family history of diabetes, prevalence of hyperinsulinemia was found to be almost 100%. Knowing that hyperinsulinemia is an antecedent to type 2 diabetes, it is clear that the epidemic of diabetes will become even more widespread among increasingly younger individuals in the years to come.

While there appears to be no difference in diabetes pathophysiology among ethnic populations compared with Caucasians, it is clear that there is a difference in the prevalence of obesity among many of the ethnic populations. This is a significant influence in hyperinsulinemia and, thus, a key risk factor for the development of diabetes.

RISK FACTORS

While the pathophysiology of diabetes in ethnic populations does not appear to differ from that in Caucasians, ethnic groups seem to have metabolic abnormalities, such as insulin resistance, hyperinsulinemia and impaired glucose tolerance (IGT), at higher rates than other populations. Given these abnormalities, all of which are associated with obesity, the most significant risk factors facing these populations are:

- Over-nutrition
- Content of the diet (high saturated fat, high in simple carbohydrates, low fibre)
- Low level of physical activity.

All of these are prime environmental factors that lead to early obesity and an increased risk of diabetes at a younger age. For example, Mexican–American children report eating higher than recommended amounts of fat, and lower than the recommended number of servings of fresh fruits and vegetables. It is also reported that children of some minority groups engage in less physically active pastimes, both at home and at school, than non-Latino whites[25].

Sedentary lifestyles among adults are also a problem. Even though there are no large-scales studies assessing physical activity and its relationship to diabetes, the level of physical activity has been examined in several Hispanic-Latino populations in the NHANES survey. NHANES showed that the prevalence of type 2 diabetes in Mexican–Americans declined with increasing occupational physical activity after controlling for age and obesity[26].

While there is no question that genetics plays an important role, we have yet to decipher what that role is and its significance among ethnic groups. One example of a genetic link has been found in the Pima Indians. Until the early 1940s Pima Indians suffered very little type 2 diabetes. In fact, researchers such as Dr E. Joslin were very interested in studying the Pima tribe to see why they were protected from diabetes. However, over the next few decades, 'westernization' caught up with the Pimas; their diet changed, weight increased and sedentary lifestyle became a problem. Within 50 years, the Pimas went from the lowest incidence of diabetes to the highest in the USA.

While the driving force behind the increasing prevalence of diabetes appears to be obesity, particularly android and central obesity, other metabolic variables must also be considered. Among participants in the San Antonio Heart Study, which compared Mexican–Americans with non-Hispanic whites who were non-diabetic at baseline, the 8-year risk factor of developing type 2 diabetes was strongly associated with level of body mass index (BMI), along with sub-scapular-to-triceps ratio, fasting and 2 h plasma glucose level, fasting serum insulin, triglycerides, systolic and diastolic blood pressure, pulse pressure (defined as the difference between systolic and diastolic blood pressure), hypertension, and low levels of HDL cholesterol[27]. However, when these variables were entered in a single stepwise multiple logistic regression model, only fasting and 2 h plasma glucose, BMI, HDL cholesterol, and pulse pressure remained significantly associated with the incidence of type 2 diabetes[28].

COMPLICATIONS

Microvascular complications

The rate of microvascular complications in high-risk ethnic populations is disproportionately higher than in Caucasians. Among Native Americans, diabetic retinopathy occurs in 18–24% of patients with diabetes. Within the same population, the rate of ESRD is six times higher than in the general Caucasian population. Amputation rates among Native

Americans are 3–4 times higher than in the general population[29].

African–Americans are twice as likely to suffer from diabetes-related blindness and up to twice as likely to suffer from lower limb amputations. In addition, African–Americans with diabetes are 2.6–5.6 times more likely to suffer from end-stage renal disease (ESRD), with > 4000 new cases being diagnosed each year[29]. The prevalence of diabetic retinopathy in Mexican–Americans is 32–40% and Mexican–Americans with diabetes are 4.5–6.6 times more likely to suffer from ESRD.

Macrovascular complications

For many years it was believed that myocardial infarction (MI) was less prevalent in minority populations. This belief was supported by the literature. In fact, the San Antonio Heart Study showed an increased prevalence of MI in Mexican–Americans compared with Caucasians[27]. More recently, Hanis reported an increased rate of MI among Mexican–Americans in Starr County, Texas[30].

Similar findings have been demonstrated in African–Americans with type 2 diabetes. This population is at an increased risk of heart disease and cerebro-vascular accidents when compared with those without diabetes[31]. ESRD is also a significant problem, and controlling hypertension and the use of agents proven to decrease the problem are imperative for the prevention of this devastating complication in African– Americans.

Relationship between complications and glycemic control

Prospective studies in type 1 and type 2 diabetes have demonstrated a relationship between glycemic control and reduction of microvascular and macrovascular complications[32–34]. Although both the Diabetes Control and Complications Trial (DCCT) and UK Prospective Diabetes Study (UKPDS) studied primarily Caucasian subjects, the same relationship between glycemia and complications has been shown to exist within ethnic populations. Studies have shown that, given similar glucose control, there is no difference between Latinos, African (Caribbean) patients and Caucasians in the development and/or severity of complications[35,36]. In short, good glycemic control makes a difference in all patients with diabetes.

Unfortunately, most Americans with type 2 diabetes – both Caucasian and ethnic populations – have unacceptable levels of glycemic control[26]. In the NHANES III Trial, conducted in the USA from 1988 to 1994, the study sample of ethnic minorities with a diagnosis of type 2 diabetes included only 490 African–Americans and 450 Mexican–Americans, with no mention of other Latino groups or ethnicities. Given these small numbers, it is difficult to fully assess the level of glycemic control within the high-risk ethnic populations. However, data from the San Antonio Heart Study clearly showed higher fasting levels of glycemia, as well as higher postprandial glucose in Mexican–Americans compared with Caucasians[27]. The study showed that approximately 50% of Latinos had postprandial glucose levels > 300 mg dL^{-1}, whereas approximately 25% of Caucasians showed similar postprandial levels.

Data on glycemic control in African–Americans are not as clear. However, available information does show a disparity between African–Americans and Caucasians in glycemic control[37].

TREATMENT AND PREVENTION

Treatment

Other chapters in this book cover treatment strategies; scientific evidence shows no reason to intervene differently with high-risk ethnic populations compared with Caucasians – achievement of normoglycemia (ADA < 7%, ACE < 6.5%) and management of diabetes risk factors should be pursued in all patient groups, regardless of ethnicity.

Prevention

Data from the Diabetes Prevention Program clearly showed that type 2 diabetes can be prevented in individuals who have IGT – often the precursor of type 2 diabetes. The trial, which included a large percentage of high-risk ethnic populations, demonstrated the importance of early intervention, as well as hygienic measures such as better nutrition, increased physical activity and moderate weight loss[38]. In one arm of the study, which employed diabetes education, nutritional intervention and a program to improve physical fitness, an overall reduction of diabetes development of almost 60%, across all age groups was demonstrated. Subjects in the second arm (treated with metformin) showed a reduction of slightly more than 30%, with little or no effect in the population aged 60 and older. Thus one must conclude that, when properly analyzed, the data in younger people will significantly improve. This is clearly relevant to high-risk populations, where individuals are being diagnosed at earlier ages.

Results from the DPP further support data from Harris *et al.*, who found that the prevalence of type 2 diabetes in Mexican–Americans declined with increasing occupational physical activity after controlling for age and obesity[39].

BARRIERS TO CARE

Healthcare provider perspectives and misperceptions

Unfortunately, disparities in control and complications continue in our high-risk ethnic populations. It is believed that these disparities come not only from suboptimal access to healthcare services, but also from inappropriate treatment practices. There is a misperception that patients who belong to certain ethnic populations cannot afford the most appropriate medications or services, and/or that they will not adhere to the prescribed regimens. In studies in African–Americans, fewer patients from this population were on oral agents than Caucasians. In addition, it was shown that African–American patients received fewer hours of diabetes education than Caucasian patients. Among Latinos, where up to 25% of patients are Spanish-speaking only, the disparities in therapies and care are further compounded.

This problem has been substantiated by studies which have shown that, in virtually every measure of quality, there is a sharp division between the healthcare experiences of Caucasians and ethnic minority Americans. Whether this division is a result of healthcare provider perceptions, communication issues, or a combination of both these factors is unclear. Nevertheless, as the US population grows increasingly diverse, these findings send a clear warning that there is a distinct and troublesome disparity in healthcare quality, which will have significant consequences in the future.

Patient perspectives and cultural issues

A key challenge encountered by the healthcare team is overcoming patient attitudes that hinder adherence to care. Many Latino patients tend not to take diabetes seriously until they face complications. Or they may believe that their diabetes is an 'act of God' and feel that treating their diabetes is hopeless. In addition, stories and recommendations from family and friends strongly influence patient behavior. In many instances this influence can be problematic, particularly when it relates to insulin treatment. In some cultures, alternative treatments or medications from abroad are often used. Patients will seldom volunteer this information.

It is also important to note the influence of family dynamics. In Latino families, the mother, grandmother or mother-in-law directs the healthcare-related matters of family members. Latino families often come as a group to the office visit, which can enhance adherence to treatment plans, with the family providing valuable reinforcement and emotional support to the patient. Conversely, family dynamics can also have a negative impact on health. For women with diabetes, family obligations can inhibit effective self-care. In many cultures it is believed that the woman's needs are secondary to the good of her family. As a result, expenditures for diabetes medications and supplies may be perceived as being less important than other family necessities[40].

Communicating with the healthcare team

Latinos, Asians and African–Americans are more likely than Caucasians to have difficulty communicating with physicians and the rest of the healthcare team. Latinos in the USA, the fastest growing minority, were more than twice as likely as whites – 33% versus 16% – to cite communication problems, such as failing to understand the doctor or feeling the doctor did not listen to them. Twenty-seven percent of Asians and 23% of African–Americans said they have experienced similar communication problems[41]. In general, members of ethnic minorities, particularly Latinos, tend to see communication as more of a barrier than economics to healthcare.

Many members of the Latino and Asian populations believe they would receive better care if they were of a different race. A survey was taken by Princeton Survey Research Associates, utilizing telephone interviews, of a random nationally representative sample of 6722 people aged 18 and older[42]. The sample included 3488 whites, 1153 Latino/Hispanic, 1037 African–Americans and 669 Asians. The error margin for the total sample was ± 1.5 percentage points. One in six African–Americans, one in seven Hispanics and one in ten Asians said they felt they would receive better healthcare if they were of a different race. Both African–Americans and non-Hispanic whites reported getting more preventive care than Latinos and Asians.

MOVING TOWARD A SOLUTION

Type 2 diabetes mellitus affects ethnic minorities to such an extent that it can be viewed as nothing less than a national health problem. Not only have we seen an absolute increase in type 2 diabetes, but we are also seeing more cases of diabetes diagnosed at a much earlier age. However, when considering the disproportionately high incidence of pre-diabetes and gestational diabetes among high-risk ethnic populations, most of whom will go on to develop type 2 diabetes, the long-term problem is staggering.

In addition, the human and financial impact of diabetic complications such as retinopathy and ESRD, which are known to affect these high-risk ethnic groups in much higher proportions than Caucasians, must also be considered. Even in those groups that, historically, have been somewhat protected from cardiovascular disease, that protection is waning. Without question, diabetes is epidemic among high-risk ethnic populations. Clinicians need to be culturally sensitive to the unique needs and concerns of these populations. Listed below are some 'action steps' to consider.

Healthcare provider focus

Encourage and support culturally sensitive diabetes education in the community
Most diabetes programs are not culturally sensitive, nor are they at the level where patients can obtain the required benefits. Unless we are willing to deliver appropriate education in a way that fully addresses the cultural differences of our high-risk populations, we will continue to blame the patient for 'poor compliance', while our patients and society suffer the consequences of poor clinical outcomes.

Employ bilingual staff
This will facilitate better communications and more trusting relationships between healthcare providers and their patients, resulting in better adherence and improved outcomes.

Learn about the impact of family dynamics within the various ethnic populations
It is often beneficial (and vital, in some cases) to get the whole family involved.

Support universal access to care
It is important to make the system more accessible and usable for all patient populations.

Patient focus

Ask more questions
Learn about your patients' fears, beliefs, treatment obstacles and any other therapies (folk therapies) they may be using. Also, find out about the practicality of the regimens you prescribe. Many patients work two jobs so don't have time to exercise.

Address the cultural characteristics of the patient and his/her family

Clinicians may even want to consider treating the entire family, even if not all are covered by insurance.

Obtain and distribute low-literacy and bilingual educational materials that are appropriate to the educational and socioeconomic status of your ethnic populations

Having pleasant surroundings as well as culturally sensitive educational materials will help. Taking the time and inviting the significant family members to participate may not only improve patient compliance and control, but could also help delay the appearance of diabetes in younger members of the family.

Prescribe qualified, culturally sensitive diabetes education

Use the skills of both nurses and dietitians.

Be aggressive in promoting effective management of all diabetes risk factors

The attitudes and beliefs of clinicians strongly influence the adequacy of treatment. Effective intervention improves outcomes and quality of life for the patient, and presents a 'window of opportunity' for diabetes prevention in family members.

CONCLUSIONS

With the projected increases in high-risk ethnic populations over the next 25 years, driven by the sharp and continuing increase in obesity throughout all populations, diabetes has become a significant threat to all Americans. To counter this threat, clinicians must find ways to be more effective and aggressive in both the prevention and treatment of type 2 diabetes in all American populations. Studies have shown that we have the potential to prevent type 2 diabetes. Studies have also shown that, armed with new pharmacological agents and monitoring technologies, we can achieve tighter glycemic control and effectively manage other risk factors of this disease, resulting in improved outcomes. We must work together to develop and implement programs that are accessible and of excellent quality, so that every person with diabetes can obtain the best care possible.

REFERENCES

1   US Department of Health and Human Services. News release, 2002. http://www.hhs.gov/news/press/2002pres/20020327.html (Accessed April, 2002).

2   Mokdad AH, Ford ES, Bowman BA *et al*. Diabetes trends in the US: 1990–1998. *Diabetes Care* 2000;23:1278–83.

3   Amos AF, McCarty DJ, Zimmet P. The rising global burden of diabetes and its complications: estimates and projections to the year 2010. *Diabet Med* 1997;14 (Suppl 5):S1.

4   *Diabetes in America*, 2nd edition. National Diabetes Data Group, National Institutes of Health National Institute of Diabetes and Digestive and Kidney Diseases NIH Publication No. 95–1468, 1995.

5   International Diabetes Federation. E-Atlas 2003. http://www.idf.org/e-atlas/home (Accessed January, 2003).

6   Centers for Disease Control and Prevention (CDC). National Diabetes Fact Sheet. http://www.cdc.gov/diabetes/pubs/factsheet.htm (Accessed January, 2003).

7   Haffner SM, Stern MP, Hazuda HP *et al*. Hyperinsulinemia in a population at high risk for non-insulin-dependent diabetes mellitus. *N Engl J Med* 1986;315:220–4.

8   Garth-Powell-Peterson Productions, 505 Park Ave, NY, 1996.

9   Haffner SM, Hazuda HP, Mitchell BD *et al*. Increased incidence of type II diabetes mellitus in Mexican Americans. *Diabetes Care* 1991;14:102–8.

10   Baxter J, Hamman RF, Lopez TK *et al*. Excess incidence of known non-insulin dependent diabetes (NIDDM) in Hispanics compared with non-Hispanic whites in the San Luis Valley, Colorado. *Ethn Dis* 1993;3:11–21.

11   US Bureau of the census, 2000.

12   Knowler WC, Pettitt DJ, Savage PJ, Bennett PH. Diabetes incidence in Pima Indians: contributions of obesity and parental diabetes. *Am J Epidemiol* 1981;113:144–56.

13   US Bureau of the Census, 2000.

14   Flegal KM, Ezzati TM, Harris MI *et al.* Prevalence of diabetes in Mexican Americans, Cubans and Puerto Ricans from the Hispanic Health and Nutrition Examination Survey, *Diabetes Care* 1991;14:628–38.

15   Haddock L, Torres de Conty I. Prevalence rates for diabetes in Puerto Rico. *Diabetes Care* 1991;14 (Suppl 3): 676–84.

15   American Diabetes Association. Basic Diabetes Information. http://www.diabetes.org/main/application/commerce (Accessed January, 2003).

16   American Diabetes Association. Clinical Practice Recommendations. Diabetes Care 1999;22(Suppl. 1).

17   Centers for Disease Control. http://www.cdc.gov/od/oc/media/pressrel/r2k1027a.htm, visited 6th November 2002.

18   http://www.cdc.gov/diabetes/projects/cda2.htm, visited 6th November 2002.

19   Fajans SS. Maturity onset diabetes of the young (MODY). *Diabetes Metab Rev* 1989;5:579–606.

20   American Diabetes Association. *Complete guide to diabetes*. Alexandria, VA: American Diabetes Association, 1997.

21   Consensus Development Conference of the American Diabetes Association. *Diabetes Care* 1997.

22   Haffner SM, D'Agostino R Jr, Mykkanen L *et al.* Insulin sensitivity in subjects with type 2 diabetes. Relationship to cardiovascular risk factors: the Insulin Resistance Atherosclerosis Study. *Diabetes Care* 1999;22:562–8.

23   Turner NC, Clapham JC. Insulin resistance, impaired glucose tolerance and non-insulin-dependent diabetes, pathologic mechanism and treatment: current status and therapeutic possibilities. *Prog Drug Res* 1998;51:33–94.

24   American Diabetes Association. Consensus Development Conference on Insulin Resistance. *Diabetes Care* 1998;21:310–4.

25   Marshall JA, Hamman RF, Baxter J. High-fat, low carbohydrate diet and the etiology of non-insulin-dependent diabetes mellitus: The San Luis Valley Diabetes Study. *Am J Epidemiol* 1991;134:590–603.

26   Kant AK. Consumption of energy-dense, nutrient-poor foods by adult Americans: nutritional and health implications. The third National Health and Nutrition Examination Survey, 1988–1994. *Am J Clin Nutr* 2000;72;929–936

27   Mitchell BD, Hazuda HP, Haffner SM *et al.* Myocardial infarction in Mexican Americans and non-Hispanic whites: The San Antonio Heart Study. *Circulation* 1991;83:45–51.

28   Stern MP, Morales PA, Valdez RA *et al.* Predicting diabetes: moving beyond impaired glucose tolerance. *Diabetes* 1993;42:706–14.

29   American Diabetes Association. Basic Diabetes Information. http://www.diabetes.org/main/application/commerce (Accessed January, 2003).

30   Steffen-Batey L, Nichaman MZ, Goff DC Jr *et al.* Change in level of Activity and risk of all-cause mortality or reinfarction: The Corpus Christi Heart Project. *Circulation* 2000;102:425–438.

31   Shafer SQ et al. Brain infarction risk factors in black New York City stroke patients. *J Chron Dis* 1990;27:127–33.

32   The DCCT Research Group. The effect of intensive treatment of diabetes on the development and progression of long-term complications in insulin-dependent diabetes mellitus. *N Engl J Med* 1993;329:977–86.

33   The UKPDS Study Group. Intensive blood-glucose control with sulphonylureas or insulin compared with conventional treatment and risk of complications in patients with type 2 diabetes (UKPDS 33) *Lancet* 1998;352:837–53.

34   Stratton IM, Adler AI, Neil HA *et al.* Association of glycaemia with macrovascular and microvascular complications of type 2 diabetes (UKPDS 35): prospective observational study. *Br Med J* 2000;321:405–12.

35   Hamman RF, Franklin GA, Mayer EJ *et al.* Microvascular complications of NIDDM in Hispanics and non-Hispanic whites. *Diabetes Care* 1991;14(suppl 3):655.

36   Cruickshank JK, Alleyne SA. Black West Indian and matched white diabetics in Britain compared with diabetics in Jamaica: body mass, blood pressure, and vascular disease. *Diabetes Care* 1987;10:170.

37   Rabb MF, Gagliano DA, Sweeney HE. Diabetic retinopathy in blacks. *Diabetes Care* 1990;13 (Suppl4):1202–6.

38   Knowler WC, Barrett-Connor E, Fowler SE *et al.* Diabetes Prevention Program Research Group. Reduction in the incidence of type 2 diabetes with lifestyle intervention or metformin. *N Engl J Med* 2002;346:393–403.

39   Harris MI. Epidemiologic correlates of NIDDM in Hispanics, Whites, and Blacks in the US population. *Diabetes Care* 1991;14 (Suppl. 3):639–48.

40   Lipton RB, Losey LM, Giachello A *et al. Diabetes Educ* 1998;24:67–71.

41   Commonwealth Fund, 2002

42   Princeton Survey Research Associates, 2002.

30

Diabetes mellitus secondary to drugs, hormones and other endocrinopathies

M James Lenhard

INTRODUCTION

All forms of diabetes are manifested by hyperglycemia. Most of the time, diabetes can be classified, based on defined criteria, as type 1, type 2, or gestational diabetes. Diabetes or glucose intolerance that develops in association with illnesses, genetic syndromes, drugs and other conditions is referred to as *secondary diabetes*. This implies that eliminating the condition associated with the new onset of diabetes will allow a return to normal glucose tolerance. While this is often the case, the distinction is not always clear.

CLASSIFICATION

The American Diabetes Association has classified diabetes into type 1, type 2, gestational and 'other specific types'[1]. The classification of diabetes due to other specific causes is shown in Table 30.1. In some situations, glucose intolerance is caused by over-production of other hormones. In other situations, complex genetic syndromes, drugs or other medications, or diseases that affect the pancreas, induce glucose intolerance. Pancreatic insufficiency is analogous to type 1 diabetes and will not be addressed. Some of the systemic genetic diseases that are associated with hyperglycemia and diabetes are discussed elsewhere. This chapter will focus on secondary diabetes that is due to:

- Drugs and medications
- Hormones and other endocrine diseases.

DIABETES SECONDARY TO DRUGS AND MEDICATIONS

Pharmaceutical advances have been dramatic in the last decade. An increasing array of drugs is available, and many of them affect glucose tolerance. Many of the newer drugs have not been rigorously tested regarding their ability to affect carbohydrate metabolism. The drugs that can induce glucose intolerance may have an effect by decreasing insulin secretion, decreasing insulin action, or both. The drugs that will be discussed are listed in Table 30.2. Additional drugs[2,3] have been found to cause hyperglycemia. Their effects are often modest, or idiosyncratic in nature.

Anti-hypertensive drugs

The medications used to treat hypertension have been associated with the development of diabetes. A variety of metabolic and epidemiological studies, and clinical trials have suggested a causal link between the use of thiazide diuretics and beta-blockers and the development of diabetes[4], although many of the studies have been criticized for a variety of reasons.

The connection between the use of antihypertensive medication and the subsequent development

---

Table 30.1 Etiologic classification of diabetes (from Reference 1): other specific types

Genetic defects of beta-cell function
Chromosome 12, HNF-1alpha (MODY3)
Chromosome 7, glucokinase (MODY2)
Chromosome 20, HNF-4alpha (MODY1)
Mitochondrial DNA
Others

Genetic defects in insulin action
Type A insulin resistance
Leprechaunism
Rabson–Mendenhall syndrome
Lipoatrophic diabetes
Others

Diseases of the exocrine pancreas
Pancreatitis
Trauma/pancreatectomy
Neoplasia
Cystic fibrosis
Hemochromatosis
Fibrocalculous pancreatopathy
Others

Endocrinopathies
Acromegaly
Cushing's syndrome
Glucagonoma
Pheochromocytoma
Hyperthyroidism
Somatostatinoma
Aldosteronoma
Others

Drug- or chemical-induced
Vacor

Pentamidine
Nicotinic acid
Glucocorticoids
Thyroid hormone
Diazoxide
Beta-adrenergic agents
Thiazides
Dilantin
Alpha-interferon
Others

Infections
Congenital rubella
Cytomegalovirus
Others

Uncommon forms of immune-mediated diabetes
'Stiff-man' syndrome
Anti-insulin receptor antibodies
Others

Other genetic syndromes sometimes associated with diabetes
Down's syndrome
Klinefelter's syndrome
Turner's syndrome
Wolfram's syndrome
Friedreich's ataxia
Huntington's chorea
Laurence–Moon–Biedl syndrome
Myotonic dystrophy
Porphyria
Prader–Willi syndrome
Others

---

of type 2 diabetes was examined in the Atherosclerosis Risk in Communities Study (ARCS)[5]. Type 2 diabetes was almost 2.5 times as likely to develop in subjects with hypertension as in subjects with normal blood pressure. After adjust-ing for confounding variables, it was determined that subjects taking thiazide diuretics, angiotensin-converting enzyme (ACE) inhibitors, or calcium-channel antagonists did not have a greater risk for developing diabetes than patients who were not

Table 30.2 Drugs with potential adverse effects on glucose homeostasis

Anti-hypertensive drugs
Beta-blockers
Thiazide diuretics
Calcium-channel blockers
Apha agonists
Minoxidil
Diazoxide

Lipid-lowering agent
Niacin

Sympathomimetics
Beta-adrenoreceptor agonists
Xanthines

Drugs used to treat HIV disease
Pentamidine
Nucleoside reverse transcriptase inhibitors
(Didanosine)
Protease inhibitors
Megestrol acetate

Antipsychotic agents/psychiatric agents
Clozapine
Risperidone
Olanzapine
Quetiapine
Lithium

Immunosuppressive and immunomodulating drugs
Cyclosporine
L-asparaginase
Interleukins
Tacrolimus

Hormones
Somatostatin
Oral contraceptives

Miscellaneous
Arsenic
Etanercept
Cyanide
Dioxin
Danazol
Phenytoin
Vacor

taking any antihypertensive medication. In contrast, patients taking beta-blockers had a 28% greater risk of developing diabetes (see Figure 30.1).

Beta-blockers

Beta-blockers, along with thiazide diuretics, have been recommended as first-line agents in the treatment of hypertension[6]. Caution was advised when considering the use of beta-blockers in patients with diabetes, because of their ability to cause glucose intolerance, precipitate overt diabetes in nondiabetic individuals and worsen glycemic control in established diabetic patients. These drugs worsen glucose tolerance because they inhibit insulin secretion, increase insulin resistance, and alter lipid metabolism. Since insulin secretion is partially mediated via $beta_2$-receptors, beta-blockers, especially non-selective ones, may impair insulin secretion[7]. Beta-blockers have also been shown to cause a deterioration in glycemic control, without any changes in fasting or post-challenge insulin levels, presumably by interfering with insulin action[8].

Thiazide diuretics

Shortly after their introduction in the 1950s, reports describing glucose intolerance or new diabetes in hypertensive patients treated with thiazide diuretics were published. Thiazides cause hyperglycemia through a combination of decreased insulin secretion and increased insulin resistance. While thiazides have no significant direct effect on insulin secretion, some studies have shown an association between decreased insulin secretion and hypokalemia, which may result from administration of thiazide diuretics[9]. Thiazides have also been shown to cause peripheral resistance to insulin[10]. Of note, the large prospective study by Gress et al.[5] failed to show any extra risk of developing diabetes for hypertensive individuals treated with thiazide diuretics. In addition to the thiazide diuretics, the loop diuretics furosemide, bumetanide and ethacrynic acid can also cause impaired glucose tolerance (IGT), although the effect seems to be less pronounced.

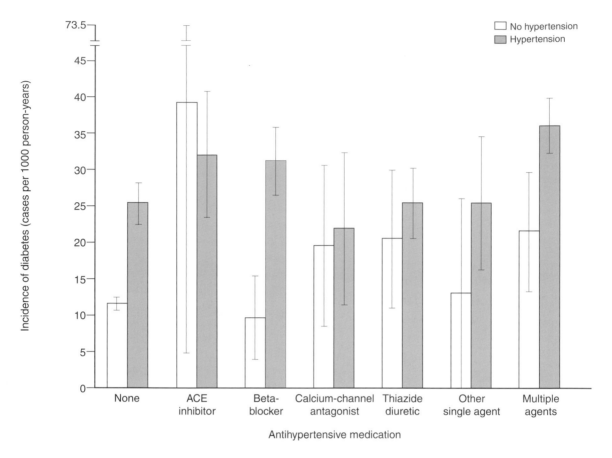

Figure 30.1 Incidence of type 2 diabetes among 12 550 adults on blood pressure and antihypertensive drug treatment. In this prospective study, use of beta-blockers was associated with an increased risk of developing diabetes, while ACE inhibitors, calcium-channel antagonists and thiazide diuretics were not. (Reprinted with permission from ref. 5)

Calcium-channel antagonists
Since the calcium ion is an important regulator of insulin secretion from the beta cell, there is a theoretical reason for concern that pharmacological blockers of calcium channels could lead to IGT. In practice, the calcium-channel antagonists do not seem to cause significant glucose intolerance in diabetic or nondiabetic subjects.

Alpha-agonists
Clonidine has been most frequently associated with causing modest glucose intolerance and has been shown to decrease insulin secretion in isolated islets and perfused pancreas, as well as inhibiting both basal and glucose-stimulated insulin responses in hypertensive subjects.

Studies have shown clonidine to cause negligible to small deterioration in glycemic control[11].

Minoxidil
There is a report of new diabetes developing in one patient with hypertension treated with minoxidil, as well as worsening of glycemic control in two other patients with known diabetes.

Sympathomimetics

Beta-agonists are another class of drugs that can cause hyperglycemia. While the beta-agonist class of drugs leads to increased insulin secretion, hyperglycemia can be seen if the beta-adrenergic mediated effects of enhanced glycogenolysis and lipolysis predominate.

Beta-adrenoceptor agonists

Most of the reports of glucose intolerance caused by beta-adrenoceptor agonists come from the obstetric literature. Beta$_2$-receptor agonists are used as tocolytic agents to treat premature labor. Pregnancy is an inherently insulin-resistant state, and when these agents are added, some women develop hyperglycemia. Salbutamol, terbutaline, and ritodrine have similar effects and may cause hyperglycemia in pregnant women with preterm labor. Terbutaline has a more pronounced hyperglycemic effect than ritodrine, because it is a less selective beta$_2$-agonist. The mechanism whereby these drugs cause glucose intolerance is mediated through the beta$_2$-agonist effects on the liver and peripheral tissue. The beta-agonists cause an increase in hepatic glucose output due to enhanced glycolysis and glycogenolysis, as well as by increasing peripheral insulin resistance[12].

Xanthines

Xanthines, such as theophylline, dyphylline and caffeine, may cause hyperglycemia, although this effect is only seen in overdose situations. The mechanisms may involve increased catecholamine concentrations, metabolic acidosis, and hypokalemia[13].

Lipid-lowering agents

Niacin (Figure 30.2)

There are multiple reports of niacin precipitating diabetes, as well as deterioration of glycemic control in patients with diabetes. In one study of heart transplant patients, 88% of the diabetic subjects needed to drop out of the study due to hyperglycemia. The mechanism for the hyperglycemia seen with niacin treatment is related to the 'rebound lipolysis' when the drug effect wanes. The increase in free fatty acids (FFA) following the waning of the antilipolytic effects of niacin may be in the order of 50–100% above baseline[14]. The result of this increase in FFA is inhibition of glycogen synthase, augmented gluconeogenesis and hepatic glucose output, together with decreased glucose oxidation and peripheral insulin sensitivity.

One randomized, placebo-controlled trial examined the effects of crystalline niacin at doses up to 3000 mg day^{-1} on lipids and glycemic

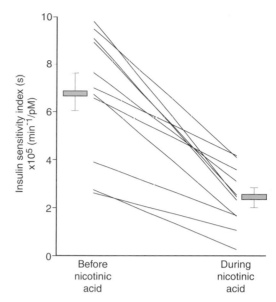

Figure 30.2 Short-term administration of niacin can lead to a decrease in insulin sensitivity in normal men.

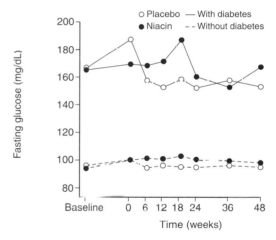

Figure 30.3 A controlled 48-week trial of niacin revealed a transient rise in glucose levels followed by normalization. The effect was more prominent in subjects with diabetes. (Reprinted with permission from ref. 15.)

control. The expected improvements in lipid parameters were observed. The average plasma glucose levels were increased modestly by 8.7 and 6.3 mg dL^{-1} (0.4 and 0.3 mmol L^{-1}), in participants with and without diabetes, glycosylated hemoglobin (HbA1c) levels were unchanged[15]. This trial suggests that niacin does cause hyperglycemia, although the effect may be modest (see Figure 30.3).

Drugs used to treat HIV disease

Within the last 5 years, reports of metabolic side effects from drugs used to treat HIV have surfaced. In addition to hyperglycemia, changes in lipid levels, adipose redistribution, and weight gain, have been described. The drugs used to treat HIV that have metabolic side effects are listed in Table 30.3.

Pentamidine

Glucose intolerance, diabetes and ketoacidosis have been observed in these patients using pentamidine. The mechanism involves a direct toxic effect of pentamidine in the beta cell. A biphasic response has been observed, with initial hypoglycemia in the first few days of treatment, which may be severe and life-threatening in some cases. The hypoglycemia is associated with increased insulin levels and beta-cell lysis. This may be accompanied by overt pancreatitis. Several days to several months later, permanent diabetes associated with beta-cell destruction may occur[16]. However, not all patients treated with pentamidine develop beta-cell lysis.

Nucleoside reverse transcriptase inhibitors (didanosine)

The nucleoside reverse transcriptase inhibitors include the drugs zidovudine (AZT) and didanosine (DDI). While zidovudine does not appear to have any deleterious effects on glucose tolerance, there are reports of hyperglycemia in at least 82 patients treated with didanosine. These include reports of pancreatitis and hyperosmolar, hyperglycemic syndrome (HHS)[17]. The mechanism whereby didanosine causes diabetes is unclear. Since pancreatitis has been reported with didanosine use, there may be a direct toxic effect on the beta cells. Other mechanisms are also possible; didanosine has also been shown to cause hypokalemia.

Table 30.3 Drugs used in the treatment of HIV/AIDS that may cause changes in glucose metabolism

Class of drug	Generic name	Metabolic side effect	Other side effects
Anti-protozoal	Pentamidine	Hyperglycemia Hypoglycemia	Pancreatitis, GI upset
Nucleoside reverse transcriptase inhibitors	Didanosine	Hyperglycemia	Pancreatitis, peripheral neuropathy
Protease inhibitors	Ritonavir	Hyperglycemia Hypertriglyceridemia	GI upset, pancreatitis, hepatitis, peripheral neuropathy
	Indinavir	Hyperglycemia Hypertriglyceridemia	GI upset, nephrolithiasis
	Saquinavir	Hyperglycemia Hypertriglyceridemia	GI upset
	Nelfinavir	Hyperglycemia Hypertriglyceridemia	GI upset
	Amprenavir	Hyperglycemia Hypertriglyceridemia	GI upset, anemia, rash
	Lopinavir/Ritonavir	Hyperglycemia Hypertriglyceridemia	Pancreatitis, GI upset, diarrhea, rash

Protease inhibitors

Protease inhibitors (PI) are potent inhibitors of HIV replication that improve morbidity and mortality in HIV-infected persons. Potential toxic side effects of the PI have emerged as the number of both potential recipients and the number of available PI has increased dramatically (see Table 30.3).

Most cases of glucose intolerance and diabetes associated with the use of PI have occurred in the context of the lipodystrophy syndrome. Metabolic features of the lipodystrophy syndrome associated with PI use include hypertriglyceridemia; hypercholesterolemia; insulin resistance and hyperinsulinemia; type 2 diabetes and IGT; peripheral lipoatrophy; and central adipose accumulation. The change in body habitus due to the reapportionment of adipose is often a very prominent feature, and some investigators have alternatively named this phenomenon the fat redistribution syndrome. In one of the largest longitudinal studies of 111 men receiving PI, 83% (92) exhibited evidence of fat redistribution, compared with 4% (one) of 28 PI-naïve controls. While HIV infection itself can lead to an elevation of triglycerides, PI therapy is a risk factor for developing significant elevations in triglycerides[18]. Hypercholesterolemia has also been reported as frequent sequelae of PI therapy. In one study of 44 patients receiving PI, 33% (44) had elevated lipid concentrations, with mean fasting triglyceride and cholesterol levels of 1194 and 310 mg dL^{-1}, respectively.

The US Food and Drug Administration (FDA) issued a public health advisory in June 1997, describing 83 cases of new diabetes or a deterioration in glycemic control for pre-existing diabetes in patients taking PI. Twenty-seven patients required hospitalization, five developed ketoacidosis, and six had blood glucose levels of approximately 1000 mg dL^{-1}. The prevalence of insulin resistance among PI-treated patients has been estimated to be 25–62%, with a prevalence of overt diabetes found in 8–10%. The mechanism whereby PI may cause glucose intolerance is not clear. It may be an indirect effect, resulting from alterations in fat and lipid metabolism, or there could be a direct effect of PI on insulin secretion or sensitivity. A recent study of 11 HIV-infected subjects treated with indinavir included oral and intravenous glucose tolerance tests. Over 8 weeks of treatment, both a decrease in insulin sensitivity and a decrease in beta-cell response were observed.

All patients that are taking PI should have blood glucose levels measured periodically and be instructed to notify their healthcare provider if symptoms of hyperglycemia develop[19].

Megestrol acetate (Megace)

Megestrol acetate is an oral progestational agent initially used in the treatment of breast and endometrial carcinoma, and more recently for the treatment of AIDS-related cachexia. Cases of reversible diabetes and hyperglycemia have been reported. The drug appears to have glucocorticoid-like activity, which may lead to peripheral insulin resistance and increased caloric intake, as well as a Cushingoid state[20].

Antipsychotic agents/psychiatric drugs

The risk of developing diabetes is increased in patients with psychiatric illness. Reports have described the prevalence of diabetes in patients with schizophrenia as 8.8% in Japan, 15.8% in Italy, and 24.5% in the USA. Diabetes was found in 9.9% of hospitalized patients with bipolar (manic depressive) disorder, and there seems to be a correlation with other mood disorders as well. Some of the medications used to treat these disorders appear to increase the risk of diabetes. To date, there are no large controlled trials to quantitate the risk or prevalence of glucose intolerance in patients receiving the newer atypical antipsychotic agents (clozapine, risperidone, olanzapine, and quetiapine)[21].

Clozapine

There are multiple case reports of new onset diabetes during treatment with clozapine, including cases of ketoacidosis. Uncontrolled trials have reported a rate of new diabetes or glucose intolerance that is 2–3 times higher in patients treated with clozapine compared with conventional neuroleptics. A 5 year observational study without a control group revealed a rate of 37% for new diabetes. Treatment with clozapine has been associated with significant weight gain and lipid abnormalities, although not all cases of new diabetes are found in patients who gained weight while taking clozapine. The mechanism for hyperglycemia remains unclear[21].

Risperidone

This atypical antipsychotic agent has been associated through case reports with glucose intolerance and diabetes. A meta-analysis of published literature suggested that a 2.1 kg weight gain occurs at a mean of 13 weeks of treatment, which can decrease insulin sensitivity.

Olanzapine

Cases of ketoacidosis and reversible diabetes associated with olanzapine have been published. The rate of new diabetes (defined as a fasting glucose above 140 mg dL^{-1}) in patients treated with olanzapine were as high as 33% in observational studies. As with the other agents in this class, increases in weight and triglycerides have been described[21].

Quetiapine

This drug is chemically similar to clozapine and olanzapine; reports of new onset diabetes, and weight gain are therefore not surprising.

Lithium

There is no consensus on the effects of lithium on glucose tolerance. As noted, patients with manic depressive disorder, where lithium may be prescribed, are at an increased risk of developing diabetes. In a review of the literature, Lazarus concluded that there was no clinically significant effect of lithium upon glucose tolerance in humans[22].

Immunosuppressive and immunomodulating drugs

Corticosteroids are often used as an adjunct to immunosuppressive and immunomodulating agents, which has confounded the ability to measure their effects on glucose tolerance. It does appear that the immunosuppressive agents have an independent effect on glucose tolerance.

Cyclosporine

The incidence of new diabetes or IGT in patients treated with cyclosporine is 13–47%. There is evidence that cyclosporine-induced glucose intolerance involves both insulin resistance and beta-cell toxicity. The effects seem to be dose-dependent[23].

L-asparaginase

Infrequently, L-asparaginase has been associated with decreased glucose tolerance, worsening of glycemic control in pre-existing diabetes, and pancreatitis. The mechanism is not well understood, but decreased insulin levels due to either direct beta-cell toxicity or depletion of amino acids essential for insulin synthesis may be involved[23].

Interleukin

New and reversible diabetes has been described with the use of interleukin-6, interleukin-2, and a combination of interferon alpha and beta. These cases occurred in the setting of ketonuria and islet cell autoantibodies. The proposed mechanism involves the induction of interleukin-induced autoimmunity.

Tacrolimus

Tacrolimus-induced cases of hyperglycemia and new diabetes have been reported in children and adults, with rates of 6–45%. The mechanism is felt to involve a direct effect on beta-cell function.

HORMONES

Several hormones have important roles in glucoregulation, and some act as insulin antagonists. Three of these, growth hormone, corticosteroids, and thyroid hormone are addressed under the section of diabetes caused by endocrinopathies. Hyperglycemia may also be seen with the clinical use of somatostatin and oral contraceptives.

Somatostatin

Somatostatin is a peptide expressed in nerve and endocrine-like cells in many parts of the body. Its actions are widespread and diverse, and include the inhibition of virtually every known endocrine and exocrine secretion. A long-acting somatostatin analogue, octreotide acetate, has been used for the treatment of hormone-producing tumors, carcinoid tumors, orthostatic hypotension, variceal bleeding, diarrhea and intestinal dysmotility. Since somatostatin may inhibit insulin secretion, diabetes has been described as a potential side effect. More commonly, however, a mild impairment of glucose tolerance is noted, with only a slight rise in postprandial glucose levels[24]. Even in the very rare case of a somatostatinoma, the hyperglycemia that is observed is minimal.

Oral contraceptives

Hormonal oral contraceptives (OC) were shown to alter carbohydrate metabolism in 1969. Observational studies from the 1970s confirmed that women using OC with both estrogens and progestogens for up to 4 years had a greater risk of IGT, but not overt diabetes[25]. Prospective studies from the 1980s suggested that OC users have a greater incidence of IGT (16% versus 8% in the control group). It has been argued that much of the older literature on OC is no longer applicable. The dosages of estrogens and progestogens have decreased over time, and the formulations of the individual components have been replaced with newer agents that have fewer effects on glucose metabolism[25].

The proposed mechanism for the decrease in glucose tolerance has included decreased insulin sensitivity, impaired plasma insulin response, and altered counterregulatory hormonal responses.

Progestogens may have important effects on glucose tolerance. Numerous studies have shown a deleterious effect of progestogens upon glucose tolerance. The effect appears to be related to both dose and potency, especially for norgestrel. Consensus supports impaired tissue insulin sensitivity as the mechanism of the hyperglycemia[26]. Women who use OC that contain only progesterone should have their glucose levels monitored for the first several months of treatment.

Studies involving combined estrogen–progesterone OC have mirrored the results listed above. Epidemiological studies involving higher dose OC have revealed IGT and hyperinsulinemia, while studies with newer, low-dose OC have shown minimal effects on glucose tolerance.

MISCELLANEOUS

Many other drugs have been shown to cause hyperglycemia in specific populations or idiosyncratic manifestations[2,3,26]. Arsenic can be toxic to beta cells, and people who live in areas with elevated levels in the water or soil have an increased prevalence of diabetes, as do people with occupational exposure to arsenic. Since tumor necrosis factor-alpha (TNF-alpha) has been implicated in the development of type 1 diabetes and diabetic complications, the report of a single case of new diabetes in a 7-year-old girl treated with etanercept, a TNF-lowering drug, is of interest. Chronic exposure to cyanide may cause peripheral neuropathy, as well as carbohydrate intolerance. Epidemiological studies have suggested a link between the time of exposure to the herbicide Agent Orange, and its contaminant dioxin, and the likelihood of developing type 2 diabetes. The testosterone-derivative danazol has been associated with reversible diabetes. Although it is now rarely used, the rat poison vacor remains a classic example of a drug that can cause diabetes through its direct toxic effect on the beta cell. Other drugs have also been shown to cause occasional hyperglycemia.

ENDOCRINOPATHIES

There are a variety of endocrine disorders that can cause glucose intolerance (see Table 30.4). The majority of these are the result of an imbalance of one of the counter-regulatory hormones

---

Table 30.4 Causes of secondary diabetes due to endocrine diseases

Acromegaly

Cushing's syndrome

Glucagonoma

Pheochromocytoma

Hyperthyroidism

Aldosteronoma

Other (hyperparathyroidism, gastrinoma syndrome, hyperprolactinemia, POEMS syndrome)

involved in glucose homeostasis. This may be due to a state of endogenous over-production of the hormone, or to exogenous administration. The diabetes that may result from the effects of these hormones is usually reversible when the underlying disorder is successfully treated.

Growth hormone and acromegaly

Metabolic effects

Growth hormone (GH) has many diverse effects on carbohydrate, protein and fat metabolism. It is a 191 amino acid, 22 kD single-chain peptide secreted from the anterior pituitary in pulses, with a relatively short half-life. Many of the growth-promoting effects of GH are caused by a family of growth factors produced by the liver in response to GH, with the most prominent effects being mediated by insulin-like growth factor I (IGF-I), also known as somatomedin C[27]. The metabolic effects of GH, and its second messenger IGF-I, can be either acute or chronic. The acute response of increasing GH to pharmacologic levels in normal subjects is a transient insulin-like effect, with hypoglycemia and increased glucose utilization, inhibition of lipolysis and protein anabolism. These effects are transient and, after a few hours, the tissues become refractory to GH and glucose utilization is reduced. Subsequently, GH infusion into the brachial arteries of normal volunteers in normal physiologic amounts resulted in insulin resistance.

Acromegaly and diabetes

GH is known to have an effect on carbohydrate metabolism. The classic studies by Houssay in the 1930s showed that hyperglycemia and glucosuria could be reduced in diabetic patients by hypophysectomy. Acromegaly results from excessive production of GH. It is a rare disease, with a reported prevalence of 5.5–6.6 per 100 000, and an incidence of 0.3–0.4 per 100 000. While diabetes occurs in 10–30% of patients with acromegaly, glucose intolerance occurs in up to 60%[28]. Hyperinsulinemia and resistance to insulin in the peripheral tissues are very common, and increased hepatic glucose output has also been described. Patients with overt diabetes in the setting of acromegaly clearly have a subnormal insulin reserve, in addition to the peripheral resistance to insulin. Consequently, the successful treatment of acromegaly results in normalization of insulin sensitivity and insulin levels in patients with GH-induced IGT, while those with GH-induced overt diabetes often have lasting defects.

GH treatment and diabetes

Cutfield and colleagues examined data from an international pharmacoepidemiological survey of children treated with GH[29]. The incidence of type 2 diabetes in this study was 34.4 cases per 100 000 years of GH treatment, which was sixfold higher than children who were not treated with GH. Only five of the 18 children were obese, based on body mass index (BMI) calculations. The authors speculated that the high frequency of type 2 diabetes with GH treatment might reflect acceleration of the disorder in predisposed individuals. There are few studies of glucose tolerance in GH-deficient adults treated with exogenous GH. Since increased levels of nocturnal GH secretion are felt to be responsible for the dawn phenomenon of fasting hyperglycemia, the development of impaired fasting glucose is not surprising.

Cortisol and Cushing's syndrome

Metabolic effects

Glucocorticoids have a wide array of metabolic effects, including diminishing glucose tolerance. Glucocorticoids can decrease insulin sensitivity and enhance hepatic glucose production. Patients with endogenous cortisol excess due to Cushing's disease have decreased sensitivity to insulin at the level of skeletal muscle and adipose[30]. In the liver, glucocorticoids act to enhance gluconeogenesis. In addition, glucocorticoids enhance glucagon secretion and augment glucagon action, to stimulate hepatic gluconeogenesis and glycogenolysis. While insulin inhibits hormone sensitive lipase, glucocorticoids promote the activation of this enzyme, resulting in lipolysis. Clearly, glucocorticoids act via multiple mechanisms to contribute to impaired glucose homeostasis.

Cushing's syndrome and diabetes

Diabetes and glucose intolerance is found with endogenous hypercortisolism so frequently that this is part of the definition of the disease. Overt diabetes can be found in 5–30% of patients with Cushing's syndrome, while IGT may be seen in 50–95%[31]. Virtually all patients with Cushing's syndrome have both basal and stimulated hyperinsulinemia. Patients with abnormally low insulin secretion are more likely to develop type 2 diabetes in the setting of Cushing's syndrome.

Glucocorticoid treatment and diabetes

Glucocorticoids are administered to patients who require the immunosuppressive or anti-inflammatory effects of these agents, and therefore IGT would be expected to be more common at baseline. The addition of glucocorticoids, however, does lead to deterioration in glucose tolerance. Analogous to the incidence observed with Cushing's syndrome, 5–10% of patients treated with glucocorticoids can be expected to develop overt diabetes, and 30–50% may develop IGT. With chronic administration of glucocorticoids, hyperinsulinemia is universal, and those individuals without adequate beta-cell reserve can be expected to develop diabetes.

Glucagonoma

This rare tumor of the pancreas is most often malignant, and frequently is accompanied by hypersecretion of other pancreatic polypeptides[32]. While glucose intolerance is almost universal with the glucagonoma syndrome, insulin resistance is not a major feature. Enhanced hepatic glucose output in response to the hyperglucagonemia causes the hyperglycemia. Peripheral insulin levels are normal or increased, correlating with the glucose levels. Ketoacidosis is rare, and probably reflects an underlying insulin-deficiency state.

Pheochromocytoma and catecholamines

Metabolic effects

The catecholamines epinephrine, norepinephrine and dopamine have profound metabolic effects. Pathophysiologic effects from excessive catecholamines may be manifested through both alpha- and beta-adrenergic receptors. Carbohydrate intolerance may be seen with both alpha- and beta-adrenergic receptor effects.

The exact mechanism whereby catecholamines induce glucose intolerance is complex and has not been fully explained. The alpha-adrenergic effect contributing to glucose intolerance is primarily from the inhibition of basal insulin secretion[33]. Alpha-receptor stimulation also leads to glucagon secretion and enhanced glucose output and glycogenolysis, via a cAMP independent mechanism. Beta-adrenergic effects include enhanced adipose tissue lipolysis, enhanced muscle tissue glycogenolysis and diminished glucose uptake by skeletal muscle. In addition, beta-adrenergic receptor stimulation leads to increased hepatic glucose output.

Pheochromocytoma and diabetes

IGT occurs in at least 30% of patients with pheochromocytoma[34]. The mechanism of the glucose intolerance in pheochromocytoma can be inferred from the metabolic effects of catecholamines, which include decreased insulin release, enhanced glucose output, peripheral insulin resistance, and increased lipolysis. The fasting glucose level is often normal, with a blunted post-challenge insulin response being observed. A return to normal glucose tolerance can be achieved by administration of an alpha-adrenergic receptor antagonist, such as phenoxybenzamine, and by surgical removal of the tumor. While insulin secretion is normalized fairly quickly after surgery, peripheral insulin sensitivity may be blunted for up to a month postoperatively.

Catecholamine treatment and diabetes

All three catecholamines are utilized clinically for a variety of physiologic derangements. Epinephrine has the most profound effects on glucose intolerance. The effects of norepinephrine are minimal in comparison. Peripheral insulin resistance is due to a postreceptor defect and increased FFA from enhanced lipolysis. As might be expected, the hyperglycemic effects of epinephrine are greater in patients with type 2 diabetes and intercurrent illness.

Hyperthyroidism

Hyperthyroidism has been associated with multiple metabolic abnormalities, including increased glycogenolysis and gluconeogenesis, lipolysis and proteolysis. In addition, the insulin clearance rate has been reported to be increased by close to 40%[35]. Glucose intolerance in the setting of hyperthyroidism is usually mild to moderate. The incidence is listed as 7–50%; overt diabetes is rare. In Maxon's 12-year study of thyrotoxic individuals, diabetes or glucose intolerance was detected in 68% of subjects at baseline. Fifty percent of previously diabetic subjects (four of eight) returned to normal glucose tolerance after treatment of their thyrotoxicosis, and remained normal for 12 years[36]. Hyperthyroidism should be considered in patients with new glucose intolerance, or in diabetic patients with worsening of glycemic control.

Hyperaldosteronism

Conn's original description of the hyperaldosteronism syndrome from 1955 includes hypertension and hypokalemia, with the presence of glucose intolerance in 50% of patients[37]. Long-term follow-up of the glucose tolerance in patients with hyperaldosteronism is not available, but the incidence is likely to be somewhat lower than 50%. The glucose intolerance is usually mild, and is likely to be due to potassium depletion, although correction of the hyperaldosteronism does not always reverse the glucose intolerance.

Hyperandrogenism

The prototypical syndrome describing a relationship between hyperandrogenism and insulin resistance is the polycystic ovary syndrome (PCOS)[38]. There is much evidence to support an association between elevated androgen levels and insulin resistance. The mechanism likely involves a decrease in insulin sensitivity at the level of the skeletal muscles. Similarly, abuse of anabolic steroids by non-diabetic weight lifters and as therapy for aplastic anemia has been associated with elevations in post-challenge glucose and insulin levels.

Other endocrinopathies

Hyperparathyroidism

Insulin hypersecretion and insulin resistance have been demonstrated in patients with primary hyperparathyroidism. A similar response has not been found in secondary hyperparathyroidism[39]. It is unclear if this is related to hypercalcemia, or to hypophosphatemia.

Gastrinoma syndrome

Occasional glucose intolerance has been reported with the gastrinoma syndrome, or the Zollinger–Ellison syndrome. The mechanism of this glucose intolerance is not clear.

Prolactin

Hyperinsulinemia and decreased post-challenge glucose tolerance has been described in hyperprolactinemia. Hypersecretion of other pituitary hormones and drugs that alter prolactin levels were screened for in these studies. Prolactin can increase FFA, and the resultant decrease in peripheral glucose uptake has been hypostulated to be part of the mechanism[40].

POEMS syndrome

POEMS is an acronym for polyneuropathy, organomegaly, endocrinopathy, monoclonal gammopathy and skin changes. It is a very rare plasma-cell disorder. Glucose intolerance or diabetes may be seen in about half of the cases[41].

REFERENCES

1 Report of the expert committee on the diagnosis and classification of diabetes mellitus. *Diabetes Care* 1998;21(Suppl. 2):B1–B167.

2 Pandit MK, Burke J, Gustafson AB *et al.* Drug-induced disorders of glucose tolerance. *Ann Intern Med* 1993;118:529–39.

3 Chan JCN, Cockram CS, Critchley AJH. Drug-induced disorders of glucose metabolism. Mechanisms and management. *Drug Safety* 1996;15:135–57.

4 Burt VL, Whelton P, Roccella EJ *et al.* Prevalence of hypertension in the US adult population: results from the Third National Health and Nutrition Examination Survey, 1988–1991. *Hypertension* 1995;25:305–13.

5 Gress TW, Nieto FJ, Shahar E *et al.* Hypertension and antihypertensive therapy as risk factors for type 2 diabetes mellitus. *N Engl J Med* 2000;342: 905–12.

6 Joint National Committee on Prevention, Detection, Evaluation and Treatment of High Blood Pressure. The sixth report of the Joint National Committee on Prevention, Detection, Evaluation and Treatment of High Blood Pressure. *Arch Intern Med* 1997;157:2413–36 [Erratum *Arch Intern Med* 1998;158:573].

7 Dornhorst A, Powell SH, Pensky J. Aggravation by propranolol of hyperglycaemic effect of hydrochlorothiazide in type II diabetics without alteration of insulin secretion. *Lancet* 1985;1: 123–6.

8 Lithell HO. Effect of antihypertensive drugs on insulin, glucose, and lipid metabolism. *Diabetes Care* 1991;14:203–9.

9 Murphy MB, Kohner E, Lewis PJ *et al.* Glucose intolerance in hypertensive patients treated with diuretics: fourteen-year follow-up. *Lancet* 1982;ii:1293–5.

10 Helderman JH, Elahi D, Anderson DK *et al.* Prevention of the glucose intolerance of thiazide diuretics by maintenance of body potassium. *Diabetes* 1983;32:106–11.

11 Guthrie GP Jr, Miller RE, Kotchen TA, Koenig SH. Clonidine in patients with diabetes and mild hypertension. *Clin Pharmacol Ther* 1983;34:713–17.

12 Spellacy WN, Cruz AC, Buhi WC, Birk SA. The acute effects of ritodrine infusion on maternal metabolism: Measurements of levels of glucose, insulin, glucagon, triglycerides, cholesterol, placental lactogen, and chorionic gonadotropin. *Am J Obstet Gynecol* 1978;131:637–42.

13 Parr MJ, Anaes FC, Day AC *et al.* Theophylline poisoning—a review of 64 cases. *Intens Care Med* 1990;16:394–8.

14 Kahn SE, Beard JC, Schwartz MW *et al.* Increased β-cell secretory capacity as mechanism for islet adaptation to nicotinic acid-induced insulin resistance. *Diabetes* 1989;38:562–8.

15 Elam MB, Hunninghake DB, Davis KB *et al.* Effect of niacin on lipid and lipoprotein levels and glycemic control in patients with diabetes and peripheral arterial disease. The ADMIT study: a randomized trial. *JAMA* 2000;284: 1263–70.

16 Anderson R, Boedicker M, Mam M. Adverse reactions associated with pentamidine isethionate in AIDS patients: recommendations for monitoring therapy. *Drug Intell Clin Pharm* 1986;20: 862–8.

17 Munshi MN, Martin RE, Fonseca VA. Hyperosmolar nonketotic diabetic syndrome following treatment of human immunodeficiency virus infection with didanosine. *Diabetes Care* 1994;17:316–17.

18 Visnegarwala F, Krause KL, Musher DM. Severe diabetes associated with protease inhibitor therapy. *Ann Intern Med* 1997;127:349.

19 Kaul DR, Cinti SK, Carver PL, Kazanjian PH. HIV protease inhibitors: advances in therapy and adverse reactions, including metabolic complications. *Pharmacotherapy* 199;19:281–98.

20 Henry K, Rathgaber S, Sukkivan C, McCabe K. Diabetes mellitus induced by megestrol acetate in a patient with AIDS and cachexia. *Ann Intern Med* 1992;116:53.

21 Gupta S, Lentz B, Lockwood K, Frank B. Atypical antipsychotics and glucose dysregulation: a series of 4 cases. *Prim Care Comp J Clin Psychiatry* 2001;3:61–5.

22 Lazarus JH. *Endocrine and metabolic effects of lithium.* New York: Plenum Medical Book Co., 1986.

23 Boudreaux JP, McHugh L, Cunetax DM *et al.* The impact of cyclosporine and combination immunosuppression on the incidence of post-transplant diabetes in renal allograft recipients. *Transplantation* 1987;44:376–81.

24 Patel YC. Somatostatin. In: Becker KL, eds. *Principles and practice of endocrinology and metabolism.* 2nd edn. Philadelphia: Lippincott Williams and Wilkins, 1995: 1436–46.

25 Spellacy WN. A review of carbohydrate metabolism and the oral contraceptive. *Am J Obstet Gynecol* 1969;104:448–60.

26 Bressler P, DeFronzo RA. Drug effects on glucose homeostasis. In: Alberti, Zimmet and DeFronzo, editors. *International textbook of diabetes mellitus.* 2nd edn. Chichester: John Wiley and Sons Ltd, 1997: 213–54.

27 Press M. Growth hormone and metabolism. *Diabet Metab Rev* 1988;4:391–414.

28 Bratusch-Marrian PR, Smith D, DeFronzo RA. The effect of growth hormone on glucose metabolism and insulin secretion in man. *J Clin Endocrinol Metab* 1982;55:973–82.

29 Cutfield WS, Wilton P, Bennmarker H *et al.* Incidence of diabetes mellitus and impaired glucose tolerance in children and adolescents receiving growth-hormone treatment. *Lancet* 2000;355:610–13.

30 Nosadini R, Del Prato S, Tiengo A. Chichester Insulin resistance in Cushing's syndrome. *J Clin Endocrinol Metab* 1983;57:529–36.

31 Bowes SB, Benn JJ, Scobie IN *et al.* Glucose metabolism in patients with Cushing's syndrome. *Clin Endocrinol* 1991;34:311–20.

32 Stacpoole PW. The glucagonoma syndrome: clinical features, diagnosis, and treatment. *Endocr Rev* 1980;2:347–61.

33 Stenström G, Sjöström L, Smith U. Diabetes mellitus in phaeochromocytoma: fasting blood glucose levels before and after surgery in 60 patients with phaeochromocytoma. *Acta Endocrinol* 1984;106:511–15.

34 Hamaji M. Pancreatic α- and β-cell function in pheochromocytoma. *J Clin Endocrinol Metab* 1979;49:322–5.

35 Foss MC, Paccola GMGF, Saad MJA *et al.* Peripheral glucose metabolism in human hyperthyroidism. *J Clin Endocrinol Metab* 1990;70: 1167–72.

36 Maxon HR, Kreines KW, Goldsmith RE, Knowles HC Jr. Long-term observations of glucose tolerance in thyrotoxic patients. *Arch Intern Med* 1975;135:1477–80.

37 Conn JW. Hypertension, the potassium ion and impaired carbohydrate tolerance. *N Engl J Med* 1965;273:1135–43.

38 Chang RJ, Nakamura RM, Judd HL, Kaplan SA. Insulin resistance in non-obese patients with polycystic ovarian disease. *J Clin Endocrinol Metab* 1983;57:356–9.

39 Yasuda K, Hurukawa Y, Okuyama M *et al.* Glucose tolerance and insulin secretion in patients with parathyroid disorders. Effects of serum calcium on insulin release. *N Engl J Med* 1975;292:501–4.

40 Foss MC, Paula ZFJA, Paccola GMGF, Piccinato CE. Peripheral glucose metabolism in human hyperprolactinemia. *Clin Endocrinol* 1995;43: 721–6.

41 Bardwick PA, Zvaifler NJ, Gill GN *et al.* Plasma cell dyscrasia with polyneuropathy, organomegaly, endocrinopathy, M protein, and skin changes: the POEMS syndrome. Report of two cases and a review of the literature. *Medicine* 1980;59:311–22.

31

New devices and drugs on the horizon

Jeffrey I Joseph and Barry J Goldstein

NEW DEVICES FOR DIABETES MANAGEMENT

Innovative devices are being developed to more effectively match insulin levels with the immediate metabolic needs of the diabetic patient. Unfortunately, no technology has been able to mimic the rapid response and closed-loop features of nondiabetic physiology. All current methods of glucose control require a great deal of vigilance, interpretation and active management by the patient, physician and diabetes educator[1].

The success of self-monitoring of blood glucose (SBGM) has shifted the focus of daily blood glucose control to the patient. Devices, therefore, need to be safe and effective when used in the home environment of the diabetic patient[2]. The narrow therapeutic window of insulin therapy and the varied educational background of the diabetic patient make this task a formidable clinical challenge. A small group of well-motivated and educated patients are able to combine frequent SBGM, oral hypoglycemia agents, and insulin therapies, to tightly control fasting and post-prandial glucose levels. Many patients in this group are able to achieve tight long-term control (glycosylated hemoglobin (HbA1c) < 7.0%) with a low incidence of hypoglycemia and weight gain[3,4].

Data from the Diabetes Control and Complications Trial (DCCT) illustrate the limitations of current methods of glucose monitoring and drug delivery. Only a small percentage of type 1 diabetic patients attempting tight control (intensive-treatment group) were able to lower their mean blood glucose and HbA1c levels into the normal range. Although the majority of patients were able to achieve an improvement in HbA1c levels, they experienced a threefold increase in the incidence of hypoglycemia. Even modest improvements in HbA1c required a level of day-to-day commitment not found in the average patient with diabetes[3].

Physicians routinely recommend aggressive monitoring and insulin delivery strategies for patients with type 1 diabetes; in contrast, a less aggressive therapeutic approach has been recommended for many patients with type 2 diabetes[5,6]. Primary-care physicians and general internists often lack the time, resources, funding, and expertise in their offices to provide the education and close medical supervision required for intensive glucose control. Modern technology has great potential for decreasing the everyday burden of diabetes management. An automated or semi-automated system would allow patients to live near-normal lives without the fear of hypoglycemia.

All current methods of glucose monitoring and drug delivery require constant patient intervention (open-loop control)[1,3,4,7]. Closed-loop systems are being developed that integrate a real-time glucose sensor, insulin pump, and computer-control algorithm to tightly control blood glucose without patient supervision or intervention[8,9]. Although originally developed for patients with type 1 diabetes, many devices have direct application in type 2 diabetics with absolute or relative insulin deficiency[10]. The following is a brief review of this evolving field. The reader is referred to the journal *Diabetes Technology and Therapeutics* (www.liebertpub.com) and the website Diabetes Mall (www.diabetesnet.com) for updated information.

PERSONAL METERS FOR SBGM LEVELS

Frequent SBGM correlates closely with improved long-term blood glucose control, and decreased risk of hypoglycemia in patients with type 1 diabetes[6]. The clinical benefit of frequent SBGM in type 2 diabetics managed with diet and oral agents remains controversial[4,7]. HbA1c levels decline when type 2 diabetics SBGM more than once per day and aggressively self-regulate their doses of insulin[11]. Current recommendations of the American Diabetes Association (ADA) call for SBGM at least 3–4 times each day for individuals with type 1 diabetes, and at least once daily for patients with type 2 diabetes treated with insulin or oral agents[2,5]. In actual clinical practice, as many as 56% of type 2 diabetics never practice SBGM. Eight to nine percent practice SBGM only once per week, 15–22% practice SBGM 1–6 times per week, and 11–17% practice SBGM more than 1 time per day[12]. Reasons for infrequent self-monitoring include fingerstick pain, inconvenience, cost, and lack of knowledge about the importance of SBGM for tight glucose control.

Older blood glucose (BG) meters did not consistently achieve either the ADA or the Food and Drug Administration's goals for BG meter accuracy[5,13]. Modern meters provide a more accurate measurement, and require a much smaller sample volume (0.3–5 μL). Recent alternative site meters allow sampling from the forearm to decrease pain. Controversy continues regarding a circulatory time delay and bias when SBGM forearm measurements are compared with fingertip measurements; however, the differences are small and are not considered to be clinically significant[14].

Several devices have simplified the process of SBGM by integrating the test strip and lancet into a miniature hand-held device. Advances in meter design allow a smaller sample volume and more consistent sample delivery to the site of assay, use membrane technology to minimize the effects of interfering substances, and give rapid measurement times. Modern meters have the capacity to store hundreds of blood glucose measurements. Data can be downloaded to a personal computer, displayed, and forwarded to a clinician for trend analysis. Strowig *et al.* demonstrated that HbA1c could be lowered by 0.5% by merely providing the diabetic patient with accurate SBGM trend data from a meter memory[15]. Software has been developed for palm-sized computers that simplifies the process of data collection, display, and trend analysis.

Hand-held laser systems have been developed to perforate the skin, in place of using a lancet, to obtain a blood sample prior to SBGM measurement. While this has been heralded as a painless approach, many patients still experience some discomfort from the procedure[16].

Non-invasive SBGM technology

It is thought that eliminating the discomfort of fingerstick sampling would result in patients SBGM more frequently. To be clinically useful, non-invasive glucose monitoring systems would have to be small, lightweight, portable, safe, and accurate. A variety of optical methods have been devised to measure glucose in blood, interstitial fluid, and eye fluid[17,18]. The prototype devices require sophisticated optics and electronics, for stability and high signal-to-noise ratios. Unfortunately, there continues to be great variability in the optical signal when the light source and detector are coupled to the sample tissue. Complex signal processing and analytical techniques are required to extract the glucose information from the optical spectra. Some of the most promising recent technologies involve shining a near-infrared light through the tongue (transmission spectroscopy)[17] and measuring the change in light polarization across the anterior chamber of the eye (optical rotation)[18].

DEVICES FOR INSULIN DELIVERY

Insulin pens

Insulin pens provide increased convenience, improve accuracy of dose, and overall safety. One-half unit incremental dosing is now possible. The most common therapeutic regimen using pens consists of multiple daily injections of rapid-acting insulin (prior to meals) and intermediate-acting insulin at bedtime[19].

Needle-free insulin delivery system

Needle-free systems inject insulin through the skin using a high-pressure jet injector. Insulin is supplied in a disposable ampule, and a manual piston or cartridge supplies the driving force. Rapid and consistent insulin absorption has been demonstrated. Although reported as painless, many patients do experience discomfort and irritation at the injection site with these devices.

External insulin pumps—continuous subcutaneous insulin infusion

External insulin pumps have gained popularity because of increased flexibility of dosing in relation to meals and exercise[20]. Basal and bolus doses of rapid-acting insulin (insulin lispro or insulin aspart in the USA) can be delivered into the subcutaneous tissue with great precision. Modern pumps are small, light-weight, water-resistant, reliable, and highly programmable.

Because failure to deliver the shorter-acting rapid insulins, due to pump malfunction, catheter occlusion, disconnection, or malplacement, can rapidly lead to hyperglycemia and ketosis, patients need to be reminded about the importance of frequent self-monitoring[2,3]. Ketoacidosis can develop within hours following complete absorption of the subcutaneous insulin depot, which may consist of only 2–4 U[3,21]. Although their effect resolves more rapidly than regular insulin, plasma levels of the rapidly acting insulins still do not return to basal levels for several hours following a meal. Hypoglycemia and weight-gain continue to pose significant clinical challenges[22]. Glycemic control using continuous subcutaneous insulin

infusion (CSII) has generally been thought to be at least equal to, if not better than, multiple daily injections of insulin[23].

In attempts to overcome some of the limitations of the subcutaneous delivery of insulin, a novel system has been developed by Disetronic Medical Systems (www.disetronic-usa.com) that delivers insulin from an external pump directly into a catheter in the peritoneal cavity, for portal vein absorption (Figure 31.1). Another potential improvement has involved the use of tissue-engineering techniques to grow a capillary network adjacent to the tip of the infusion catheter. This has been shown to provide rapid and complete absorption of insulin, and overcomes some of the pharmacokinetic limitations of subcutaneous delivery[24].

The use of insulin pumps and CSII therapy in the management of type 2 diabetes has been more controversial. Frequent SBGM monitoring, carbohydrate counting, and careful control of

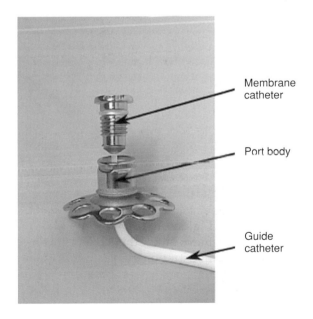

Figure 31.1 Long-term implantable intraperitoneal insulin infusion catheter from Disetronic Medical (Diaport). Insulin is delivered from an external insulin pump to the peritoneal cavity through the removable inner membrane catheter. The port body remains implanted within the subcutaneous tissue with a percutaneous exit site.

caloric intake are required to avoid hypoglycemia and excessive weight gain. Excellent glycemic control has been achieved in type 2 diabetics where there is insulin resistance and progressive beta-cell dysfunction[10,25].

Implantable insulin pumps—continuous peritoneal insulin infusion

The safety and efficacy of continuous peritoneal insulin infusion (CPII) therapy using a programmable implantable insulin pump have been demonstrated in patients with type 1 and type 2 diabetes. An external programmer is used to control the basal rate and timing/amount of a regular insulin bolus infused prior to meals. Peritoneal insulin delivery significantly reduces the risk of hypoglycemia, an advantage that may be due to portal delivery of insulin and a more physiological ratio of portal to systemic insulin levels. The subcutaneous pump reservoir can be easily refilled (with U-400 insulin) every 2–3 months in the physician's office (Figure 31.2)[26].

Inhaled insulin

Inhaled insulin therapy appears to be safe and effective, at least in short-term studies. Dry

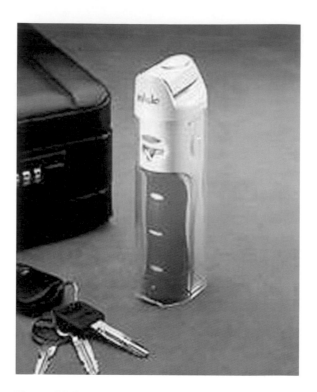

Figure 31.3 Hand-held insulin inhaler developed by Inhale Technologies.

powder or liquid insulin formulations are aerosolized within the inhaler, and delivered during non-turbulent airflow. Insulin molecules are deposited deep within the lung for alveolar absorption (Figure 31.3). Inhaled insulin can be given immediately before meals because the peak glucose-lowering effect occurs in around 60 min. Studies in type 2 diabetics demonstrate post-prandial BG control similar to subcutaneous lispro insulin[27]. However, the long-term health effects of delivering large doses of insulin deep in the lung are unknown. Only 30% of the inhaled dose is bioavailable, and some of the potential adverse effects include reduced lung volumes and pulmonary thromboses.

CONTINUOUS GLUCOSE MONITORING (REAL-TIME SENSORS)

It is not possible to perform SBGM frequently enough to accurately identify all major blood glucose excursions (Figure 31.4). Real-time

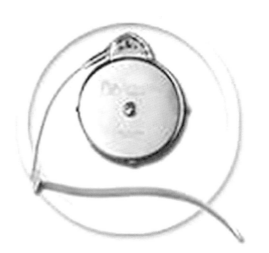

Figure 31.2 Implantable programmable insulin infusion pump and catheter system (Medtronic-MiniMed Corp.).

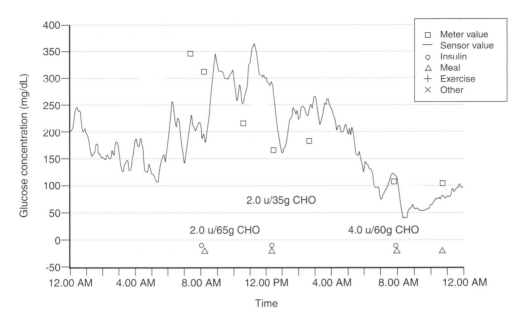

Figure 31.4 Twenty-four-hour glucose profile using the Medtronic-MiniMed Continuous Glucose Monitoring System (CGMS). Note dynamic nature of glucose fluctuations and relationship between continuous sensor measurements and intermittent fingerstick self-monitoring capillary blood glucose (SMBG) measurements.

glucose monitoring systems have great potential to direct drug therapy and for providing alarms for impending hypo- and hyperglycemia[32]. More aggressive drug therapy can be initiated to lower fasting, post-prandial, and HbA1c levels without the risk of hypoglycemia. Frequent glucose data can be used by the patient, physician, and diabetes educator to enhance blood glucose control, through a better understanding of the relationship between meals, exercise, and sleep and the amount/timing of insulin and oral hypoglycemic drug therapy[28].

Non-invasive glucose sensor using reverse iontophoresis

Cygnus Corporation (Redwood, CA, USA, www.cygn.com) has developed a non-invasive, interstitial fluid glucose monitoring system called the Glucowatch Biographer. The system resembles a wristwatch, and uses dual electrodes and reverse iontophoresis (electric current) to extract glucose-containing interstitial fluid from the skin. Tissue fluid is collected

within a gel pad, and analyzed for glucose using a standard enzyme, electrochemical technique. The system provides glucose data in real-time for patient interpretation, and includes programmable alarms to warn against low or high glucose levels. The technology is limited by a long extraction time (20 min), long warm-up period (2 h), short gel-pad lifetime (12 h), and irritation of the skin[29].

Needle-type glucose sensor

Miniature needle-type glucose sensors are inserted across the skin into the subcutaneous adipose tissue. This classic electrochemical glucose sensor uses a glucose oxidase enzyme to covert interstitial fluid glucose to hydrogen peroxide. This generates electrons and a current that is correlated with a glucose measurement by a two-point calibration, performed by the patient. Sensitivity and specificity for glucose are excellent over the physiological range (40–400 mg dL[-1]). The electrodes and glucose oxidase enzyme are protected beneath a porous

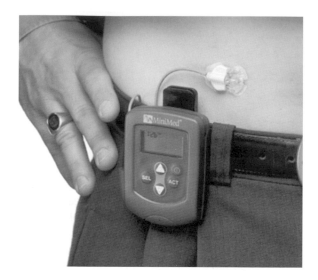

Figure 31.5 Continuous glucose monitoring system (CGMS) developed by Medtronic MiniMed Corp. Needle-type sensor is attached to an electronics module with a flexible cable. Interstitial fluid glucose measurements are automatically recorded every five minutes for three days (864 data points). Future models will include a graphical display and alarms to warn of impending hypo and hyperglycemia.

membrane that is permeable only to small molecules, such as oxygen and glucose.

Following insertion, however, the pores of the membrane become fouled with white blood cells and protein, causing an immediate loss of sensitivity (decreased sensor output in response to a change in glucose concentration). Drift of the signal from the sensor necessitates multiple SBGM measurements per day to maintain calibration. Long-term sensor function is limited due to foiling of the underlying enzyme. The risk of infection necessitates placement of a new sensor at an alternative location every 2–4 days.

Medtronic-MiniMed's continuous glucose monitoring system (CGMS) measures the concentration of interstitial fluid glucose every 5 min (www.medtronic-minimed.com, Northridge, CA, USA). Sensor drift necessitates four or more SBGM measures per 24 h, followed by a retrospective calibration. The system is designed to store 72 h of glucose data in the hand-held device for future interpretation by a physician (Figure 31.5)[30]. Forthcoming devices will provide real-time data for patient interpretation, including alarms for hypo- and hyperglycemia. Clinical experience with the CGMS in diabetic patients has revealed a high incidence of previously unrecognized post-prandial hyperglycemia, as well as nocturnal hypoglycemia[31].

Interstitial fluid glucose sensor using skin poration

The minimally invasive glucose monitoring system developed by Spectrex (Norcross, GA, USA, www.spectrx.com) uses a hand-held laser to form four small holes in the epidermis. Interstitial fluid flows from the skin into an external gel-pad containing the enzyme glucose oxidase. Glucose is measured every few minutes using a standard electrochemical sensor technique. Epidermal pores are reported to provide ample tissue fluid for more than 2 days (Figure 31.6).

Dialysis-type glucose sensor

Dialysis-type sensors consist of a miniature dialysis catheter inserted through the skin into the subcutaneous adipose tissue. A glucose-free solution (dialysate) is infused into the catheter and allowed to equilibrate with the interstitial fluid. Glucose-containing fluid is pumped from the in-dwelling catheter to an enzyme-based electrochemical sensor external to the body. Sensor drift is less of a problem because the enzyme and electrodes are not in direct contact with the tissues of the body. Limitations include a long sample acquisition time (15 min) and risk of infection.

Disetronic has developed a novel dialysate solution that changes viscosity according to the glucose concentration. Sensor stability and accuracy are improved by measuring inflow and outflow dialysate pressure and viscosity.

ARTIFICIAL ENDOCRINE PANCREAS (FOR AMBULATORY PATIENTS)

An artificial endocrine pancreas consists of a real-time glucose sensor, an insulin infusion

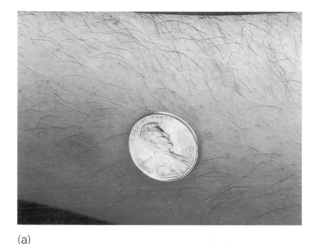

(a)

(b)

Figure 31.6 SpectRx Glucose Monitoring System. Small pores are formed within skin using a hand-held laser. Interstitial tissue fluid is continuously collected by the external sensor head for the real-time monitoring of glucose levels. Patient-worn electronics module provides data display with programmable alarms.

pump, and a computer control algorithm (controller)[32]. An integrated system can automatically determine the appropriate dose and timing of insulin, based upon absolute glucose measurements, recent glucose trends, and the recent dose of insulin given. Predictive and adaptive control algorithms use a model of patient physiology and insulin pharmacokinetics/dynamics to determine the appropriate dose of insulin for subsequent delivery. Glucose trends, including the onset of hypoglycemia, can be predicted with accuracy[8]. Simpler controllers have been developed and validated in human volunteers[9]. Closed-loop algorithms are designed to automatically regulate the delivery of insulin without patient intervention. Semi-closed-loop algorithms require data input from the patient regarding meal timing/composition and the onset of exercise.

EXTERNAL ARTIFICIAL ENDOCRINE PANCREAS

The ADICOL project (Advanced Insulin Infusion with a Control Loop), led by Disetronic, has integrated an external glucose sensor (dialysis-type or needle-type), an external insulin pump (CSII or CPII using rapid-acting insulin), and a computer to provide closed-loop control of blood glucose levels in ambulatory patients with type 1 diabetes. Similar systems have achieved near-normal glucose control, without hypoglycemia, in a small number of diabetic animals and ambulatory humans[8,9]. Issues related to sensor calibration, time delays resulting from the sensor and insulin delivery, and algorithm robustness, remain obstacles to routine clinical application.

IMPLANTABLE ARTIFICIAL ENDOCRINE PANCREAS

Medtronic-MiniMed has developed a glucose sensor with the potential for long-term implantation. The system resembles a pacemaker with a subcutaneous electronics module and a catheter for placement within the superior vena cava. The catheter tip contains glucose oxidase enzyme and dual oxygen sensors. Blood glucose is calculated by measuring the oxygen concentration adjacent to the enzyme (decreased due to oxidation of glucose) compared with the ambient oxygen concentration. Excellent accuracy and sensor stability have been demonstrated. Membrane fouling, enzyme degradation, and clot formation are common causes of premature sensor failure. A study was recently initiated in diabetic humans to demonstrate feasibility of a combined implantable insulin pump and vena cava sensor system.

Animas Corporation (www.animas.com, Fraser, PA, USA) has developed a long-term implantable sensor that uses near-infrared spectroscopy to measure the concentration of glucose in blood. The system resembles a pacemaker with a subcutaneous electronics/optical module and a miniature sensor head mounted around a blood vessel. A universal calibration algorithm has been developed that allows glucose to be accurately predicted from the optical spectra. The system may overcome the biocompatibility limitations of other electrochemical sensors, because near-infrared light can easily pass through any layer of cells and protein that coats the optical windows following implantation. To date, the feasibility of the sensor head design has been demonstrated long-term in an animal model[33].

ARTIFICIAL ENDOCRINE PANCREAS (FOR HOSPITALIZED PATIENTS)

In a landmark study, van Den Berghe and colleagues demonstrated that control of glucose to near normal levels (90–110 mg dL^{-1}) decreases morbidity and mortality following surgery and major illness in hospitalized patients[34]. Current hospital methods require frequent bedside glucose monitoring and careful titration of an intravenous insulin infusion to achieve tight blood glucose control. Despite these precautions, the incidence of wide swings in blood glucose and episodes of hypoglycemia remains high. The artificial pancreas systems developed in the 1970s (Biostator), primarily for research studies, successfully automated the process of glucose monitoring and insulin delivery. The devices were large, required frequent sensor recalibration, and caused 200 mL phlebotomy per day.

A compact flow-through glucose sensor was recently developed by Metracor Technologies (www.metracor.com, San Diego, CA, USA) that samples the blood, measures the glucose level, and returns the blood to the patient with a small volume flush, as frequently as every 5 min for up to 72 h[35]. This method avoids the loss of blood observed with other methods of venous sampling. A modern artificial pancreas system is under development that combines the Metacor sensor, an infusion pump, and a computer to provide closed-loop control of blood glucose levels in hospitalized patients.

NEW DRUGS FOR TYPE 2 DIABETES ON THE HORIZON

Recent advances in our understanding of the disease processes that cause type 2 diabetes have led to the identification of new targets for drug therapy[36]. This, in turn, has paved the way for the development of novel pharmaceuticals to help control blood glucose levels[37]. Strategies for normalizing blood glucose levels are aimed at various components of the pathophysiological triad that contributes to the diabetic state:

- Glucose disposal into skeletal muscle and adipose tissue
- Hepatic glucose production
- Pancreatic insulin secretion.

To gain acceptance into the marketplace, a new pharmaceutical agent would be expected to be more efficacious than currently available agents, while limiting untoward side-effects that may restrict its use in the aggressive management of diabetes, especially hypoglycemia and weight gain.

The section below will briefly introduce a number of new targets that are currently being explored as candidates for novel therapeutics that may ultimately find a role in the future management of diabetes.

TARGETING INSULIN RESISTANCE IN SKELETAL MUSCLE AND ADIPOSE TISSUE

Resistance to the action of insulin in glucose disposal is a key component of type 2 diabetes.

Much of this insulin resistance is associated with obesity, especially abdominal or visceral adiposity. Although the cellular defects leading to the observed resistance to insulin signaling have not been fully elucidated, an increasing body of evidence points to factors secreted from adipose tissue, including free fatty acids (FFA) and adipocytokines, such as tumor-necrosis factor-alpha (TNF-alpha), interleukin-6 (IL-6) and adiponectin[38]. The mechanism by which these circulating mediators affect insulin signaling is the subject of much ongoing research.

Insulin signaling is transmitted by the tyrosine kinase activity of the receptor that triggers a downstream cascade of protein tyrosine phosphorylation on receptor substrate proteins[36]. FFA and the inhibitory adipocytokines (TNF-alpha and IL-6) block post-receptor signaling by stimulating a variety of cellular enzymes that can inhibit the tyrosine phosphorylation cascade responsible for the activation of the insulin signal in the cell. Knowledge of some of the defects that occur in this signaling system in patients with type 2 diabetes has provided a framework for the development of new therapeutic compounds.

The thiazolidinediones, ligands for the PPAR-gamma receptor, have proven to be of substantial benefit in the treatment of type 2 diabetes[39]. These drugs target the underlying insulin resistance, and not only help to lower blood glucose levels, but also ameliorate a variety of cardiovascular defects found in patients with the 'metabolic syndrome'. The mechanism of thiazolidinedione action appears to involve activation of the PPAR-gamma nuclear receptor in adipose tissue, which lowers circulating FFA and affects the secretion of adipocytokines, which secondarily enhances insulin signal transduction in skeletal muscle and liver tissue[40]. The beneficial effect of thiazolidinediones on beta-cell insulin secretion is also postulated to result from a reduction in systemic lipid availability and levels of tissue triglycerides in the beta-cells themselves[41]. Newer pharmaceuticals that improve on the currently available thiazolidinediones might have enhanced glucose-lowering capacity, possibly with a reduction in troubling side-effects, including weight gain and fluid retention[42]. Characterization of the cellular proteins whose abundance is modulated by stimulation

with PPAR-gamma ligands may also help to identify new targets for the future development of diabetes drugs[37].

PPAR-alpha, the major cellular target for lipid-lowering fibrate drugs, has received interest as a target for therapy of the mixed hyperlipidemia often found in type 2 diabetes. Novel drugs with combined PPAR-gamma and PPAR-alpha binding activity, and with enhanced lipid-lowering effects, have been sought by several pharmaceutical companies[43]. The discovery of selective modulators of nuclear hormone receptors, including members of the PPAR family, may be a successful strategy for the development of new drugs that can effectively manage hyperglycemia, dyslipidemia and endothelial dysfunction, possibly with fewer untoward effects on adipose redistribution and fluid retention than observed with the currently available agents[44].

A glucocorticoid-metabolizing enzyme in adipose tissue has recently been identified as a novel potential target for ameliorating the metabolic defects found in the insulin resistance syndrome. The striking phenotypic similarities between Cushing's syndrome and type 2 diabetes, involving central obesity, insulin resistance, hypertension and glucose intolerance, has provided an impetus for seeking a pathophysiological link between these two disorders. The enzyme 11-beta-hydroxysteroid dehydrogenase type 1 (11-betaHSD1) catalyzes the tissue conversion of cortisone to the active glucocorticoid, cortisol, and is increased in obese humans[45]. Mice that over-express 11-betaHSD1 selectively in adipose tissue develop visceral obesity exaggerated by a high-fat diet, along with insulin-resistant diabetes and hyperlipidemia, a condition similar to type 2 diabetes[46]. Since 11-betaHSD1 expression is suppressed by treatment with thiazolidinediones[47], inhibition of 11-betaHSD1 may effectively prevent some of the manifestations of the metabolic syndrome, and serve some benefit in the treatment of type 2 diabetes.

ACTIVATION OF THE INSULIN-RECEPTOR TYROSINE PHOSPHORYLATION CASCADE

In another novel approach, it has recently been shown that non-peptide small molecules can selectively activate the insulin receptor, opening the way for the possibility that an oral, non-peptide drug might stimulate the receptor in the same way as insulin[48,49].

An alternative approach to the direct activation of the insulin receptor is to inhibit cellular enzymes that deactivate the receptor. Receptor activation and early post-receptor signal transduction depends on the phosphorylation of specific tyrosine residues in the receptor and its cellular substrate (IRS) proteins[50]. The specific protein-tyrosine phosphatase enzymes (PTPases) that dephosphorylate these proteins and negatively regulate the early insulin-receptor signaling cascade have been targeted for pharmaceutical intervention[51]. One cellular PTPase, PTP1B, has been identified as a major regulator of insulin signaling, as well as obesity. Mice lacking expression of PTP1B are not only more insulin-sensitive, but also resistant to weight gain with high fat feeding, apparently due to increased energy expenditure[52,53]. Given the potential additional benefit of PTP1B inhibition to affect glucose metabolism and weight regulation, this enzyme has been an attractive target for new drug development. The approaches to PTP1B inhibition have involved oral enzymatic inhibitors, as well as a novel anti-sense oligonucleotide reagent taken orally, which significantly reduces tissue expression of PTP1B and enhances insulin action[54].

INHIBITING NEGATIVE REGULATORS OF INSULIN METABOLIC SIGNALING

Other putative negative regulators of insulin signaling have recently been targetted for drug development. Glycogen synthase kinase-3 (GSK-3) is an enzyme in the downstream cellular signaling cascade that inhibits the activation of glycogen synthase and opposes the action of insulin in muscle. Recent animal studies with selective GSK-3 inhibitors demonstrated an enhancement of insulin action[55].

Other downstream kinases have been implicated in the negative regulation of the insulin-signaling pathway, possibly activated by FFA, hyperglycemia or TNF-alpha, including I-kappa-B kinase[56,57] and protein kinase C-theta[58].

AMP-activated kinase (AMPK) is an enzyme activated by reduced cellular energy charge that is involved in insulin-independent activation of glucose transport[59]. Activation of AMPK with an allosteric enzyme activator, the adenosine analog AICAR, has been shown to inhibit hepatic glucose output and increased muscle glucose uptake, raising the possibility that it could be the target of new drug development[60]. Recently, AMPK has also been implicated in the mechanism of metformin inhibition of hepatic glucose production[61].

Adiponectin is a relatively abundant plasma protein secreted from adipose tissue whose blood levels are negatively correlated with insulin resistance and atherosclerosis[62]. In obese, insulin-resistant subjects, and those with coronary artery disease, adiponectin levels are reduced, and administration of adiponectin has been shown to reduce hepatic glucose in mice and to improve endothelial function[63]. Adiponectin also appears to induce tissue fatty acid oxidation, with a reduction of triglycerides and FFA in animal models, suggesting that a pharmaceutical agent that can stimulate the adiponectin signaling pathway might have beneficial effects on a variety of abnormalities in patients with the metabolic syndrome[64,65].

TARGETS FOR REDUCING EXCESSIVE HEPATIC GLUCOSE PRODUCTION

Glucagon receptor

Glucagon enhances glycogenolysis and gluco-neogenesis, and the excessive glucagon secretion found in type 2 diabetes contributes markedly to hyperglycemia. Blocking the action of glucagon at the receptor itself has been identified as a target that might be susceptible to small-molecule pharmaceutical development[66].

Amylin

Amylin is a 37 amino-acid polypeptide that is co-secreted with insulin from the pancreatic beta-cells in response to nutrient stimuli. In type 2 diabetes, amylin levels are more variable, but tend to be decreased in the later stages of the disease[67]. Infusion of pharmacological concentrations of amylin, or a more stable analog called pramlintide, inhibits gastric emptying and decreases glucagon secretion, possibly mediated by interference with vagal nerve activity[68]. Thus, amylin tends to enhance glucose control in patients with diabetes via several complementary mechanisms.

Glycogen breakdown and gluconeogenesis

Inhibition of hepatic glycogen phosphorylase has been identified as another target of drug therapy[69]. Since glucose-6-phosphatase is the final biosynthetic step prior to release of glucose into the bloodstream from the liver, drugs blocking this enzyme, or one upstream in the gluconeogenic cascade, would be expected to inhibit hepatic glucose production[70,71]. Potential concerns with these approaches might include hypoglycemia, since liver glucose release could be affected in an uncontrolled manner. The transcriptional coactivator PGC-1 has recently been shown to be a key mediator of increased hepatic glucose production in animal models of relative insulin deficiency, suggesting that it may be a target for drug intervention in type 2 diabetes. PGC-1 is induced in liver-cell cultures by cyclic AMP and glucocorticoids, and mediates a complex program of gluconeogenic enzyme expression that results in increased glucose output[72].

TARGETS FOR ENHANCING GLUCOSE-STIMULATED INSULIN SECRETION

There is clearly a current need for drugs that will enhance the secretion of insulin in a manner more closely dependent on the ambient glucose concentration, without promoting excessive insulin secretion. This would avoid the hypoglycemia that is a major limiting factor with the aggressive use of sulfonylureas and related insulin secretagogs. Other drawbacks of current therapy with insulin secretagogs include weight gain, possibly exacerbated by episodic hypoglycemia, and secondary failure over time[73].

New strategies may take advantage of the effects of the incretin peptides: gut-derived hormones that potentiate insulin secretion and

normally enhance insulin secretion in response to oral delivery of nutrients to the gut[74]. Endogenous incretins that might be useful as pharmaceutical agents to enhance glucose-coupled insulin secretion include glucagon-like peptide-1 (GLP-1) and gastric inhibitory peptide (GIP)[75]. GLP-1 has the additional potential advantages of inhibiting gastric emptying and reducing glucagon secretion. Besides the administration of GLP-1 or peptide derivatives by injection or buccal absorption, a novel approach to enhancing the effects of these agents has been to target dipeptidylpeptidase–IV (DPP-IV), a plasma enzyme that rapidly degrades these peptides in the circulation. Pharmaceutical inhibition of DPP-IV improves metabolic control, apparently by the relatively specific enhancement of the effects of GLP-1[76]. Exendin-4 is a modified GLP-1 analog that is relatively resistant to DPP-IV and has prolonged activity *in vivo*[77].

CONCLUSIONS

Since the worldwide epidemic of obesity and type 2 diabetes shows no signs of abating, there will be an increased need in the coming years for new approaches to pharmacologic therapies for this disorder. In addition to therapies directed at improving glucose metabolism and the lipid profile, there is a clear need for safe drugs that will help to manage obesity and prevent the weight gain that underlies much of the current epidemic of the metabolic syndrome.

Recent studies have identified multiple targets in various tissues that may eventually provide novel approaches to the management of type 2 diabetes and its concomitant cardiovascular risk profile. We can anticipate that new treatments will eventually become available that can be used in combination with currently available agents, or supplant them entirely, as we become more aggressive in managing patients towards appropriate clinical goals affecting glycemic control, lipid, blood pressure, and emerging, less traditional, cardiovascular risk factors.

REFERENCES

1 Klein R, Klein BE, Moss SE, Cruikshanks KJ. The medical management of hyperglycemia over a 10-year period in people with diabetes. *Diabetes Care* 1996;19:744–50.

2 American Diabetes Association. Self-monitoring of blood glucose (Consensus statement). *Diabetes Care* 1996;19(Suppl 1):562–6.

3 The Diabetes Control and Complications Trial Research Group. The effect of intensive treatment of diabetes on the development and progression of long-term complications in insulin-dependent diabetes mellitus. *N Engl J Med* 1993;329:977–86.

4 UK Prospective Diabetes Study (UKPDS) Group. Intensive blood-glucose control with sulfony-lureas or insulin compared with conventional treatment in patients with type 2 diabetes (UKPDS 33). *Lancet* 1998;352: 837–53.

5 American Diabetes Association. Standards of medical care for patients with diabetes mellitus. *Diabetes Care* 2001;23(Suppl 1):S33–S34.

6 Edelman SV. Importance of glucose control. *Med Clin N Am* 1998;82:665–87.

7 Faas A, Schellevis FG, van Eijk JT. The efficacy of self-monitoring of blood glucose in NIDDM subjects: a criteria-based literature review. *Diabetes Care* 1997;20:1482–6.

8 Rebrin K, Fischer U, von Woedtke T *et al.* Automated feedback control of subcutanous glucose concentration in diabetic dogs. *Diabetologia* 1989;32:573–6.

9 Shichiri M, Sakakida M, Nishida K, Shimoda S. Enhanced, simplified glucose sensors: long-term clinical application of wearable artificial endocrine pancreas. *Artif Organs* 1998;22:32–42.

10 Turner RC, Cull CA, Frighi V, Holman RR, for the UK Prospective Diabetes Study Group (UKPDS). Glycemic control with diet, sulfonylurea, metformin, or insulin in patients with type 2 diabetes mellitus. Progressive requirement for multiple therapies (UKPDS 49). *J Am Med Assoc* 1999;281:2005–12.

11 Franciosi M, Pellegrini F, De Berardis G *et al.* The impact of blood glucose self-monitoring on metabolic control and quality of life in type 2 diabetic patients. *Diabetes Care* 2001;24:1870–7.

12 Harris MI, Eastman RC, Cowie CC *et al.* Racial and ethnic differences in glycemic control of adults with type 2 diabetes. *Diabetes Care* 1999;22:403–13.

13 Food and Drug Administration. Review criteria assessment of portable blood glucose monitoring in-vitro diagnostic devices using glucose oxidase, dehydrogenase or hexokinase methodology. Draft guidance document, 1997 (www.fda.gov).

14 Feldman B, McGarrraugh G, Heller A *et al.* A small-volume electrochemical glucose sensor for home blood glucose testing. *Diabetes Technol Ther* 2000;2:221–9.

15 Strowig SM, Raskin P. Improved glycemic control in intensively treated type 1 diabetic patients using blood glucose meters with storage capacity and computer-assisted analyses. *Diabetes Care* 1998;21:1694–8.

16 Yum SI, Roe J. Capillary blood sampling for self-monitoring of blood glucose. *Diabetes Technol Ther* 1999:1;29–37.

17 Burmeister JJ, Arnold MA, Small GW. Non-invasive blood glucose measurements by near-infrared transmission spectroscopy across human tongues. *Diabetes Technol Ther* 2000;2:5–16.

18 Cameron B, Gorde H, Satheesan B, Cote G. The use of polarized laser light through the eye for noninvasive glucose monitoring. *Diabetes Technol Ther* 1999;1:135–43.

19 Wikby A, Stenstrom U, Andersson PO, Hornquist J. Metabolic control, quality of life, and negative life events: a longitudinal study of well-controlled and poorly regulated patients with type 1 diabetes after changeover to insulin pen treatment. *Diabetes Educator* 1998;24:61–6.

20 Farkas-Hirsch R, Hirsch IB. Continuous subcutaneous insulin infusion: a review of the past and its implementation for the future. *Diabetes Spec* 1994;7:136–8.

21 Reichel A, Rietzsch H, Kohler HJ *et al.* Cessation of insulin infusion at night-time during CSII-therapy: comparison of regular insulin and insulin lispro. *Exp Clin Endocrinol Diabetes* 1998; 106:168–72.

22 Herbel G, Boyle PJ. Hypoglycemia—pathophysiology and treatment. *Endocrinol Clin N Am* 2000;29:725–43.

23 Hayward RA, Manning WG, Kaplan SH *et al.* Starting insulin therapy in patients with type 2 diabetes: effectiveness, complications, and resource utilization. *J Am Med Assoc* 1997;278: 1663–9.

24 Dziubla TD, Torjman MC, Joseph JI *et al.* Evaluation or porous networks of poly (2-hydroxyethyl methacrylate) as interfacial drug delivery devices. *Biomaterials* 2001;22:2893–9.

25 Jennings AM, Lewis KS, Murdoch S *et al.* Randomized trial comparing continuous subcutaneous insulin infusion and conventional insulin therapy in type II diabetic patients poorly controlled with sulphonylureas. *Diabetes Care* 1991;14:738–44.

26 Saudek CD. Novel forms of insulin delivery—current therapies for diabetes. *Endocrinol Metab Clin N Am* 1997;26:599–610.

27 Weiss SR, Berger S Cheng S *et al.*, for the Phase II Inhaled Insulin Study Group. Adjunctive therapy with inhaled human insulin in type 2 diabetic patients failing oral agents: A multi-center phase II trial. *Diabetes* 1999;48 (Suppl 1):A12.

28 Gross TM, Ter Veer A. Continuous glucose monitoring in previously unstudied population subgroups. *Diabetes Technol Ther* 2000: 2 (Supp.1);27–34.

29 Tierney MJ, Tamada JA, Potts RO *et al.* The GlucoWatch biographer: a frequent, automatic, and non-invasive glucose monitor. *Ann Med* 2000;32:632–41.

30 Mastrototaro JJ. The MiniMed continuous glucose monitoring system. *Diabetes Technol Ther* 2000; 2 (Suppl 1): S13–S18.

31 Moghissi E, Mestman J. Type 2 diabetes. *Diabetes Technol Ther* 2000; 2 (Suppl 1):S61–S65.

32 Armour JC, Lucisano JY, McKean BD, Gough DA. Application of chronic intravascular blood glucose sensor in dogs. *Diabetes* 1990;39:1519–26.

33 Joseph JI, Torjman MC, Moritz M *et al.* Long-term vessel patency following perivascular sensor implantation. *Biomaterials* 2000;1 (Suppl):S231.

34 van Den Berghe G, Wouters P, Weekers F *et al.* Intensive insulin therapy in critically ill patients. *N Engl J Med* 2001;345:1359–67.

35 Lucisano JY, Edelman SV, Quinto BD, Wong DK. Development of a biosensor-based patient-attached blood glucose monitoring system. *Science Engineering* 1997;76:564–5.

36 Saltiel AR, Kahn CR. Insulin signalling and the regulation of glucose and lipid metabolism. *Nature* 2001;414:799–806.

37 Moller DE. New drug targets for type 2 diabetes and the metabolic syndrome. *Nature* 2001;414:821–7.

38 Zick Y. Insulin resistance: a phosphorylation-based uncoupling of insulin signaling. *Trends Cell Biol* 2001;11:437–41.

39 Moller DE, Greene DA. Peroxisome proliferator-activated receptor (PPAR) gamma agonists for diabetes. *Adv Protein Chem* 2001;56:181–212.

40 Goldstein BJ. Current views on the mechanism of action of thiazolidinedione insulin sensitizers. *Diabetes Technol Ther* 1999;1:267–75.

41 Unger RH, Orci L. Lipotoxic diseases of non-adipose tissues in obesity. *Int J Obesity* 2000;24:S28–S32.

42 Parulkar AA, Pendergrass ML, Granda-Ayala R *et al.* Nonhypoglycemic effects of thiazolidinediones [review]. *Ann Internal Med* 2001;134:61–71.

43 Murakami K, Tobe K, Ide T *et al.* A novel insulin sensitizer acts as a coligand for peroxisome proliferator-activated receptor-alpha (PPAR-alpha) and PPAR-gamma. *Diabetes* 1998;47:1841–7.

44 Schoonjans K, Auwerx J. Thiazolidinediones: an update. *Lancet* 2000;355:1008–10.

45 Seckl JR, Walker BR. Minireview: 11beta-hydroxysteroid dehydrogenase type 1 – a tissue- specific amplifier of glucocorticoid action. *Clin Exp Pharmacol Physiol* 2001;142:1371–6.

46 Masuzaki H, Paterson J, Shinyama H *et al.* A transgenic model of visceral obesity and the metabolic syndrome. *Science* 2001;294:2166–70.

47 Berger J, Tanen M, Elbrecht A *et al.* Peroxisome proliferator-activated receptor-gamma ligands inhibit adipocyte 11 beta-hydroxysteroid dehydrogenase type 1 expression and activity. *J Biol Chem* 2001;276:12629–35.

48 Zhang B, Salituro G, Szalkowski D *et al.* Discovery of a small molecule insulin mimetic with antidiabetic activity in mice. *Science* 1999;284:974–7.

49 Li M, Youngren JF, Manchem VP *et al.* Small molecule insulin receptor activators potentiate insulin action in insulin-resistant cells. *Diabetes* 2001;50:2323–8.

50 White MF. The IRS-signaling system: a network of docking proteins that mediate insulin and cytokine action. *Recent Prog Horm Res* 1998;53:119–38.

51 Goldstein BJ. Protein-tyrosine phosphatase 1B (PTP1B): a novel therapeutic target for type 2 diabetes mellitus, obesity and related states of insulin resistance. *Curr Drug Targets – Immune, Endocrine Metabol Disorders* 2001;1:265–75.

52 Elchebly M, Payette P, Michaliszyn E *et al.* Increased insulin sensitivity and obesity resistance in mice lacking the protein tyrosine phosphatase-1B gene. *Science* 1999;283:1544–8.

53 Klaman LD, Boss O, Peroni OD *et al.* Increased energy expenditure, decreased adiposity, and tissue-specific insulin sensitivity in protein-tyrosine phosphatase 1B-deficient mice. *Mol Cell Biol* 2000;20:5479–89.

54 Zinker B, Xie N, Clampit J et al. Anti-diabetic effects of protein tyrosine phosphatase 1B (PTP1B) antisense treatment in a rodent model of diabetes: potential therapeutic benefit [abstract]. *Diabetes* 2001;50:1378.

55 Henriksen EJ, Johnson KW, Ring DB et al. Glycogen synthase kinase-3 inhibitors potentiate glucose tolerance and muscle glycogen synthase activity in the Zucker diabetic fatty rat [abstract]. *Diabetes* 2001;50:A279.

56 Yuan MS, Konstantopoulos N, Lee JS et al. Reversal of obesity- and diet-induced insulin resistance with salicylates or targeted disruption of IKK beta. *Science* 2001;293:1673–7.

57 Kim JK, Kim YJ, Fillmore JJ et al. Prevention of fat-induced insulin resistance by salicylate. *J Clin Invest* 2001;108:437–46.

58 Shulman GI. Cellular mechanisms of insulin resistance. *J Clin Invest* 2000;106:171–6.

59 Mu J, Brozinick JT, Jr., Valladares O et al. A role for AMP-activated protein kinase in contraction- and hypoxia-regulated glucose transport in skeletal muscle. *Mol Cell* 2001;7:1085–94.

60 Winder WW. Energy-sensing and signaling by AMP-activated protein kinase in skeletal muscle. *J Appl Physiol* 2001;91:1017–28.

61 Zhou G, Myers R, Li Y et al. Role of AMP-activated protein kinase in mechanism of metformin action. *J Clin Invest* 2001;108:1167–74.

62 Yamauchi T, Kamon J, Waki H et al. The fat-derived hormone adiponectin reverses insulin resistance associated with both lipoatrophy and obesity. *Nat Med* 2001;7:941–6.

63 Ouchi N, Kihara S, Arita Y et al. Adiponectin, an adipocyte-derived plasma protein, inhibits endothelial NF-kappaB signaling through a cAMP-dependent pathway. *Circulation* 2000;102:1296–301.

64 Fruebis J, Tsao TS, Javorschi S et al. Proteolytic cleavage product of 30-kDa adipocyte complement-related protein increases fatty acid oxidation in muscle and causes weight loss in mice. *Proc Natl Acad Scie USA* 2001;98:2005–10.

65 Combs TP, Berg AH, Obici S et al. Endogenous glucose production is inhibited by the adipose-derived protein Acrp30. *J Clin Invest* 2001;108:1875–81.

66 Connell RD. Glucagon antagonists for the treatment of type 2 diabetes. *Exp Opin Ther Patents* 1999;9:701–9.

67 Permert J, Larsson J, Westermark GT et al. Islet amyloid polypeptide in patients with pancreatic cancer and diabetes. *N Engl J Med* 1994;330: 313–18.

68 Samsom M, Szarka LA, Camilleri M et al. Pramlintide, an amylin analog, selectively delays gastric emptying: potential role of vagal inhibition. *Am J Physiol Gastrointest Liver Physiol* 2000;278:G946–G951.

69 Treadway JL, Mendys P, Hoover DJ. Glycogen phosphorylase inhibitors for treatment of type 2 diabetes mellitus. *Expert Opin Invest Drugs* 2001;10:439–54.

70 Zhang BB, Moller DE. New approaches in the treatment of type 2 diabetes. *Curr Opin Chem Biol* 2000;4:461–7.

71 Parker JC, VanVolkenburg MA, Levy CB et al. Plasma glucose levels are reduced in rats and mice treated with an inhibitor of glucose-6-phosphate translocase. *Diabetes* 1998;47:1630–6.

72 Yoon JC, Puigserver P, Chen GX et al. Control of hepatic gluconeogenesis through the transcriptional coactivator PGC-1. *Nature* 2001;413:131–8.

73 Lebovitz HE. Oral therapies for diabetic hyperglycemia. *Endocrinol Metabol Clinics N Am* 2001;30:909–33.

74 Creutzfeldt W. The entero-insular axis in type 2 diabetes—incretins as therapeutic agents. *Exp Clin Endocrinol Diabetes* 2001;109:2–S303.

75 Drucker DJ. Development of glucagon-like peptide-1-based pharmaceuticals as therapeutic agents for the treatment of diabetes. *Curr Pharm Des* 2001;7:1399–1412.

76 Ahren B, Simonsson E, Efendic S et al. Inhibition of DPPIV by NVP DPP728 improves metabolic control over a 4 week period in type 2 diabetes [abstract]. *Diabetes* 2002;50:A416.

77 Greig NH, Holloway HW, De Ore KA et al. Once daily injection of exendin-4 to diabetic mice achieves long-term beneficial effects on blood glucose concentrations. *Diabetologia* 1999;42: 45–50.

Index